Laser Therapy in Veterinary Medicine

Laser Therapy in Veterinary Medicine

Photobiomodulation

Edited by

Ronald J. Riegel

American Institute of Medical Laser Applications
Marysville, OH, USA

John C. Godbold, Jr.

Stonehaven Veterinary Consulting
Jackson, TN, USA

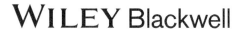

Registered Office
John Wiley & Sons Ltd, The Atrium, Southern Gate, Chichester, West Sussex, PO19 8SQ, UK

Editorial Office
1606 Golden Aspen Drive, Suites 103 and 104, Ames, Iowa 50010, USA

For details of our global editorial offices, customer services, and more information about Wiley products visit us at www.wiley.com.

Wiley also publishes its books in a variety of electronic formats and by print-on-demand. Some content that appears in standard print versions of this book may not be available in other formats.

Library of Congress Cataloging-in-Publication data applied for

Hardback ISBN: 9781119220114

Cover Design: Wiley
Cover Image: Courtesy of the Editors

Set in 10/12pt Warnock by SPi Global, Pondicherry, India

SKY10093734_121224

To my family. Cynthia for her love, tireless support, and understanding; to my parents, children, and grandchildren, without whom my life would be empty and without inspiration.

To Dr. John C. Godbold Jr., my co-editor. Without his efforts, guidance, and wisdom, the completion and the comprehensive scope of this text would not have been possible.

To all of the contributing authors of this text. Their collaboration will benefit both our profession and our patients.

To Drs. Bryan Pryor and Sean Wang. The knowledge, insight, and opportunities they have provided have allowed me to pursue this paradigm in both the veterinary and the medical fields.

To all of my clients, who have given me the honor of allowing me to work on their animals, and to all of my patients, who have provided me a life of daily education.

Ronald J. Riegel, DVM
Marysville, Ohio

To all of the contributing authors of this text. Thank you. You made this happen.

To Dr. Ronald J. Riegel, my co-editor. Your tireless work, willingness to share your knowledge, and passion for veterinary medicine inspire me.

To my parents, John and Betty. You encouraged me to be whatever I wanted to be.

To George V. Kenmore, DVM and Louis Charles "Bud" Cardinal, Jr., DVM. For as long as I can remember, I wanted to be like you.

To all who have helped me learn about laser technologies. You transformed my career and led me on a new journey.

To all of my patients. Regardless of the direction, the journey has always been about you.

To my wife Nancy, and our girls Elizabeth and Bryghte. You have always made wherever I am on the journey a good place.

John C. Godbold, Jr., DVM
Jackson, Tennessee

Contents

About the Editors

Ronald J. Riegel, DVM

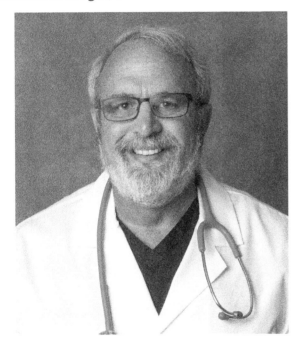

Ronald J. Riegel, DVM purchased his first therapy laser in 1979. It was a 1 mW HeNe laser. Throughout the 1980's and 90's, he observed the changes in technology, with power outputs reaching 500 mW. Laser therapy was always employed in his practice. In 2009, he co-founded the American Institute of Medical Laser Applications (AIMLA) to provide education on all types of medical laser in both the veterinary and the health care professions. His background in laser technology and applications encompasses not only companion, equine, and exotic animals, but also the human fields of non-pharmaceutical pain management, chiropractic, physical therapy, and sports medicine.

Since selling his multi-doctor private veterinary practice, he has authored more than 20 research papers, book chapters, professional articles, and books. His veterinary books include the subjects of anatomy (*Illustrated Atlas of Clinical Equine Anatomy and Common Disorders of the Horse*, Volumes I and II), utilizing physical therapy modalities (*Helping Horses Heal*), canine nutrition (*From Bones to Biscuits*), and laser therapy (*Laser Therapy for the Equine Athlete* and *Laser Therapy in the Companion Animal Practice*). The *Illustrated Atlas of Clinical Equine Anatomy and Common Disorders of the Horse*, Volume I won the Benjamin Franklin Award for Education/ Teaching/Academic Textbooks in 1999. He co-authored the human laser therapy text *Clinical Overview and Applications of Class IV Therapy Lasers*.

Dr. Riegel has spent the last decade lecturing nationally and internationally to human and veterinary health care professions. In the last 3 years, he has spoken in over 78 national, regional, state, and local venues.

He has been a Fellow of the American Society for Laser Medicine & Surgery (ASLMS) since 2012, is a Board Member of the Optical Society, and is a member of the North American Association for Laser Therapy (NAALT), the World Association for Laser Therapy (WALT), and the American Academy of Thermology (AAT).

John C. Godbold, Jr., DVM

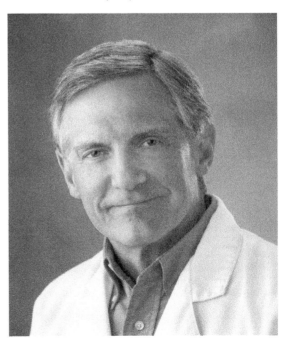

John C. Godbold, Jr., DVM graduated with honors from Auburn University School of Veterinary Medicine in 1978. In 1980, he established Stonehaven Park Veterinary Hospital in Jackson, Tennessee, where he practiced full time as a solo small-animal practitioner for 33 years. Dr. Godbold currently works full time with Stonehaven Veterinary Consulting teaching and assisting colleagues as a consultant for laser surgery and laser therapy.

Since 1999, Dr. Godbold has pursued a special interest in surgical lasers and the use of other laser modalities in small-animal practice. He has extensive experience with surgical and therapeutic lasers, has developed new surgical and therapeutic techniques, and assists equipment manufacturers with the development of new laser and laser-associated technologies.

Dr. Godbold has published numerous papers, articles, and chapters about the use of lasers in small-animal practice. His publications have appeared in the *Journal of the American Veterinary Medical Association, Clinician's Brief, Laserpoints, The Feline Patient, The Integrative Veterinary Care Journal,* and the *Newsletter of the Veterinary Surgical Laser Society.* He is a member of the Medical Advisory Board of the American Institute of Medical Laser Applications (AIMLA), the Companion Therapy Laser Veterinary Advisory Board, and the American Society for Laser Medicine & Surgery (ASLMS).

Dr. Godbold published the internationally distributed *Atlas of CO2 Laser Surgery Procedures* in 2002, with a new edition each year since. In 2009, Dr. Godbold published the *Atlas of Class IV Laser Therapy – Small Animal,* also updated with a new edition each year.

In high demand as a continuing-education speaker, Dr. Godbold has led over 500 laser workshops, wet-labs, and continuing-education meetings throughout North America and in over 21 countries around the world.

List of Contributors

Juanita J. Anders, PhD
Edward Hébert School of Medicine
Uniformed Services University of the Health Sciences
Bethesda, MD, USA

Ray A. Arza, DVM
RSA Veterinary Technologies
Taylorsville, KY, USA

Kenneth E. Bartels, DVM, MS
Professor Emeritus
Department of Veterinary Clinical Sciences
Oklahoma State University
Stillwater, OK, USA

David S. Bradley, DVM, FASLMS
K-Laser USA
Oakdale, CA, USA

Matthew W. Brunke, DVM, CCRP, CVPP, CVA
North Country Veterinary Referral Center
Queensbury, NY, USA

Steven Buijs, DVM
Dierenhospitaal Visdonk
Roosendaal, Netherlands

Debra Canapp, DVM, CCRT, CVA, DACVSMR
Veterinary Orthopedic and Sports Medicine Group
Orthobiologic Innovations
Annapolis Junction, MD, USA

Daniel M. Core, DVM
Airline Animal Health and Surgery Center
Bossier City, LA, USA

Liza Dadone, VMD
Cheyenne Mountain Zoo
Colorado Springs, CO, USA

David J. Fenoglio, DVM
Augusta Animal Clinic
Indianapolis, IN, USA

Damiano Fortuna, DVM
Imaginalis S.r.l.
Sesto Fiorentino (FI), Italy

Julie Gard, DVM, PhD, DACT
Department of Clinical Sciences
Auburn University College of Veterinary Medicine
Auburn, AL, USA

John C. Godbold, Jr., DVM
Stonehaven Veterinary Consulting
Jackson, TN, USA

Richard L. Godine, DVM
North American Association for Light Therapy
Ruckersville Animal Hospital and Veterinary Laser
Therapy Center
Ruckersville, VA, USA

Barbara R. Gores, DVM, DACVS
Veterinary Specialty Center of Tucson
Tucson, AZ, USA

Deborah M. Gross, DPT, MSPT, DABPTS, CCRP
Wizard of Paws Physical Rehabilitation for Animals
Colchester, CT, USA

Tara Harrison, DVM, MPVM, DACZM, DACVPM
North Carolina State College of Veterinary Medicine
Raleigh, NC, USA

Renaud Houyoux, CVT, LVT, CVDT, VNA
Companion Animal Health
Newark, DE, USA

Jennifer F. Johnson, VMD, CVPP
Stoney Creek Veterinary Hospital
Morton, PA, USA

Ann Kobiela Ketz, PhD, RN
Center for Nursing Science and Clinical Inquiry
Landstuhl Regional Medical Center
Landstuhl, Germany

Laura Kortelainen, Veterinary Nurse
Evidensia Finland
Järvenpää, Finland

Jennifer O. Lavallee, DVM, RSO
Cat Specialist
Castle Rock, CO, USA

Dianne Adjan Logan, RVT, CCRP
Wilmington Animal Fitness & Rehabilitation Center at
Needham Animal Hospital
Wilmington, NC, USA

Jörg Mayer, DVM, MS, DABVP (ECM), DECZM
(Small Mammal)
Department of Small Animal Medicine and Surgery
University of Georgia
Athens, GA, USA

Brenda McDuffee, CHT-V
Independent Laser Sales Representative
Ocala, FL, USA

Carolina Medina, DVM, DACVSMR, CVA, CVCH
Coral Springs Animal Hospital
Coral Springs, FL, USA

Lisa A. Miller, DVM, CCRT, CVA
Companion Animal Health by LiteCure
Newark, DE, USA

Diane J. Miller, MBA
The Animal Athlete
Newark, DE, USA

Robert D. Ness, DVM
Ness Exotic Wellness Center
Lilse, IL, USA

Erin O'Leary, DVM
HEAL Mobile Veterinary Laser Therapy
Cary, NC, USA

James Olson, DVM, DAVBP (Feline), RSO
Cat Specialist
Castle Rock, CO, USA

Sean Redman, DVM
Equine Integrated Veterinary Solutions, PLLC
Ocala, FL, USA

Ronald J. Riegel, DVM
American Institute of Medical Laser
Applications
Marysville, OH, USA

Jeffrey J. Smith, DVM, CCRP
Middletown Animal Hospital
Middletown, CA, USA

Bryan J. Stephens, PhD
SOUND (a VCA Company)
Franklin, TN, USA

Donald W. Stremme, PhD
Academy of Natural Sciences of Drexel University
and
AQUAVET & Cornell University College
of Veterinary Medicine
Cape May Beach, NJ, USA

Xingjia Wu, BS
Edward Hébert School of Medicine
Uniformed Services University of the
Health Sciences
Bethesda, MD, USA

Foreword

Meet Dixie! Dixie is not only a cat who thinks she is dog and enjoys sitting on her hind legs like a meerkat but also embodies how a good veterinarian can have a direct influence on the happiness and well-being of a whole family. I adopted Dixie from my veterinarian. She was rescued from the woods as a lone, tiny kitten, and was living at his practice.

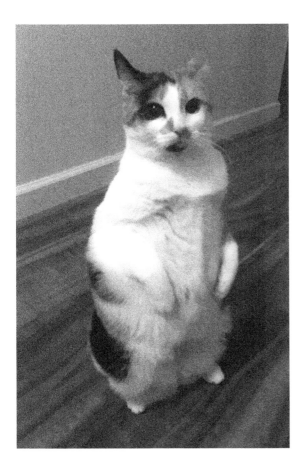

Besides sharing a love for Dixie, my veterinarian and I also shared our interest in the use of light as a therapeutic tool. He had recently acquired a laser and was introducing it into his practice. However, as is typical for the majority of veterinarians who are now using photobio-modulation therapy (PBMT), he had questions on the appropriate device and treatment parameters to be used for different conditions. He attended a number of classes on the use of lasers and other light sources in veterinary practice, but these were often manufacture-sponsored and did not present a non-biased global view.

This book fulfills this need with guidelines for effective use of laser therapy in many clinical applications in various veterinary specialties. For that reason and many others, I am honored and delighted to write this foreword. For the last 25 years, I have been involved in the development of PBMT at the basic science and translational pre-clinical levels. My research has resulted in over 50 peer-reviewed publications on light interaction with cells and tissues, and in three patents.

As the field of photonic medicine matured, veterinarians were on the forefront of adopting laser therapy into their clinical practices. The acceptance of PBMT by veterinarians and their eagerness to learn about its clinical benefits and mechanistic basis afforded me the opportunity to meet and interact with this incredible group of clinicians. The first conference I attended devoted to the use of PBMT in veterinary care was held at Colorado State University College of Veterinary Medicine and Biomedical Sciences in 2010. The veterinarians I had the pleasure to meet at that conference and at other venues impressed me with their concern for their patients, love of animals, intelligence and thoughtful questioning, and their desire to adopt new promising therapies that could help their patients.

Two of the remarkable veterinarians that I had the pleasure to meet were John C. Godbold, Jr. and Ronald J. Riegel. John and Ron, co-editors and chapter contributors for this book, were early adopters of laser technology. They have years of experience with clinical applications of laser therapy and have successfully used this technology to treat companion, equine, and exotic animals. They are active members of a number of veterinary and laser societies. To educate their colleagues and dispel the prevalent myths about laser technology, John and Ron collectively have presented, nationally and internationally, over 700 laser workshops, wet-labs, and continuing-education meetings. They are experienced authors and editors and have amassed an impressive list of national and international scientists and veterinarians from research, academia, industry, specialty practices, and general practice as chapter contributors.

This book represents a reputable source of information about laser therapy that is applicable to the diverse group of practitioners representing the veterinary community. The chapters on the history, theory, and science of laser therapy are clearly presented and serve to establish the credibility of this therapy. Furthermore, the chapters on clinical applications make this book a practical and usable clinical reference that will help practitioners use the technology effectively and therefore help their patients. It contains practical guidelines about treatment and safety and a thorough presentation of clinical applications in companion, equine, exotic, zoological, food-animal, rehabilitation, and regenerative-medicine specialties.

Another outstanding feature of the book is that it is non-commercial. Company names and logos were not allowed and the text describes treatment procedures and protocols in generic, non-commercially-specific ways. Hopefully, this book will counter some of the misinformation that has been presented in the veterinary market place.

Finally, the book supports trans-species application of research and clinical evidence and encourages veterinarians to use laser therapy in their practice by applying the basic concepts and knowledge to multiple species. I envision that this trans-species approach will provide important knowledge that will benefit a wide range of animals and inform pre-clinical research for translation of effective laser therapy to the human species. I sincerely believe that this book will prove to be an important, game-changing text for the veterinary community and will lead the way in establishing guidelines on the effective use of PBMT in many applications of veterinary care. I look forward not only to Dixie benefiting from the knowledge imparted in this book but also to the development of effective PBMT for the human members of her family.

Juanita J. Anders, PhD
Professor of Anatomy, Physiology and Genetics,
Professor of Neuroscience,
Edward Hébert School of Medicine
Uniformed Services University of the Health Sciences
Bethesda, Maryland

Preface

Parallel backgrounds led us to produce this much-needed resource on the use of lasers for therapeutic purposes in veterinary medicine. The initial focus of our independent careers was in private practice. While practicing, we developed interests in lasers and their use in practice, and became passionate about laser technology.

Our interests and passions gave us opportunities to work with those developing and supplying laser technology to veterinary medicine, and stimulated us to share knowledge and experience with colleagues through training and continuing education. We have both enjoyed working with colleagues all over the world, advancing knowledge about how to use laser technology to help patients.

Years of sharing information about therapeutic lasers and the clinical application of photobiomodulation (PBM) made us realize this textbook was needed. Our goal was to produce a reputable source of information to promote the application of photobiomodulation therapy (PBMT), help colleagues use the technology more effectively, and, in the end, help improve the quality of life of patients.

We recognized that we live in a world of rapid digital communication, filled with bullet-point information and often-confusing claims by therapeutic laser equipment vendors. The hundreds of questions colleagues ask about laser therapy require more than bullet points, and they should be answered in one place. The science and evidence should be gathered together, and should be more complete than glossy marketing claims. The shared clinical experience of thousands of practitioners, in a diversity of practice settings, should be available in one resource. This book is that place, that gathering together, and that resource.

The book was designed to be applicable to a diverse group. We understood that as the first complete publication about PBMT in veterinary medicine, it needed to be well grounded in science, yet practical and usable for clinical reference. Thus, the content covers a spectrum of background theory and science. It contains practical guidelines about treatment and safety. It contains a thorough presentation of clinical applications in companion, equine, exotic, zoological, food-animal, rehabilitation, and regenerative-medicine practice, and several chapters on integration and economics.

To give such a broad presentation required engaging a diverse, well-qualified group of contributing authors from research, academia, industry, specialty practice, and general practice. We have brought the depth of knowledge of colleagues from academia and research, and of those with specialty practice credentials, together with the practical experience of Main Street practitioners.

Contributing authors have been required to reference their chapters heavily. We recognize that in order to help the credibility of PBMT in veterinary medicine, the evidence for its use must be overwhelming. We recognize the importance of trans-species application of research and clinical evidence. The contributing authors were encouraged to facilitate what veterinarians do every day in practice: apply basic concepts and knowledge to multiple species.

As editors, we have ensured that this resource is broad-based and represents the different approaches that have historically been used to deliver PBMT. It is not specific to any therapy laser equipment, and does not have any commercial bias. The techniques described by the contributing authors reflect their experience and the success they have had with them, using a wide variety of therapeutic laser devices.

Throughout the chapters (and even in the book's title and subtitle), there is mixed use of terminology to label the technology. This reflects the current shift from the use of multiple descriptive terms for laser therapy to the use of the more accurate term "photobiomodulation therapy." The contributing authors use the terms "laser therapy" and "photobiomodulation therapy" interchangeably. Older, less descriptive terms such as "low-level laser therapy" and "cold laser therapy" have been avoided except where used in a historical context.

We have tried, where possible, to standardize the format of dose recommendations. We understand that the historical variation in the way treatment parameters and doses have been reported has been a challenge in the clinical treatment of patients. To facilitate the application of recommendations in as many different therapeutic laser devices as possible, most doses are given as joules per square centimeter (J/cm^2). In the very few instances where doses are reported using other parameters, the editors recommend consulting the general guidelines and recommendations in Part II.

We encourage those involved in research to use this book as a guide for future studies. We encourage those in industry to use it as a map for the development of veterinary-specific therapeutic laser devices. We encourage those in clinical practice to use it as a daily guide for how to treat more patients, with more conditions, more effectively. We will have succeeded with our goals if you turn to this book often. May your copy become well worn.

Ronald J. Riegel, DVM
John C. Godbold, Jr. DVM
August 1, 2016

Disclaimer

Please read the statements and therapy protocols within this text carefully before utilizing any of this information. The information and recommendations are based on previously published scientific information and years of practice, clinical, and research experience by the contributing authors.

Knowledge about laser therapy and photobiomodulation therapy (PBMT) is constantly changing through ongoing research, clinical trials, and day-to-day clinical experience. The information within this text is presented for educational purposes only and is designed to be a reference to complement formal training about laser therapy and PBMT.

This text contains neither complete nor comprehensive information about any of the conditions addressed, and each condition should be evaluated on an individual basis in each patient prior to therapy. This text is not a substitute for professional advice, care, diagnosis, or treatment. It is the sole responsibility of the veterinarian, veterinary surgeon, technician, nurse, assistant, and therapist to gain the knowledge and comply with all federal, national, provincial, state, and local laws regarding the use of therapeutic lasers for any condition. Dr. Ronald J. Riegel, Dr. John C. Godbold Jr., all of the contributing authors, and anyone involved with the publication of this text expressly disclaim any and all responsibility and legal liability for any kind of loss or risk, personal or otherwise, which is the result of the direct or indirect use or application of any of the material within this text.

Part I

The History of Laser Therapy

1

The History of Laser Therapy

Ronald J. Riegel

American Institute of Medical Laser Applications, Marysville, OH, USA

Introduction

Various forms of heliotherapy (light therapy) have been practiced around the world for centuries. Physicians and healers in Ancient Greece, Egypt, and Rome – including renowned Greek historian Herodotus in the 6th century B.C. – all realized the benefits of such therapy (Ellinger, 1957). Likewise, the Inca and Assyrian cultures worshiped the sun with the belief that it would bring them health. Around 1500 B.C., Indian medical literature described treatments combining herbal medicine with natural sunlight to treat non-pigmented skin. There are records in the Buddhist literature from around 200 A.D. and Chinese documentation from the 10th century recording similar therapeutic effects from light.

In the 17th century, Sir Isaac Newton discovered that prisms could disassemble or separate white light, a phenomenon he described in his book *Opticks,* originally printed in 1704 (Newton, 1704). He was also the first to use the word "spectrum" (Latin for "appearance" or "apparition") in 1671.

Heliotherapy in the Modern World

Niels Ryberg Finsen, a Faroese physician and scientist of Icelandic descent, is widely regarded as the original proponent of phototherapy. In 1903, he was awarded the Nobel Prize in Medicine and Physiology for the successful treatment of diseases using phototherapy; specifically, lupus vulgaris, a skin infection caused by *Mycobacterium tuberculosis* (Nobel Prize, 2014b). He also famously utilized ultraviolet light to treat smallpox lesions (Nobel Lectures, 1967).

Shortly thereafter, in 1916, Albert Einstein postulated the theory of lasers to support his Theory of Relativity. First, Einstein proposed that an excited atom in isolation can return to a lower energy state by emitting photons, a process he termed "spontaneous emission." Spontaneous emission sets the scale for all radiative interactions, such as absorption and stimulated emission. Atoms will only absorb photons of the correct wavelength; the photon disappears and the atom goes to a higher-energy state, setting the stage for spontaneous emission. Second, his theory predicted that as light passes through a substance, it stimulates the emission of more light (Hilborn, 1982).

Einstein hypothesized that photons prefer to travel together in the same state. If one has a large collection of atoms containing a great deal of excess energy, they will be ready to emit photons randomly. If a stray photon of the correct wavelength passes by (or, in the case of a laser, is fired at) an atom already in an excited state, its presence will stimulate the atom to release its photons early. The new photons will then travel in the same direction as the original stray photon, with identical frequency and phase. A cascading effect ensues: as the identical photons move through other atoms, ever more photons are emitted (Pais, 1982).

The Laser is Born

On May 16, 1960, Theodore Maiman produced the first ruby laser at the Hughes Aircraft Research Laboratory in Malibu, California, basing his new creation on Albert Einstein's explanation of stimulated emission of radiation, coupled with Townes' and Schawlow's 1958 work with optical masers (Schawlow and Townes, 1958; Itzkan and Drake, 1997).

Several years after the invention of the laser, Dr. Endre Mester – considered the founding father of laser therapy – became the first to experimentally document the healing effects of lasers. Because he used mice as

Laser Therapy in Veterinary Medicine: Photobiomodulation, First Edition. Edited by Ronald J. Riegel and John C. Godbold, Jr.
© 2017 John Wiley & Sons, Inc. Published 2017 by John Wiley & Sons, Inc.

his experimental model, this is also the first documented use of lasers to accelerate healing in veterinary medicine (Mester *et al.*, 1967). His experiments would also later prove that the acceleration of healing was a systemic – not just localized – event (Perera, 1987). Mester's work had a cascading effect, motivating other researchers in Western and Eastern Europe to recognize the value of laser therapy and initiate studies of their own.

Early in the 1970's, the use of laser therapy was documented not only in Eastern Europe, but also in China and the Soviet Union; all of the early research emanates from these geographical regions. Over the next decade, the use of laser therapy spread to Western Europe and became accepted as an effective physical therapy modality (Goodson and Hunt, 1979). Unfortunately, the lasers used were only capable of 5–50 mW of power and didn't generate the consistent clinical results that we have since witnessed with higher-powered lasers.

Yo Cheng Zhou, an oral surgeon in China, was the first to stimulate an acupuncture point with a laser. He used laser stimulation instead of standard local anesthetic protocols during routine dental extractions. A beam from a 2.8–6.0 mW helium-neon laser apparatus (Model CW-12, Chengdu Thermometer Factory) was applied for 5 minutes before the removal of a tooth (Zhou, 1984). Photonic stimulation was then applied to LI-4 Hegu. This acupuncture point has long been recognized to produce systemic analgesia.

From the mid 1970's to the early 1980's, laser therapy became an accepted physical therapy modality throughout Western European and several Asian countries. It finally appeared in the United States around 1977, but there were only a small number of therapists that understood its potential. All of the equipment in the United States during this time frame was in the 1–5 mW range, and acceptance by medical and veterinary professions was very limited due to the inconsistent clinical results.

The first Independent Institutional Review Board for Laser Acupuncture Research was established in 1993, based on research comiled by Margaret Naeser, Ph.D., Lic.Ac. through the Robert Wood Johnson Foundation of Princeton, New Jersey. This initiated the effort and motivation of several colleagues to compile enough current information and research to be in compliance with US Food and Drug Administration (FDA) regulations. Dr. Naeser is currently involved with a large number of research projects, including "Neural Networks and Language Recovery in Aphasia from Stroke victims" (Naeser, 2007). She has published papers on utilizing laser therapy in stroke cases (Naeser and Hamblin, 2011).

Three associations have formed over the years to encourage scientists and practitioners to exchange knowledge and information. The American Society for Laser Medicine and Surgery (ASLMS), formed in 1981, was the first (www.aslms.org). It was the dream of its founders that this organization be unique and include physicians, clinicians, and outstanding researchers in the areas of biophysics, biochemistry, biomedical engineering, laser biology, and laser safety. In 1994, the World Association for Laser Therapy (WALT) was formed by combining the International Laser Therapy Association (ILTA) and the International Society for Laser Applications (ISLAM) (www.waltza.co.za). The North American Association for Laser Therapy (NAALT) was established in 1998. It included the regions of Mexico, Canada and the United States of America. In 2015, NAALT changed its name to the North American Association for Photobiomodulation Therapy (www.naalt.org). All three of these organizations have the common goals of promoting research, improving the understanding of photobiological mechanisms, providing education, clinical applications, and new clinical techniques, and establishing treatment and regulatory guidelines.

The Evolution of Laser Therapy Equipment

The first laser diode, utilizing coherent light emission from a gallium arsenide (GaAs) semiconductor diode, was revealed in 1962 by two groups: Robert N. Hall at the General Electric research center (Hall *et al.*, 1962) and Marshall Nathan at the IBM T.J. Watson Research Center (Nathan *et al.*, 1962).

Later in 1962, other teams at the MIT Lincoln Laboratory, Texas Instruments, and RCA Laboratories also demonstrated the emission of light and lasing in semiconductor diodes. Early in 1963, a team led by Nikolay Basov in the Soviet Union utilized GaAs lasers to achieve emission of light (Nobel Prize, 2014a).

In 1970, the first laser diode to achieve continuous-wave (CW) emission was revealed simultaneously by Zhores Alferov and collaborators in the Soviet Union, and Morton Panish and Izuo Hayashi in the United States (Ghatak, 2009). However, it is widely accepted that Alferov and his team reached the milestone first, and they were consequently awarded the Nobel Prize in Physics in 2000.

While many types of therapeutic lasers were in use around the world, it was not until 2002 that Class IIIb lasers gained FDA approval for therapeutic purposes in the United States. These lasers are commonly referred to as "cold lasers" or "low-level laser therapy" (LLLT) devices. They are limited to 500 mW and are considered effective in the treatment of superficial conditions. The term "cold lasers" refers to the lack of a heating effect on tissue cultures in early experiments. The description

"LLLT" differentiates low-power therapeutic lasers from surgical or cutting lasers.

Class IV therapy lasers, operating above 500 mW, were approved by the FDA in 2006. This was the dawn of "high-power laser therapy" (HPLT). Delivery systems and precise dosage software have evolved through the years to allow the safe and effective delivery of 500 mW–60 W to target tissues.

Photobiomodulation: A New Name

The history of laser therapy and the evolution of laser therapy devices have produced confusing terminology. Multiple terms have been used to describe the technology. Many are more descriptive of the devices being used than of the therapy they deliver.

Recognizing that an accurate, clear, and unambiguous name was needed, 15 international participants joined in a nomenclature consensus meeting at the joint conference of NAALT and WALT in September 2014 (Anders *et al.*, 2015). Respected authorities Dr. Jan Bjordal and Dr. Juanita Anders co-chaired the meeting. The term "photobiomodulation therapy" (PBMT) was recognized as being most descriptive of a science that involves complex mechanisms, some which are stimulatory, some inhibitory. Since that meeting, the National Library of Medicine (United States) has added the term "photobiomodulation therapy" to the MeSH database (MeSH, 2016).

The committee suggested a "definition for the term photobiomodulation therapy as 'A form of light therapy that utilizes non-ionizing forms of light sources, including lasers, LEDs, and broadband light, in the visible and infrared spectrum. It is a nonthermal process involving endogenous chromophores eliciting photophysical (i.e., linear and nonlinear) and photochemical events at various biological scales. This process results in beneficial therapeutic outcomes including but not limited to the alleviation of pain or inflammation, immunomodulation, and promotion of wound healing and tissue regeneration'" (Anders *et al.*, 2015).

Older terminology continues to be used even as the term "photobiomodulation therapy" becomes more commonplace in publications and practical applications. In this text, the terms "laser therapy" and "photobiomodulation therapy" will be used interchangeably.

Conclusion

The historic development of this new technology is in the past. There has now been a wealth of scientific and clinical evidence published. Thousands of veterinary practitioners around the world have adopted laser therapy into their practices. We, as veterinarians, should be at the forefront of this scientifically and clinically proven modality. Continued collaboration and sharing of information between us is essential to the future development of this 21st-century medical technology. The previous history has been written; be a part of the history other veterinarians quote 10 years from now.

References

Anders, J. *et al.* (2015) Low-level light/laser therapy versus photobiomodulation therapy. *Photomed Laser Surg.* **33**(4):183–184.
Ellinger, F. (1957) *Medical Radiation Biology*. Literary Licensing, Springfield, IL.
Ghatak, A. (2009) *Optics*. Tata McGraw-Hill, New Delhi.
Goodson, W. and Hunt, T. (1979) Wound healing and the diabetic patient. *Surg Gynecol Obstet.* **149**(4):600–608.
Hall, R.N. *et al.* (1962) Coherent light emission from GaAs junctions. *Phys Rev Lett.* **9**(9):366–368.
Hilborn, R.C. (1982) Einstein coefficients, cross sections, f values, dipole moments, and all that. *Am J Phys.* **50**(11):982.
Itzkan, I. and Drake, E. (1997) History of laser in medicine. In: *Lasers in Cutaneous and Aesthetic Surgery*. (eds. Arndt, K. *et al.*), pp. 3–10. Lippincott-Raven, Philadelphia, PA.

MeSH. (2016) Photobiomodulation. Available from: http://www.ncbi.nlm.nih.gov/mesh/?term= photobiomodulation (accessed November 30, 2016).
Mester, E. *et al.* (1967) Effect of laser on hair growth of mice. *Kiserl Orvostud.* **19**:628–631.
Naeser, M. (2007) Neural networks and language recovery in aphasia from stroke: fMRI studies. Available from: http://www.bu.edu/naeser/aphasia/projects.html (accessed November 30, 2016).
Naeser, M. and Hamblin, M. (2011) Potential for transcranial laser or LED therapy to treat stroke, traumatic brain injury, and neurodegenerative disease. *Photomed Laser Surg.* **29**(7):443–446.
Nathan, M.I. *et al.* (1962) Stimulated emission of radiation from GaAs p-n junctions. *Appl Phys Lett.* **1**(3):62.

Newton, I. (1704) *Opticks or, A Treatise of the Reflexions, Refractions, Inflexions and Colours of Light; also Two Treatises of the Species and Magnitude of Curvilinear Figures.* Octavo, Palo Alto, CA.

Nobel Lectures. (1967) *Physiology or Medicine 1901–1921.* Elsevier, Amsterdam.

Nobel Prize. (2014a) Nicolay G. Basov – facts. Nobel Media AB. Available from: http://www.nobelprize.org/nobel_prizes/physics/laureates/1964/basov-facts.html (accessed November 30, 2016).

Nobel Prize. (2014b) Niels Ryberg Finsen – facts. Nobel Media AB. Available from: http://www.nobelprize.org/nobel_prizes/medicine/laureates/1903/finsen-facts.html (accessed November 30, 2016).

Pais, A. (1982) *Subtle is the Lord: The Science and the Life of Albert Einstein.* Oxford University Press, New York.

Perera, J. (1987) The "healing laser" comes into the limelight. *New Scientist.* March 19.

Schawlow, A.L. and Townes, C.H. (1958) Principles of the optical laser. *Phys Rev Lett.* **1**(1).

Zhou, Y. (1984). Innovations. An advanced clinical trial with laser acupuncture anesthesia for minor operations in the oro-maxillofacial region. *Lasers Surg Med.* **4**(3):297–303.

Part II

The Theory and Science of Laser Therapy

2

Fundamental Information

Ronald J. Riegel[1] and John C. Godbold, Jr.[2]

[1] *American Institute of Medical Laser Applications, Marysville, OH, USA*
[2] *Stonehaven Veterinary Consulting, Jackson, TN, USA*

Introduction

Laser therapy utilizes penetrating photonic energy to achieve physiological and biochemical changes within the targeted tissues. Also known as "photobiomodulation therapy" (PBMT), this is a form of light therapy that "results in beneficial therapeutic outcomes including but not limited to the alleviation of pain or inflammation, immunomodulation, and promotion of wound healing and tissue regeneration" (Anders *et al.*, 2015).

Understanding key, fundamental information about how lasers work, different features unique to each individual piece of laser equipment, and clinical application techniques encourages an appreciation for the versatility of this modality and the immense benefits it brings to patients.

The purpose of this chapter is to provide general, fundamental information that will aid in the understanding of the chapters that follow. It is an overview of PBMT and laser therapy basics. Each subsequent chapter will provide more specific, detailed information on its respective subject.

Nomenclature

The term "LASER" is an acronym for "light amplification by stimulated emission of radiation" (Gould, 1959). Most lasers used in the veterinary profession are medical devices for therapeutic and surgical applications. They emit light through a process of optical amplification based on the stimulated emission of electromagnetic radiation (LaserFest, 2016).

Technically, a laser that produces light should be defined as an optical oscillator rather than an optical amplifier. However, the acronym for "light oscillation by stimulated emission of electromagnetic radiation" is *LOSER*; for obvious reasons, the term was never adopted.

The original acronym, LASER, is used as a noun, and optical amplifiers have come to be referred to as laser amplifiers. Note the redundancy in that designation (Chu and Townes, 2003).

Historically, laser therapy has been described in the literature by any of the following terms: low-level laser therapy (LLLT), low-intensity laser therapy (LILT), cold laser therapy, hot laser therapy, soft laser therapy, low-power laser therapy, light therapy, phototherapy, biostimulation laser therapy, Class 3 laser therapy, Class 4 laser therapy, and high-power laser therapy (HPLT). These terms are vague and bewildering. The correct nomenclature for the application of electromagnetic radiation within the red and infrared spectrum over injuries and lesions to stimulate healing and provide pain relief within those tissues is PBMT (Anders *et al.*, 2015). Though the use of the terms "laser therapy" and "PBMT" will be interchangeable in this text, the term "photobiomodulation" (PBM) is more precise. It "distinguishes photobiomodulation therapy, which is nonthermal, from the popular use of light-based devices for simple heating of tissues as can be accomplished using near-infrared lamps, or other applications of light energy that rely on thermal effects for all or part of their mechanism of action" (Anders *et al.*, 2015).

Application of laser therapy in conjunction with regenerative therapies such as stem cell or platelet-rich plasma injections is properly termed "photobioregeneration" (Ginani *et al.*, 2015).

Therapy lasers emit energy in the form of photons, which are energy packets of electromagnetic radiation. Photons have zero resting mass, and therefore travel at the speed of light in a vacuum (Einstein, 1905). Without photons, we would have no ability to see; they are the foundation of our visual sense.

Clarification of the terms "laser therapy" and "therapy laser" is necessary, since they are often used incorrectly. A therapy laser is a medical device, whereas laser therapy is the application of the light produced by this device. Use of the newer, more accurate and descriptive term "PBMT" is now encouraged in publications and in written and verbal communication.

The verb "lase" is used to refer to the production of coherent laser light (Merriam-Webster, 2016d). When a laser is in operational mode, it is producing and emitting light; this is referred to as "lasing" or "lasering"; either is correct (e.g, "I am lasering the right hip of this patient," "I am lasing the right hip of this patient").

Basic Terminology

- **Centimeter (US spelling) or centimetre (international spelling, as used by the International Bureau of Weights and Measures, BIPM) (cm):** A unit of length in the metric system, equal to one-hundredth of a meter (BIPM, 2014). Dosages of photonic energy are expressed in joules per square centimeter (J/cm^2).
- **Coherent:** Light that radiates in a very orderly fashion from its source. Each photon moves in phase with all of the other photons emitted (Hewitt, 2001).
- **Collimated:** Tight, strong, and concentrated (as of a laser beam) (Hewitt, 2001).
- **Continuous wave (CW):** Emission of radiant energy in a constant intensity at a specific power (Siegman, 1986). When the emission is continuous, the average power output is always the setting on the laser equipment.
- **Dose (dosing):** A measure of the density of energy delivered to the surface of the target tissue. Expressed in J/cm^2. The dose describes the prescribed amount of photonic energy delivered to a precise area (Jenkins and Carroll, 2011).
- **Duty cycle:** The period of time, expressed as a percentage, that it takes for emission to complete an on-and-off cycle (Barrett and Pack, 2006).
- **Energy:** A property of objects that can be transferred to other objects or converted into different forms, but cannot be created or destroyed (Kittel and Kroemer, 1980). It is difficult to give one single comprehensive definition of energy because of its many forms.
- **Fluence:** A measure of the instantaneous power output, similar to irradiance or power density, delivered to a defined area. Fluence is measured in watts per square centimeter (W/cm^2) (Kerker, 1969; Zaini, 1995). Dose calculation algorithms require fluence data as input (Zaini *et al.*, 1996).
- **Frequency:** The number of light waves passing a fixed point in a specific time interval. Frequency is measured in hertz (Hz) (Siegman, 1986; Silfvast, 1996), or the number of cycles per second. A frequency of 1 Hz means that one light wave has passed a fixed point in 1 second. A frequency of 500 Hz means that 500 light waves have passed a fixed point in 1 second. The

frequency of the emitted laser light is one of the parameters available for selection in most therapeutic lasers. Older literature and owner manuals sometimes refer to frequency as "cycles per second."

- **Irradiance:** The density of radiation incident on a given surface, expressed as W/cm^2 (Merriam-Webster, 2016b).
- **Joule (J):** A unit of work or energy equal to the work done by a force of 1 Newton acting through a distance of 1 m (Merriam-Webster, 2016c). In reference to the application of laser therapy, the energy emitted in each individual therapy session is expressed as a total number of joules.
- **Milliwatt (mW):** One-thousandth of a watt (BIPM, 2014).
- **Monochromatic:** Composed of only one wavelength (of laser light) (Hewitt, 2001).
- **Nanometer (US spelling) or nanometre (BIPM spelling) (nm):** A unit of length in the metric system, equal to one-billionth of a meter (0.000000001 m) (BIPM, 2014).
- **Photobiomodulation therapy (PBMT):** The therapeutic use of light, absorbed by the chromophores found in the body, to stimulate non-harmful and non-thermal reactions within the cell that result in a beneficial therapeutic outcome (Anders. *et al.*, 2015; MeSH, 2016).
- **Power:** The rate at which energy is emitted (Merriam-Webster, 2016e). Power is not the total amount of energy emitted; rather, it is an expression of energy over time. When describing laser emission, power is expressed in watts (1 W = 1 J/sec).
- **Power density:** The concentration or intensity of power output. Power density is measured in W/cm^2 (Smil, 2008).
- **Pulse (pulsing):** This term is interchangeable with "frequency." Both describe a disruption of the energy flow on a predetermined basis (Siegman,1986; Silfvast, 1996; Svelto, 1998).
- **Spot size:** Technically, the radius of a laser beam. Spot size can be calculated at any distance from the optical aperture from which the beam emerges (VALUE @ Amrita, 2016). In the practical application of laser therapy, the term "spot size" is commonly used to describe the width of the laser beam at the surface of the tissue being treated.
- **Superpulse:** A pulse in which the power output is extremely high and then returns to zero within a very short time (Berger and Eeg, 2006; Bartels, 2014). The duration of a superpulse is measured in nanoseconds. A good analogy is a flashbulb: a high intensity of light, then nothing. This mode of emission results in a low average power output.
- **Watt (W):** The SI unit of power, equivalent to 1 J/sec (BIPM, 2014).

- **Wavelength:** The distance between two successive points in a wave that are characterized by the same phase of oscillation (Dictionary.com, 2016; Hecht, 1987). Different wavelengths of visible light are perceived by the eye as different colors. The wavelength of a laser determines its absorption properties. The unit of measurement of the wavelengths used in lasers for PBMT is the nanometer (nm).

The Components of a Laser

A laser has three main components: an energy source, an amplifying medium, and a resonating cavity bounded by mirrors (Figure 2.1).

Electrons are excited by the energy source from a lower resting state to a higher energy level. The excited electrons decay back to a lower energy state according to a particular time constant that characterizes the transition. When an electron decays, a photon is emitted; this is spontaneous emission. Photons are emitted randomly into an amplifying medium, which is very specific spectrally; photons of only one wavelength are emitted (Coldren *et al.*, 2012). The emitted photons then stimulate other atoms in the medium and cause them to emit their stored energy.

This produces an avalanche of photons, all originating as extracted energy from the transition of atoms from a higher to a lower energy state (Loudon, 2001). A laser, therefore, is an optical amplifier that provides an environment in which to maintain a continuous stimulated emission of photons (Scholarpedia, 2016).

The Electromagnetic Spectrum

Figure 2.2 shows the range of all wavelengths of the electromagnetic spectrum. This spectrum runs from very short gamma rays to very long radio waves. Visible light is in the ~380–400 nm (violet) to ~700–780 nm (red) range.

Therapeutic lasers emit in the 620 nm (red) to 1200 nm (near-infrared) range. Optimal penetration in tissue requires wavelengths that minimize scattering and reflection at the tissue surface and absorption by unwanted chromophores (Jacques, 2013). At the shorter wavelengths, 600–800 nm, a significant quantity of photonic energy is absorbed by melanin, hemoglobin, and oxyhemoglobin chromophores. Consequently, these wavelengths are better suited for therapy applied to superficial areas. At longer wavelengths, above 1100–1200 nm, water is the primary incidental absorber. When

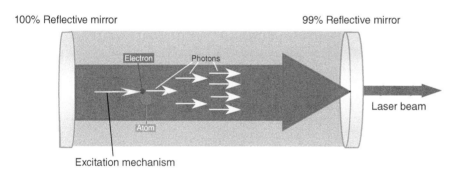

Figure 2.1 The components of a laser.

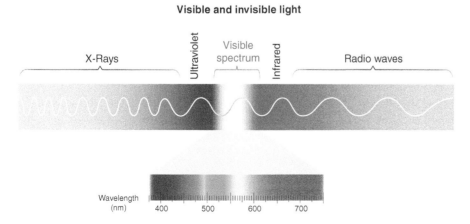

Figure 2.2 The electromagnetic spectrum.

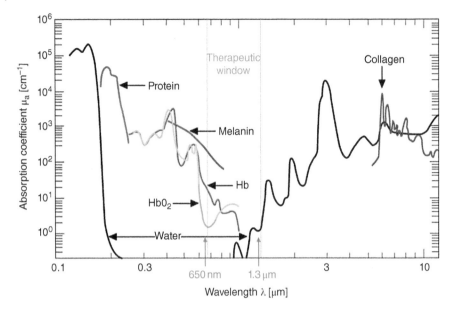

Figure 2.3 The therapeutic window for PBMT.

the photonic energy is absorbed by these incidental unwanted chromophores, it is then unavailable to cause a biological, biochemical, or physiological response.

To effectively penetrate to and treat deeper target cells, therapy lasers should emit in the 800–1000 nm range. This range is referred to as the "therapeutic" or "optical" window for PBMT (Figure 2.3). It is within this range that chromophores within tissue can absorb light. Therefore, the target tissue in which the pathological process is located and the absorption spectra of the target chromophores determine the efficacy of PBM for the wavelength being emitted.

The Three Properties of Laser Light

Laser light has three properties that allow its penetration through tissues to the cellular level. Lasers emit monochromatic (single-color wavelength), collimated (nondivergent), and coherent (in-phase wavelengths) light (Hewitt, 2001). Monochromaticity is logical, since the photons originate in a stimulated emission from one set of atomic energy levels. Collimation of the beam results from the bouncing back and forth between reflective, mirrored ends of the laser's resonant cavity. The photonic pathways, which sustain amplification, must pass between the mirrors many times and must be nearly perpendicular to the mirrors in order to be emitted. This creates the characteristic narrow beam. The coherent property is established by each photon traveling in phase with all other emitted photons.

To compare laser light to light produced by light-emitting diodes (LEDs), LEDs may emit light of a single wavelength,

but do so at much lower power than lasers. The photons are neither coherent nor collimated. Light from LEDs is much less able to penetrate tissues, yet may stimulate PBM in very superficial tissues (Craford *et al.*, 2001; Zheludev, 2007).

Laser Classifications

The basis for all four major laser classifications, or hazard categories, is the potential to cause histological damage to the eye or skin (ANSI, 2011). These classifications caution users of the optical hazards associated with their laser. They are based on output energy or power, wavelength, exposure duration, and the cross-sectional area of the laser beam at the point of interest.

Two organizations are responsible for establishing these classifications: the American National Standards Institute (ANSI) and the International Electrotechnical Institute (IEC, 2014). The ANSI Z136 series of laser safety standards is referenced by the Occupational Safety and Health Administration (OSHA), as well as many states in the United States, as the basis for the evaluation of laser safety concerns (ANSI, 2011; LIA, 2016).

Manufacturers of laser products are regulated in the United States by the Center for Devices and Radiological Health and the Food and Drug Administration (FDA). The FDA has established polices that regulate product performance. All laser products sold in the United States since August 1976 must meet product performance and safety standards, and be labeled by the manufacturer to indicate their laser hazard (safety) classification (LIA, 2016).

Class 1

This class of laser cannot emit levels of optical radiation above the exposure limits for the eye under any exposure conditions inherent in the design of the laser product. Class 1 laser products are generally exempt from radiation hazard controls during operation and maintenance (but not necessarily during service). These lasers may be high-power if they are confined within an enclosure that does not permit any exposure to the operator (FDA, 2015). Examples are CD players and laser printers.

Class 1M

Lasers in this classification are not capable of producing hazardous exposure under normal operating conditions, but may be hazardous if viewed with the aid of magnifying optical instrumentation (FDA, 2015). Optical instrumentation includes binoculars, telescopes, microscopes, and magnifying glasses (but not prescription eyeglasses).

Class 2

Class 2 lasers are limited to 1 mW CW, or more if the emission time is less than 0.25 seconds or if the light is not spatially coherent. These lasers are too dazzling to stare into for any extended period of time, and our aversion response (<0.25 seconds) will protect the eye from damage. Intentional extended viewing for longer periods is considered hazardous. There is no hazard from exposure to this diffuse radiation (FDA, 2015). Examples are retail point-of-sale scanners and some measuring instruments.

Class 2M

Class 2M lasers have the same criteria as Class 2 but are hazardous when the beam is viewed with optical instruments (FDA, 2015).

Class 3R

The output power of Class 3R lasers can be up to 5 mW. They are only a hazard if focused or viewed for an extended period. They are not a fire hazard or a hazard to the skin (FDA, 2015). Until recently, this classification was known as 3A. Most laser pointers are Class 3R.

Class 3B

Class 3B lasers can have a power output up to 500 mW and wavelengths in the range from 300 nm up to the far infrared (FDA, 2015). There is an optical hazard when there is direct or reflected viewing of the beam. Protective eyewear must be worn when operating these devices. Therapeutic lasers that have a power output between 5 and 500 mW are Class 3B.

Class 4

Class 4 is the highest and most dangerous class of laser, and includes all lasers that exceed the Class 3B accessible emission limit. By definition, a Class 4 laser has a power greater than 500 mW and can burn the skin or cause devastating and permanent eye damage as a result of direct, diffuse, or indirect beam viewing. These lasers may ignite combustible materials, and thus may represent a fire risk. Any therapeutic laser that has an average output power greater than 500 mW is within this classification (FDA, 2015). Protective eyewear must be worn when operating these devices.

Modes of Emission

Simply stated, the mode of emission is the pattern of emission over time. Therapeutic lasers can have one of two modes of emission: CW or pulsing (emitting at a frequency) (Paschotta, 2016). There are two types of pulsing: gated pulsing and superpulsing.

There are various claims suggesting ideal pulsing frequencies for specific tissues. To date, there are no published papers which provide evidence of the advantages of pulsed emissions for the reduction of pain and inflammation in humans. A 2010 literature review by Hashmi *et al.* examined CW versus pulsed light and concluded that more evidence is needed: "It was impossible to draw any meaningful correlations between pulse frequency and pathological condition, due to the wide-ranging and disparate data." The authors concluded, "there is no consensus on the effects of different frequencies and pulse parameters on the physiology and therapeutic response of the various disease states that are often treated with laser therapy" (Hashmi *et al.*, 2010).

CW emission, as illustrated in Figure 2.4, is the simplest form of output to understand. The laser system produces a constant power output over the period for which the

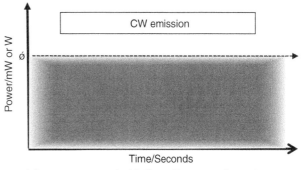

ó Average power output is the setting on equipment

Figure 2.4 CW emission produces a constant power output over the period for which a unit is activated. The average power output is the same as the power setting.

unit is activated by the therapist. The average power output, therefore, is the same as the power setting.

The terms "pulsing" and "frequency" are used interchangeably when there is an interruption of the power output. When pulsing, the laser output is turned on and off very quickly, similar to a strobe light.

The majority of veterinary therapeutic lasers provide both CW and pulsed output. Some allow the operator to select a pulse mode, while others have a fixed pulsing mode, or several pulsed modes within preset protocols. The characteristics pulsing regimes are often determined by the laser diodes in the device and the control systems and software incorporated in the user interface.

The frequency of the laser light is a function of wavelength. Pulse frequency is different, and refers to the number of pulses of light the laser emits each second. Just as when referring to the frequency of laser light, when referring to the number of pulses a laser emits each second, the unit of measurement is Hz (Merriam-Webster, 2016a): 1 Hz is one cycle per second; 500 Hz is 500 cycles per second.

If the laser is set in a gated-pulse mode, it will emit light on and off in a cycle. The result is a lower average power output. The duty cycle is the ratio of the power output when on versus off. In a 50% duty cycle, the power is on 50% of the time and off 50% of the time. Figure 2.5 illustrates the concepts of gated pulsing and a 50% duty cycle.

Think of pulsing as a way of slowing down administration of laser therapy. If there is any concern about heating the tissue, pulsing may be an option. Pulsing does not affect penetration into the tissue. In a 2015 publication that looked at the administration of photonic energy to human cadaver brain tissue, no differences in penetration were observed between pulsed and CW laser light (Tedford, 2015).

The superpulsed mode of emission is a series of extremely short, intense light pulses followed by an interval before the next pulse. The duration of each

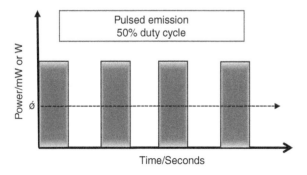

ó Average power output 50% of setting

Figure 2.5 If a laser is set in a gated-pulse mode, it will emit light on and off in a cycle. In a 50% duty cycle, the power is on 50% of the time and off 50% of the time.

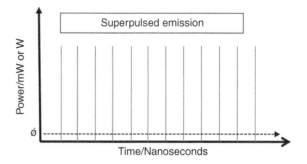

ó Average power output very low

Figure 2.6 Superpulsed emission is a series of extremely short, intense light pulses followed by an interval before the next pulse. Since each superpulse emission is very short, the average power of a series of superpulses is low.

superpulse emission is measured in nanoseconds or picoseconds; therefore, the average power of a series of superpulses is low (Berger and Eeg, 2006). The concept of superpulsing is illustrated in Figure 2.6.

Therapeutic lasers often utilize multiple modes of emission simultaneously. Different wavelengths are sometimes set at different modes of emission, resulting in a blend of wavelengths and emissions in an effort to achieve consistent clinical results.

Application Techniques

If a patient does not respond to laser therapy as expected, one of two possibilities is likely the cause. The therapy may have been administered to the wrong tissue, or the condition may have been misdiagnosed. Alternatively, insufficient photonic energy may have reached the target cells due to a blockage in the transmission of photons or an inadequate dosage.

A correct diagnosis and identification of all affected tissues is imperative. Visualize all of the anatomical structures within the target area and adapt a technique to ensure that all of the tissue – each cell, each mitochondrion – receives photonic energy. Treat not only the primary target area but also all of the secondary and tertiary areas of involvement.

Each therapy laser has its own optics design and one or more delivery handpieces. Though there are a myriad of handpieces, laser therapy is applied using one of two techniques: point-to-point or scanning. Either technique can be used with the handpiece in contact or not in contact with the tissues.

A significant amount of photonic energy is lost when treating off-contact, as both the skin and the hair reflect and absorb a percentage of the energy. When possible, treat in contact with the tissue. Fewer photons are reflected with this technique, and compression blanches the tissue, reducing incidental absorption by chromophores in blood.

Become familiar with the spot size, the power density, and the modes of emission of the device being used, and select an appropriate handpiece for each area being treated. Often, a combination of on- and off-contact techniques will be used to treat the same anatomical area. An example is treating otitis: an off-contact technique is used to treat the pinna and visible structures, and an on-contact technique is used to transcutaneously treat the more proximal portion of the ear canal.

Regardless of the administration technique, keep the handpiece perpendicular to the target tissue and, whenever possible, place the target area through a passive range of motion during treatment. Before initiating therapy, pretest the area to establish a normal, comfortable range of motion. There is often an immediate analgesic effect due to PBM, so take care not to move through a range of motion beyond the limits established before starting the treatment.

In a point-to-point technique, the handpiece is placed close to or in contact with the target treatment area and held there until the appropriate dosage is administered. If the target area is larger than the spot size, the handpiece is moved adjacent to the first treatment area, and the administration is repeated until the entire area has received the appropriate dosage.

When using the scanning technique, the handpiece is similarly placed either close to or in contact with the tissue, but it is constantly moved over the target area at a speed of 3–7 cm/sec. A repetitive scanning pattern with a series of parallel movements back and forth, alternating with a series of parallel movements at 90°, is utilized. The handpiece is aimed from every possible direction toward the target tissue, treating from 360° when possible. A border of normal adjacent tissue is also treated. Wide margins are not a concern, since the administration of photonic energy has no detrimental effect on normal cells.

The application of laser therapy is easy and the learning curve is not steep. There is almost no way to administer it improperly. Therefore, there should be no harm to the patient. The biggest concern of novices using high-power therapy lasers is a fear of heating the tissues. This is easily avoided by using a finger as a digital thermometer. When treating at a high power setting, place a trailing finger adjacent to the end of the handpiece. If the patient's skin or hair warms beyond a comfortable temperature, move the handpiece to another location.

Dosing

The amount of photonic energy applied during laser therapy is a function of the patient's individual characteristics and the location of the target tissue (Enwemeka, 2009). In veterinary medicine, no two patients are alike. All have different hair thicknesses, coat colors, body types, and skin thicknesses and colors, and each will have an individual response to therapy.

There are no global dosages appropriate for every patient. However, there are two important principles. First, if the dose is inadequate, there will not be a consistent clinical response. In fact, there may not be a clinical response at all. Second, there is a wide margin of safety. New scientific evidence is published regularly, and studies and clinical trials of dosages are increasing on a regular basis.

In 2010, the World Association for Laser Therapy (WALT) published a list of suggested dosages (WALT, 2010). Despite subsequent publication of scientific, evidence-based research, these suggested dosages have not been revised in over 5 years. Though a multi-hour discussion about dosage recommendations was held at WALT's annual combined meeting with the North American Association for Photobiomodulation Therapy (NALT) in 2014, no consensus was reached. The range of dosages mentioned varied from just a few joules applied to an entire anatomical area to research doses of several hundred J/cm^2. In both the human and the veterinary sessions at the annual meeting of the American Society for Laser Medicine & Surgery (ASLMS) in April of 2015, no paper was presented about PBM that used dosages less than $5–8\,J/cm^2$ when the target tissue was not superficial.

Though there is no standard, one-size-fits-all dosing guide, patients can be treated with doses reported as being successful in research and clinical-trial publications. Reported doses are safe starting points and can be adjusted as needed based on the patient response.

Calculating the dosage to be delivered to a patient's specific anatomical area is easy. It is the uncertainty of the penetration of that dose to the target tissue that is the challenge. Enough energy has to be delivered to the tissue surface, at the appropriate power and wavelength, frequently enough, to achieve a consistent clinical response.

As photons penetrate to the cellular target, they can be reflected, scattered, and absorbed by the different densities of tissues and incidental chromophores they encounter (Jacques, 2013). These obstacles to penetration lead to exponentially decaying intensities of light with depth. A study reporting the successful translation of *in vitro* results obtained in the Petri dish to the treatment of surgically repaired nerves *in vivo* found the optimal dose for nerve repair *in vitro* to be 97.5% less than that required when delivered on the surface of the skin (Anders *et al.*, 2014).

Concerns about correct dosages and effective penetration can be reduced by the use of newer, veterinary-specific therapy lasers. These devices have software programs that provide preset dosage protocols for a wide variety of conditions, in a variety of species. Input of

> **Box 2.1 Laser therapy dose recommendations.**
>
> **Companion Animal Species**
> Superficial tissue conditions: 1–5 J/cm^2
> Deep tissue conditions: 8–10 J/cm^2
> Chronic complex conditions: 15–25 J/cm^2
> **Equine, Food Animal, and Large Zoo Species**
> Superficial tissue conditions: 1–5 J/cm^2
> Superficial musculoskeletal conditions: 8–20 J/cm^2
> Deep musculoskeletal conditions: 15–35 J/cm^2
> **Exotic Species**
> Small mammals: 0.5–8 J/cm^2
> Avian: 0.5–5 J/cm^2
> Reptiles: 2–8 J/cm^2

patient-specific characteristics (weight, body type, skin color, and coat length and color) enables the software to deliver a protocol that ensures a correct dose is delivered with maximum photon penetration.

Chapters in this text will offer specific dosage guidelines for various conditions and applications. These guidelines will vary depending on the species, condition, and body area being treated. A general summary of current dosage recommendations is presented in Box 2.1.

Frequency of Treatment and Management Protocols

The frequency of administration of laser therapy is unique to each case and is dependent on the condition, client compliance, and the patient's response to the therapy. The three characteristic phases included in the management of conditions with laser therapy are induction, transition, and maintenance.

- **Induction Phase:** An aggressive series of treatments in which therapy is administered on consecutive days or every other day until a significant clinical response is noted. Evaluation of an acceptable response to treatment depends on the patient, the condition, and the expectations of the clinician and the owner. Many acute conditions will only require induction-phase treatments.
- **Transition Phase:** A series of treatments at gradually reducing frequency, used to establish the frequency

required to maintain the clinical response. If induction-phase treatments have been administered every other day, transition-phase treatments are recommended twice a week for several weeks, once a week for several weeks, every other week, every 2 weeks, every 3 weeks, and then as needed.

- **Maintenance Phase:** A long-term series of treatments administered as frequently as required in order to maintain the clinical response and the patient's quality of life. Most chronic conditions can be maintained with a treatment every 3–4 weeks. Frequency must be adjusted to the patient's requirements. Client involvement in determining the frequency of maintenance-phase treatments is helpful.

The effect of PBM is cumulative. After each session, there should be an improvement in the clinical condition or an increase in the duration of the response. Patient progress can be observed subjectively, scored objectively, or monitored with digital thermal imaging (Nahm, 2013; Turner, 2001). Digital thermal imaging also aids in the identification of secondary and tertiary areas that would benefit from treatment. Treatment of all affected anatomical areas simultaneously provides a more holistic approach, and often better clinical results.

If there is no response after three or four treatment sessions, re-evaluate the patient, the diagnosis, and the areas being treated. A clever and accurate maxim used by a practitioner of human laser therapy is, "better in four, or schedule no more" (www.stopchasingpain.com).

Conclusion

By developing an understanding of the fundamental principles of laser therapy, practitioners can maximize the full potential of this therapeutic modality. Knowledge of how therapeutic lasers generate and emit photonic energy that penetrates to cellular targets, resulting in a physiological and biochemical cascade of events providing a relief of pain, a modulation of the inflammatory reaction, and an increase in the microcirculation, is essential. Once this fundamental information is acquired, it can be applied while using any laser therapy device, to treat any appropriate condition, in any species.

References

Anders, J. *et al.* (2014) In vitro and in vivo optimization of infrared laser treatment for injured peripheral nerves. *Lasers Surg Med.* **46**(1):34–45.

Anders, J. *et al.* (2015) Low-level light/laser therapy versus photobiomodulation therapy. *Photomed Laser Surg.* **33**(4):183–184.

ANSI (2011) American National Standard for Safe Use of Lasers in Health Care Facilities. ANSI Z136.3 – 2011. American National Standards Institute, Washington, DC.

Barrett, S.F. and Pack, D.J. (2006) Timing subsystem. In: *Microcontrollers Fundamentals for Engineers and Scientists*, pp. 51–64. Morgan and Claypool, San Rafael, CA.

Bartels, K.E. (2014) Lasers in veterinary medicine – an introduction to surgical lasers. In: *Current Techniques in Small Animal Surgery*, 5 edn., pp. 35–36. Teton NewMedia, Jackson, WY.

Berger, N.A. and Eeg, P.H. (2006) General principles. In: *Veterinary Laser Surgery: A Practical Guide*, p. 17. Wiley-Blackwell, Hoboken, NJ.

BIPM. (2014) SI brochure: the International System of Units (SI) [8th edition, 2006; updated in 2014]. Available from: http://www.bipm.org/en/publications/si-brochure/(accessed November 30, 2016).

Chu, S. and Townes, C. (2003) Arthur Schawlow. *Biographical Memoirs*. **83**:202.

Coldren, L.A. *et al.* (2012). *Diode Lasers and Photonic Integrated Circuits*, 2 edn. John Wiley and Sons, Hoboken, NJ.

Craford, M. *et al.* (2001) In pursuit of the ultimate lamp. *Scientific American*. **284**(2):62–67.

Dictionary.com. (2016) Wavelength. Available from: http://dictionary.reference.com/browse/wavelength (accessed November 30, 2016).

Einstein, A. (1905) On a heuristic point of view concerning the production and transformation of light. Available from: http://einsteinpapers.press.princeton.edu/vol2-trans/100 (accessed November 30, 2016).

Enwemeka, C.S. (2009) Intricacies of dose in laser phototherapy for tissue repair and pain relief. *Photomed Laser Surg*. **27**(3):387–393.

FDA. (2015). Laser hazard classes. Available from: http://www.fda.gov/radiation-emittingproducts/radiationemittingproductsandprocedures/homebusinessandentertainment/laserproductsandinstruments/default.htm (accessed November 30, 2016).

Ginani, F. *et al.* (2015) Effect of low-level laser therapy on mesenchymal stem cell proliferation: a systemic review. *Lasers Med Sci*. **30**(8):2189–2194.

Gould, G.R. (1959) *The LASER, Light Amplification by Stimulated Emission of Radiation*. The Ann Arbor Conference on Optical Pumping, The University of Michigan. June 15–18, Ann Arbor, MI.

Hashmi, J.T. *et al.* (2010) Effect of pulsing in low-level light therapy. *Lasers Surg Med*. **42**(6):450–466.

Hecht, E. (1987). *Optics*, 2 edn. Addison Wesley, Boston, MA.

Hewitt, P. (2001) *Conceptual Physics*, 9 edn. Addison Wesley, Boston, MA.

IEC. (2014) *Safety of Laser Products – Part 1: Equipment Classification and Requirements*, 3 edn. IEC 60825-1:2014. International Electrotechnical Commission, Geneva.

Jacques, S.L. (2013) Optical properties of biological tissues: a review. *Phys Med Biol*. **58**(11):R37–R61.

Jenkins, P.A. and Carroll, J.D. (2011) How to report low-level laser therapy (LLLT)/photomedicine dose and beam parameters in clinical and laboratory studies. *Photomed Laser Surg*. **29**(12):785–787.

Kerker, M. (1969) *The Scattering of Light*. Academic Press, New York.

Kittel, C. and Kroemer, H. (1980) *Thermal Physics*. W.H. Freeman, New York.

LaserFest. (2016) Laser definition. Available from: http://laserfest.org/lasers/how/laser.cfm (accessed November 30, 2016).

LIA. (2016) Laser safety information. Available from: https://www.lia.org/subscriptions/safety_bulletin/laser_safety_info/(accessed November 30, 2016).

Loudon, R. (2001) *The Quantum Theory of Light*, 3 edn. Oxford University Press, New York.

Merriam-Webster. (2016a) Hertz. Available from: http://www.merriam-webster.com/dictionary/hertz (accessed November 30, 2016).

Merriam-Webster. (2016b) Irradiance. Available from: http://www.merriam-webster.com/dictionary/irradiance (accessed November 30, 2016).

Merriam-Webster. (2016c) Joule. Available from: http://www.merriam-webster.com/dictionary/joule (accessed November 30, 2016).

Merriam-Webster. (2016d) Lase. Available from: http://www.merriam-webster.com/dictionary/lase (accessed November 30, 2016).

Merriam-Webster. (2016e) Power. Available from: http://www.merriam-webster.com/dictionary/power (accessed November 30, 2016).

MeSH. (2016) Photobiomodulation. Available from: http://www.ncbi.nlm.nih.gov/mesh/?term=photobiomodulation (accessed November 30, 2016).

Nahm, F.S. (2013) Infrared thermography in pain medicine. *Korean J Pain*. **26**(3):219–222.

Paschotta, R. (2016) Modes of laser operation. Available from: https://www.rp-photonics.com/modes_of_laser_operation.html (accessed November 30, 2016).

Scholarpedia. (2016) Optical amplification. Available from: http://www.scholarpedia.org/article/Optical_amplification (accessed November 30, 2016).

Siegman, A.E. (1986). *Lasers*. University Science Books, Sausalito, CA.

Silfvast, W.T. (1996) *Laser Fundamentals*. Cambridge University Press, Cambridge.

Smil, V. (2008) *Energy in Nature and Society: General Energentics of Complex Systems*. MIT Press, Cambridge, MA.

Svelto, O. (1998) *Principles of Lasers*, 4 edn. Springer Science+Business Media, New York.

Tedford, C.E. (2015). Quantitative analysis of transcranial and intraparenchymal light penetration in human cadaver brain tissue. *Lasers Surg Med*. **47**(4):312–322.

Turner, T.A. (2001) Diagnostic thermography. *Vet Clin North Am Equine Pract*. **17**(1):95–113.

VALUE @ Amrita. (2016) Laser beam divergence and spot size. Available from: http://vlab.amrita.edu/?sub=1&brch=189&sim=342&cnt=1 (accessed November 30, 2016).

WALT. (2010) WALT dosage recommendations. Available from: http://waltza.co.za/documentation-links/recommendations/dosage-recommendations (accessed November 30, 2016).

Zaini, M. (1995) Measuring the fluence of clinical electron beams. Ph.D. thesis. The University of Wisconsin – Madison. *Dissertation Abstracts International.* **56-12**(B):6617.

Zaini, M. *et al.* (1996) Measuring the electron fluence of clinical accelerators. *Radiation Meas.* **27**(3):511–521.

Zheludev, N. (2007) The life and times of the LED – a 100-year history. *Nat Photon.* **1**(4):189–192.

3

Laser Physics in Veterinary Medicine

Bryan J. Stephens

SOUND (a VCA Company), Franklin, TN, USA

Introduction

Crucial to you getting the most out of the rest of this book is your understanding of some very basic properties of light. The more you understand about the complete set of characteristics of the magic that comes out of your therapy laser, the better equipped you will be to tailor your treatment protocols and enhance the clinical efficacy of your therapy. You are going to read chapters that tell you about *in vitro* experiments that demonstrate the enhancement of cellular mechanisms, followed by even more real-world data that show a broad range of clinical usefulness based on these mechanisms. Within this stockpile of evidence, there will be some basic recommendations on dose prescriptions, power settings, pulse frequency characteristics, and treatment periodicity. These will be necessarily broad, to account for patient and condition variations, but also because the parameters used throughout both the anecdotal reports and the well-controlled experiments are quite mixed. My goal in this chapter is to have an informal conversation (rather than an encyclopedic lookup) that identifies what can be tweaked, explains its significance, and gives you a glimpse of its clinical implications.

Why Use Light?

Simply put, we use light because it can penetrate into the body and then cause a physiological change once it gets inside. An eighth-grader may not agree with that, since he cannot see through his own hand, and when he shines a flashlight on his arm he does not start to grow another. However, you are not so naïve. You have seen x-rays that have allowed you to peer inside the body. And you can read these pages, so you accept the idea (however unconsciously) that light gets absorbed by the cones in your eyes, which causes chemical reactions that lead to electrical signals that affect your chemistry and even your mood, your behavior, and your health. Yes, ducking when you see a baseball coming towards your head is a health-altering effect of light's interaction with your biological self.

However, visible light does not penetrate very well into our bodies, and your eyes cannot see x-rays. So what is the difference between these and the other flavors of light you are here to read about?

Flavors of Light

Despite the wide range of interactions and applications of light, there is literally only one fundamental difference between any two types: wavelength. To understand what this means, we first need to know what light *is* – an oscillating electric and magnetic field that travels in a straight line and at a constant speed (the speed of light). This is why the technical term for light is "electromagnetic radiation." What it *does* is much more complex, and we will dive into some of that in this chapter, but that is all that light *is*. So, since light always travels at the same speed, the structure of its oscillation can be described equivalently either by the distance between its peaks (and valleys) or by how many peaks (or valleys) it has in a given time. We call these values the "wavelength" and "frequency," respectively. This is not to be confused with pulse frequency or repetition rate. That has to do with turning light on and off periodically. We will get to that later.

Going forward, I will refer to the different types of light by either of these characteristics, but you will know that they refer to the same thing, and that is this one-dimensional scale of the oscillating electromagnetic wave we call light. My favorite A.M. sports radio station growing up broadcasted using light at 660 kHz (frequency), I heated up my coffee in the microwave this morning with light at 2.45 GHz (also frequency), but my favorite color is 450 nm (the wavelength of blue light). Indeed, these are all just different colors of light; the

Laser Therapy in Veterinary Medicine: Photobiomodulation, First Edition. Edited by Ronald J. Riegel and John C. Godbold, Jr.

human eye only evolved to contain cones that can detect wavelengths from about 390 to 700 nm, which is what we call the visible part of the spectrum. The near-infrared spectrum spans from about 700 to 1100 nm.

If you were clever, you would have hesitated when I said "one-dimensional scale," since you know we experience three dimensions. In fact, the electric and magnetic fields that make up light are always at 90° from each other, so there are the other dimensions for you. This brings about two characteristics of light you may have heard referenced: polarization, which simply means the alignment of the electric (or magnetic) fields of light, and coherence, which means that the peaks and valleys of two different pieces of light are lined up. However, these values (and these other two dimensions) only matter when whatever you are shining the light on is structured enough to make a difference. Biological matter, in general, is not; but we are jumping ahead a little. First, we have to define the interactions, and then things will clear up a bit.

Wait, one more fundamental property of light: it turns out that the energy of light is directly proportional to its frequency (and therefore inversely proportional to its wavelength). The amount of energy any "piece" of light carries is discrete or "quantized." Therefore, in a sense, light is made up of individual packets of light, called "photons." No reason to explore the wave–particle duality of light here, but it was important to mention, since it will affect how we talk about light a little later. Figure 3.1 illustrates the fundamental structure of an electromagnetic wave and the relationship between wavelength, frequency, and energy.

So, how does this one fundamental property of light (frequency or wavelength or energy, however you want to refer to it) lead to such different effects in the different regions of the spectrum? In other words, why do different colors of light interact differently with matter?

Interactions

In the region of the electromagnetic spectrum that concerns this book (the visible and near-infrared), there are two basic interactions: absorption and scatter. But before we get to these, we have to understand what we are shining the light on: biological matter. The body seems rigid enough, and it is at the scale of a baseball. However, when you are using light, you have to see things at the scale of light, which we see in Figure 3.1 is on the order of hundreds of nanometers. When you zoom in that closely, you will see that we are made up of molecules. If you

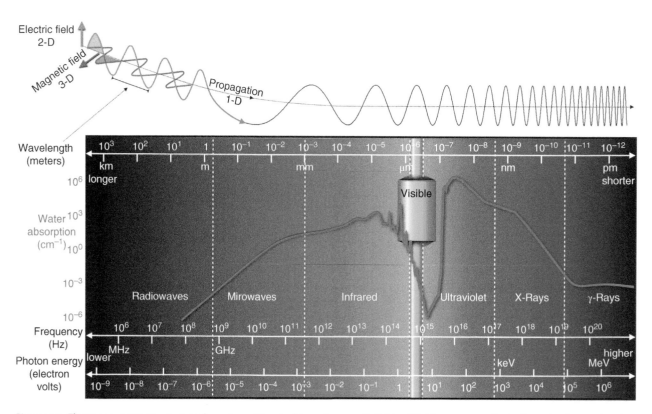

Figure 3.1 Electromagnetic structure and spectrum. The electric and magnetic fields of light are perpendicular to each other and to the direction of propagation. The name and effect of the radiation vary by wavelength (top axis), and equivalently by frequency and energy (bottom axes). The blue curve represents the absorption of water throughout the spectrum (Hale and Querry, 1973; Segelstein, 1981; Zolotarev *et al.*, 1969).

zoomed in further, you would see atoms, but that would fall in the realm of x-rays (with wavelengths below 10 nm); visible and near-infrared light does not interact very strongly with objects that small.

Intra- and intermolecular bonds, however, are just the right size and so interact very well in this region. These bonds are nothing more than shared electron clouds (moving, charged particles), but they effectively act as springs between the constituent atoms. When charged particles are subject to an electric and magnetic field (like when you shine light on them), they experience forces, and since the field is oscillating, so do the bonds; and like strings on a guitar, they each have their own natural frequency.

Absorption

Absorption happens when the frequency of light is close to this natural frequency. Just like pushing someone on a swing or a mass on a spring, if you push in rhythm with the natural rhythm, you can transfer the most energy of your push to the system. In the visible and near-infrared region of the spectrum on biological tissue, photons of light either impart all of their energy to what they strike or bounce off; they are completely absorbed or they scatter. So, in effect, light is absorbed by bonds that have just the right frequency, which makes it clear to see why absorption is wavelength- and tissue-dependent. Different tissues have different constituents, made up of bonds with different frequencies.

When these bonds absorb the light, they do what any excited spring does: bend, twist, expand, contract, and any combination of these. What this does, in effect, is change the shape of the molecule or chain of molecules. This is chemistry at its very core. You have to understand, the main way chemistry works (i.e., the way that two molecules combine) is a very sensitive, physical lock-and-key mechanism. Things that fit together nicely (both spatially and electrically) tend to bond together. If they do not fit, they do not bond. By changing the shape of one part of a molecule, even slightly and even on a very short time scale, you can cause the molecule to shed parts of itself or grab on to new things. What magical biochemical effects come from these absorption events is the topic of later chapters.

For those of you who have worked with surgical lasers (or kitchen microwaves, for that matter), you will realize that if you use enough light in a wavelength (or frequency) range that coincides with bonds that are prevalent in the tissue, these vibrations will reinforce themselves, create a lot of heat, and eventually shake molecules apart. Most of the time, the target molecules are water, and this boiling of water in the tissue either heats your food in a general way (if diffuse) or ablates the tissue in a very efficient, localized way (if focused).

In either case, absorption allows the targeting of molecules by light with the "right" frequency. However, statistically speaking, the majority of light bounces off something before it is absorbed.

Scatter

In the visible and near-infrared, virtually all of the scatter is elastic – photons retain their energy and simply bounce off particles in their path that do not have the "right" frequency to be absorbed (and even when they do, there is always a non-zero probability of each interaction). Which direction the photon travels after the bounce depends on what it bounced off: mostly the size of the particle. Scattering of light by particles smaller than about 1/10th the wavelength of light is referred to as "Rayleigh scattering." Scattering by particles larger than that is referred to as "Mie scattering." The result of Rayleigh scattering is isotropic; the scattered light has equal intensity in all directions (except for at around 90°). Mie scattering, on the other hand, is very much forward pointing, and the extent to which it points forward is represented by a number called the "anisotropy factor." Little do you care that this is defined as the average cosine of the scattering angle, but a value of 1 means forward scattering (the incoming and outgoing light are going in exactly the same direction), a value of 0 means scattering at 90°, and a value of −1 means complete reflection. Values for the near-infrared on biological tissue are in the 0.75–0.90 range, so this is what I mean by forward pointing.

How Much of Each

We do not talk about absorption and scattering on an individual basis, simply because there are more of these events in the first millimeter of skin than all of humanity could count in a lifetime. Instead, we talk about macroscopic quantities like absorption coefficients, μ_a, and reduced-scattering coefficients, μ_s', both of which have units of 1/length. These give you the average amount of absorption or scattering along the path of light and yield the shape of an exponential decay curve that describes the attenuation of light intensity with depth. Inversely (i.e., if you take one divided by these quantities), you are left with what is called the "mean free path," which tells you the average distance between absorption and scattering events. Each of these quantities depends on both wavelength and tissue, since for absorption it is all about matching the frequency of light with the frequency of bonds, and for scatter the size and number of the scattering particles (i.e., tissue composition and density) dictate the storyline.

Absorption coefficients are easy to understand, because either a photon is absorbed or it is not. Therefore, we use absorption coefficients along with depth from the surface to understand total absorption (and therefore the total relative intensity that is left in the beam). The blue curve in the background of Figure 3.1 shows the absorption coefficient of water throughout nearly the entire spectrum for reference.

Scattering is a bit trickier because the direction the light bounces depends on what it bounced off. In addition, the path length of the light is never the same as (and is usually a lot more than) the depth, because of all the little bounces in different directions. Still, we do not track each bounce, but rather treat this directionality on average. This is why you saw me refer to the *reduced* scattering coefficient, which incorporates the anisotropy into its calculation. Basically, the reduced scattering coefficient gives you a directionally corrected scattering coefficient that makes calculations simpler and lets you use the depth (which you know, or at least want to know) rather than individual path length of every light ray (which you do not know nor care about). Therefore, the inverse, or reduced mean free path, gives you the average depth between scattering events.

These two quantities combine to form an effective attenuation coefficient, which is a generalized way of describing the loss of original beam intensity. With this, we can now understand how much light, relative to how much we started with, gets to what depth. Figure 3.2 illustrates the idea of attenuation in each of its mechanisms. Again, intensity is an exponentially decaying quantity, meaning that the deeper you go, the less light remains than in the original beam. That sounds simple enough. Just give me μ_a and μ_s' of a tissue, and I will tell how much light gets to that joint you are trying to treat.

Not so fast! In any target treatment area, there are many different amounts and types of tissue, which are not sliced and stacked neatly on top of on one another like deli meat in its packaging. So tracking the amount of absorption, type of scattering, and direction of scattering along the wide variety of interactions as light bounces around inside the body becomes a complicated mess. We can make some generalizations to help, though.

First, once inside the body, scattering is by far the dominant interaction in biological tissue, with its effect being strongest at shorter wavelengths. As some perspective, this means that the average depth of a scattering event is at most every half millimeter (and usually less). At the skin, absorption and scattering play about equal roles, and there are a lot of both. Though the skin is not the

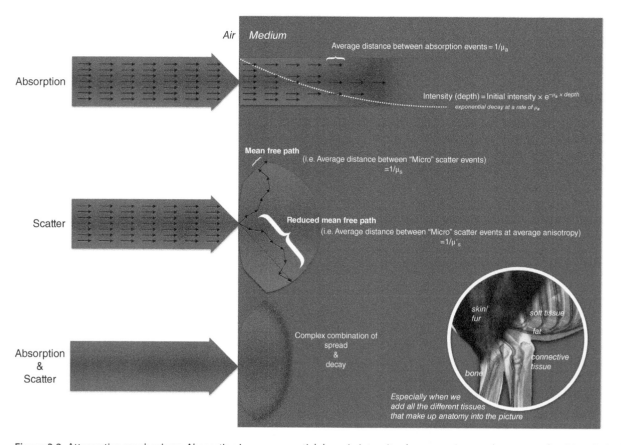

Figure 3.2 Attenuation mechanisms. Absorption is an exponential decay in intensity along any given path at a rate of μ_a. Many "micro" scattering events are often characterized by their average distance and angle, i.e., "macro" information, which is combined in the reduced scattering coefficient μ_s'. Combined, these processes lead to a general "mushrooming" of the beam, i.e., a decay in intensity and spread of the beam with depth inside the patient.

ironclad barrier to the outside world like it is for, say, water, it is an obstacle for light. But, since the anisotropy factor of visible and near-infrared light incident on biological tissue is very close to 1, on average these scattering events point the light even deeper into the patient.

Second, even though absorption is smaller in magnitude inside the body (a factor of 200–5000 times smaller than scattering coefficients), with absorption events taking place along the windy path the light ends up bouncing along inside the body, virtually all of the light that gets in is absorbed somewhere inside (Jacques, 2013). You do not see the animal glowing with near-infrared light as you treat them, even with an infrared camera. If you had a very sensitive detector, you would definitely find some light coming out, but the majority is absorbed by the body. In addition, a small fraction of absorption of a lot of photons still gives a lot of total absorption. How much are we talking about?

Units You Have Heard Of (Hopefully)

We measure the energy of an individual photon in a unit called an electron volt (eV), with the energy of a photon equal to 1240 divided by the wavelength in nanometers. Therefore, a photon of red light at 620 nm carries 2 eV of energy. However, we measure the energy of a beam of light in a unit called joules (J). For reference, 1 J of energy is equal to 6 242 000 000 000 000 000 eV. So, 1 J of red light consists of 3 121 000 000 000 000 000 photons. Now you see what I meant when I said a small fraction of a big number is still a big number.

For another reference, 1 J of energy is how much it takes to lift a baseball 28 inches up off the ground. At the same time, when you drop a baseball from 28 inches, it hits the ground with 1 J of energy. So why does your patient not feel like they are being bombarded with baseballs when you shine light at them? The reason is the flexibility of the molecular bonds in the body that we have been talking about. The body is not rigid when it comes to light, like it is with incoming baseballs. The energy absorbed (and we determined that the majority of the light you shine on the patient is absorbed by them) is transferred to the three-dimensional configuration of the billions of molecules and bonds in the treatment area on an individual basis and at varying depths within the tissue. Most of the absorbed vibrations turn into heat, which quickly dissipates as the bonds come back to rest in their equilibrium states.

However, to say that you delivered 1 J of energy is meaningless. Did you expose the entire body to that energy, or just one part? Did you deliver that energy over the span of an hour or in a fraction of a second? Remember that photons move very fast (at the speed of light) and their absorption events are virtually instantaneous, so the time scale is very important.

For this reason, we like using the quantity called "power," which is defined as energy per time, and is usually given in units of watts (W; 1 W = 1 J/sec). This gives a more accurate picture of the scale of interaction, because while we will see that the accumulation of light–tissue interactions is important, the body is living and moving, and so the amount of light delivered on any given time scale is important. As a clinician, you are not naïve enough to think that if you were to give 1 J of light to a patient once per day, by the time you had given them 100 J of energy their tissue or symptoms or overall condition would still be the same as when you started. If you delivered that same energy in 1 minute, it is very reasonable to assume that not much would have changed. However, we still have not answered the question relating to the size of the treatment area. Again, you know better than to think that 100 J across the whole animal would give the same clinical impact as if you only exposed the paw.

Therefore, while total energy and power are easy to calculate, they do not tell the whole story. This is important and dangerous, because without context, these quantities can be warped and used to manipulate the truth. The two quantities that give a more complete picture are *energy density* and *power density*, and they are simply the total energy and power per unit area, respectively.

As you deliver light to a patient and accumulate energy in a treatment area, you are forcing more light–tissue interactions in that area. Decades of research have shed the tiniest bit of light (pun definitely intended) on what biological, physiological, and clinical implications these interactions can initiate and sustain. Equally important has been the study of the time scale of these effects. So, while energy density, which we call *dose* (energy per area, usually given in units of J/cm^2) and power density (power per unit area, in W/cm^2) are better descriptors, one without the other still falls short of being explanatory because of the element of time. Dose is a description of deposition (how much), while power density describes exposure (how quickly). These are hugely important when combined, yet they are dangerously hollow independently. More on the idea of reciprocity later.

Deciding Dose

There is only one way to determine how much dose is best for a given treatment: precise science (trial and error). However, there are two places to start, both of which are important and independently necessary. First, you can start with the individual cells. Much of the research in the past 2 decades falls into this category, where people expose cells in a very controlled environment to different amounts of light and measure the magnitude of cellular effects, which can range from mitochondrial activity to adhesion to glass, luminescence, DNA replication rates, and much more. These studies have the benefit of being controlled, in that virtually all parameters other than the one you wish to change can be held fixed, and so individual mechanisms and their dose dependencies can be tracked. They are at the same time limited by their weak relation to real-world situations, where cell signaling and the transport of nutrients, wastes, and heat in a three-dimensional matrix of the cells that make up tissue are vastly different than in a monolayer of cells living on glass.

Nonetheless, for the determination of optimal dose, this is the cleanest method. Once you find the peak in the response curve, you then need to estimate the percentage of the light that reaches the cells that are at the heart of the condition you are treating. After reading the sections on absorption and scatter, you should be well-convinced that there is an enormous difference between what you expose to the surface and what actually reaches an internal structure. Penetration studies have been sprinkled within the literature (too sparsely, if you ask me) and lend some assistance in estimating this exposure-to-delivery ratio. This is fundamentally the best strategy for an accurate dose prescription model.

However, we really care about the clinical efficacy, and so if the results do not follow from this prescription, we are forced to use the second starting point: the clinical version of trial and error, where we vary the dose over a sample of patients and see what works best. This can be very scientific or anecdotal; in the coming chapters, you will see results of both versions. If you do care to be true scientists about this, the right path is to get your starting point from the fundamental calculations, then tweak them based on a combination of clinical and anecdotal literature and more fundamental science. So, what else can you tweak, and which are the intelligent ways to do so?

Knobs to Turn

There are three knobs that virtually every laser has, whether they are physical knobs or not: spot size, power, and time. Combined, these knobs determine the dose and power density of treatment. Two can change without the third. Doubling the time and halving the power keeps the dose unchanged, and doubling the power and doubling the treatment area keeps the power density unchanged, which, given the same time, keeps the dose the same.

Advice about which to change for a given treatment should (and, in later chapters, will) come from clinicians, but the meaningful limits of each are more fundamental than that, and mostly have to do with power density. Use a too-low power density and you might as well prescribe walks in the park for the animal, because the sun exposes your patient to about $33\,\mathrm{mW/cm^2}$ of near-infrared light (ASTM, 2008). Use too-high power density and heat will be deposited in the patient faster than the body can dissipate it, and so will accumulate, causing first pain, then eventually irreversible tissue damage when the tissue reaches a temperature of about $45\,°C$ ($113\,°F$). The threshold for pain is very much patient-dependent (and tissue- and wavelength-dependent, since different combinations absorb at different strengths), but a ballpark figure is that $1–2\,\mathrm{W/cm^2}$ of near-infrared light will begin to hurt after a few seconds, and more than that will begin to hurt immediately. The body has a built in safety net, though: pain comes well before any serious damage can be done (unless you are working well above this power density). As long as you are not treating while the patient is writhing in pain, odds are you have not done any serious damage. Nevertheless, within this window of usefulness and comfort, there are knobs to turn.

Spot Size

Spot size is limited by the optical engineering of the light source. Obviously, too small a spot size will simply take too long to deliver an adequate dose, unless you use lots of power, which will probably set your power density over the threshold. An instance where a small spot size is useful is in the practice of laser acupuncture, where the light can be used to stimulate qi meridians, where apparently not much energy is needed (I have already gone beyond my sphere of knowledge; I will defer to the experts of later chapters). In general treatment, however, the lower limit of spot size is determined by the practicality of covering the entire treatment area in a clinically feasible time. The upper limit is determined by the optical coupling of the light source to the patient. We spoke about scatter microscopically earlier, but macroscopically, scatter is very much angle-dependent. Administering light perpendicular to the surface minimizes scatter from the surface, with the amount of scatter increasing super-linearly with angle (the bigger the angle, the less light gets inside the patient). Therefore, the upper limit of the spot size is about the size of the handpiece from which the light originates; any larger than that, and the light on the edges of the treatment area will no longer be perpendicular to the surface, and the amount of light delivered inside the patient will be substantially diminished.

A quick aside on types of light sources. Lasers and light-emitting diodes (LEDs) are among the most popular light sources in the therapeutic world, and they have two fundamental differences, one that matters and one that likely does not: divergence and coherence. While technically both light sources produce somewhat divergent light, light from lasers is in general inherently much more collimated. LEDs, on the other hand, are virtually isotropic light sources, which means they emit light in all directions. This is not to say that the light emitted from either cannot pass through some focusing optics to produce similar beams of light. If it did, then their only difference would be that the light from the laser would be coherent (the peaks and valleys of all the constituent light would be aligned), but as discussed earlier, this only really matters when the light is shone on something that is structured enough to resolve it: usually crystalline lattices and metals. But LEDs without any spherical or parabolic mirrors to reflect and focus the emitted light do not expose the patient to the total amount of light they produce; much of the light is not even pointed at the patient, but rather in the opposite or peripheral directions.

Power

Combined with spot size (and, obviously, wavelength), power dictates the real time state of the laser. We just identified the upper and lower limits of power density, and since the spot size of your laser is usually fixed (or at least, fixed for any given treatment), the window of useful power output is set for you. The two principle reasons for changing power are to decrease your treatment time and to increase your penetration during a set treatment time.

"Whoa, whoa, whoa. Hold on. I thought wavelength determines the penetration?" Correct. Mostly. We talked about how both absorption and scattering lead to exponentially decaying intensities of light with depth inside the patient. And yes, the shape of these curves (how quickly the intensity drops) is dependent on the combination of wavelength and tissue type. If you start with more light, then you are left with more light at each depth. In fact, any percentage increase of power will lead to the same percentage decrease in treatment time required to deliver the same dose to the same depth. Refer to Figure 3.3 as we explain. Suppose the goal is to deliver 20 J of energy to a depth A. We can see from the curve that only 50% of the beam's surface intensity remains at this depth. Thus, the 2 W laser would have to treat for 20 seconds to build up the desired dose, while the 8 W laser could deliver the exact same dose to the exact same depth in only 5 seconds (a quarter of the time, since the laser is four times as powerful).

To think of it from another perspective, one that really gets at the heart of this power-versus-penetration issue, let us consider the example of treating for a fixed amount of time and calculate the depth to which each laser will deliver the same dose. As before, treating for 20 seconds with a 2 W laser will deliver 20 J of energy to A. Now, even though the transmission percentage is four times lower at depth B (12.5%), since we start off with four times more photons with the higher-powered laser, the same 20 J of energy can be delivered to this deeper target (B vs. A) in the same treatment time. Again, the lower-powered laser can eventually accumulate the same amount of dose, but only with longer treatment time. The depth scale of this figure is exaggerated, and so the distance between A and B might be quite small (in highly attenuating tissue), but the concept that higher power in a fixed treatment time yields deeper penetration holds, in general.

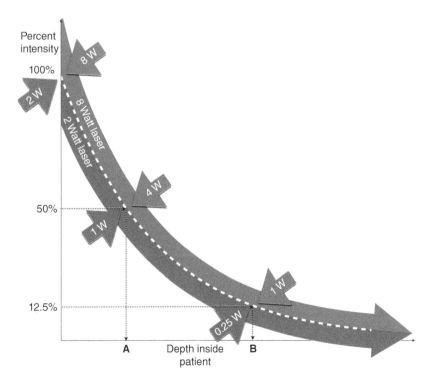

Figure 3.3 Comparison of penetration between lasers of different power output. To a given depth, a higher-powered laser delivers a dose in less time. In a given time, a higher-powered laser delivers the same dose to a greater depth.

Time

Where does the optimal treatment time come from? Realistically, the main factor is clinical feasibility. Nobody has time to treat each patient for an hour. In fact, any more than a few minutes begins to strain the animal's and the laser administrator's attention span. The better answer is that we start from dose; we know how much dose we want at the target, back-calculate how much dose we need at the surface, and then set the power to whatever it needs to be to deliver that many joules in whatever we call a "feasible treatment time." However, that is still not an unbiased, scientifically grounded answer.

More than Just Dose

In general, reciprocity is a serious question. Is the accumulation of dose (irrespective of the delivery method) a sufficient predictor of clinical effect? In particular, on the time scale of treatment (both intra- and intertreatment), should a treatment that aims to deliver $2\,J/cm^2$ of light take 2 minutes, or 20 minutes, or 2 hours? Should those treatments be repeated every hour, every day, or every week? Or does it matter at all? Will all of these situations produce the same clinical effect as long as they deliver the same total dose?

These are ultimately clinical questions, but I can tell you that the literature suggests that while reciprocity does not seem to hold across the board (Hashmi *et al.*, 2010; Karu *et al.*, 1996), there are certain windows within the broad treatment spectrum where you can be reasonably confident that slight tweaks (because a pet owner could not get to the clinic that morning, or because you have the chance to deliver a second treatment since the animal is being boarded overnight) will not severely impact your standard expectation of therapeutic outcome.

A quick, but related aside having to do with this same idea of dose accumulation is the determination of treatment axis. We have covered enough about scatter to convince you that in the near-infrared spectrum and in biological tissue, the treatment beam does not look like a beam once it gets in the body. Instead, the beam sort of "mushrooms" once it passes the skin and spreads out, but principally inside the body. The clinicians again will have much to say about what gaps, in what joints, and along which nerve routes and lymphatic paths to point the laser, but one thing to keep in mind is that dose, in the short term (on the order of seconds to minutes), is a cumulative quantity. There are many joints in the body that are more or less equidistant from two surfaces. It is often very useful to treat along different axes, always pointing at the same internal structure, in order to accumulate more dose at the intersection of axes than is delivered along any individual path. In radiation oncology with x-rays that encounter much less scatter,

this technique is used in virtually every radiation treatment plan to spare benign tissues unnecessary dose while building up a toxic amount within the planned treatment volume. Granted, much more scatter is involved in the infrared, but in smaller geometries like the shoulders, hips, and more distal sites in the extremities, treating from under a leg or an arm can be a good adjunct, especially since the hair and fur (strong scatterers) are much less dense there.

Still, most of the advice you seek about the time scale of treatments will come from the clinicians in later chapters. But what about on a shorter time scale, like milliseconds?

On and Off (and On and Off)

We talked about heat macroscopically, but while bulk tissue takes seconds to dissipate joules of energy, that translates to individual cells dissipating microjoules of energy (small fractions of the total beam) in microseconds. Therefore, if you can turn the beam on and off in around the same time it takes cells to return to equilibrium, you can mitigate the heat. In fact, you may even enhance the effect of your therapy. This is the pulse frequency or repetition rate I referred to earlier and warned you not to confuse with the frequency of light, which is equivalent to wavelength and energy.

If we can pulse the light source (turn it on and off periodically) at a frequency that coincides with the thermal dissipation rates of individual cells, then perhaps we can make the most out of the absorption events. If we pulse too quickly (or do not pulse at all) and we deliver more energy per time than the cells can dissipate, then we may actually be wasting a lot of the cellular energy and diminishing our clinical effect. If we pulse too slowly, then we are not taking full advantage of the cell's potential.

By this logic, it is reasonable to assume that since different types of cell have different densities (mostly due to differences in water content), each will have different average thermal dissipation rates and therefore respond optimally to different pulse frequencies

Beyond avoiding bulk thermal saturation, pulsing can be used to modify chemistry periodically. There are several intracellular processes, called redox (reduction-oxidation) reactions, that play a crucial role in the effect of laser therapy, as well as cellular metabolism in general. Two such reactions (which will be covered at greater length in Chapter 5) involve cytochrome c oxidase (CCO) and nicotinamide adenine dinucleotide phosphate-oxidase (Hamblin and Demidova, 2006; Karu *et al.*, 2008). In both cases (and in these redox reactions in general), electrons are passed back and forth between two molecules: reduction is the gain of electrons (which reduces the oxidation state) and oxidation is the loss of electrons (which increases the oxidation state). There is a ton of biochemistry involved here, but important for you is the fact that light has been shown to predictably change the redox states of these molecules in a bilateral way. That is, if the enzyme is in a relatively oxidized state, light absorption can cause a transient reduction – and the converse holds true, if the enzyme is in an initial reduced state (Karu *et al.*, 2008). This means that for the cyclical reactions in our cells (both within the mitochondria and on the cell membrane), light can trigger the process both in the forward direction (to produce something, such as adenosine triphosphate (ATP) or an intercellular signal) and in the backward direction (to reset the structure so that it can produce that something again). Since these processes are virtually identical in most tissues, this may lead to the idea that there are some "universal" frequencies (or dose domains) where a biostimulatory effect could be expected (Karu *et al.*, 1997).

There is much at play here, and most of it is beyond the scope of this book, but suffice it to say that pulsing the light in your therapy can elicit some effects that continuous exposure cannot. Unfortunately, the clinical attempts to determine which are the appropriate parameters for which applications have been widely inconsistent, often due to bad reporting of data (Hashmi *et al.*, 2010), but more generally because clinicians simply do not have access to the large sample sizes needed to really isolate any optimizations. Scientists who have dug into the fundamentals, however, and who use biology laboratories with virtually limitless sample sizes (you can grow thousands of cell cultures without too much added expense), have uncovered several effects (by way of several isolated mechanisms) that are elicited from pulsed light and not from continuous-wave (CW) irradiation (Karu *et al.*, 1996, 1997).

With that comes some more nomenclature, though. *Frequency* tells you how many times the beam is on then off per second, but an important quantity that people often overlook is the *duty cycle*. This is the percentage of time the *beam* is on versus off. By definition, then, CW irradiation refers to 100% duty cycle. Two different pulse structures can lead to the same or very different average powers (the total amount of energy delivered per second). Figure 3.4 illustrates this idea.

With respect to pulsing, it is clear that the rule of reciprocity (that total exposure or dose determines clinical effect) does not hold across the board. The beneficial nature of pulsing relies on a specific timing of

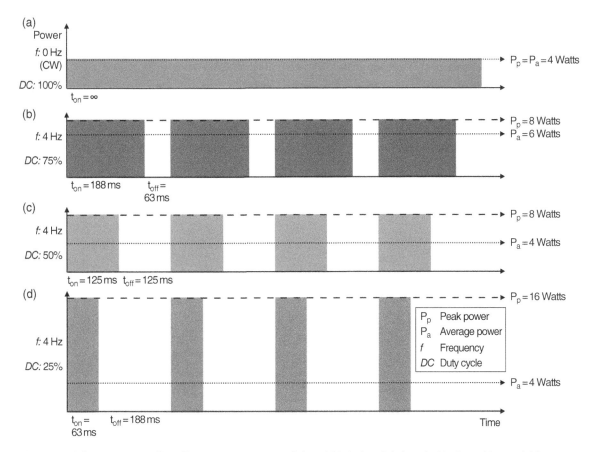

Figure 3.4 Pulse structure and its effect on average power. Pulse width (t_{on}) and dark period (t_{off}) combine to yield more common parameters – frequency and duty cycle – which, combined with peak power (P_p), can be used to calculate average power (P_a). Careful, though: these parameters alone can be misleading, as different combinations can lead to the same (a, c, and d) or different (b and c or d) average outputs.

pulses – either in the time the light is on during a pulse, or in the time the light is off between pulses. Therefore, it is clear that if you modified the pulse structure (e.g., by decreasing the peak power but increasing the pulse width proportionally), you could expect a very different intratissue effect, even though the total energy per pulse, and therefore delivered dose, would be identical. Your new pulse might be too long to allow the cells to return to thermal equilibrium, or there might not be sufficient dark time before the next pulse to allow the redox reaction to reset. That said, it might coincide with some different reaction rate or resonant effect. Alternatively, your changes might have been too subtle to make a difference. The point is, the pulse structure has at least some impact on the biological effect; if not, why are we pulsing at all? We still have much to learn here, but again, the goal is to bridge the gap between what scientists continue to uncover in cell culture and what advantages clinicians might be able to exploit in the treatment of their patients.

Conclusion

I have told you a story that is made up of lots of little stories that do not tell the whole story. Why? To confuse you (more than the last sentence did)? No. I just think that understanding a little about all of the factors involved makes you better prepared to prescribe and administer an appropriate therapy. You are going to read a lot in the coming chapters about treating all sorts of injuries with a variety of clinical presentations, each with a variety of treatment prescriptions. The good news is that all that follows is based on the fact that laser therapy works, to some degree or another. My goal for this chapter was to arm with you a more technical vocabulary so that you can participate in the protocol development and selection conversation. You should now have some idea of how these protocols have emerged and, more importantly, how you might modify them based on fundamental ideas in order to enhance your treatments and the efficacy they induce.

References

ASTM. (2008) *Standard Tables for Reference Solar Spectral Irradiances: Direct Normal and Hemispherical on 37° Tilted Surface*. ASTM Standard G173-03. ASTM International, West Conshohocken.

Hale, G.M. and Querry, M.R. (1973) Optical constants of water in the 200 nm to 200 μm wavelength region. *Appl Opt.* **12**(3):555–563.

Hamblin, M.R. and Demidova, T.N. (2006) Mechanisms of low level light therapy. *Proceedings of SPIE – The International Society for Optical Engineering.* **6140**(61001):1–12.

Hashmi, J. *et al.* (2010) Effect of pulsing in low-level light therapy. *Lasers Surg Med.* **42**(6):450–466.

Jacques, S. (2013) Optical properties of biological tissues: a review. *Phys Med Biol.* **58**(11):R37–R61.

Karu, T.I. *et al.* (1996) Different sensitivity of cells from tumor-bearing organisms to continuous-wave and pulsed laser light (632.8 nm) evaluated by chemiluminescence test. *Lasers Life Sci.* **7**(3):141–156.

Karu, T.I. *et al.* (1997) Nonmonotonic behavior of the dose dependence of the radiation effect on cells in vitro exposed to pulsed laser radiation at 820 nm. *Lasers Surg Med.* **21**(5):485–492.

Karu, T.I. *et al.* (2008) Absorption measurements of cell monolayers relevant to mechanisms of laser phototherapy: reduction or oxidation of cytochrome c oxidase under laser radiation at 632.8 nm. *Photomed Laser Surg.* **26**(6):593–599.

Segelstein, D.J. (1981) The complex refractive index of water. M.S. thesis. Department of Physics, University of Missouri – Kansas City.

Zolotarev, V.M. *et al.* (1969) Dispersion and absorption of liquid water in the infrared and radio regions of the spectrum. *Opt Spectrosc.* **27**:430–432.

4

Therapy Laser Safety

Kenneth E. Bartels

Professor Emeritus, Department of Veterinary Clinical Sciences, Oklahoma State University, Stillwater, OK, USA

Introduction

The discussion regarding safe use of the laser began at the time a ruby laser was first developed in 1960. Theodore Maiman, working at the Hughes Research Laboratory in California, is credited for the announcement and publication of work shining a high-power pulsed flash lamp on a ruby rod with silver-coated surfaces to produce laser light – high-power light energy that is collimated, intense, and has a marked narrowing of the wavelength. The concept of stimulated emission, whereby a ground-state energy level is excited to produce an intense beam of light energy, was studied for potential uses that had been mostly considered science fiction for many years. Other physicists and engineers, including Charles Townes, Charles Schalow, Peter Sorokin, Mirek Stevenson, Ali Javen, William Bennett, Donald Harriott, and Robert Hall, from research and development companies including IBM, Bell Labs, and General Electric, were also involved in the concept of "a solution looking for a problem." In other words, there was tremendous interest in potentially using this new technology to advance communication, industrial applications, medical devices, and weapon systems. In the development of these technologies, concepts of energy absorption, transmission, reflection, and material ablation to minimize potential harm to operators or patients were considered potentially serious limiting problems (Bartels, 2002; Fry, 2002).

Many veterinarians, including new graduates, have had little or no training regarding the clinical and safe use of medical lasers. The curricula of most veterinary schools until the last several years often did not cover this topic, and current content in core didactic course work is still minimal. To that end, many veterinarians begin using this technology following limited exposure during corporate-sponsored weekend short-courses, or at state, regional, national, or international continuing-education meetings that include a minimum of "hands-on" experience and a brief discussion of medical laser safety. Safety hazards associated with improper use of medical lasers need to be understood and observed, since they are related to many state, national, and international mandated guidelines (Barat, 2014a). The safe use of medical lasers is essential for the use of high-power surgical lasers (Sliney, 1995). It also is an essential aspect of using medical lasers designated for photobiomodulation therapy.

Function of the American National Standards Institute and the Laser Institute of America

Laser safety is a part of the multi-mission task of the American National Standards Institute (ANSI). Founded in 1918, ANSI remains a private, non-profit membership organization supported by both private industry and public-sector organizations. It helps to facilitate specific American National Standards by working with constituent groups composed of organizational bodies and individuals from manufacturers, government agencies, medical institutions, and the academic community. It maintains basic requirements for openness, balance, consensus, and due process in order to develop voluntary national consensus standards that relate to products, processes, services, systems, and safety. It ensures that standards undergo public review. Consensus must be reached by representatives from affected businesses and companies. Comments from the consensus body and public review must be reported in good faith, and an appeals process is a requirement. An estimated 10,000 American National Standards exist today. ANSI promotes standardization efforts in the United States, but also advocates for these policies and technical positions to the international community as international standards are adopted (ANSI, 2014).

The Laser Institute of America (LIA) was founded in 1968, as the professional society for laser applications and safety. Its mission is to foster lasers as a useful technologic advancement, encourage useful laser applications, and promote laser safety worldwide. It represents the core of the profession and includes a group of academic scientists, engineers, physicist, manufacturers, and medical specialists who are passionate about growing the technology, as well as turning it into a viable industry that is both safe and efficacious for many uses. Further, to enhance this mission, it serves as the secretariat and publisher of the ANSI Z136 series of laser safety standards (www.lia.org). Its standards are the foundation of laser safety programs throughout the United States and in most of the world.

The American Veterinary Medical Association (AVMA) saw the need for the veterinary profession to become a part of the ANSI group in 1999, to ensure the profession met the standards for safe use of medical lasers and to collaborate in the standardization of safety guidelines by the ANSI Z136 Laser Safety Committee. This membership has been crucial in ensuring veterinary medicine has been included in discussions over the writing of new guidelines as the technology has grown, including the use of high power surgical lasers and, more recently, the use of therapy lasers in photobiomodulation therapy.

The ANSI documents are definitive in outlining the safe use of lasers in veterinary medicine (ANSI, 2011a, 2014). The Z136 guidelines represent general agreement among manufacturers, sales personnel, and users regarding the best current practices. ANSI Z136.3 addresses the "Safe Use of Lasers in Health Care Facilities," whereas ANSI Z136.1, "American National Standard for Safe Use of Lasers," covers the much broader topic of laser safety in general, including in industrial and research environments. These standards are guidelines (not regulations) for the safe use of laser systems. Currently, use of medical lasers in veterinary medicine is included in both standard sections and as an appendix within the Z136.3 guideline. It must also be assumed that the Occupational Safety and Health Administration (OSHA) and state regulatory agencies will use these same guidelines as safety issues arise in veterinary medicine. It is up to the veterinary profession to be proactive and to provide the safest possible use of medical lasers, both for the sake of patient care and for the health of the veterinarian and technical assistants. Both of these laser safety documents are continuously under review, and it is highly likely that a new version of Z136.3 will be released in the next 3 years.

Additional federal regulations regarding lasers as medical devices fall under the authority of the Food and Drug Administration (FDA) Center for Devices and Radiological Health (CDRH) via enforcement of the Federal Laser Product Performance Standard and the Medical Devices Amendment to the Food, Drug, and Cosmetic Act (FDA, 2015a). All laser products sold in the United States since August 1976 must be certified by the manufacturer as meeting safety standards, and each laser must bear a label indicating compliance with the standards and giving its laser hazard classification (Class 1–4). Operating manuals must be included with the device and must contain adequate instructions for assembly, calibration (especially for Class 3 and 4 lasers), operation, and maintenance, including necessary precautions to avoid potentially hazardous exposure to direct laser and collateral radiation.

Laser Hazard Classification

The ANSI standard laser hazard classifications are used to indicate the level of hazard associated with a laser system and the degree of safety control required. Lasers are classified based on the ability of the beam to cause histologic damage to the eye and skin. The relevant parameters include laser output energy or power, radiation wavelengths, exposure duration, and the cross-sectional area of the laser beam at the tissue target area. Laser hazard classification is also based on the accessibility of the laser radiation or accessible emission limit within a particular laser hazard class.

A Class 1 laser system (Class 1/1 M) is considered not able to produce tissue damage during operation, so is exempt from control measures. Class 1 M laser systems are considered incapable of producing a hazardous beam exposure during normal operation unless the beam is viewed with an optical eye-loupe or telescope. The safety goal is to prevent potentially hazardous optically aided viewing. Examples of Class 1 lasers are grocery store price-scanning devices and laser printers (LIA 2000).

A Class 2 laser system (Class 2/2 M) emits a visible portion of the light spectrum (400–700 nm). Ocular protection is usually provided by the aversion response, which includes the blink reflex (<0.25 seconds), eye or head movement, and pupillary constriction. A Class 2 M laser system also emits a similar visible light spectrum and is considered hazardous if viewed with optical aids. In considering this laser classification, the concept of maximum permissible exposure (MPE) is introduced. MPE is defined as the level of laser radiation to which an unprotected person may be exposed without adverse biological changes in the eye or skin. In the case of a Class 2 M system, MPE equals the 0.25 second eye-aversion response time (LIA, 2000).

Class 3 laser systems (3R/3B) are not considered a fire hazard or a significant hazard to the skin. Class 3B laser systems (medium-power lasers) can be dangerous under direct and indirect or specular (mirror-like) viewing conditions, but are usually not a hazard through diffuse reflection or a fire hazard.

Class 4 laser systems (high-power visible and invisible wavelengths) are potentially an acute hazard to the eye and skin on direct intrabeam exposure and on diffuse or scattered reflection. Class 4 lasers also potentially present a hazard for ignition (fire) and byproduct production via ablated (vaporized) laser-generated airborne contaminants (LGACs), which include gaseous toxic compounds, dead and live cellular components, and viruses (ANSI, 2011a; LIA, 2000).

For the ANSI Z136.1 and Z136.3 guidelines, the ANSI 136 Committee made an extreme effort to have classification guidelines be identical or as close as possible to the FDA Code of Federal Regulations Title 21, Part 1040 – Performance Standards for Light-Emitting Products (FDA, 2015c) and Part 878 – Medical Devices: General and Plastic Surgery Devices (FDA, 2015a), FDA guidance regarding low-level laser systems for aesthetic use (FDA, 2011), FDA laser hazard classes (FDA, 2015b), the International Electrotechnical Commission guidelines (FDA, 2007), and OSHA regulations regarding laser hazards (OSHA, 2015).

Though some US states and the international community may rewrite them to include a different approach, including laser registration processes, the ANSI guidelines usually are closely utilized to "harmonize" documents so as not to create confusion among laser users and institutional entities, such as national laboratories and universities. In the past few years, the major change that has been considered is a reclassification of laser classes to align with ocular hazards related to actual hazards detectable from beams enclosed in a protective housing, as well as to include classes of lasers that may be hazardous under direct or specular reflection but pose minimal hazard for fire or do not generate LGACs.

Laser Beam-Related Hazards and Hazard Prevention

Primary hazard assessment of medical lasers includes concerns over eye safety and skin exposures (Winburn, 1990). MPE values have been calculated based on laser wavelength for both skin and eye exposures (Henderson and Schulmeister, 2004b). MPEs are dependent upon laser wavelength, exposure time, and mode of delivery: continuous-wave (CW) or pulsed repetition. Values are expressed as either radiant exposure (J/cm^2), also known as "fluence," or as irradiance (W/cm^2), also known as "power density." Values for each laser are published in the ANSI documents. Any value higher than the MPE can cause tissue damage. In general, the longer the laser wavelength, the higher the MPE, and the longer the exposure time, the lower the MPE (ANSI, 2011a, 2014).

Eye Hazards

Laser bioeffect hazards to the eye associated with high-power surgical lasers and therapy lasers consist of corneal and lenticular opacities and retinal damage, both of which are dependent upon laser wavelength, expressed in nanometers (Sliney and Freasier, 1973). Other factors that also affect the amount and type of tissue damage include tissue volume and circulation, beam energy, and length of exposure (LIA, 2000).

Visible-wavelength energy (400–780 nm) and near-infrared (IR-A; 780–1400 nm) will pass through the cornea and lens and directly induce thermal damage to the retina, causing loss of color vision, night blindness, and potentially complete loss of vision. As a result, visible and near-infrared wavelengths are known as the "retinal hazard region" of the light spectrum. Neodymium-doped yttrium aluminum garnet lasers (1064 nm) and some diode wavelength lasers (808 and 980 nm), utilized in veterinary medicine in both high-power and therapy lasers, may induce retinal damage, resulting in decreased vision or potential blindness. This damage is increased with longer-duration exposures and pupillary dilation. Within the retinal hazard zone (440–1400 nm), the retina is 100 000 times more vulnerable to injury than the skin (LIA, 2000).

Near-ultraviolet wavelengths (UV-A; 315–400 nm) pass through the cornea and are absorbed by the lens, resulting in photochemical denaturation of lens proteins, which potentially causes cataract formation. Far-ultraviolet wavelength energy (UV-B, UV-C; 100–315 nm) will be absorbed by the corneal epithelium, resulting in photokeratitis due to denaturation of corneal proteins. Conjunctivitis is also a possible result. Far-infrared wavelengths (IR-B, IR-C; 1400–10 600 nm) will result in corneal damage due to selective tissue water absorption inducing protein denaturation on the corneal surface, which results in corneal burns. Wavelengths from 1400 to 3000 nm may penetrate deeper and lead to cataracts, due to heating of lens proteins. Minimal temperature rise is necessary for these changes to occur (LIA, 2000).

In deciding what type of eye protection is needed, two important factors must be determined: laser wavelength and the maximum viewing duration for the specific procedures. MPE limits are used to determine guidelines for protecting personnel from three types of viewing conditions: (i) unintentional accidental exposure to a visible beam where the MPE may exceed 0.25 seconds – the blink-aversion reflex; (ii) unintentional, accidental viewing of a near-infrared laser beam for up to 10 seconds; and (iii) intentional viewing of diffuse reflection for up to 600 seconds. In order to choose the most appropriate set of safety glasses for a specific device designed for a specific procedure, optical density (OD) should be employed. OD is a mathematical–physics logarithmic calculation that factors attenuation of the laser beam input radiance divided by the transmittance radiance. Tabular values are provided in ANSI guidelines and other references. The bottom line is that the OD of the filtration medium (glass or polycarbonate plastic) should match the exposure condition for diffuse or intrabeam viewing conditions.

For safe use of medical lasers, eyewear must match the conditions of potential exposure during treatment (Barat, 2014b). Most manufacturers of both high-power and therapy devices provide appropriate eyewear for diffuse, accidental beam exposure. Specifically for therapy lasers, an essential understanding of power (laser class) and wavelength is required to avoid potential accidents to the operator, assistant, and patient. Class 3B and 4 devices are of major safety concern. Instructions provided by the manufacturer and ANSI guidelines must be followed. As explained previously, Classes 1 through 3R lasers need to be used with care to avoid direct exposure to the eye, but Classes 3B and Class 4 devices can and will damage the eye if used carelessly and safety guidelines are ignored.

Design of laser-safe eyewear is a factor that must be considered in order to afford the best compliance for proper use. If eyewear is heavy, uncomfortable, or restricts visualization of the target tissue due to the color of the optical filter, its use may be ignored. Even with newer designs of glasses and goggles designated for specific devices, administrative controls or requirements implemented by the practice or institution for appropriate use must be seriously applied. The choice between glass and plastic (polycarbonate) lenses should be considered: glass-lensed eyewear is heavier and more expensive, but usually more robust and resistant to scratches and breakage. For laser therapy, and even high-power laser surgery, eyewear is designed with appropriate OD requirements to protect the wearer against specular reflection but not direct beam impact. Side shields are also recommended, to protect against unnoticed reflection, which could potentially cause ocular damage (Figure 4.1).

With the tunability of some surgical lasers and the manufacture of laser therapy devices with multiple wavelength availability, special caution must be considered when selecting safe eyewear for clinical use. A pair of single-wavelength protective eyewear is obviously not appropriate for multiple-wavelength delivery. Most

manufacturers providing proper eyewear for their own product take care to supply dual-wavelength protection, but it is still the operator's responsibility to ensure the appropriate laser-safe eyewear has been provided. All laser eyewear must be distinctly marked on the bows, frames, or lenses regarding the protective OD designation and the wavelengths covered (LIA, 2000) (Figure 4.2).

Laser-safe eyewear must be properly fitted (Henderson and Schulmeister, 2004a). It should be maintained to protect against breakage and scratches. If utilized appropriately, laser-safe eyewear can provide many years of use. It always needs to be carefully examined prior to laser therapy and surgery. If it is damaged in anyway (broken frames, scratched or cracked lenses), it must be replaced.

Patient eye protection is also essential. Potential options for shielding include saline-moistened sponges, pieces of black felt, wavelength-specific laser eye-shields, corneal shields, and laser-safe eyewear fitted for animals (Fry, 2002; Riegel, 2008).

Class 2 and 3R lasers powered by AAA and AA batteries marketed as laser pointers are restricted within the United States to 0.1–0.5 mW of laser radiation. Used improperly, laser pointers are potentially hazardous; even with an aversion response, temporary flash blindness or "welder's glare" can result. Instances of permanent damage to the retina can potentially occur from direct beam viewing of Class 3R laser pointers. Some illegally imported laser pointers have visible wavelengths ranging from 532 nm green light to 690 nm red light generate in excess of 0.5 mW. These are classified as Class 3B, and require additional considerations regarding eye safety.

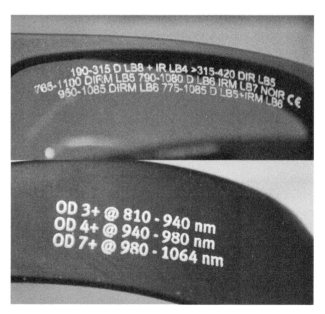

Figure 4.2 Specification of wavelength and OD on the lens (top) and frame (bottom).

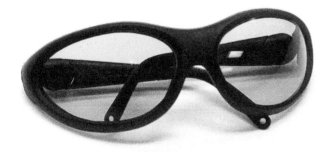

Figure 4.1 Laser-protective glasses.

Skin Hazards

Far-ultraviolet radiation (UV-B, UV-C) falls in the actinic or photochemical ultraviolet zone. Exposures may result in erythema or blistering of skin due to epidermal absorption. A common source of UV-B is sunlight, which has been implicated in skin carcinogenesis. Devices emitting the shorter wavelengths of ultraviolet light (180–200 nm) are used for their potential germicidal effects in some laser therapy devices. Skin effects may occur in all regions of the infrared spectrum (IR-A, IR-B, IR-C), being influenced by hyperpigmentation and photosensitization from certain drugs. With extreme exposure, they can include blistering or charring of the tissue.

Skin hazards need to be considered with higher-powered visible or infrared lasers (Class 4), which includes all surgical lasers and some laser therapy devices. Lower-power lasers (Classes 1–3B), though potentially hazardous to the eye, are not usually considered as hazardous to the skin. Some Class 4 therapy laser devices have potential to cause photothermal skin injury if not used according to manufacturer's recommendations. Even then, factors such as the laser power emitted, the beam diameter of the delivery device, pulsed versus CW beam delivery, the patient's skin pigmentation, hair length, and color, and the depth of beam penetration can potentially cause blistering and perhaps photothermal skin necrosis. There are many recommendations regarding treatment regimens for multiple conditions, including pain relief and wound healing, that must be considered on an individual patient basis in order to ensure appropriate exposure and medical benefit.

Laser therapy protocols are recommended from many sources, including research papers and case reports, as well as technical representatives of companies. Computerized programs installed in some devices, as well as manuals provided with the devices, make the use of therapeutic lasers seem easy for most amenable conditions. Treatments provided to animals that are not anesthetized or lightly sedated may cause them to react to uncomfortable photothermal sensitivity, providing the operator with the necessary reaction to adjust the dosage appropriately. The potential advantages of using higher-power therapeutic laser devices include providing treatment protocols using higher radiant energy during a shorter time interval and, potentially, allowing deeper penetration of that energy. However, the operator must be aware that a "set recipe" treatment protocol for a specific condition may not be appropriate for every patient treated for that specific condition. Close clinical observation of the patient and the use of the laser as an extension of the veterinarian's other treatment modalities is most prudent.

Laser Use Environment

Use of high-power medical lasers (Class 4) of various wavelengths and in different operational modes (CW vs. pulsed) for tissue vaporization presents a very different spectrum of beam hazards compared to therapy lasers. Therapy lasers (Classes 1–4) vary from low-power (Class 1–3B), sometimes called "cold lasers," to high-power (Class 4), and include wavelengths ranging from the ultraviolet to the infrared, as previously outlined.

The nominal hazard zone (NHZ) is defined by ANSI as the space within which the level of direct-beam, reflected, or scattered laser radiation during treatment (especially Class 3B or 4) exceeds the applicable MPE and presents potential detrimental laser effects to the laser operator, surgical assistants, and casual observer. Even with use of Classes 1 M, 2, 2 M, and 3R lasers, if there is potential for any direct beam exposure, proper signage should be considered. In practice, the NHZ is considered the room in which the procedure is performed. Often, therapy lasers are used in a treatment or exam room, which can be acceptable if proper warning signage is used and any potential observation windows are blocked with an opaque laser-safe material or appropriate filter glass (which is often quite expensive). Another option is to use portable laser-safe barriers or curtains, which can be purchased from laser manufacturers.

Appropriate laser radiation warning signage for use on doors or access areas for laser therapy treatment zones needs to be in accordance with ANSI Z535.2 – "Environmental and Facility Safety Signs" (ANSI, 2011b). Understanding the need for warning signs is essential (Barat 2006a; Henderson, 1997). Laser manufacturers should, and usually do, provide the appropriate signage with the device. The warning sign needs to conform to the specifications designated for the class of laser, as given by the ANSI Z136.1 or ANSI Z136.3 guidelines, which also comply with the OSHA Technical Manual for Laser Hazards (OSHA, 2015). Some laser surgery or therapy areas may have illuminated signage that is used when laser radiation is being emitted. More common is temporary signage, removed after laser therapy, which is adhered to the entry door of the laser treatment area. The sign should clearly indicate the danger of laser radiation, the eye safety requirements, the wavelength of laser light, and the highest power emission available with the specific device (Figure 4.3).

In some rare cases, especially with high-power Class 4 surgical or industrial lasers, safety interlocks may be used to interrupt laser emission if the entry door is opened during a procedure. Their use is somewhat problematic, however, since interrupting a procedure could be detrimental to the patient's health and safety.

Operating room protocol should never be casual, particularly when a laser is in use. Laser warning signs

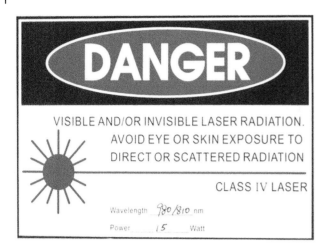

Figure 4.3 Laser safety temporary warning/danger sign with laser classification and precautions for use with all Class 3B and 4 lasers. The sign is removed from the laser control environment after the procedure is completed.

should be in full view on the doors, and all windows and doors need appropriate laser-safe covers. Prior to laser activation, the attending clinician should announce, "laser on," so that no one is uncertain about beam activation. When not in use, standby modes are appropriate to avoid inadvertent laser radiation exposure.

Non-Beam Hazards

Electrical Hazards

Since most lasers utilize high-voltage power supplies, the possibility of electric shock does exist. Medical laser manufacturers are required to build in many safety features to reduce the chances of shock, electrocution, or inadvertent laser beam exposure, and to comply with FDA manufacturer guidelines. These features include protective housings, key control, laser door interlocks, shutters or attenuators, radiation emission indicators, error-sensing programs, fail-safe circuitry and shutter design, power output monitoring, and appropriate classification labeling. Other features include guarded foot or hand switches to prevent inadvertent laser exposure, low-power visible lasers (diode or helium neon devices) that emit aiming beams to ensure accurate tissue targeting, and emergency off (kill) switches (Fry, 2002).

The probability of electrical shock is minimal if operation is in compliance with instructional manuals and common precautions are exercised with any electrical device. However, removal of the exterior housing for servicing may dramatically increase the risk of serious injury. Only authorized professional service personnel should ever attempt to remove the housing and perform maintenance on the laser.

Respiratory Hazards (Laser-Generated Airborne Contaminants)

Use of Class 4 medical lasers for tissue ablation creates a laser plume (smoke), which has been shown to contain a wide array of dangerous LGACs that have deleterious effects on both humans and animals (Sliney, 1995). Control of the plume is primarily achieved with the use of smoke evacuators with appropriate filters. However, use of Class 4 therapy laser devices at the recommended power and pulse settings should alleviate most of concerns. In rare instances, ignition of the hair in the target area is possible. This phenomenon only occurs when proper application techniques are not utilized.

Fire Hazards and Controls

As with concern over LGACs, the likelihood of fire hazard due to the thermal effects of therapy laser devices is minimal. However, if there is a malfunction of a laser therapy handpiece, an undetected broken laser fiber or cable, or accidental laser beam exposure due to improper use, especially with a Class 4 device used at maximum power, the potential for ignition of protective drapes or other accessories becomes possible, though still extremely unlikely. The availability of a fire extinguisher should always be considered, in case a fire does occur.

Administrative Controls

Each veterinary facility that utilizes any medical laser should appoint a laser safety officer (LSO) with primary responsibility for all aspects of the institution's laser safety program (Barat, 2006b; Oleson, 2016). In a general practice or private specialty practice, the LSO's duties may be fulfilled by either a veterinarian or a technician. The LSO is responsible for laser system classification (Classes 1–4), hazard evaluation, control measures, standard operating procedure development, protective equipment use, appropriate signage and labels, and facility modification to follow manufacturer's guidelines for safe laser installation. Of utmost importance for the LSO, is the establishment and maintenance of laser safety training programs for all individuals in the practice. The programs should ensure that all Class 3B and 4 laser users and observers are properly instructed and know how to maintain personnel and patient safety. Familiarity with established guidelines, local, state, and federal regulations, advisory standards, and professional recommended practices is extremely important. Though clinical experience with one class of medical laser can be beneficial, it is important that a laser user be familiar with each specific device, especially regarding its wavelength and absorption characteristics.

Conclusion

Medical laser safety is a critical component in any laser therapy program. Used improperly, therapeutic lasers have the potential to be hazards to the eyes and skin. For these reasons, each laser user has an obligation to establish and comply with a laser safety program, as outlined by ANSI and implemented by the facility's LSO. It is essential, even with therapeutic laser devices, that potential beam hazards be recognized and precautions be taken to ensure the use of laser-safe eyewear and the establishment of a controlled laser operational environment, with appropriate signage and security precautions.

References

ANSI. (2011a) *American National Standard for Safe Use of Lasers in Health Care Facilities ANSI Z136.3 – 2011.* American National Standards Institute, Washington, DC.

ANSI. (2011b) *American National Standard for Environmental and Facility Safety Signs ANSI Z535.2 – 2011.* American National Standards Institute, Washington, DC.

ANSI. (2014) *American National Standard for Safe Use of Lasers ANSI Z136.1 – 2014.* American National Standards Institute, Washington, DC.

Barat, K. (2006a) Warning signs and labels. In: *Laser Safety Management*, p. 58. Taylor & Francis, Boca Raton, FL.

Barat, K. (2006b) Laser safety officer or advisor. In: *Laser Safety Management*, p. 9. Taylor & Francis, Boca Raton, FL.

Barat, K. (2014a) Laser safety – where are we? In: *Laser Safety: Tools and Training*, 2 edn., pp. 1–2. CRC Press, Boca Raton, FL.

Barat, K. (2014b) Laser eyewear In: *Laser Safety: Tools and Training*, 2 edn., pp. 243–262. CRC Press, Boca Raton, FL.

Bartels, K. (2002) Lasers in veterinary medicine – where have we been, and where are we going? *Vet Clin North Am Small Anim Pract.* **32**(3):495–515.

FDA. (2007). Laser Products – Conformance with IEC 60825-1 and IEC 60601-2-22 (Laser Notice No. 50). Available from: http://www.fda.gov/MedicalDevices/DeviceRegulationandGuidance/GuidanceDocuments/ucm094361.htm (accessed November 30, 2016).

FDA. (2011) Guidance for Industry and FDA Staff – Class II Special Controls Guidance Document: Low Level Laser System for Aesthetic Use. Available from: http://www.fda.gov/RegulatoryInformation/Guidances/ucm251260.htm (accessed November 30, 2016).

FDA. (2015a) Federal Laser Product Performance Standard and the Medical Devices Amendment to the Food, Drug, and Cosmetic Act. FDA 21 CFR Part 878. Available from: https://www.accessdata.fda.gov/scripts/cdrh/cfdocs/cfcfr/CFRSearch.cfm?fr=878.4810 (accessed November 30, 2016).

FDA. (2015b) Laser hazard classes. Available from: http://www.accessdata.fda.gov/scripts/cdrh/cfdocs/cfcfr/CFRSearch.cfm?FR=1040.10 (accessed November 30, 2016).

FDA. (2015c) Performance Standards for Light Emitting Products. FDA 21 CFR Part 1040. Available from: https://www.accessdata.fda.gov/scripts/cdrh/cfdocs/cfCFR/CFRSearch.cfm?CFRPart=1040 (accessed November 30, 2016).

Fry, T. (2002) Laser Safety. *Vet Clin North Am Small Anim Pract.* **32**(3):535–547.

Henderson, A.R. (1997) Signs and warning labels. In: *A Guide to Laser Safety*, pp. 26–27. Bioptica, Cambridge.

Henderson, A.R. and Schulmeister, K. (2004a) Eye protection. In: *Laser Safety*, pp. 403–419. Taylor & Francis, New York.

Henderson, A.R. and Schulmeister, K. (2004b) The concepts of exposure limits (MPE). In: *Laser Safety*, pp. 74–101. Taylor & Francis, New York.

LIA. (2000) *LIA Guide for the Selection for Laser Eye Protection*, 5 edn. Laser Institute of America, Orlando, FL.

OSHA. (2015) Occupational Safety and Health Administration Section III: Chapter 6, Laser Hazards. Available from: https://www.osha.gov/dts/osta/otm/otm_iii/otm_iii_6.html (accessed November 30, 2016).

Oleson, S. (2016) Laser safety officer information. Available from: https://www.lia.org/subscriptions/safety_bulletin/laser_safety_info/#The Laser Safety Officer (accessed November 30, 2016).

Riegel, R. (2008) *Laser Therapy in the Companion Animal Practice*, pp. 39–43. LiteCure, Newark, NJ.

Sliney, D.H. (1995) Laser safety. *Lasers Surg Med.* **16**(3):215–225.

Sliney, D.H. and Freasier, B.C. (1973) Evaluation of optical radiation hazards. *Appl Opt.* **12**(1):1–24.

Winburn, D.C. (1990) Laser damage mechanisms. In: *Practical Laser Safety*, 2 edn., p.16. Marcel Dekker, New York.

5

Basic Principles of Photobiomodulation and Its Effects at the Cellular, Tissue, and System Levels

Juanita J. Anders[1], Ann Kobiela Ketz[2], and Xingjia Wu[1]

[1] Edward Hébert School of Medicine, Uniformed Services University of the Health Sciences, Bethesda, MD, USA
[2] Center for Nursing Science and Clinical Inquiry, Landstuhl Regional Medical Center, Landstuhl, Germany

Photobiomodulation: Nomenclature History

Dr. Theodore Maiman developed the first working laser at Hughes Research Laboratory, and published his paper describing its operation in *Nature* in 1960 (Maiman, 1960). By 1963, pioneering experiments were being done on surgical applications of the laser (McGuff *et al.*, 1963, 1964). Dr. Endre Mester is believed to have been the fourth physician to use lasers in medical applications, and he was the first to publish results suggesting that low-power lasers could have a stimulating effect on cells (Mester *et al.*, 1968a, 1968b).

Surgical applications of lasers were, and still are, widely accepted due to a number of factors. The mechanisms behind how they work were identified, easily understood, and accepted. It was believed that the surgical use of lasers represented an improvement over the traditional scalpel by providing accurate cutting, coagulation, decontamination, and faster healing. Furthermore, the terminology used to describe the surgical applications of lasers was consistent and unified. In contrast, the use of low-powered lasers to alter cellular and tissue function was met with skepticism, for a number of reasons. The beneficial effects were subtle and difficult to study and measure, and the mechanistic basis for how photons could interact with cells to cause a positive therapeutic outcome was not known (Mick, 2016).

Another factor that added to the confusion surrounding this emerging field was inconsistent terminology. In Mester's 1968 publication, he used the phrase "low power laser rays" (Mester *et al.*, 1968a), and he introduced the term "biostimulation" in 1985 (Mester, 1985). A number of other terms were also introduced, such as "cool laser," "cold laser," "cold low-level laser therapy," "soft laser," and "low-power laser therapy." These terms were primarily industry-driven, in an attempt to distinguish these lasers from surgical lasers (Calderhead, 1991). As pointed out by Calderhead (1991), all these terms were "hardware-related," and ignored the effect of the lasers on the tissue. Many were not accurate, since a high-powered surgical laser such as a carbon dioxide (CO_2) laser could be used as a low-power device if the beam was spread to a large spot size (Calderhead, 1991).

The most important factor in selecting a term for this scientific and therapeutic field is the interaction of light with the target tissue, leading to a cascade of photon driven cellular effects. A number of terms have been introduced to capture the light–tissue interaction, including "light therapy" or "phototherapy," "low reactive-level laser treatment," and "low level-laser therapy" (LLLT). It is interesting to note that it is now commonly thought that LLLT refers to the power of the laser. However, when this term was introduced by Calderhead (1991), it referred to the level of tissue reaction to the dose of light delivered. Thus, LLLT was defined as a dose of light that is below the level of the damage threshold and causes cellular photoactivation (Figure 5.1) (Calderhead, 1991).

Mester reviewed his 20 years of clinical and experimental use of lasers in 1985 (Mester, 1985). Though he notes in his abstract that "Low-energy laser radiation was found to have a stimulating effect on cells, and high-energy radiation had an inhibiting effect," the tremendous amount of data demonstrating stimulatory effects led him to propose the term "biostimulation."

Around the time (1988–89) that the first edition of the journal *Laser Therapy* was published, Calderhead recalls debating the use of the terms "photobiostimulation," "photobiomodulation," and "photobioactivation." The journal rejected the use of "photobiostimulation" because of the inhibitory effects observed with LLLT (e.g., decrease in collagen III synthesis in the prevention or

Figure 5.1 Tissue reaction to light, related to the parameters used. "High-level laser therapy" (HLLT) refers to the response of tissue to treatment parameters that are above the survival threshold, such as in surgical applications. "Medium-level laser therapy" (MLLT) is the response of tissue to laser parameters that are above the damage threshold but below the survival threshold. "Low-level laser therapy" (LLLT) is the modulation of functions of cells and tissues to parameters that are below the damage threshold. Adapted with permission from an illustration by Calderhead (1991).

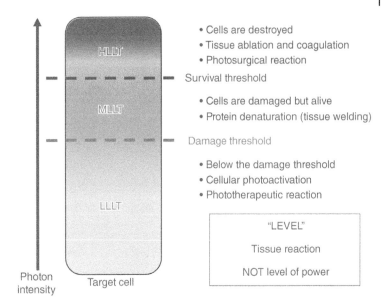

remodeling of hypertrophic scars). "Photobioactivation" was chosen over "photobiomodulation" "because we felt it conveyed more accurately the overall effect on a target organism and its components" (Calderhead, pers. comm.). The term "photobioactivation" appeared in the subheading on the front cover and in the editorial of the pilot issue of *Laser Therapy* (Ohshiro, 1989). In 1991, Calderhead expanded on the concept that light can cause stimulation or inhibition in relation to its dose, as well as on the selection of the term "photobioactivation" (Calderhead, 1991).

The first formal reported use of "photobiomodulation" in the PubMed literature dates back to 1997 (Yu *et al.*, 1997a), though it had been used colloquially for several preceding years. In 2002, in conjunction with the Defense Advanced Research Projects Agency (DARPA) program entitled "Persistence in Combat," which focused on the use of light to accelerate wound healing, a meeting was held at Uniformed Services University of the Health Sciences in Bethesda, MD, which included Drs. Tiina Karu, Ronald Waynant, Ilko Ilev, Kurt Henry, and Juanita Anders. At this meeting, it was decided that the term "photobiomodulation" should be used exclusively for this discipline. In 2003, Dr. Anders formally requested that the American Society for Laser Medicine & Surgery (ASLMS) change the name of their Biostimulation abstract session to "Photobiomodulation." A major effort was made by many leaders in the field to use this term and to encourage others to do the same.

A nomenclature consensus meeting was organized under the auspices of the joint conference of the North American Association for Light Therapy and the World Association for Laser Therapy in 2014. It was attended by 15 international participants and co-chaired by Drs. Jan Bjordal and Juanita Anders. "Photobiomodulation" was considered by the majority of the participants to be

the term of choice to describe the mechanistic and scientific basis for this photonic specialty, and "photobiomodulation therapy" the term for its therapeutic application. However, a major limitation to the adoption of this term was that "photobiomodulation therapy" was not a MeSH term of the National Library of Medicine (NLM)'s controlled vocabulary thesaurus. A request was submitted to the MeSH Section at the NLM, thanks to the efforts of Dr. Praveen Arany, and "photobiomodulation therapy" was added to the MeSH database's 2016 version as an entry term for the existing record of "laser therapy, low-level."

In summary, "photobiomodulation therapy" is an accurate and specific term for this effective and important therapeutic application of light. Universal use of "photobiomodulation" (PBM) and "photobiomodulation therapy" (PBMT) will eliminate confusion in the field and in the scientific, clinical, and lay literature. A suggested definition for PBMT was published in a recent editorial: "A form of light therapy that utilizes non-ionizing forms of light sources including lasers, LEDs, and broadband light, in the visible and infrared spectrum. It is a non-thermal process involving endogenous chromophores eliciting photophysical and photochemical events at various biological scales" (Anders *et al.*, 2015).

Making Sense of Commonly Used Device and Treatment Parameter Terminology

Besides the confusion that surrounded the name for this photonic science and therapy, a brief review of the PBM and PBMT literature will convince you of the non-standardized and often confusing use of device parameters

Table 5.1 Summary of terms commonly used to report device and treatment parameters.

Term	Definition	Abbreviation (SI unit)	Formula	Synonym
Watt	Unit of power (Jenkins and Carroll 2011)	W	$W = J/time(t)$	Radiant power
Joule	Unit of work and energy (Jenkins and Carroll 2011)	J	$J = W \times t$	Radiant energy
Fluence	The radiant energy received by a surface per unit area (Jenkins and Carroll 2011)	J/m^2, J/cm^2	J/cm^2	Radiant exposure; radiant fluence; energy density
Irradiance	The power received by or crossing a surface per unit area	W/m^2, W/cm^2	W/cm^2	Intensity; power density
Fluence rate	W/m^2 seen by an absorber inside a medium (Anders *et al.*, 2014) It is only equal to irradiance when the beam is orthogonal to the surface (Mester *et al.*, 1971)	W/cm^2	W/cm^2	

and treatment terms. Table 5.1 is a summary of terms commonly used to report device and treatment parameters, their definitions and abbreviations, and synonyms.

Another problem plaguing the PBM and PBMT community is the lack of a complete description of the device and treatment parameters used in a laboratory or in clinical studies (Jenkins and Carroll, 2011). A comprehensive list of desirable parameters to provide was published in 2011 (Jenkins and Carroll, 2011). Not every parameter described in this report may be relevant to a specific experiment or treatment. For example, if an *in vivo* PBM treatment is targeting deep tissue with the handpiece in contact with the skin, then beam spot size and area irradiated at the depth of the target may be unknown. However, every parameter that can be measured should be included in the report.

Another error in describing treatment parameters that many scientists and clinicians still make is to report only the total joules (J) delivered. This parameter is useless on its own. The output power of the device, time of treatment, and spot size or treatment area are essential in order for the total joules delivered to be useful, repeatable data. Based on research from our laboratory, 65 J delivered transcutaneously to the transected peroneal nerve in a white New Zealand rabbit injury model either inhibited nerve regeneration or significantly increased the rate of regeneration, depending on the output power and treatment time (Anders *et al.*, 2014). The parameters used in this study were: control group (received no laser treatment), 2 W group (980 nm wavelength, continuous-wave (CW), output power: 2.0 W, treatment time: 32 seconds, 8 cm² area, 65 J), and 4 W group (output power: 4.0 W, treatment time: 16 seconds, 8 cm² area, 65 J) (Anders *et al.*, 2014). The fact that total joules reported on its own is a useless parameter was discussed by Calderhead (1991). It is disheartening that 25 years later, many scientists and clinicians, including veterinarians, are still only reporting total joules delivered.

PBM Device and Treatment Parameters Based on Location of Target Tissue

Mester *et al.* (1971) reported that a dose of 1 J/cm² from a ruby laser caused significant stimulation of healing of cutaneous wounds and burns in a mouse model. In his *in vitro* and animal experiments, Mester tested the effects of fluences ranging from 0.05 (Mester *et al.*, 1968c) to 4.0 J/cm² (Mester, 1985; Mester *et al.*, 1968a, 1968c, 1971). These reported fluences had a significant impact on *in vitro* and pre-clinical animal studies. Indeed, a review of the literature on PBM effects on the proliferation of cultured cells concluded that a fluence of 0.5–4.0 J/cm² and a visible spectrum ranging from 600 to 700 nm enhanced the proliferation rate of various cell lines (AlGhamdi *et al.*, 2012). Similarly, a review of the literature on *in vivo* rat and mouse animal studies of wound healing identified that use of red or near-infrared wavelengths at a range of fluences with a median of 4.2 J/cm² resulted in significant improvement in wound healing (Peplow *et al.*, 2010a).

Therefore, many experiments supported the validity of Mester's original parameters for superficial applications. However, when clinicians began to use PBM to treat structures that were located deeper in the body, they persisted in using these parameters, with negative results. This led to the publication of a number of negative studies and the conclusion that there was inadequate evidence to recommend PBM for clinical use (Basford, 1993, 1995; Basford *et al.*, 1998). It is now obvious that the negative studies were the result of incorrect device and treatment parameters (Tuner and Hode, 1998). Recently, two important advances have been made in PBMT: a broadening of the clinical application of this therapy to transcutaneous treatment of tissues and organs within the body, and the recognition that optimization of the therapeutic parameters should be based on the photonic dose reaching the target tissue (Anders *et al.*, 2014; Weersink *et al.*, 2007).

The wavelength of light used governs its depth of penetration into a tissue. Both the absorption and the scattering coefficients of living tissues are higher at shorter wavelengths, meaning near-infrared light penetrates more deeply than red light (Gardner and Welch, 2001). In 2005, we examined transcutaneous light penetration to the level of the spinal cord in adult, anesthetized Sprague–Dawley rats (Byrnes *et al.*, 2005a). An incoherent broadband white light was applied to the surface of the skin over the thoracic vertebrae. A tissue-activated optical fiber probe was inserted sequentially into the skin, subcutaneous connective tissue layer, deep connective tissue layer, dorsal muscle mass, and spinal cord within the vertebral column. At each of these layers, a transmission spectrum in the range of 500–1200 nm was collected. Analysis of the transmission spectra revealed the range of penetration was highest through all tissue layers overlying the spinal cord and through blood between the 770 and 850 nm wavelengths, with a peak at 810 nm. The 810 nm wavelength was minimally absorbed by blood and water. These data demonstrate that 810 nm wavelength light is within the optimal range for light penetration to tissues deep in the body (Byrnes *et al.*, 2005a).

Experiments in our laboratory also established that transcutaneous treatment parameters for a specific wavelength of light could be determined initially using *in vitro* models to identify effective laser parameters at the cellular level, and that these parameters could then be translated to pre-clinical research and clinical practice (Anders *et al.*, 2014). The translation of dose from *in vitro* to *in vivo* was accomplished by adjusting the *in vitro* parameters based on light penetration measurements. On average, 2.45% of infrared light (980 nm wavelength) applied to the skin reached the depth of the peroneal nerve in anesthetized white New Zealand rabbits. Based on our calculations, the following treatment parameters were used on the injured peroneal nerve: 980 nm wavelength, CW, output power: 1.5 W, treatment time: 43 seconds, scanned over an 8 cm^2 area, 65 J. This resulted in a significant improvement in the toe-spread reflex test compared to controls (Anders *et al.*, 2014).

Photoacceptors

Knowledge of the fundamental tenets of photobiology is essential to understanding the mechanistic basis of PBM and PBMT. The First Law of Photochemistry states that light must be absorbed for photochemistry to occur (Smith, 1991). Therefore, for PBM to occur, there must be a molecule capable of absorbing light: a photoacceptor.

Upon light absorption, an electronically excited state occurs, which alters the primary molecular processes that lead to biological effects at the cellular level by secondary biochemical reactions and cellular signaling (Passarella and Karu, 2014). What wavelengths a photoacceptor will absorb can be determined by its absorption spectrum (Smith, 1991).

The electron transport chain, which is embedded in the inner membrane of eukaryotic mitochondria, consists of four large membrane protein complexes. The function of the electron transport chain is to produce a transmembrane proton electrochemical gradient through redox reactions (Murray *et al.*, 2003). Two of the protein complexes contain photoacceptors: NADH dehydrogenase and cytochrome c oxidase (CCO). NADH dehydrogenase is located in complex 1, which is the first enzyme of the electron transport chain (Brandt, 2006), and absorbs light in the violet to blue spectral region, with absorption maxima at 272, 372, and 448 nm wavelengths (Wakao *et al.*, 1987).

Mitochondrial CCO

CCO is located in complex IV of the electron transport chain, and its oxidized and reduced forms have absorption spectra in the red and near-infrared region (Figure 5.2) (UCL, 2016). It is a complex enzyme, consisting of a large number of polypeptide subunits (Figure 5.3). Subunits I, II, and III are mitochondrially encoded, and I and II are the catalytic core of the enzyme. Subunit I contains two heme groups (heme a, heme a3) and a redox-active copper site, Cu_B; subunit II contains another redox-active copper site, Cu_A, and the cytochrome c binding site (Cooper *et al.*, 1991). Cytochrome c is the small protein that delivers electrons to CCO. CCO uses the metal ions to reduce molecular oxygen to water (Tsukihara *et al.*, 1995; Voet and Voet, 2010).

Karu defined the action spectra for the DNA and RNA synthesis rate, adhesive properties, and proliferation rate of HeLa cells, and generated a generalized action spectrum in the range of 580–860 nm. This action spectrum had defined maxima at 620, 680, 760 and 820 nm (Karu, 1998). Based on the premise that the action spectrum approximates the shape of the absorption spectrum of the photoacceptor (Hartmann, 1983), Karu proposed that the bands of the generalized action spectrum may be related to CCO (Karu 1998). In fact, Karu had previously proposed that the photoacceptor for PBM was a component of the mitochondrial respiratory chain (Karu, 1987). Based on comparative analysis of the generalized action spectrum and the spectroscopic data for CCO, Karu and Afanas'eva hypothesized that the 820 nm band correlated with the oxidized CU_A, the 760 band with the reduced Cu_B, the 680 band with the oxidized CU_B, and the 620 band with the reduced CU_A (Figure 5.3)

(a)

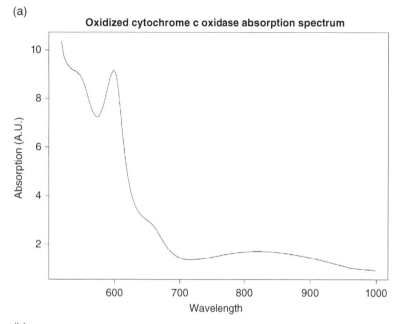

(b)

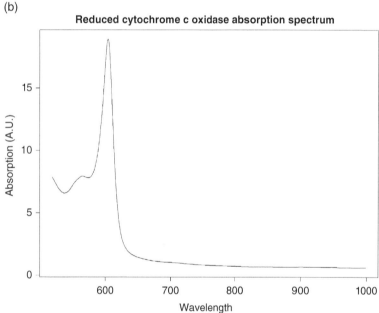

Figure 5.2 Oxidized (a) and reduced (b) CCO absorption spectra (converted to absorbance from extinction spectra data by Xingjia Wu).

(Karu and Afanas'eva, 1995). An experiment looking at the effect of 632.8 nm light on the purified CCO enzyme caused an increase in the oxidation of the enzyme and increased electron transfer, thus supporting Karu's conclusion (Pastore *et al.*, 2000).

Cellular Signaling Molecules

Excitation of CCO leads to an electronically excited state and acceleration of electron transfer reactions in mitochondria, which eventually leads to alteration of molecular and cellular changes through cellular signaling reactions. Increases in three signaling molecules are implicated in PBM activation of cellular signaling cascades. These molecules are adenosine triphosphate (ATP), reactive oxygen species (ROS), and nitric oxide (NO) (Hamblin and Demidova, 2006; Karu, 2010).

Adenosine Triphosphate

ATP is a nucleotide that performs many essential roles in the cell. It provides the energy for most of its energy-consuming activities and regulates many biochemical

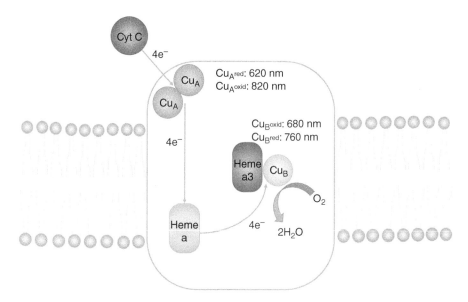

Figure 5.3 Subunit components of CCO and the wavelength maxima that correlate with the oxidized and reduced forms of the copper sites, as suggested by Karu. CCO uses the metal ions to reduce molecular oxygen to water. Subunit I contains heme a, heme a3, and a redox-active copper site, Cu_B; Subunit II contains the redox-active copper site (Cu_A) and the cytochrome c binding site. Cytochrome c is the small protein that delivers electrons to CCO.

pathways. ATP levels control the level of cyclic adenosine monophosphate (cAMP)- and ATP-driven carriers for ions such as Na^+/K^+ ATPase and calcium ion pumps. ATP stimulates intracellular pathways such as mitogen-activated protein kinases (MAPKs), and can act in conjunction with growth factors such as fibroblastic growth factor 2 (FGF2), epidermal growth factor (EGF), and nerve growth factor (NGF) to elicit biological responses. Therefore, ATP levels can have profound effects on almost every important biochemical process (Hamblin and Demidova, 2006; Karu, 2010).

In 1984, Passarella demonstrated that irradiation of isolated rat liver mitochondria with 632.8 nm light increased ATP synthesis, mitochondrial membrane potential, and the electrochemical proton gradient (Passarella *et al.*, 1984). Increased ATP syntheses induced by various wavelengths of light have been reported not only in isolated mitochondria but also in various cells types (Karu, 2007; Passarella and Karu, 2014). Therefore, increasing cellular ATP and cellular metabolism can have beneficial effects on injured and diseased cells and tissues in which cellular metabolism is suppressed (Karu, 2010).

It is now known that ATP is also an important intercellular signaling molecule (Burnstock, 2009; Karu, 2010; Khakh and Burnstock, 2009; Novak, 2003;). The release of ATP from cells can affect the ATP-releasing cells or adjacent cells through purinergic receptors. A wide variety of purinergic receptors associated with many different cell types is now known (Novak, 2003).

In 1978, Burnstock proposed that specific G-protein-linked receptors mediate the physiological effects of ATP, such as calcium mobilization and second messenger activation (Burnstock, 1978). Abbracchio and Burnstock (1994) proposed that two families of purinoceptors be established: (i) a P2X family, which mediates fast receptor responses linked to an ion channel, and (ii) a P2Y family, which mediates slower responses through G-proteins. They further proposed that the P2-purinoceptors (ATP/ADP) that are G-protein-coupled should be incorporated into the P2Y family (Abbracchio and Burnstock, 1994). G-protein-coupled receptors represent the largest superfamily of proteins in the body, with over 1000 different receptors identified. Interestingly, G-protein-coupled receptors mediate exogenous stimuli such as light, smell, and taste (Gether, 2002). In 2008, our laboratory reported that P2Y receptors were involved in light-mediated neurite outgrowth of normal human neuronal progenitor cells (Figure 5.4). In this study, we used 810 nm-wavelength light and demonstrated that neurite outgrowth stimulated by PBM was caused by increased ATP acting as a signaling molecule through the P2Y receptors (Anders *et al.*, 2008). These findings suggest that G-protein-coupled membrane receptors may play a critical role in the response of cells to light.

Reactive Oxygen Species

Oxygen metabolism produces chemically reactive, oxygen-containing molecules known collectively as ROS (Chung *et al.*, 2012). High concentrations of ROS produced by chronic inflammatory processes, toxic chemical exposure, and environmental stresses can cause oxidative cell damage. However, in lower concentrations,

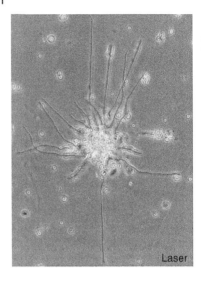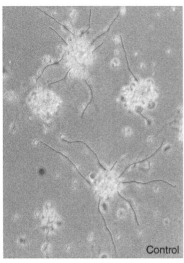

Laser   Control

Figure 5.4 Photomicrographs of normal human progenitor cells (208×). Laser panel shows cells treated with a CW, 810 nm-wavelength diode laser with an output power of 150 mW at an irradiance of 50 mW/cm^2, an exposure time of 4 seconds, and a fluence of 0.2 J/cm^2. The control panel shows cells that were handled exactly like the laser-treated cells, except the laser was off. Neurite extensions are marked in pink using Neuron J in Image J (http://rsb.info.nih.gov/ij/). Note that the irradiated cells have more neurites and longer total neurite length.

these molecules (including peroxides, superoxide, hydroxyl radical, and singlet oxygen) have beneficial effects (Chung *et al.*, 2012; Farivar *et al.*, 2014; Tafur and Mills, 2008). ROS have been shown to promote cell proliferation (Burdon, 1995; Burdon *et al.*, 1995; Callaghan *et al.*, 1996; Murrell *et al.*, 1990), induce neuronal differentiation (Suzukawa *et al.*, 2000), protect cardiac cells (Das, 2001; Vanden Hoek *et al.*, 1998), and serve as important signaling molecules for gene expression, cell growth, and transcription factor activation (Rhee, 1999; Suzuki and Ford, 1999).

ROS production *in vitro* by both visible and near-infrared light has been reported by various laboratories. Lubart and colleagues used a 780 nm-wavelength diode laser to stimulate proliferation of cultured normal human keratinocytes with a single dose of 0.45–0.95 J/cm^2 and reported an increase in cell number and cell division. To determine the role of ROS in keratinocyte proliferation, they added a variety of ROS scavengers and antioxidants, which resulted in differing levels of reduction in proliferation (Grossman *et al.*, 1988; Lubart *et al.*, 2005). Experiments with skin fibroblasts have had similar results. In an elegant study carried out in conjunction with colleagues at the Food and Drug Administration (FDA), we used a specially designed nanoprobe to measure real-time transient ROS kinetics in fibroblasts exposed to 832.8 nm-wavelength light. We found an increase in ROS production that was dependent on both laser intensity and total energy dose (Pal *et al.*, 2007). Using confocal laser-scanning microscopy, Alexandratou *et al.* (2002) illuminated single human fetal foreskin fibroblast cells with a 647 nm-wavelength laser and reported ROS generation as monitored by specific fluorescent vital probes. Using both 810 and 980 nm-wavelength light, the Hamblin laboratory reported dose-dependent ROS production in mouse embryonic

fibroblasts; 0.03–0.3 J/cm^2 resulted in a positive effect, while 30 J/cm^2 reduced ROS production (Chen *et al.*, 2011).

Cells respond to ROS in a variety of ways, maintaining the tight balance between moderate oxidative stress and cytotoxic high concentrations of ROS. Various molecules with ROS-detection systems can initiate signal transduction pathways via transcription factors, resulting in production of scavenger antioxidants, protein modification, and gene expression (Chen *et al.*, 2011). Some of the transcription factors that are regulated by these changes in mitochondrial respiration are redox factor 1 (Ref-1), dependent activator protein 1 (AP-1) (a heterodimer of c-Fos and c-Jun), nuclear factor kappa B (NF-KB), p53, activating transcription factor/cAMP response element-binding protein (ATF/CREB), hypoxia inducible factor 1 (HIF-1), and HIF-like factor (Chung *et al.*, 2012; Farivar *et al.*, 2014). Activation of these factors leads to synthesis of proteins that play roles in cell proliferation, tissue oxygenation, and cytokine modulation, as well as growth factors and other inflammatory mediators (Chung *et al.*, 2012; Hamblin and Demidova, 2006).

Nitric Oxide

Robert F. Furchgott first described the relaxation of endothelial cells in blood vessels mediated by light in 1968 (Hamblin and Demidova, 2006). His work led to the discovery of NO, a potent vasodilator that plays an important role in CCO activity. NO is a free-radical gas that regulates circulation and acts as an essential neurotransmitter (Hamblin and Demidova, 2006). It is generated from the amino acid L-arginine by the enzyme nitric oxide synthase (NOS), which has three isoforms.

Two main pathways have been proposed to explain the ability of light to increase local production and release of

NO (Chung *et al.*, 2012). The first is disassociation of NO from CCO by PBM. NO is well known to inhibit mitochondrial respiration through its competitive displacement of oxygen with the reduced binuclear center CuB/a3 of CCO (Farivar *et al.*, 2014). The "NO hypothesis" proposes that near-infrared light can cause NO to disassociate from CCO heme iron and copper centers, resulting in an increase in oxygen binding and leading to increased respiration (Hamblin and Demidova, 2006).

Karu *et al.* (2005) were the first to provide evidence for the involvement of NO in PBM. They irradiated suspensions of HeLa cells with either 600–860 nm-wavelength light or an 820 nm-wavelength diode laser, then, after a 30-minute incubation, recorded the number of cells attached to the glass matrix. They added NO donors to the suspensions before or after irradiation, and demonstrated that the addition of NO donors affected CCO binding by the NO molecules, and that the effect was dependent on both the wavelength and the fluence of the irradiation (Karu *et al.*, 2005).

Increased NO has also been reported in *in vivo* studies using a 780 nm-wavelength laser to stimulate bone healing in rats (Guzzardella *et al.*, 2002) and an 804 nm-wavelength laser to promote cardioprotection and angiogenesis following heart attacks in mice (Tuby *et al.*, 2006).

The second pathway that might explain the increase in NO bioavailability in response to PBM was proposed by Ball and colleagues, who demonstrated nitrite reductase enzymatic activity regulation by CCO in biological conditions where the oxygen concentration was low, such as in many disease states (Ball *et al.*, 2011; Poyton and Ball, 2011; Poyton *et al.*, 2009). Conversely, other investigators reported reduced levels of NO in local tissues in response to PBM, and proposed that PBM in these cases reduced one of the isoforms of NOS (Leung *et al.*, 2002; Moriyama *et al.*, 2005). Research elucidating the different mechanisms of NO related to PBMT continues.

The NO produced by these proposed pathways can have effects both intracellularly, where it is involved in hypoxic signaling, and extracellularly (Ball *et al.*, 2011; Karu *et al.*, 2005; Poyton *et al.*, 2009). Beneficial effects of NO include pain relief, resolution of edema, improved lymphatic drainage, and improved wound healing via angiogenesis (Hamblin, 2008).

PBMT Effects at the Molecular, Organelle, Cellular, and System Level

Molecular Level: Alteration of Gene Expression

There have been a number of reports on the effects of PBM on gene expression. It has been reported that red light increases expression of a number of growth factors by cells *in vitro*, including FGF-2, insulin-like growth factor (IGF), NGF, and vascular endothelial growth factor (VEGF) (Peplow and Baxter, 2012). Gene expression profiles of normal human fibroblasts exposed to 632.8 nm-wavelength light were examined using a cDNA microarray (Zhang *et al.*, 2003), and 111 genes were altered by the light. This group included an up-regulation of genes related to energy metabolism and the respiratory chain, and cell proliferation. Other genes were down-regulated, including stress-induced phosphoprotein. Red light (660 nm wavelength) also caused an up-regulation of the genes coding for the subunits of enzymes involved in complexes I and IV of the mitochondrial electron transport chain and ATP synthase in *in vitro* fibroblasts (Masha *et al.*, 2013).

We examined the effects of PBM on gene expression in olfactory ensheathing cells (OECs) (Byrnes *et al.*, 2005b). OEC transplantation has been under investigation as a treatment for spinal cord injury. OECs were purified from adult rat olfactory bulbs and exposed to 810 nm-wavelength light. Analysis of gene expression revealed statistically significant up-regulation of brain-derived neurotrophic factor (BDNF), glial-derived neurotrophic factor (GDNF), and collagen expression. These results demonstrate that PBM up-regulated neurotrophic growth factors and extracellular matrix (ECM) proteins known to support neurite outgrowth.

We also investigated gene expression in a rat model of spinal cord injury (dorsal hemisection at vertebral level T9 in adult female rats). The PBMT parameters used for the laser-treated group were: 810 nm wavelength CW diode laser, 150 mW output power, treatment time = 49 minutes, 57 seconds, spot size = 0.3 cm^2, fluence = 1589 J/cm^2. The treatment was done daily for 14 consecutive days. For microarray analysis, microarrays with over 1200 genes were run at 1, 6, and 48 hours post-injury and light treatment, or post-lesion and sham treatment. Expression of over 200 genes was significantly altered after PBMT and spinal cord injury. Many of the altered genes were involved in decreasing the inflammatory response, increasing receptor expression for neurotrophic factors, decreasing receptor expression for glutamate and gamma-amino butyric acid (GABA) (which can induce cell death), and decreasing cell proliferation. Based on reverse transcription polymerase chain reaction (RT-PCR) analysis (Figure 5.5), PBMT caused suppression of interleukin 6 (IL6) expression at 6 hours (IL6's peak), suppression of tumor necrosis factor alpha (TNFα) expression at 6 hours (peak at 1 hour), suppression of IL1β at 6 hours (IL1β's peak), and an increase in expression of transforming growth factor beta (TGF-β) at 1 and 6 hours. TGF-β normally peaks at 7 days post-injury and is responsible for decreasing the inflammatory response. In summary, there was suppression of RNA expression of pro-inflammatory cytokine genes

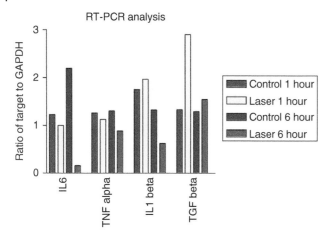

Figure 5.5 Bar graph showing the ratio of target to glyceraldehyde 3-phosphate dehydrogenase (GAPDH) based on RT-PCR analysis of control and irradiated injured spinal cord tissue at 1 and 6 hours post-injury. PBM caused a suppression of RNA expression of pro-inflammatory cytokine genes (TNFα, IL1β, and IL6) and an increase in RNA expression of the anti-inflammatory gene TGF-β.

(TNFα, IL1β, and IL6) and an increase in RNA expression of the anti-inflammatory gene TGF-β. Our previous experiments established that PBMT increases axonal regrowth following injury and decreased inflammatory cell invasion/activation (Byrnes *et al.*, 2005a). These data demonstrate that PBMT also has a significant effect on altering gene expression in the injured spinal cord.

Organelle Level: Mitochondrial Function

The structure and function of mitochondria are affected by irradiation with visible and near-infrared light. Functional changes that occur in response to irradiation relate to oxidative phosphorylation, including modulation of the mitochondrial membrane potential and metabolism and calcium intake (Passarella and Karu, 2014).

The effect of irradiation on membrane potential was first reported by the Passarella laboratory in 1984 (Passarella *et al.*, 1984). *In vitro* rat liver mitochondria irradiated with a HeNe laser ($15\,mW/cm^2$, $5\,J/cm^2$) caused an increase in membrane potential and proton gradient difference compared to non-irradiated samples. However, Passarella and Yu further demonstrated that high membrane potential alone does not account for the effects of PBM (Passarella *et al.*, 1984, 1988; Yu *et al.*, 1997b). Further studies with $660\,nm$-wavelength light demonstrated increased oxygen consumption, phosphate potential, energy charge, and electron chain enzymatic activity (Hermann and Shaw, 1988).

Of the mitochondrial processes responsive to PBM, several involve Ca^{2+} activity, including modifying the shape of cytosolic Ca^{2+} pulses, oxidative phosphorylation rate, induction of the mitochondrial permeability transition, and possibly apoptotic cell death (Passarella

and Karu 2014). Investigators have attempted to determine the role of Ca^{2+} in response to PBM. Lubart and colleagues (Breitbart *et al.*, 1996; Lubart *et al.*, 1997) tested to see whether PBM could influence Ca^{2+} transport across the mitochondrial membrane. They irradiated digitonin-treated spermatozoa or plasma membrane vesicles with a HeNe laser (fluence rate: $0.3–10.0\,mW/cm^2$; fluence: $0.04–0.8\,J/cm^2$) and measured Ca^{2+} uptake. For these experiments, cells were incubated in a medium with Ca^{2+} and immediately irradiated. The investigators determined that PBM at lower power caused an increased uptake of Ca^{2+} by mitochondria but not by membrane vesicles, while higher-power irradiation inhibited Ca^{2+} uptake (Breitbart *et al.*, 1996). Lubart also reported that irradiation with $780\,nm$-wavelength light inhibited Ca^{2+} uptake by mitochondria, indicating the importance of dosing. Passarella reported increased mitochondrial membrane potential, along with increased cytosolic free Ca^{2+} and c-fos expression changes, when isolated hepatocytes were mixed with Ca^{2+} and irradiated with a HeNe laser (fluence rate: $12\,mW/cm^2$; fluence: $0.24\,J/cm^2$) (Vacca *et al.*, 1997).

Cellular Level

Cellular responses to PBMT have been determined using *in vitro* and *in vivo* models. They include increases in metabolism, proliferation, migration, synthesis, and secretion of proteins. This section will focus on cell proliferation in the treatment of tendinopathies and wound healing, to highlight these two important clinical PBMT applications. *In vitro* studies have demonstrated the proliferative effect of PBMT in a variety of human and animal cell types, including fibroblasts, keratinocytes, endothelial cells, lymphocytes, muscle cells, and stem cells (Hamblin and Demidova, 2006; Peplow *et al.*, 2010b). Though the mechanisms for each cell type are not completely understood, in general, the increase of ROS by irradiated cells results in the expression of transcription factors such as NF-KB, which then activate a form of NOS and lead to proliferation (Alexandratou *et al.*, 2002; Lubart and Breitbart, 2000).

PBMT has been used clinically to treat a variety of tendinopathies (Doyle *et al.*, 2016; Haslerud *et al.*, 2015; Nogueira and Júnior Mde, 2015), and one potential mechanism is the proliferation of tenocytes (Tsai *et al.*, 2012, 2014). Tenocyte migration and proliferation are largely responsible for the deposition of the extracellular matrix (ECM) required in the regenerative phase of tendon repair (Chen *et al.*, 2009). *In vitro* rat tenocytes were used to test the effects of PBMT on cellular proliferation in response to irradiation with $660\,nm$-wavelength light (output power: $50\,mW$; energy densities: 1.0, 1.5, 2.0, or $2.5\,J/cm^2$) (Tsai *et al.*, 2014). These dosing parameters were similar to those used to increase Achilles tendon fibroblast proliferation in other experiments by the same investigators (Chen *et al.*, 2009). Proliferation was significantly elevated compared to controls in these studies.

PBMT has also been effectively used to accelerate wound healing; proliferation of fibroblasts and epithelial cells plays an important role in the multi-step wound-healing process. After the inflammatory phase of healing, fibroblast division and collection at wound edges occur, as fibroblasts are essential in the synthesis of connective-tissue proteins, such as collagen (Reddy, 2004). Fibroblast proliferation has been demonstrated in response to PBMT for several decades, with the first experiments, performed by Hardy *et al.* (1967), reporting a fivefold increase in mouse fibroblasts *in vitro* when irradiated by pulsed ruby laser, as compared to non-irradiated controls. More recently, Lucroy irradiated mouse fibroblasts and endothelial cells with a range of wavelengths: visible red light from 625–675 nm (KTP pumped tunable dye laser) and near-infrared light at 810 nm with a diode laser (power density: 5 mW/cm^2; energy density: 10 J/cm^2) (Moore, 2005). They measured proliferation 72 hours post-irradiation using a colorimetric assay for viable cells. Compared to control cells, irradiated fibroblasts had increased proliferation in all visible red wavelengths studied, but near-infrared 810 nm-wavelength light resulted in inhibition. Maximum proliferation was measured in those fibroblasts irradiated with red light. In endothelial cells, proliferation was recorded in all red and near-infrared wavelengths, with the maximum proliferation at 655 nm (Moore, 2005). This study and others highlight the importance of well-designed PBM parameters and serve as precursors to pre-clinical and clinical studies (Peplow *et al.*, 2010b).

Recent results from our laboratory demonstrate that effective *in vitro* parameters can be translated into optimized parameters for pre-clinical wound-healing experiments (Wu *et al.*, 2015). An *in vitro* hyperglycemic, diabetic model of primary human dermal fibroblasts (HDFs) was irradiated with an organic light-emitting diode (OLED) (623 nm peak wavelength at either 7 or 10 mW/cm^2, with fluences of 0.2, 1.0, or 5.0 J/cm^2). The effects on ATP production, mitochondrial metabolism, and HDF proliferation were measured. Groups treated with 10 mW/cm^2 at all three fluences showed significant HDF proliferation compared to controls. The 5 J/cm^2 energy density was chosen for the *in vivo* experiments based on positive results in cell proliferation and mitochondrial metabolism. The Zucker diabetic fatty (ZDF) rats were used for the pre-clinical study. An 8 mm full-thickness biopsy punch wound was made on the left and right flanks. The right-side wounds were treated by direct contact with the OLED device or laser (635 nm wavelength) and the left-side wounds were untreated

controls. Measures of wound closure were obtained at regular intervals, histological scoring was conducted using skin samples from day 13 post-injury, and immunohistochemistry was performed to measure macrophages (ED1) and FGF2. FGF2 was used to measure cell proliferation. The OLED- and laser-treated wounds had significantly higher percentages of wound closure than control wounds; histological scores were also significantly higher in the treated groups compared to controls. Additionally, OLED-treated wounds had significantly more macrophage (ED1) labeling and FGF2 expression than non-treated controls (Wu *et al.*, 2015).

System Level

The broad systemic effects of PBMT make it an ideal therapy to use to promote wound healing, resolve inflammation, and treat pain (Chung *et al.*, 2012). This section will focus on the effect of PBM on inflammation and pain.

Decreased Inflammation

The immunological process of inflammation is controlled by a variety of mediators, including cytokines and chemokines, which regulate the process using complex signaling mechanisms (Viegas *et al.*, 2007). Immune cells can be triggered by certain wavelengths of light, resulting in the release of inflammatory mediators (Chung *et al.*, 2012). Inflammation plays an important role in wound healing, pain management, and peripheral and central nervous system (CNS) injuries, and multiple other disease processes.

Muscle repair following acute injury involves regulation by inflammatory cytokines. PBMT has been used to speed recovery, presumably by modulation of the inflammatory process. The proinflammatory cytokine IL1β was decreased in PBM-treated groups (660 nm wavelength, 20 mW, 5 J/cm^2) of male Wistar rats with cryoinjury, but not in injured rats without PBM treatment 1 week after injury (Fernandes *et al.*, 2013).

The effect of PBMT on inflammatory joint diseases has been investigated. Following subplantar muscle-tissue carrageenan injection of rat paws, PBM with 660 or 684 nm wavelength (30 mW, 7.5 J/cm^2) resulted in increased mRNA expression of IL1β, TNFα, and IL6 3 hours after treatment (Albertini *et al.*, 2008). Another study reported the IL1β, TNFα, and IL6 response to PBMT following papain solution (4%) injection into knee joints of male Wistar rats (osteoarthritis model). Two dose groups of 808 nm-wavelength light were compared, a 50 and a 100 mW group. The 50 mW group had a power density of 1.78 W/cm^2, while the 100 mW group had a power density of 3.57 W/cm^2; both groups had a total energy of 4 J and an energy density of 142.4 J/cm^2. The 50 mW group had decreased cellular inflammation, as assessed by histological analysis, and, more significantly, decreased IL1β and IL6 expression compared to the 100 mW group (Alves, 2013).

The effect of PBMT on inflammatory markers in neuropathic pain animal models has been investigated. Masoumipoor *et al.* (2014) investigated the effect of PBM (660 nm-wavelength light) on inflammatory markers in a neuropathic pain model (chronic constriction injury) in adult male Sprague–Dawley rats. Hsieh *et al.* (2012) reported a decrease in pro-inflammatory markers (TNF, IL1β, HIF-1α) at the injury site (sciatic nerve) in PBMT-treated animals compared to non-treated-injured animals. Both studies provide evidence that PBMT effectively modulates the inflammatory response following nerve injury.

PBMT also altered microglial phenotypes across the M1/M2 spectrum *in vitro* in a dose-dependent manner (von Leden *et al.*, 2013). Primary microglia and a microglial cell line were exposed *in vitro* to 808 nm-wavelength light. Higher energy densities (4–30 J/cm^2) induced expression of the M1 (pro-inflammatory) phenotype, whereas lower densities (0.2–10.0 J/cm^2) induced M2 (anti-inflammatory) marker expression. Fernandes *et al.* (2015) demonstrated that both 660 and 780 nm-wavelength light could reduce TNFα and inducible NOS (iNOS) expression and TNFα and cyclooxygenase 2 (COX-2) production in J774 cells activated to the M1 (pro-inflammatory) macrophage phenotype.

Immunohistochemistry and Western blot were used to characterize changes in activated macrophages promoting cytokine production following nerve injury. Treated animals also had reduced production of TNFα and IL1, reduced macrophage activation, and decreased accumulation of HIF-1α-positive cells compared to non-treated injured animals (Hsieh *et al.*, 2012). The reduction in these pro-inflammatory cytokines implicated in neuropathic pain initiation and maintenance may elucidate a mechanism for the effectiveness of PBM treatment in decreasing neuropathic pain and should be carefully characterized. Peripheral nerve injury caused region-specific macrophage and microglia activation along spinothalamic and dorsal-column medial lemniscus pathways. There was no difference between treated and non-treated groups in the expression of Iba-1, a general macrophage and microglial cell-surface protein. However, the pro-inflammatory microglial marker CD86 was expressed in the spinal cord of injured rats in contrast to the PBM-treated and sham groups. Additionally, the PBM-treated dorsal root-ganglion macrophages expressed the anti-inflammatory macrophage marker CD206 (Ketz *et al.*, 2016).

Decreased Pain

PBMT has been used to reduce pain and improve function in a variety of musculoskeletal and neuropathic pain conditions. Evidence from animal studies and clinical trials provides insight into the multiple potential mechanisms involved in treating both acute and chronic pain. It is likely that multiple mechanisms are at play when treating complex issues such as pain.

Based on several studies, it has been proposed that local vasodilation and increased microcirculation from release of NO contribute to musculoskeletal pain relief (Cidral-Filho *et al.*, 2014; Mitchell and Mack, 2013; Samoilova *et al.*, 2008). Other groups have hypothesized that PBMT increases the nociceptive threshold by inhibiting Aδ and C nerve fibers, as evidenced by a group of studies demonstrating slowed conduction velocity in peripheral nerves. A systematic review of 44 studies indicated that PBM has a range of inhibitory neural effects across different peripheral nerve experimental models of pain (Chow *et al.*, 2011). Other data suggest that PBMT may increase endorphins, activate endogenous opioids, and recruit opioid-containing leukocytes to the site of injury (Cidral-Filho *et al.*, 2014). In one study utilizing the plantar incision model of postoperative pain in adult male Swiss mice, the animals were treated with a 950 nm-wavelength light-emitting diode (LED) device (spot size: 1 cm^2; irradiance: 80 mW/cm^2; dose: 9 J/cm^2; time: 153 seconds) under different conditions. The investigators assessed the involvement of opioid receptors, recruitment of opioid-containing leukocytes to inflamed tissue, and activation of the L-arginine/NO pathway by injecting agonist or antagonist solutions intrathecally prior to LED treatment. Pain behavior was measured using mechanical hypersensitivity via von Frey filament. The results of behavioral testing indicated that pre-administration of L-arginine prevented the analgesic effect of the LED therapy. They also provided evidence that activation of peripheral, but not central, opioid receptors, along with recruitment of opioid-containing leukocytes to the injury site, is involved in the efficacy of LED therapy in decreasing mechanical hypersensitivity in this model (Cidral-Filho *et al.*, 2014).

Hsieh *et al.* (2012, 2015) investigated the effect of PBM on neuropathic pain and functional recovery in rats with a chronic constriction injury. They treated four spots (spot size 0.2 cm^2) transcutaneously over the constriction site with a CW 660 nm-wavelength laser beginning 7 days after injury. Each spot was treated for 60 seconds with an energy density of 9 J/cm^2, daily for 7 consecutive days. Mechanical allodynia was assessed with an electronic von Frey filament and functional recovery was assessed using walking patterns. PBM-treated animals demonstrated significant improvements in neuropathic pain measures and functional recovery.

Two other studies compared different parameters for 660, 830, and 980 nm-wavelength light on pain outcome measures in male Wistar rats. Bertolini *et al.* (2011) found that animals that received five daily treatments of

830 nm-wavelength light at doses of 4 and 8 J/cm^2 following chronic constriction injury had significant improvements in the rat knee-joint incapacitation test. Another group compared control, 660 nm-wavelength light, and 980 nm-wavelength light for chronic constriction injury. The 660 nm-wavelength irradiation group received 4 J/cm^2 (0.354 W/cm^2) and the 980 nm wavelength group received 4 J/cm^2 (0.248 W/cm^2). Both treatment groups were effective at reducing mechanical allodynia (Masoumipoor *et al.*, 2014).

Our laboratory has conducted a series of pilot studies using the spared nerve injury model to optimize laser parameters and treatment schedules for PBMT in neuropathic pain (unpublished). Parameters were selected based on results from light-penetration experiments and previous *in vivo* and *in vitro* experiments using 980 nm-wavelength light, and used in a study to characterize the activation of macrophages and microglia along ascending somatosensory pathways related to neuropathic pain. Adult male Sprague–Dawley rats underwent a spared nerve injury (SNI) model and were randomly assigned to three groups: sham injury, SNI with no treatment, and SNI with PBMT. Light was applied to affected hind paw (output power: 1 W; 20 seconds; 41 cm above skin; power density: 43.25 mW/cm^2; dose: 20 J), dorsal root ganglia (output power: 4.5 W; 19 seconds; in skin contact; power density: 43.25 mW/cm^2; dose: 85.5 J), and spinal cord (output power: 1.5 W; 19 seconds; in skin contact; power density: 43.25 mW/cm^2; dose: 28.5 J) regions every other day from day 7–30 postoperatively. Mechanical hypersensitivity was measured by electron von Frey device, and immunohistochemistry was used to characterize macrophage and microglial activation. Injured groups demonstrated mechanical hypersensitivity 1–30 days postoperatively. PBM-treated animals began to recover after two treatments; at day 26, mechanical sensitivity reached baseline (Ketz *et al.*, 2016). Though treatment parameters and behavioral measurements differ between these studies, the findings suggest that PBMT can be effective in decreasing neuropathic pain behavior and altering the inflammatory process associated with peripheral nerve injury (Hsieh *et al.*, 2012).

Conclusion

Since Mester's discovery in the 1960's that low-level light produces biostimulatory effects on cells, an incredible amount of work has been done to elucidate the mechanisms behind PBM. Though much is yet to be discovered, great strides have been made in understanding the effects of light on the primary photoacceptor, along with its effects at the molecular, organelle, cellular, and system levels. To further strengthen the science, future work must focus on a deeper understanding of molecular mechanisms and the biological contexts of treating conditions (Arany, 2012). Of paramount importance is the establishment of device and dosing parameters to achieve desired clinical outcomes.

Acknowledgements

The opinions expressed herein are those of the authors and are not to be construed as reflecting the opinions of the Uniformed Services University of the Health Sciences, Landstuhl Regional Medical Center, the United States Department of Defense, or the United States Army, Navy, or Air Force.

References

Abbracchio, M.P. and Burnstock, G. (1994) Purinoceptors: are there families of P2X and P2Y purinoceptors? *Pharmacol Ther.* **64**(3):445–475.

Albertini, R. *et al.* (2008) Cytokine mRNA expression is decreased in the subplantar muscle of rat paw subjected to carrageenan-induced inflammation after low-level laser therapy. *Photomed Laser Surg.* **26**(1):19–24.

Alexandratou, E. et al. (2002) Human fibroblast alterations induced by low power laser irradiation at the single cell level using confocal microscopy. *Photochem Photobiol Sci.* **1**(8):547–552.

AlGhamdi, K.M. *et al.* (2012) Low-level laser therapy: a useful technique for enhancing the proliferation of various cultured cells. *Lasers Med Sci.* **27**(1):237–249.

Alves, A.C. (2013) Effect of low-level laser therapy on the expression of inflammatory mediators and on neutrophils and macrophages in acute joint inflammation. *Arthritis Res Ther.* **15**(5): R116.

Anders, J.J. *et al.* (2008) Light supports neurite outgrowth of human neural progenitor cells: the role of P2Y receptors. *IEEE J Sel Top Quantum Electron.* **14**(1):118–125.

Anders, J.J. *et al.* (2014) In vitro and in vivo optimization of infrared laser treatment for injured peripheral nerves. *Lasers Surg Med.* **46**(1):34–45.

Anders, J.J. *et al.* (2015) Low-level light/laser therapy versus photobiomodulation therapy. *Photomed Laser Surg.* **33**(4):183–184.

Arany, P.R. (2012) Photobiomodulation: poised from the fringes. *Photomed Laser Surg.* **30**(9):507–509.

Ball, K.A. *et al.* (2011) Low intensity light stimulates nitrite-dependent nitric oxide synthesis but not oxygen consumption by cytochrome c oxidase: Implications for phototherapy. *J Photochem Photobiol B.* **102**(3):182–191.

Basford, J.R. (1993) Laser therapy: scientific basis and clinical role. *J Orthop.* **16**(5):541–547.

Basford, J.R. (1995) Low intensity laser therapy: still not an established clinical tool. *Lasers Surg Med.* **16**(4):331–342.

Basford, J.R. *et al.* (1998) A randomized controlled evaluation of low-intensity laser therapy: plantar fasciitis. *Arch Phys Med Rehabil.* **79**(3):249–254.

Bertolini, G.R. *et al.* (2011) Low-level laser therapy, at 830 nm, for pain reduction in experimental model of rats with sciatica. *Arq Neuropsiquiatr.* **69**(2b):356–359.

Brandt, U. (2006) Energy converting NADH:quinone oxidoreductase (complex I). *Annu Rev Biochem* **75**:69–92.

Breitbart, H. *et al.* (1996) Changes in calcium transport in mammalian sperm mitochondria and plasma membrane irradiated at 633 nm (HeNe laser). *J Photochem Photobiol B.* **34**(2–3):117–121.

Burdon, R.H. (1995) Superoxide and hydrogen peroxide in relation to mammalian cell proliferation. *Free Radic Biol Med.* **18**(4):775–794.

Burdon, R.H. *et al.* (1995) Hydrogen peroxide and the proliferation of BHK-21 cells. *Free Radic Res.* **23**(5):471–486.

Burnstock, G. (1978) A basis for distinguishing two types of purinergic receptor. In: *Cell Membrane Receptors for Drugs and Hormones: A Multidisciplinary Approach*, pp. 107–118. Raven Press, New York.

Burnstock G. (2009) Purines and sensory nerves. *Handb Exp Pharmacol.* **194**:333–392.

Byrnes, K.R. *et al.* (2005a) Light promotes regeneration and functional recovery and alters the immune response after spinal cord injury. *Lasers Surg Med.* **36**(3):171–185.

Byrnes, K.R. *et al.* (2005b) Low power laser irradiation alters gene expression of olfactory ensheathing cells in vitro. *Lasers Surg Med.* **37**(2):161–171.

Calderhead, R.G. (1991) Watts a joule: on the importance of accurate and correct reporting of laser parameters in low reactive-level laser therapy and photobioactivation research. *Laser Ther.* **3**(4):177–182.

Callaghan, G.A. *et al.* (1996) Reactive oxygen species inducible by low-intensity laser irradiation alter DNA synthesis in the haemopoietic cell line U937. *Lasers Surgery Med.* **19**(2):201–206.

Chen, C.H. *et al.* (2009) Low-level laser irradiation promotes cell proliferation and mRNA expression of type I collagen and decorin in porcine Achilles tendon fibroblasts in vitro. *J Orthop Res.* **27**(5):646–50.

Chen, A.C. *et al.* (2011) Low-level laser therapy activates NF-kB via generation of reactive oxygen species in mouse embryonic fibroblasts. *PloS One.* **6**(7):e22453.

Chow, R. *et al.* (2011) Inhibitory effects of laser irradiation on peripheral mammalian nerves and relevance to analgesic effects: a systematic review. *Photomed Laser Surg.* **29**(6):365–381.

Chung, H. *et al.* (2012) The nuts and bolts of low-level laser (light) therapy. *Ann Biomed Eng.* **40**(2):516–533.

Cidral-Filho, F.J. *et al.* (2014) Light-emitting diode therapy induces analgesia in a mouse model of postoperative pain through activation of peripheral opioid receptors and the L-arginine/nitric oxide pathway. *Lasers Med Sci.* **29**(2):695–702.

Cooper, C.E. *et al.* (1991) Cytochrome c oxidase: structure, function, and membrane topology of the polypeptide subunits. *Biochem Cell Biol.* **69**(9):586–607.

Das, D.K. (2001) Redox regulation of cardiomyocyte survival and death. *Antioxid Redox Signal.* **3**(1):23–37.

Doyle, A.T. *et al.* (2106) The effects of low-level laser therapy on pain associated with tendinopathy: a critically appraised topic. *J Sport Rehabil.* **25**(1):83–90.

Farivar, S. *et al.* (2014) Biological effects of low level laser therapy. *Lasers Med Sci.* **5**(2):58–62.

Fernandes, K.P. *et al.* (2013) Effect of photobiomodulation on expression of IL-1beta in skeletal muscle following acute injury. *Lasers Med Sci.* **28**(3):1043–1046.

Fernandes, K.P. *et al.* (2015) Photobiomodulation with 660-nm and 780-nm laser on activated J774 macrophage-like cells: effect on M1 inflammatory markers. *J Photochem Photobiol B.* **153**:344–351.

Gardner, G. and Welch, A.J. (2001) Optical and thermal response of tissue to laser radiation. In: *Lasers in Medicine*, pp. 27–45. CRC Press, Washington, DC.

Gether, U. (2002) Uncovering molecular mechanisms involved in activation of G protein-coupled receptors. *Endocr Rev.* **21**(1):90–113.

Grossman, N. *et al.* (1988) 780 nm low power diode laser irradiation stimulates proliferation of keratinocyte cultures: involvement of reactive oxygen species. *Lasers Surg Med.* **22**(4):212–218.

Guzzardella, G.A. *et al.* (2002) Laser stimulation on bone defect healing: an in vitro study. *Lasers Med Sci.* **17**(3):216–220.

Hamblin, M.R. (2008) The role of nitric oxide in low level light therapy. *Proc of SPIE.* **6846**(684602).

Hamblin, M.R. and Demidova, T.N. (2006) Mechanisms of low level light therapy. *Proc of SPIE.* **6140**(612001):1–12.

Hardy, L.B. *et al.* (1967) Effect of ruby laser radiation on mouse fibroblast culture. *Fed Proc.* **26**:668.

Hartmann, K.M. (1983) Action spectroscopy. In: *Biophysics*, pp. 115–134. Springer-Verlag, Berlin.

Haslerud, S. *et al.* (2015) The efficacy of low-level laser therapy for shoulder tendinopathy: a systematic review and meta-analysis of randomized controlled trials. *Physiother Res Int.* **20**(2):108–125.

Hermann, G.J. and Shaw, J.M. (1988) Mitochondrial dynamics in yeast. *Annu Rev Cell Dev Biol.* **14**:265–303.

Hsieh, Y.L. *et al.* (2012) Low-level laser therapy alleviates neuropathic pain and promotes function recovery in rats with chronic constriction injury: possible involvements in hypoxia-inducible factor 1alpha (HIF-1alpha). *J Comp Neurol.* **520**(13):2903–2916.

Hsieh, Y.L. *et al.* (2015) Fluence-dependent effects of low-level laser therapy in myofascial trigger spots on modulation of biochemicals associated with pain in a rabbit model. *Lasers Med Sci.* **30**(1):209–216.

Jenkins, P.A. and Carroll, J.D. (2011) How to report low-level laser therapy (LLLT)/photomedicine dose and beam parameters in clinical and laboratory studies. *Photomed Laser Surg.* **29**(12):785–787.

Karu, T. (1987) Photobiological fundamentals of low-power laser therapy. *IEEE J Quantum Electron.* **23**(10):1703–1717.

Karu, T. (1998) Primary and secondary mechanisms of the action of monochromatic visible and near infrared radiation on cells. In: *The Science of Low Power Laser Therapy*, pp. 53–94. Gordon and Breach Science Publishers, London.

Karu, T. (2007) *Ten Lectures on Basic Science of Laser Phototherapy*. Prima Books AB, Grängesberg.

Karu, T. (2010) Mitochondrial mechanisms of photobiomodulation in context of new data about multiple roles of ATP. *Photomed Laser Surg.* **28**(2):159–160.

Karu, T.I. and Afanas'eva, N.I. (1995) Cytochrome c oxidase as the primary photoacceptor upon laser exposure of cultured cells to visible and near IR-range light. *Dokl Akad Nauk.* **342**(5):693–695.

Karu, T.I. *et al.* (2005) Cellular effects of low power laser therapy can be mediated by nitric oxide. *Lasers Surg Med.* **36**(4):307–314.

Ketz, A.K. *et al.* (2016) Characterization of macrophage/microglial activation and effect of photobiomodulation in the spared nerve injury model of neuropathic pain. *Pain Med.* doi:10.1093/pm/pnw144.

Khakh, B.S. and Burnstock, G. (2009) The double life of ATP. *Sci Am.* **301**(6):84–92.

Leung, M.C. *et al.* (2002) Treatment of experimentally induced transient cerebral ischemia with low energy laser inhibits nitric oxide synthase activity and up-regulates the expression of transforming growth factor-beta 1. *Lasers Surg Med.* **31**(4):283–288.

Lubart, R. and Breitbart, H. (2000) Biostimulative effects of low-energy lasers and their implications for medicine. *Int J Drug Dev Res.* **50**(3–4):471–475.

Lubart, R. *et al.* (1997) Changes in calcium transport in mammalian sperm mitochondria and plasma membranes caused by 780 nm irradiation. *Lasers Surg Med.* **21**(5):493–499.

Lubart, R. *et al.* (2005) Low-energy laser irradiation promotes cellular redox activity. *Photomed Laser Surg.* **23**(1):3–9.

Maiman, T.H. (1960) Stimulated optical radiation in ruby. *Nature.* **187**(4736):493–494.

Masha, R.T. *et al.* (2013) Low-intensity laser irradiation at 660 nm stimulates transcription of genes involved in the electron transport chain. *Photomed Laser Surg.* **31**(2):47–53.

Masoumipoor, M. *et al.* (2014) Effects of 660- and 980-nm low-level laser therapy on neuropathic pain relief following chronic constriction injury in rat sciatic nerve. *Lasers Med Sci.* **29**(5):1593–1598.

McGuff, P.E. *et al.* (1963) Studies of the surgical applications of laser (light amplification by stimulated emission of radiation). *Surg Forum.* **14**:143–145.

McGuff, P.E. *et al.* (1964) Surgical applications of laser. *Ann Surg.* **160**(4):765–777.

Mester, E. (1985) The biomedical effects of laser application. *Lasers Surg Med.* **5**(1):31–39.

Mester, E. *et al.* (1968a) The stimulating effect of low power laser rays on biological systems. *Laser Rev.* **1**:3.

Mester, E. *et al.* (1968b) The effect of laser beams on the growth of hair in mice. *Radiobiol Radiother Berl.* **9**(5):621–626.

Mester, E. *et al.* (1968c) On the effect of laser beams on bacterial phagocytosis of leukocytes. *Acta Biol Med Ger.* **21**(3):317–321.

Mester, E. *et al.* (1971) Effect of laser rays on wound healing. *Am J Surg.* **122**(4):532–535.

Mick, J. (2016) Study silences controversy, illuminates the biochemistry of laser healing. Available from: http://www.dailytech.com/Study+Silences+Controversy+Illuminates+the+Biochemistry+of+Laser+Healing/article34991.htm (accessed November 30, 2016).

Mitchell, U.H. and Mack, G.L. (2013) Low-level laser treatment with near-infrared light increases venous nitric oxide levels acutely: a single-blind, randomized clinical trial of efficacy. *Am J Phys Med Rehabil.* **92**(2):151–156.

Moore, P. (2005) Effect of wavelength on low-intensity laser irradiation-stimulated cell proliferation in vitro. *Lasers Surg Med.* **36**(1):8–12.

Moriyama, Y. *et al.* (2005) In vivo study of the inflammatory modulating effects of low-level laser therapy on iNOS expression using bioluminescence imaging. *Photochem Photobiol.* **81**(6):1351–1355.

Murray, R.K. *et al.* (2003) *Harper's Illustrated Biochemistry*, 26 edn., p. 693. McGraw-Hill Medical, New York.

Murrell, G.A *et al.* (1990) Modulation of fibroblast proliferation by oxygen free radicals. *Biochem J.* **265**(3):659–665.

Nogueira, AC Jr. and Júnior Mde, J. (2015) The effects of laser treatment in tendinopathy: a systematic review. *Acta Ortop Bras.* **23**(1):47–49.

Novak, I. (2003) ATP as a signaling molecule: the exocrine focus. *News Physiol Sci.* **18**(1):12–17.

Ohshiro, T. (1989) *Editorial. Laser Ther.* **1**(1):5.

Pal, G. *et al.* (2007) Effect of low intensity laser interaction with human skin fibroblast cells using fiber-optic nano-probes. *J Photochem Photobiol B.* **86**(3):252–261.

Passarella, S. *et al.* (1984) Increase of proton electrochemical potential and ATP synthesis in rat liver mitochondria irradiated in vitro by helium-neon laser. *FEBS Lett.* **175**(1):95–99.

Passarella, S. *et al.* (1988) Increase in the ADP/ATP exchange in rat liver mitochondria irradiated in vitro by helium-neon laser. *Biochem Biophys Res Commun.* **156**(2):978–986.

Passarella, S. and Karu, T. (2014) Absorption of monochromatic and narrow band radiation in the visible and near IR by both mitochondrial and non-mitochondrial photoacceptors results in photobiomodulation. *J Photochem Photobiol B.* **140**:344–358.

Pastore, D. *et al.* (2000) Specific helium-neon laser sensitivity of the purified cytochrome c oxidase. *Int J Radiat Biol.* **76**(6):863–870.

Peplow, P.V. and Baxter, G.D. (2012) Gene expression and release of growth factors during delayed wound healing: a review of studies in diabetic animals and possible combined laser phototherapy and growth factor treatment to enhance healing. *Photomed Laser Surg.* **30**(11):617–636.

Peplow, P.V. *et al.* (2010a) Laser photobiomodulation of wound healing: a review of experimental studies in mouse and rat animal models. *Photomed Laser Surg.* **28**(3):291–325.

Peplow, P.V. *et al.* (2010b) Laser photobiomodulation of proliferation of cells in culture: a review of human and animal studies. *Photomed Laser Surg.* **28**(Suppl. 1): S3–S40.

Poyton, R.O. and Ball, K.A. (2011) Therapeutic photobiomodulation: nitric oxide and a novel function of mitochondrial cytochrome c oxidase. *Discov Med.* **11**(57):154–159.

Poyton, R.O. *et al.* (2009) Mitochondria and hypoxic signaling: a new view. *Ann N Y Acad Sci.* **1177**:48–56.

Reddy, G.K. (2004) Photobiological basis and clinical role of low-intensity lasers in biology and medicine. *J Clin Laser Med Surg.* **22**(2):141–150.

Rhee, S.G. (1999) Redox signaling: hydrogen peroxide as intracellular messenger. *Exp Mol Med.* **31**(2):53–59.

Samoilova, K.A. *et al.* (2008) Role of nitric oxide in the visible light-induced rapid increase of human skin microcirculation at the local and systemic levels:

II. Healthy volunteers. *Photomed Laser Surg.* **26**(5):443–449.

Smith, K.C. (1991) The photobiological basis of low level laser radiation therapy. *Laser Ther.* **3**(1):19–24.

Suzukawa, K. *et al.* (2000) Nerve growth factor-induced neuronal differentiation requires generation of Rac1-regulated reactive oxygen species. *J Biol Chem.* **275**(18):13 175–13 178.

Suzuki, Y.J. and Ford, G.D. (1999) Redox regulation of signal transduction in cardiac and smooth muscle. *J Mol Cell Cardiol.* **31**(2):345–353.

Tafur, J. and Mills, P.J. (2008) Low-intensity light therapy: exploring the role of redox mechanisms. *Photomed Laser Surg.* **26**(4):323–328.

Tsai, W.C. *et al.* (2012) Low-level laser irradiation stimulates tenocyte migration with up-regulation of dynamin II expression. *PloS One.* **7**(5):e38235.

Tsai, W.C. *et al.* (2014) Low-level laser irradiation stimulates tenocyte proliferation in association with increased NO synthesis and upregulation of PCNA and cyclins. *Lasers Med Sci.* **29**(4):1377–1384.

Tsukihara, T. *et al.* (1995) Structures of metal sites of oxidized bovine heart cytochrome c oxidase at 2.8 A. *Science.* **269**(5227):1069–1074.

Tuby, H. *et al.* (2006) Modulations of VEGF and iNOS in the rat heart by low level laser therapy are associated with cardioprotection and enhanced angiogenesis. *Lasers Surg Med.* **38**(7):682–688.

Tuner, J. and Hode, L. (1998) It's all in the parameters: a critical analysis of some well-known negative studies on low-level laser therapy. *J Clin Laser Med Surg.* **16**(5):245–248.

UCL. (2016) Tissue spectra. Available from: http://www.ucl.ac.uk/medphys/research/borl/intro/spectra (accessed November 30, 2016).

Vacca, R.A. *et al.* (1997) The irradiation of hepatocytes with He-Ne laser causes an increase of cytosolic free calcium concentration and an increase of cell membrane potential, correlated with it, both increases taking place in an oscillatory manner. *Int J Biochem Mol Biol.* **43**(5):1005–1014.

Vanden Hoek, T.L. *et al.* (1998) Reactive oxygen species released from mitochondria during brief hypoxia induce preconditioning in cardiomyocytes. *J Biol Chem.* **273**(29):18 092–18 098.

Viegas, V.N. *et al.* (2007) Effect of low-level laser therapy on inflammatory reactions during wound healing: comparison with meloxicam. *Photomed Laser Surg.* **25**(6):467–473.

Voet, D. and Voet, J.G. (2010) *Biochemistry*, 4 edn., p. 1520. John Wiley & Sons, New York.

von Leden, R.E. *et al.* (2013) 808 nm wavelength light induces a dose-dependent alteration in microglial polarization and resultant microglial induced neurite growth. *Lasers Surg Med.* **45**(4):253–263.

Wakao, H. *et al.* (1987) Purification and properties of NADH dehydrogenase from a thermoacidophilic archaebacterium, Sulfolobus acidocaldarius. *J Biochem.* **102**(2):255–262.

Weersink, R. *et al.* (2007) Light dosimetry for low-level laser therapy: accounting for differences in tissue and depth. *Proc of SPIE.* **6428**(642803).

Wu, X. *et al.* (2015) Organic light emitting diode improves diabetic cutaneous wound healing in rats. *Wound Repair Regen.* **23**(1):104–114.

Yu, W. *et al.* (1997a) Improvement of host response to sepsis by photobiomodulation. *Lasers Surg Med.* **21**(3):262–268.

Yu, W. *et al.* (1997b) Photomodulation of oxidative metabolism and electron chain enzymes in rat liver mitochondria. *Photochem Photobiol.* **66**(6):866–871.

Zhang, Y. *et al.* (2003) cDNA microarray analysis of gene expression profiles in human fibroblast cells irradiated with red light. *J Invest Dermatol.* **120**(5):849–857.

Part III

Practical Applications of Laser Therapy

6

General Principles of Laser Therapy

Jeffrey J. Smith

Middletown Animal Hospital, Middletown, CA, USA

Introduction

Laser therapy has three broad effects on animal tissue: it decreases inflammation, it decreases pain, and it accelerates healing. When training staff, using the mnemonic reminder of pointing two fingers down (decreased inflammation and pain) and the thumb upward (increased healing) is an easy way to keep the entire team conveying the same information. Further, these effects are not the result of heating or warming the tissue (photothermal). Instead, they are the result of a photobiochemical change akin to the events that occur with photosynthesis or vitamin D synthesis: biological changes in chemistry at the cellular level, caused by light.

"Photobiomodulation" is the best term to describe the effects of near-infrared laser light in tissue (Anders *et al.*, 2015), since some parts of the healing process are accelerated (organization and proliferation), while other parts are diminished (inflammation). The initial effect of near-infrared laser light is stimulation of production of adenosine triphosphate (ATP), reactive oxygen species (ROS), and nitric oxide (NO) (Farivar *et al.*, 2014; Karu, 2010; Sommer, 2014; Sommer *et al.*, 2014). In turn, these bioactive substances cause the cascade of effects for each of the three mechanisms of action involving inflammation, pain, and healing (Chung *et al.*, 2012). These cascades are well documented, and are summarized in Chapter 5.

Therapeutic Dosing

Much of the successful evolution of laser therapy is the direct result of understanding the dose-dependent nature of tissue response to infrared light. In other words, tissue must receive the appropriate target dose of light energy to manifest the effects of laser therapy. This phenomenon is analogous to dosing tissue with antibiotics (mg/kg) or radiation ($J/kg = Gy$), but for laser therapy the dosing is in joules per square centimeter (J/cm^2). If suboptimal doses are administered, then the effects will also be suboptimal, or may even not be apparent.

Multiple current publications indicate that proper dosing for most superficial tissue is in the $1–4 J/cm^2$ range (Peplow *et al.*, 2010), while dosing for most deep tissue is in the $8–20 J/cm^2$ range (Bjordal *et al.*, 2003; Roberts *et al.*, 2013).

To facilitate delivering proper doses of laser therapy, power, wavelength, and pulsing must be understood (Sommer *et al.*, 2015). Doses are affected by tissue type, anatomic site, tissue depth, species, coat color and length, skin color, and body condition score (Anders *et al.*, 2014; Enwemeka, 2009; Weersink, 2007). Effective dosing intervals (again, just like with antibiotic or radiation therapy) are critical to achieving positive clinical outcomes. Factors such as patient preparation, application techniques, frequency of administration, and proper patient management are also essential for optimal results.

Therapeutic Dosing Parameters

To understand accurate dosing of infrared light, one must understand the physical characteristics of light. These include wavelength, power, and frequency. One must also understand how the light is delivered to the target tissue.

Wavelengths between 800 and 1100 nm (all near-infrared) are able both to penetrate into deep tissue and to stimulate photobiomodulation. No particular wavelength has any unique biological effects, though there are small differences in absorption depending on the amount of pigment present in the treated tissue. Though numerous studies have been published using multiple wavelengths, there is no consensus that one wavelength of light has an optimal effect. The main chromophore for photobiomodulation is cytochrome c oxidase (CCO), which is a class of hemoprotein found in the mitochondria of cells (Kim, 2014; Passarella and Karu, 2014).

The power of therapeutic lasers is measured in watts (W), where 1 W = 1 J/sec. This means that a 1 W laser can deliver 60 J/min, while a 10 W laser can deliver 600 J/min. Power does not determine depth of penetration (that is a function of wavelength) but does determine the number of photons reaching the depth to which a particular wavelength can penetrate, in a particular tissue, in a fixed amount of time.

Power determines the rate of delivery. Utilizing higher power settings allows for the application of the target dosage in a more reasonable and efficient amount of time. For example, a laser set to deliver 1 W would take 100 minutes to deliver 6000 J, while a laser set to deliver 15 W would only take 6 minutes 40 seconds to deliver the same amount of energy. Reducing treatment time by using higher power settings is particularly relevant when treating larger areas or larger animals.

The frequency or pulsing of therapeutic infrared light was at one time thought to have an effect on the different mechanisms of photobiomodulation. A comprehensive recent review of literature publications indicates that there is little consensus about the effect of pulsing in different clinical conditions (Hashmi *et al.*, 2010). To many laser therapists, this review supports the concept that light should be delivered continuously (continuous wave, CW). This intuitively makes sense, since the cellular effect is the direct result of photons stimulating CCO, and not the result of some spacing or "blinking" of the photons as they arrive at the mitochondria. In addition, any pulsing (whether at 50 or 5000 Hz) results in the laser light being on some of the time and off some of the time. The amount of time the laser spends emitting while pulsing is referred to as the "duty cycle" (Barrett and Pack, 2006).

Pulsing means that more time is required to deliver the same dose. Thus, to treat a large dog's lumbar region with 6000 J of energy would take 10 minutes with a 10 W laser in CW, but would take 20 minutes with a 10 W laser pulsing with a 50% duty cycle. This is not only inefficient, it is an added cost to the client, since most laser therapy fees are based on the amount of time a therapy session requires.

The delivery method is an often overlooked component of the therapeutic dose, because many laser therapy devices only offer a non-contact delivery method. When a handpiece is placed in contact with the tissue and used to introduce the light to deep tissues, significantly more photons can be delivered to those deeper structures (Enwemeka, 2009). This enhanced delivery is accomplished by reducing reflection, reducing the distance to the target tissue by compression, and parting or pushing the hair coat out of the way. Since hemoglobin is a main absorber of light in the dermis, blood absorption is a barrier to photon penetration (Lister *et al.*, 2012). The pressure of contact of the handpiece with the tissue produces blanching and improves light penetration to deeper target tissues. In addition, using a handpiece in contact with the tissue delivers an added, independent, massaging benefit that stimulates myofascial trigger points.

General Therapeutic Doses

As stated previously, most tissue doses can be categorized as either superficial (the lesions or tissues are visible to the eye) or deep (the lesions or tissues are below the skin or mucosa) dosing. The doses are different not because the cells in those locations require different dosages, but because there is a loss of light energy in the interposing tissue on the way to the deeper target tissues due to reflection, scatter, and absorption (Lister *et al.*, 2012).

Proper dosing for most superficial tissue is in the $1-4 \text{ J/cm}^2$ range, while dosing for most deep tissue is in the $8-20 \text{ J/cm}^2$ range (Bjordal *et al.*, 2003; Roberts *et al.*, 2013).

An important concept in proper dosing is the inclusion of all of the tissue associated with a lesion or area, and not just the visible or suspected pathology. For example, when treating pyotraumatic dermatitis, one should include a wide margin around the visible lesion, which in most cases nearly doubles the size of the area being treated. Similarly, if one is treating the hip, it is important to treat all of the associated anatomical structures (such as the iliopsoas muscle) around the entire hip joint. This means treating the joint from 360° and at least half the distance to the stifle and all the way to the midline.

Manual Dose Calculation

It is helpful to conceptualize laser therapy dosing by calculating or confirming dosing manually. A $7.5 \times 12.7 \text{ cm}$ index card or a CD is almost exactly 100 cm^2, and because 100 is an easy multiplier, one can determine approximate dosages by visualizing the area to be treated relative to one of these objects. For example, if one wanted to treat the hip of a dog (360° around the joint), and the area approximated that of five index cards, one would multiply the dose (10 J/cm^2) by the area (500 cm^2) to calculate the total amount of energy to be delivered (5000 J). On the other hand, if a pyotraumatic dermatitis lesion was half the size of an index card, one would multiply the dose (4 J/cm^2) by the area (50 cm^2) to calculate the total amount of energy to be delivered (200 J). Most people's flattened hand approximates the area of an index card (compare your own hand to one), which provides a good visual marker for gauging treatment areas.

The inverse of this concept is also helpful. When given a dose to administer, an understanding of what area to administer that dose to can be helpful. For example, for deep tissue being dosed at $10\,\mathrm{J/cm^2}$, every $1000\,\mathrm{J}$ should be spread over an area of $100\,\mathrm{cm^2}$. Therefore, a dose of $4500\,\mathrm{J}$ would be administered over an area of 4.5 index cards. For superficial tissue being dosed at $4\,\mathrm{J/cm^2}$, every $400\,\mathrm{J}$ should be administered over an area $100\,\mathrm{cm^2}$. Therefore, a superficial dose of $200\,\mathrm{J}$ would be administered over an area of half an index card.

Software Dose Calculation

Fortunately, many lasers are now programmed with very specific and detailed dosing information in their software. Operators enter patient-specific data and anatomical information, and the software calculates the dose according to the science and experience incorporated in its algorithms. Software-calculated doses are usually in the accepted $1-4\,\mathrm{J/cm^2}$ range for superficial conditions, with the majority of lesions being treated with $4\,\mathrm{J/cm^2}$. Software-calculated doses for deep-tissue conditions typically fall in the $8-20\,\mathrm{J/cm^2}$ range, with the majority of lesions being treated with $10\,\mathrm{J/cm^2}$.

Adjusting Calculated Doses

Software in newer-generation therapy lasers provides a starting point for most conditions, and the dosing delivered will be successful in the majority of cases. Still, it is important to have a working knowledge of how dosing is calculated, in much the same way that it is important to understand the readings on patient monitoring devices. Some patients and conditions require adjustment of the dose for best effect on an individual case-to-case basis.

Lesions that have both a superficial and a deep component, like degloving injuries, postsurgical fractures, and advanced otitis, should be treated with a higher dose. Superficial target tissues within this treatment area will be treated simultaneously.

Refractory conditions often respond to higher dosing. For example, if a canine patient has a particularly bad coxofemoral arthritis that is not responding to $10\,\mathrm{J/cm^2}$, then doubling the dose to $20\,\mathrm{J/cm^2}$ will often achieve a better outcome. A dose of $37.5\,\mathrm{J/cm^2}$ has been validated in the application of laser therapy for chronic lower back pain in humans (Vallone *et al.*, 2014).

Practicing clinicians have noted that certain difficult conditions or lesions may require higher doses in order to see consistent clinical responses. These include lick granulomas ($30-40\,\mathrm{J/cm^2}$), degenerative myelopathy ($25-45\,\mathrm{J/cm^2}$), equine spinal structures ($20\,\mathrm{J/cm^2}$), and feline eosinophilic complex lesions ($30-40\,\mathrm{J/cm^2}$).

Dosing Intervals

Though therapy laser software provides the proper dosing for most conditions, it does not provide any information about the interval between treatments. Determining and prescribing the number and frequency of laser therapy sessions is the responsibility of the prescriber. Most conditions fall into one of three categories: post-procedure, acute, or chronic. Less frequently are acute-on-chronic or relapsed conditions that warrant additional consideration. In addition, multimodal management, as opposed to laser therapy alone, will have an effect on dosing intervals (AAHA, 2015).

Post-Procedure Conditions

Post-procedure treatments are applied once or twice with the goal of mitigating or managing postoperative or post-traumatic pain and swelling. Since these treatments are not sustained over a long period of time, no increase in healing times is necessarily expected. Nonetheless, laser therapy should be part of a multimodal pain management plan according to the new 2015 American Animal Hospital Association (AAHA)/American Association of Feline Practitioners (AAFP) Pain Management Guidelines for Dogs and Cats (AAHA, 2015). Laser therapy will dramatically reduce edema, pain, self-mutilation, and acute inflammation. These treatments are typically very short and are applied during the anesthetic recovery period. If animals are hospitalized overnight, they benefit from a second application the following day. The cost of these treatments is often incorporated into the procedure or pain-management fees for the patient.

Acute Conditions

Acute conditions are typically treated daily or every other day, and then at decreasing intervals until resolution of the condition. In addition to the post-procedure benefits, wounds will heal and resolve noticeably faster (Avci *et al.*, 2013) and the pain-modulating effect will be more sustained. In most cases, the more acute the injury or inflammation, the more important it is to try to treat daily. In some cases, treating daily for 3 days and then every other day until the condition resolves is efficacious. When pets are hospitalized, daily treatments are both very beneficial and practical. If owners have their pets treated on an outpatient basis, then sometimes a compromise between ideal medical care (daily treatments) and reasonable client compliance (every 2–3 days) must be worked out. In the majority of cases, treating more than once a day does not provide substantially improved outcomes. The fees for treating these conditions are usually based on the treatment time.

Chronic Conditions

Chronic conditions are more complicated to treat than post-procedure or acute conditions. In general, one should expect chronic conditions to respond "chronically" (after a series of treatments), unlike acute conditions, which usually respond "acutely" (after one or two treatments). Chronic conditions are managed in three phases:

1) **Induction phase:** Up to 12 treatments, administered two to three times a week.
2) **Transition phase:** One or two treatments a week for 4 weeks.
3) **Maintenance phase:** One treatment every 2–4 weeks.

Patients will often show significant improvement after three treatments and remarkable improvement after six treatments, but induction should continue until improvement plateaus for two or three treatments. Some particularly advanced conditions will require the entire induction period to show significant improvement.

Be careful to evaluate improvement from both lameness and mobility perspectives. For example, the author treated a 14-year-old German shorthair pointer named Reba that had severe bilateral elbow arthritis. After 11 treatments, Reba appeared to be moving no differently than before her laser sessions. When the owner was asked about this, she said, "Reba is doing fantastic! Following me into the garden. Walking up the stairs. Much more like her old self!" In this case, Reba could not move her elbows any differently (she was still lame), but was much more comfortable and mobile than before her therapy.

There will also be cases where the owner does not perceive the patient's gradual improvement over a 4-week period, and they will have to be reminded, or shown a "before" video, in order to see the improvement in their own pet.

Like fees for acute conditions, fees for treatment of chronic conditions are based on the treatment time.

Acute-on-Chronic Conditions

Some conditions will manifest both acute and chronic components. Examples are degloving injuries, post-tibial-plateau-leveling osteotomy surgery, and intervertebral disk disease (IVDD). In cases like these, address the acute component first by following an acute dosing protocol (daily or every other day). Once the acute component of the injury or condition is managed (typically in six to ten treatments), transition to a chronic condition protocol (three times a week) until the chronic component is managed or resolved.

Relapsed Conditions

Patients that have done well with laser therapy can exacerbate their controlled condition with a burst of overactivity, such as a day or two of duck hunting. These pets can sometimes be rescued with a series of three to six daily or every-other-day treatments. Another scenario is the pet that responded well to laser therapy, but has stopped returning for its maintenance therapy. Often, after several months without laser therapy, the pet's symptoms will begin to recur. In these cases, the patient needs to restart the entire chronic condition protocol (induction phase first) in order to control their symptoms. This is an important point to make clients aware of in order to keep them compliant with the maintenance phase of their pet's laser therapy.

Multimodal Management versus Laser Therapy Alone

Laser therapy is a very effective modality, but it is even more effective when used as a component of a multimodal management strategy. There are many excellent pharmaceutical and non-pharmaceutical options when treating pain and delayed healing. New standards of care call for incorporating multiple modalities for maximum effectiveness and minimum side effects.

When laser therapy is used as a sole modality, it is likely to require use that is more frequent and that delivers less optimal results, especially with advanced conditions and pathology. When multiple modalities are used to manage pain, inflammation, and healing at different points along the healing and pain pathways, superior outcomes are the logical and scientifically proven result (AAHA, 2015).

Preparation for Laser Therapy

The impulse to get started treating a patient needs to be balanced with the benefits of being well prepared to administer laser therapy. Following the same routine or checklist every time will ensure proper technique, positive outcomes, and a pleasant experience for the patient and client. Laser therapy is unique among the services that veterinarians offer to clients in that the clients usually remain with the pet during the treatment. Furthermore, the pet has a less fearful experience because it is not experiencing anything painful like an injection, a blood draw, or a nail trim. As a result, clients and pets can have an entirely new experience at the veterinarian's office, which leads to clients becoming very bonded to the practice.

Laser Therapy Treatment Procedure

Laser therapists should develop a routine that ensures all appropriate steps are included in sessions (Box 6.1). Begin by preparing the client and the patient. Explain

---

Box 6.1 Fifteen-step laser therapy treatment procedure.

1) Briefly explain to the owner what laser therapy does.
2) Communicate the expectations for the laser therapy.
3) Instruct the owner about their role in the patient's restraint and positioning.
4) Take a few 4–5-second videos of the patient moving, if they are lame.
5) Position the patient comfortably in the laser therapy treatment environment.
6) Program the laser and enter the patient's details into the laser software.
7) Provide protective eyewear to all people in the room or area.
8) Provide protective goggles or eye protection (soft black Elizabethan collars) to the patient.
9) Take a few photos of the patient wearing their goggles.

10) Allow the owner to feel what the laser therapy is like. Briefly apply the laser to their forearm or hand to give them the assurance that the laser treatment will be comfortable. This will help prevent questions and concerns from developing mid-treatment.
11) Approach the patient briefly with the handpiece without turning the laser on. This allows the patient to adapt to the sensation of the handpiece prior to the addition of laser therapy itself.
12) Activate the laser and apply the laser therapy.
13) Pause as needed.
14) Treat all of the prescribed treatment areas.
15) Record the laser therapy treatment and relevant progress notes.

---

why laser therapy is being prescribed, and outline the expected results. Instruct the owner about his or her role in the pet's restraint and positioning.

Take a few 4–5-second videos of the pet moving or trotting, if they are lame. When incorporated into the patient's record, these videos can be an important reference for evaluating progress during future sessions.

If the therapy laser software has an individual record-keeping system, enter the patient's pertinent information. If the software has condition-specific protocols, select the prescribed protocol and prepare for the administration of therapy. If the therapy laser does not have software, or has only limited software, calculate the number of joules to be administered.

Provide protective eyewear to all people in the room or area and explain why protection is required. Likewise, provide protective goggles or eye protection (black, soft Elizabethan collars are an excellent alternative) for the pet. Take several images of the patient wearing their goggles for the owner to share with friends and their online community.

Allow the owner to feel what laser therapy is like. Briefly apply the laser to their forearm or hand. This reassures the owner that the laser is comfortable and prevents questions or concerns from developing during the treatment.

Approach the patient briefly without turning the laser on to allow them to adapt to the sensation of the hand-piece prior to the addition of laser therapy itself. Activate the laser and administer the laser therapy. Pause as needed during the treatment to reposition and allow the patient to reposition. Proceed sequentially through the prescribed areas to be treated. After the treatment is completed, record treatment parameters, observations, and progress notes in the patient's record.

Record Keeping

Good record keeping is important for all of the same reasons as for other medical procedures. The most important information to record is the dose administered, in J/cm^2, and the total number of joules administered to any specific area. Other information like application method, power (wattage), frequency (if using pulsed emission), treatment response, pain score, and owner comments can also be included.

Records can be in electronic or written form. Some lasers will record (and export) treatment records. These lasers have the added benefit of allowing quick, repeatable access to previous treatments, which provides added efficiency and reproducibility.

Photos, Videos, Radiographs, and Digital Thermal Images

Records can also include visual formats like photographs, videos, radiographs, and digital thermal images. These types of imaging are helpful to both the veterinarian and the owner, as they provide excellent before-and-after documentation of the progress being made with the laser therapy. Photographs are particularly valuable for wounds, incisions, and dermatitis. Videos are very helpful for lameness and neurologic conditions. Radiographs are appropriate for fractures and boney lesions. Digital thermal imaging is a simple and effective method of producing an image that reveals changes in temperature and circulation in injured and healing tissue (Figure 6.1).

(a)

(b)

(c)

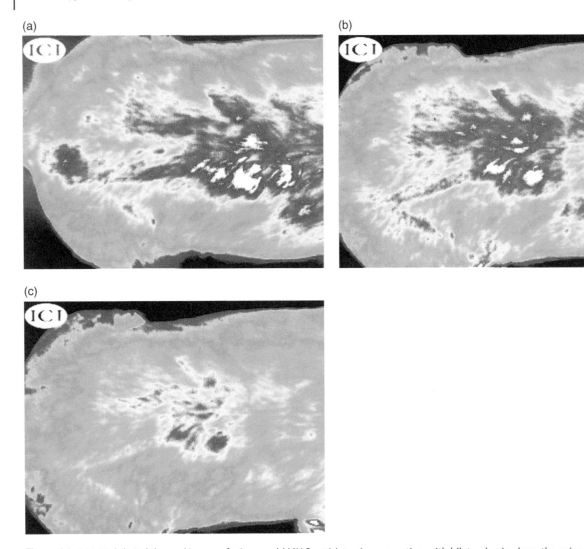

Figure 6.1 (a) Initial digital thermal image of a 9-year-old MN Scottish terrier presenting with bilateral pain along the spine. The white and red areas in the image are areas of increased thermal gradient. Using a combination of 810 and 980 nm, 8 J/cm^2 of laser therapy was administered with a contact scanning technique. No medication was administered. (b) Digital thermal image taken 24 hours after the initial laser therapy. Clinically, the patient was not in as much pain and was moving a great deal more easily. This image indicates a drop in thermal gradient of 34%. This is a very close approximation of the progress of the therapy and is a guide as to where to direct the next therapy session. Laser therapy was repeated with a slightly higher dose to all areas still exhibiting higher thermal gradients. (c) Digital thermal image taken 72 hours after the initial therapy and 48 hours after the second treatment, depicting a 92.5% decrease within the initial increased thermal gradients. Clinically, the patient was not in pain on palpation and was ready to play.

Extra mention should be made of the benefit of photographing the patient with their safety goggles on. Most owners are overcome with amusement when they see their pet in these "sunglasses." Use the photos as part of your own internal promotions and online presence, and provide them to the owners to share with their friends via social networks. Printed and electronic digital thermal images are similarly loved by owners.

Preparing the Laser Therapy Room

Ideally, the laser therapy room should be a quiet, separate, relaxing space designed for the comfort of the patient, as well as the owner and therapist (Figure 6.2). In the limited confines of some hospitals, this is not possible, and other rooms may be tasked to serve a dual function. Many post-procedure treatments can be performed in the treatment or surgery room. In mobile practices, laser therapy can be performed in a huge variety of settings, though these sometimes present extra challenges.

The room should be equipped with either two large (60 × 120 cm) dog beds or a single large (120 × 200 cm) platform table to make the therapy sessions both comfortable and ergonomic. A couple of small, low, rolling stools can also be very helpful. In most cases, the pets will assume a prone position for laser therapy, though positioning is ultimately a question of patient comfort and compliance.

Figure 6.2 Laser therapy-appropriate room with appropriate bedding. Client, patient, and laser therapist are all comfortable, and the patient can easily be moved to access treatment areas.

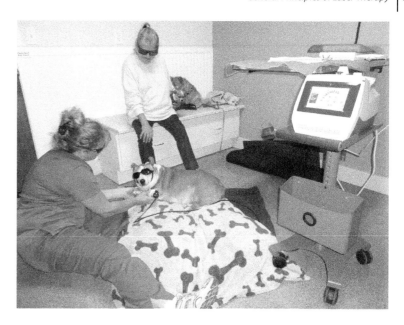

Preparing for Laser Safety

Safe operation of the laser equipment is a function of good training, and of compliance with that training. Regulators require two main safety measures: appropriate eye protection for humans and patients, and "Laser in Use" signage (ANSI, 2011a, 2011b). See Chapter 4 for a complete discussion of laser therapy safety.

Other than eye safety, the central objective in applying laser therapy safely is to introduce the energy into the tissues without excessive or uncomfortable warming. This is accomplished primarily by proper choice of delivery handpiece, proper movement of the handpiece, and proper choice of power (often determined by the laser's software). When appropriate, monitoring the patient's skin temperature with a trailing finger is good practice. If a temperature other than a pleasant, gentle warming is detected, the speed of movement of the handpiece should be increased.

Preparing the Laser Equipment

The laser itself should be prepared and programmed in advance, if possible. In addition, the cleanliness, integrity, and functionality of the laser should be checked.

Preparing the Patient for Laser Therapy

On rare occasions, patients require sedation, but most pets come to accept and appear to enjoy their laser therapy sessions. Naturally soothing or calming methods such as dog-appeasing pheromone dispensers, feline pheromone diffusers, quiet music, special treats, and low lighting are preferred, and are quite beneficial.

Anesthesia

Patients will sometimes be under anesthesia when laser therapy is administered, and this requires extra attention to be paid to the warmth of the tissue being treated. Since an unconscious patient cannot respond to excessive warmth, continually checking the tissue temperature with a trailing finger or using a lower power setting is appropriate.

Hair Coat Challenges

The coat of an animal can provide a significant impediment to the penetration of light into deeper tissues. This effect can be significantly reduced with the use of a contact handpiece, which also provides enhanced dosing of deeper tissues. In cases where the coat is excessively long or thick, wetting or misting the hair can be an effective method of reducing interference. Water will not significantly reduce laser therapy penetration, so treatments can be administered to pets emerging from underwater treadmill therapy, as well. If the coat is matted, crusted, or dirty, then clipping, debriding, or cleaning may be needed.

Bandages, Splints, Casts, and Pet Clothing

Laser therapy should not be administered through any sort of clothing, bandage, splint, or cast. The amount of light scattered by these materials is so variable, and in some case so complete, that the dose of light reaching the target tissue is unknown, and therefore unreliable. Remove any clothing the pet is wearing. If a bandage is being used, administer laser therapy when the bandage is changed. If a splint or cast is being used, create a window over the area to be treated, and cover the window with material that can be easily removed for successive laser therapy treatments (Figure 6.3).

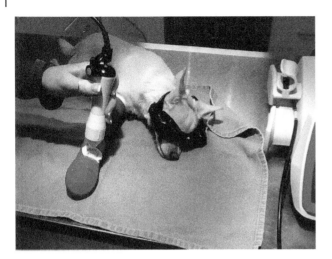

Figure 6.3 Use of a window in a cast to allow for laser therapy treatment.

Laser Therapy Application Techniques

Proper application of laser therapy is not technically difficult, but it does require attention to be paid to basic technical principles, which can have profound effects on the success of treatment of the targeted tissue or area. Often, a lack of attention to these details is responsible for suboptimal outcomes.

General Application Techniques

Maintain Movement

Early in the use of lasers for therapeutic purposes, a point-to-point treatment technique was employed. With this technique, the handpiece was placed close to or in contact with a "point" in the target area and held in one place. If the target area was larger than the spot size, the handpiece was moved adjacent to the first treatment area, and the administration was repeated until multiple points had been treated.

With better understanding of required target doses and the development of lasers that can deliver those doses to large areas of tissue within relevant amounts of time, a scanning or moving technique can now be used. The laser handpiece should always be kept moving at 2–7 cm/sec, since this prevents excessive heat from accumulating in the tissue. Do not hold the handpiece stationary and do not merely vibrate or wobble the light back and forth in the same area. The laser light beam should move over the target tissue, as well as a margin of adjacent normal tissue.

Treat All Locally Affected Tissue

Treat all affected and associated tissue. This means treating a large area around a wound or a joint, since most pathology affects a larger area than the visible pathology itself. An area around a wound equal to the area of the wound should be treated. If treating a joint, the area around, proximal, and distal to the joint should be treated. For example, the dorsolateral area of an arthritic hip might look the most painful on an x-ray, but joint pain from the hip emanates from the entire joint capsule, and thus the hip and associated soft tissues should be treated from dorsolateral, dorsocranial, dorsocaudal, and ventral directions.

Treat All Distant Affected Tissue

Be aware of two targets that can improve outcomes. First, innervating spinal nerve root segments can become involved in wind-up pain and contribute significantly to the discomfort of an area in a remote location. Treating the involved nerve root segments (commonly the lumber or cervical area) is frequently beneficial. Second, compensating joints or muscles can also be stressed and painful from abnormal or unnatural movement caused by a painful area. Often, animals with hip pain will have back pain, iliopsoas muscle pain, or both. Similarly, pets with knee pain will often have hip or back discomfort. Treating these compensating tissues can often lead to greater success.

Treat in a Grid-like Pattern

Movement of the handpiece should be in a grid-like or crosshatched pattern. Avoid circles, curly-q's, or random scribbling with the handpiece, because these lead to inconsistent and non-uniform saturation of the target tissue. When treating any large or awkwardly shaped area, the area should be divided into halves, thirds, or quarters to facilitate easier application of the total dose.

Treat Perpendicular to the Tissue Surface

Keep the handpiece perpendicular to the surface of the tissue to minimize reflection and maximize penetration. This can create awkward or difficult movements unless the treatment areas are divided into smaller sections. This is often a challenging concept to new laser technicians.

Treat from 360°

When possible, treat tissues from 360°, or from both medial and lateral sides. This allows the entire associated anatomy to be treated and provides superior results to a focused or limited application. For example, treat a hip laterally, caudally, cranially, and medially. As a second example, treat a mouth while both open and closed.

Maintain Distance when Using Non-Contact Treatment

Treat the tissue from 2–5 cm away when using a non-contact handpiece.

Treat through Passive Range of Motion

Move the targeted tissue through a passive range of motion (try for at least two different positions) when treating extremities and joints, in order to reach all aspects. At the start of a course of therapy, the patient may be in great pain, and movement of the area being treated may not be possible during the first few laser sessions. In these cases, it is best first to treat in a passive position, and then to attempt gentle movement for passive range of motion during subsequent treatments.

Therapy Laser Settings

Options are available in the software of many laser therapy devices to select patient-specific parameters regarding coat color, skin color, body condition, and coat length. When available, the selection of the proper parameters will allow the software to adjust the wavelength and power for optimal dosing.

Pause When Required

Whenever it is necessary to reposition or rest the patient or the laser technician, it is prudent to pause the treatment. Ideally, this can be done from a switch on the laser handpiece, rather than by returning to the operational screen.

Laser Handpiece Selection

Select the proper laser handpiece, or handpiece adapter, for the condition being treated (contact or deep-tissue versus non-contact or superficial tissue).

Contact, On-Contact, or Deep-Tissue Application

A contact handpiece should be used for any pathology that is not visible to the eye or is below the skin or mucosa. Examples are musculoskeletal conditions, abdominal conditions, thoracic conditions, middle- or inner-ear conditions, and conditions within the closed mouth. Handpieces designed to be in contact with the tissue surface can also be designated as deep-tissue applicators if the lens introduces the light directly into the tissue (Figure 6.4). These applicators can deliver significantly more photons to deep-tissue structures than can non-contact applicators (Enwemeka, 2009). This phenomenon is the result of decreased interference from hair (the end of the handpiece parts and pushes hair out of the way), decreased reflection from the skin surface, decreased distance to the target tissue from compression, and decreased interference from hemoglobin (compression-induced blanching),

Non-Contact, Off-Contact, or Superficial Tissue Application

Handpieces designed not to be in contact with the tissue surface are designated for superficial conditions (those conditions where the pathology is visible to the eye, or is not below the skin or mucosa) (Figure 6.5). These applicators are preferred for infected, moist, painful, sterile, and difficult-to-access conditions. Examples are dermatitis, wounds, incisions, the outer ear, the open mouth, and intraoperative applications.

Combination Contact and Non-Contact Application

Ears, mouths, and some extensive wounds like degloving injuries benefit from a combination of both superficial and deep-tissue treatment, since they have components of both pathologies. For example, when treating ears, use non-contact application for the pinnae and outer ear, then change to contact application for the middle and inner ear and the surrounding tissue. When treating the mouth, use non-contact application to treat the visible structures and

Figure 6.4 Proper positioning for treatment with a handpiece designed for deep-tissue treatment. The handpiece is perpendicular to and in contact with the tissue surface.

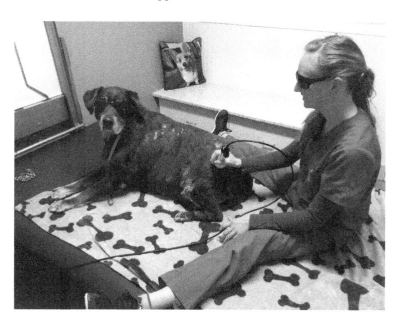

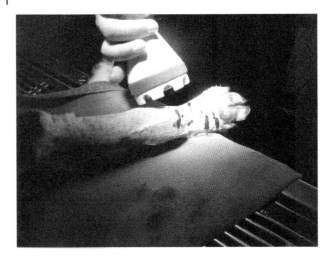

Figure 6.5 Treatment with a handpiece designed for non-contact treatment of superficial tissue conditions.

pathology, then change to contact application to treat the intramandibular space, buccal mucosa, temperomandibular joint, and surrounding tissue. When treating extensive wounds, use non-contact application to treat the open wound and contact application to treat the surrounding area of injured, inflamed, and painful tissue.

Large- versus Small-Diameter Handpieces

Many higher-powered (>5 W) therapy lasers come with a choice of handpiece sizes, or a choice of small or large handpiece adapters, in both contact and non-contact designs. Others have handpieces that allow for manual adjustment of the diameter of the emitted laser beam. These choices improve application ergonomics and allow the option of spreading higher-power laser beams over a larger area of application.

As a general rule, handpieces or adapters that produce a beam diameter <2 cm should be used with a power of 3 W or less. These are most useful when treating small patients or small areas at those lower power settings.

Larger handpieces or adapters that produce a beam diameter >2 cm can be used with any power setting (0.5–15.0 W), since they spread the energy over a much larger area than the small versions. When a higher power setting is selected, some therapy laser software will provide a warning to use a handpiece or adapter that emits a larger beam diameter.

Ergonomics

As in dentistry, operator comfort is important for long-term success and contentment in applying laser therapy. As mentioned before, large dog beds or a raised (45 cm) 120 × 200 cm treatment platform are the standard recommendations for use during longer musculoskeletal treatments. In addition, a couple of small, low rolling stools

can be helpful. Lasers that can be repeatedly activated and deactivated from the handpiece are also very beneficial when repositioning, resting, or pausing during therapy.

Patients often learn that laser therapy is a pleasant, pain-relieving experience once they have completed two or three treatments. Therapy sessions tend to proceed more quickly as the therapy progresses. Extra patience and time should be allowed for the initial therapy sessions while that process develops.

Training and Expertise

All laser therapists should be fully trained in the safe and effective delivery of therapeutic treatments. Each practice should develop a training protocol, and trainees should finalize a training checklist prior to treating patients (Box 6.2).

After initial training, there are three levels of expertise in the application of laser therapy. It takes most therapists about 10 treatments to become comfortable and about 100 treatments to become thoroughly competent. After 1000 treatments, the therapist should be an expert.

- **Level one:** The therapist is able to apply laser therapy following all of the guidelines given in this chapter.
- **Level two:** The therapist is able to treat deep-tissue conditions with a contact handpiece that also stimulates myofascial trigger point release. Using a combination of laser therapy and massaging technique to provides a combined benefit, the therapist is able to increase pain relief and stimulation of recovery.
- **Level three:** The therapist is able to treat all presenting conditions and to monitor the patient's soreness or comfort during treatment. The therapist is able to interpret the way the patient moves away from or into the laser therapy handpiece and the patient's pain and sensitivity. These observations allow the therapist to report to the veterinarian the patient's progress or response to laser therapy.

Laser Therapy Treatment Plans

Treatment plans should incorporate all of the information provided in this chapter. It is helpful to "under promise" and "over deliver" when creating expectations for laser therapy. Photos, videos, and digital thermal imaging will often help the owner see the progress being made with therapy and enforce the validity of the treatment plan.

Six, Nine, and Twelve Packs

For acute and chronic conditions, laser therapy should be prescribed as six to twelve treatments. Like antibiotics,

---

Box 6.2 Therapy laser training checklist.

Equipment Care

– Assembly and disassembly of the laser for travel
– Proper care and insertion of the fiber into the laser
– Proper cleaning of the end of fiber optic cable
– Proper cleaning of handpiece and attachments
– Application of the emission and fiber caps
– Maximum bending radius for the fiber and handpiece
– Shutdown of the laser device

General Laser Therapy Guidelines

– Versatility and goals of laser therapy in practice
– Software safety features and messages
– Proper recording of laser therapy treatments in the patient record

Safety First

– Safety features of the laser device
– Emergency shutdown switch or icon
– Standby, ready, and emission modes
– Safety Interlock
– Power on/off visual indicator
– Laser emission indicator
– Eye protection
– Device-specific safety glasses for humans
– Patient eye protection: goggles, dark cloth, dark soft Elizabethan collars, therapist's hand
– "Laser in Use" safety sign
– Pigment levels in hair, skin, and tattoos
– Safe location for use of the laser device
– Contraindications, special considerations, and precautions

General Therapy Protocols

– Correct dosage for a given area and condition
– Calculation of dosage for therapy
– Positioning of the patient for the administration of the therapy
– Handpiece selection
– Non-contact handpiece for superficial tissue conditions
– Contact handpiece for deep-tissue conditions
– Maximum power for small versus large handpieces or beam diameters
– Treatment settings concerning skin and coat color
– Number and frequency of therapy sessions required for therapeutic outcomes:
  • **Post-procedure:** 1–2 treatments
  • **Acute conditions:** 3–6 treatments, daily or every other day
  • **Chronic conditions:** Open-ended number of treatments through three phases:
    ○ **Induction phase:** Up to 12 treatments, every other day or three times a week
    ○ **Transition phase:** Gradual reduction in frequency of treatments
    ○ **Maintenance phase:** Treatments as needed to maintain effect

General Treatment Principles

– Holding handpiece perpendicular to tissue
– Treatment from 360° or multiple directions
– Movement of handpiece at 2–7 cm/sec
– "Grid-like" or "spray paint" application pattern
– Treatment of joints through range of motion
– Avoid splint, casting, and bandage material

---

a full course of therapy is commonly needed to achieve the desired outcome, so providing treatments one at a time can be counterproductive. Most owners will see satisfying progress after a few sessions, so compliance is generally very high.

Expectations and Progress

Generally, patients should show noticeable improvement after three treatments, and significant improvement after six treatments. If this is not the case, review of the diagnosis, dose, application technique, and secondarily involved tissues is indicated. In more severe chronic cases, this timeline may be extended and owners should be well prepared to complete an entire 12 induction phase treatments. It is good practice to incorporate a veterinarian consultation and re-check after every six laser treatments (whether in the induction, transition, or maintenance phase) to gauge progress and modify therapy as indicated.

Conclusion

Mastering the techniques of laser therapy is like mastering the techniques of dental prophylaxis. Attention to the principles and methods described in this chapter will optimize outcomes, improve consistency, and ensure both safety and efficiency. Like dentistry, laser therapy is largely a technician-administered modality that offers veterinarians the opportunity to provide a service that produces excellent results, endears strong client bonding, and adds an entirely new revenue stream.

References

AAHA (2015). 2015 AAHA/AAFP Pain Management Guidelines for Dogs and Cats. Available from: https://www.aaha.org/professional/resources/pain_management.aspx (accessed November 30, 2016).

Anders, J.J. *et al.* (2014) In vitro and in vivo optimization of infrared laser treatment for injured peripheral nerves. *Lasers Surg Med.* **46**(1):34–45.

Anders, J. *et al.* (2015) Low-level light/laser therapy versus photobiomodulation therapy. *Photomed Laser Surg.* **33**(4):183–184.

ANSI. (2011a) *American National Standard for Safe Use of Lasers in Health Care Facilities ANSI Z136.3 – 2011.* American National Standards Institute, Washington, DC.

ANSI. (2011b) *American National Standard for Environmental and Facility Safety Signs ANSI Z535.2 – 2011.* American National Standards Institute, Washington, DC.

Avci, P. *et al.* (2013) Low-level laser (light) therapy (LLLT) in skin: stimulating, healing, restoring. *Semin Cutan Med Surg.* **32**(1):41–52.

Barrett, S.F. and Pack, D.J. (2006) Timing subsystem. In: *Microcontrollers Fundamentals for Engineers and Scientists*, pp. 51–64. Morgan and Claypool, San Rafael, CA.

Bjordal, J. *et al.* (2003) A systematic review of low level laser therapy with location specific doses for pain from chronic joint disorders. *Aust J Physiother.* **49**(2):107–116.

Chung, H. *et al.* (2012) The nuts and bolts of low-level laser (light) therapy. *Ann Biomed Eng.* **40**(2):516–533.

Enwemeka, C.S. (2009) Intricacies of dose in laser phototherapy for tissue repair and pain relief. *Photomed Laser Surg.* **3**:387–393.

Farivar, S. *et al.* (2014) Biological effects of low level laser therapy. *J Lasers Med Sci.* **5**(2):58–62.

Hashmi, J. *et al.* (2010) Effect of pulsing in low-level light therapy. *Lasers Surg Med.* **42**(6):450–466.

Karu, T. (2010) Mitochondrial mechanisms of photobiomodulation in context of new data about multiple roles of ATP. *Photomed Laser Surg.* **28**(2):159–160.

Kim, H.P. (2014) Lightening up light therapy: activation of retrograde signaling pathway by photobiomodulation. *Biomol Ther (Seoul).* **22**(6):491–496.

Lister, T. *et al.* (2012) Optical properties of human skin. *J Biomed Opt.* **17**(9):90901.

Passarella, S. and Karu, T. (2014) Absorption of monochromatic and narrow band radiation in the visible and near IR by both mitochondrial and non-mitochondrial photoacceptors results in photobiomodulation. *J Photochem Photobiol B.* **140**:344–358.

Peplow, P.V. *et al.* (2010) Laser photobiomodulation of wound healing: a review of experimental studies in mouse and rat animal models. *Photomed Laser Surg.* **28**(3):291–325.

Roberts, D.B. *et al.* (2013) The effectiveness of therapeutic class IV (10 W) laser treatment for epicondylitis. *Lasers Surg Med.* **45**(5):311–317.

Sommer A.P. (2014) On the mechanism of photobiostimulation. In: *Proceedings of the International Conference on Laser Applications in Life Sciences*, p. 149. June 29–July 2, 2014. Ulm.

Sommer, *et al.* (2014) Tuning the wheel of life with light. In: *Proceedings of the International Conference on Laser Applications in Life Sciences*, p. 145. June 29–July 2, 2014. Ulm.

Sommer, A.P. *et al* (2015) Tuning the mitochondrial rotary motor with light. *Ann Transl Med.* **3**(22):346.

Vallone, F. *et al.* (2014) Effect of diode laser in the treatment of patients with nonspecific chronic low back pain: a randomized controlled trial. *Photomed Laser Surg.* **32**(9):490–494.

Weersink, R. (2007) Light dosimetry for low level laser therapy: accounting for difference in tissue and depth. *Proc of SPIE.* **6428**:642803.

7

Contraindications, Special Considerations, and Precautions

John C. Godbold, Jr.[1] and Ronald J. Riegel[2]

[1] Stonehaven Veterinary Consulting, Jackson, TN, USA
[2] American Institute of Medical Laser Applications, Marysville, OH, USA

Introduction

Since Endre Mester and his colleagues first reported what we now know as photobiomodulation (PBM) in 1968 (Mester *et al.*, 1968), those using lasers for therapeutic purposes have sought to use them safely. Researchers, industry, and laser therapists have published contraindications for laser therapy in an effort to "do no harm." Texts and journal articles have published lengthy lists of contraindications (Houghton *et al.*, 2010; Navratil and Kymplova, 2002; Tuner and Hode, 2010), some of which have been reproduced in veterinary therapy laser user manuals.

Significant inconsistency remains among the recommendations in publications, texts, and user manuals. The historical contraindications for PBM have been not been appropriately re-evaluated in light of the significant number of publications that have appeared as laser therapy has become more widely used and analyzed in numerous bench-top studies, animal-model studies, and clinical trials. Some conditions originally considered contraindication for PBM now require special consideration before treatment. Some simply require precaution when treating. Other conditions are no longer contraindications.

Proper training is a requirement for treating veterinary patients with a therapy laser. Only with proper training and knowledge can contraindications, special considerations, and precautions be evaluated and appropriately applied in each patient's treatment.

Contraindications

The list of absolute contraindications for exposure to therapeutic laser light is remarkably short, with only one item (Box 7.1).

Eye Exposure

The one absolute clinical contraindication for laser therapy is direct or reflected exposure through the pupil on to the retina. The hazards inherent in laser interaction with ocular structures are the historical basis for laser classifications by regulatory bodies, and present the greatest threat to the laser therapist, support staff, patient, and those who accompany the patient.

As is well addressed in Chapter 4 and in international and national safety standards (ANSI, 2011; IEC, 2014; OSHA, n.d.; Standards Australia, 2004), it is mandatory that eyes be protected by wavelength-specific safety eyewear or other shielding devices. Safety eyewear for humans will be supplied by any responsible veterinary therapy laser manufacturer. The patient's eyes can be protected by wavelength-specific goggles made for animals, dark soft Elizabethan collars, or covering with a dark cloth or a hand. The patient should not be allowed to investigate the target area while the treatment is being administered. Food treats or attention should be used to distract the patient, or restraint, when required.

One can adapt the environment in which the therapy laser is used to reduce the possibility of direct or reflected accidental laser beam exposure of eyes. Reflective surfaces, like stainless steel veterinary treatment tables, should be covered with patient-comfortable, non-reflective material. Mirrors, jewelry, and other potential sources of reflected laser energy must also be evaluated for potential harm.

Optical exposure is a stringent contraindication. The hazard comes from the therapy laser beam penetrating the cornea and pupil, and being focused by the lens on the retina. Scattered photons reaching the retina after transmission through other tissues do not pose an optical hazard. Thus, careful laser therapy application to

---

Box 7.1 Laser therapy contraindications, special considerations, and precautions.

Absolute Contraindication

- Eye exposure

Special Considerations

- Locally injected medication
- Malignancy
- Pregnancy

Precautions

- Active epiphyses
- Hemorrhage
- Testicles
- Thyroid gland

False Contraindications

- Hyperpigmentation and tattoos
- Implants
- Microbial infection
- Photosensitizing medications

---

periorbital tissues is possible, as long as direct or reflected beam penetration through the pupil is avoided.

Special Considerations

Historically, a lack of knowledge and a healthy dose of prudence resulted in a long list of conditions being considered contraindications to laser therapy. Increased knowledge of the mechanisms of PBM brings an increased understanding that most of those conditions are not absolute contraindications. Rather, some are conditions that merit special consideration before being treated (see Box 7.1).

Patients with special consideration conditions will most often not be appropriate candidates for therapy. These are patients with conditions for which the risk of laser therapy, or the perceived risk, outweighs the benefit. Properly trained and knowledgeable veterinary laser therapists will evaluate each patient, communicate the special considerations to the patient's owner, obtain owner consent, and then deliver laser therapy treatment only when appropriate.

Locally Injected Medication

Laser therapy should not be applied over local vaccine or medication injection sites until sufficient time has passed for the injected substance to be absorbed and translocated from the site. Laser-induced vasodilation may alter pharmacologically ideal absorption and translocation rates, and no information exists about how various wavelengths of light might interact with vaccine components or medications.

If an injection is going to be made, and the area is going to be treated with laser therapy, first treat with laser therapy, and then administer the injection.

A good understanding of the pharmacodynamics of any vaccine or medication will help the veterinarian properly schedule therapy laser treatments. If, for example, a medication administered by intramuscular injection induces a myositis, and if that medication is renally cleared in 24 hours, then laser therapy of the myositis is appropriate after 24 hours.

Malignancy

A significant number of contradictory data exist concerning the effect of laser therapy on malignant tissue.

Most of the data come from *in vitro* studies using malignant human cell lines.

Using various wavelengths and parameters, laser application has been demonstrated to induce increased proliferation in human leukemic cells (Dastanpour *et al.*, 2015) and increased proliferation and invasion in human oral squamous cell carcinoma (SCC) cells (Gomes *et al.*, 2014). Seemingly contradictory is the demonstration of laser application having no significant effect on human breast adenocarcinoma cells (Cialdai *et al.*, 2015) and having a selective cytotoxic effect on human oral cancer cells (Liang *et al.*, 2015). A recent study analyzed the effect of PBM on the modulation of the osteoclastogenic potential of a cell line derived from human lingual SCC (Dias Schalch *et al.*, 2016). Using parameters for mucositis treatment, the study demonstrated a reduced osteoclastogenic effect on the tumor cells and suggested that PBM might represent a potential useful side effect while treating mucositis.

To date, no similar studies have been conducted using malignant cells from animal models. The effect of laser therapy on the malignant tissue of veterinary patients is not known. Until data specific to veterinary species are available, laser therapy should not be applied over a malignancy or the surgical site from which a malignancy has been removed.

Special consideration should be given to a surgical site from which a malignancy has been removed and surgical margins have been submitted for histopathological review. A positive margin report is an obvious contraindication for laser therapy and an indication for further surgical resection. Less obvious is whether laser therapy is appropriate after a negative or clear margin report. In generating negative margin reports, pathologists look at a very small percentage of the entire margin, and there is often not a standard definition of how wide a negative margin has to be. Thus, even with a negative margin report, a possibility remains that some malignant cells have not been removed. That possibility should be discussed with the owner before instituting laser therapy.

Consideration must also be given to the safety of treating sites in close proximity or distant to a malignancy. A pilot study indicated an improved quality of life when PBM was used in the management of radiation dermatitis in human breast cancer patients (Censabella *et al.*, 2016). Though PBM does result in some systemic effects, current data indicate it is safe to apply laser therapy to veterinary patients in areas distant to known malignancies. The safety of treating at a distant site is illustrated by the use of laser therapy to treat chemotherapy-induced oral mucositis in human cancer patients (Ottaviani *et al.*, 2013).

Another special consideration regarding laser therapy and malignancy exists for terminal veterinary patients. PBM can be effective in reducing the pain and inflammation in tissue around a malignancy, so it should be considered a part of hospice management for terminal cancer patients. Owners should be involved in the decision to add laser therapy for pain management in terminal malignancies, after being informed about the potential effect on the malignancy. Anecdotal reports from practitioners support the concept that laser therapy can increase the duration and quality of the lives of veterinary hospice patients with terminal malignancy.

The special considerations required for the application of PBM in the presence of malignancy are very likely to change as further evidence emerges. A 2012 systematic literature review presented existing data on the potential application of PBM in the treatment of solid tumors (Santana-Blank *et al.*, 2012a). This review proposed that PBM might help restore homeostasis and homeokinesis in cancer patients. It suggested that by re-establishing physiological rhythms and inducing physiologically reparative effects for disease reversal in cancer and other complex diseases, PBM might, with minimal or no adverse effects, provide significant improvements in quality of life, even in patients with advanced neoplasms.

In a more recent publication, Santana-Blank *et al.* (2016) described what has been a paradigm shift or "quantum leap" in the understanding and use of light. Based on existing evidence, they argued that PBM can raise the standard of care and improve the quality of life of patients with cancer and other complex diseases. They noted strong arguments made within the past few years for a new understanding of the role of PBM in the treatment of cancer (Karu, 2010; Lanzafame, 2011; Santana-Blank *et al.*, 2012b).

Pregnancy

Applying laser therapy over a gravid uterus is almost always listed as a contraindication. The historical basis for pregnancy being a contraindication is lack of knowledge of the potential effect on the fetus, in addition to studies demonstrating changes in chicken embryo tissue after application of visible red laser wavelengths through a window opened in the eggshell (Avila *et al.*, 1999).

A rational analysis would indicate that fetal tissue within a gravid uterus will not be harmed by visible or near-infrared light photons. These wavelengths lack any mutagenic or teratogenic effect. Further, the fetus is well protected from exposure to photons, being surrounded by a significant thickness of tissues rich in the chromophores that most readily absorb the wavelengths being used.

Yet, despite evidence to the contrary, unless a special consideration exists that warrants direct treatment over a gravid uterus, the prudent veterinary laser therapist will avoid such treatment. As with some other modalities used during pregnancy, no proof exists of potential harm to the fetus. But, no proof exists that there is not a potential harm. Absence of proof does not legally constitute proof of absence. Thus, if laser therapy is applied over the gravid uterus, and an unrelated pregnancy complication or fetal deformity occurs, the burden of proof will be on the veterinarian to demonstrate that laser therapy did not cause the complication (Tuner and Hode, 2010).

A valid consideration is whether pregnant veterinary laser therapists (or other pregnant females present during treatment) are at risk. Clothing reflects, scatters, and absorbs visible and infrared photons, significantly reducing the number reaching underlying skin. Thus, clothing gives an additional layer that blocks photons from reaching the fetus. There is no evidence that the well-protected fetus of a pregnant and clothed female is at risk during a veterinary therapy laser application.

Precautions

Veterinary patients often present with conditions mentioned as contraindications for laser therapy for which strong evidence now indicates the risk, or the perceived risk, is significantly outweighed by the benefits of therapy. These conditions require precautions in prescribing and administering laser therapy (see Box 7.1).

Active Epiphyses

Epiphyses and open fontanels have been listed as contraindications because these are areas of rapid growth, with rapidly dividing cells. The reasoning has been that if metabolic rate is increased by laser therapy, and osteogenesis is stimulated, then perhaps premature closure or asynchronous bone growth might occur.

Dozens of studies demonstrate that laser light has a stimulatory effect on osteogenesis (Jawad *et al.*, 2013; Son *et al.*, 2012). Yet, confusing data exist about the effect of laser therapy on active epiphyses. Studies have demonstrated different effects depending on wavelength and different treatment parameters in animals.

Daily application for 21 days of $10 J/cm^2$ of 830 nm laser light to the distal epiphysis of rat femurs negatively influenced growth plates and reduced longitudinal length (Oliveira *et al.*, 2012). Application every other day for 20 days of 5 and $15 J/cm^2$ of 830 nm laser light induced changes in epiphyseal cartilage, and increased the number of chondrocytes present, but the changes were insufficient to induce changes in bone length (Cressoni *et al.*, 2010). Daily application for 10 days of 4, 8, and $16 J/cm^2$ of 670 nm laser light induced no changes in the epiphyseal cartilage or final bone length of rat tibias (de Andrade *et al.*, 2012).

Common to these studies is multiple applications of laser light over a period of several weeks. What these studies do not suggest is that application of laser therapy over a few days, for acute conditions in the area of active epiphyses, will induce the same negative consequences.

Prudent application of laser therapy, several times over 3–4 days, to an acute epiphysitis would be below the parameters used in the studies mentioned, and is indicated. Prolonged and repeated treatment over multiple weeks is not indicated.

Another consideration is the possible effect that laser therapy will have on an epiphysis if applied in close proximity. Though systemic effects are noted with laser therapy, animal studies indicate that while there is a local biostimulative effect on bone in the area being treated, the effect is not observed distant to the treated area (Batista *et al.*, 2015).

Hemorrhage

It has been clearly demonstrated, using a variety of wavelengths, energy densities, and delivery modes, that laser therapy induces a transient vasodilation (Chung *et al.*, 2012; Larkin *et al.*, 2012; Maegawa *et al.*, 2000). Since any induced vasodilation is unwanted during active hemorrhage, laser therapy should not be applied to tissue that is bleeding.

This precaution does not apply to tissue in which active hemorrhage is no longer present. No data suggest laser therapy will reactivate hemorrhage. Anecdotal reports from veterinary practices using laser therapy during and after invasive procedures, and for treatment of wounds, confirm that hemorrhage is not reactivated once hemostasis has been achieved.

Testicles

Though application of laser therapy to the testes has been listed as a possible contraindication in some sources, treatment in the area of the testes and of scrotal skin should be considered safe. The wavelengths of light used for veterinary laser therapy are not mutagenic.

In vitro studies have demonstrated increased motility in human sperm after irradiation with 830 and 905 nm laser light (Firestone *et al.*, 2012; Salman *et al.*, 2014). In an *in vivo* study using an animal model, a cumulative dose of approximately $28 J/cm^2$ of 830 nm laser light over 15 days resulted in increased spermatogenesis, while a cumulative dose of approximately $47 J/cm^2$ over the same time had a destructive effect on the seminiferous epithelium (Taha and Valojerdi, 2004).

These studies suggest that normally recommended doses of laser therapy light applied to the skin of the scrotum or the tissues around the testicles will, at worst, increase spermatogenesis and sperm motility. They also suggest that excessively high doses should not be applied directly into the testicle.

Thyroid Gland

Early animal studies on the effect of laser irradiation of the thyroid gland demonstrated increased mitotic activity of follicular cells and changes in the thyroid parenchyma (Parrado *et al.*, 1990, 1999). Using 904 nm laser light, these studies delivered cumulative doses of up to $140 J/cm^2$ over 10 sessions. Understandably, reports like these suggest that laser therapy application over the thyroid glands should be contraindicated.

Subsequent studies indicated that lower total doses, delivered with fewer applications, result in no histological changes in the thyroid parenchyma. Three daily applications of 780 nm laser light at $4 J/cm^2$ produced no morphological alteration in the thyroid glands of mice (Azevedo *et al.*, 2005). This study also demonstrated that irradiation of the thyroid has a stimulatory effect on thyroid hormone levels.

Even more recent studies suggest that laser therapy can be used for chronic autoimmune thyroiditis in humans, reducing dependence on medication (Höfling *et al.*, 2010, 2013).

An objective analysis indicates that repetitive, high-dose treatment directly over the glands should be avoided. It also indicates that occasional inadvertent exposure of the thyroid glands when treating nearby tissue is not contraindicated.

As more is learned about dosing, frequency of treatment, and effect on the thyroid gland in animal-model studies, it is possible that laser therapy may be indicated for veterinary species that experience reduced thyroid function.

False Contraindications

Conditions once thought to be contraindications for laser therapy that have been clearly disproved are false contraindications (see Box 7.1). Veterinary laser therapists should be able to explain to patients' owners why these conditions are no longer contraindicated.

Hyperpigmentation and Tattoos

Increased presence of pigments in the form of melanin or tattoo pigment is not a contraindication for laser therapy. Increased pigments will result in more superficial photon absorption, so when pigments are increased, treatment parameters need to be adjusted accordingly (Anderson and Parrish, 1981).

Patients with darker skin and hair coats should be treated with longer wavelengths in the therapeutic spectrum when possible, and the total dose conditions are treated with should be increased to ensure proper dosing for deep-tissue conditions. When using higher power density, monitoring the patient's skin temperature with a trailing finger is good practice. If a temperature other than a pleasant, gentle warming is detected, the speed of movement of the handpiece should be increased. Faster movement of the laser beam across the surface of the tissue can help avoid accumulation of unpleasant warmth, even when using veterinary therapy lasers that deliver a higher power-density laser beam.

Implants

Therapy laser wavelengths do not have a detrimental effect on metal or synthetic implants, suture material, or tissue adhesives used in veterinary medicine. Use when implants are present is not contraindicated.

PBM has been demonstrated to improve the health of soft tissue around implants in a number of animal models and in human dental patients (Aoki *et al.*, 2015; Tang and Arany, 2013). Since implant success is dependent on the health of the surrounding soft tissue, laser therapy may actually improve the chances of implant success.

The presence of a reflective metal implant does change the recommended parameters of treatment when the implant is only covered by a thin layer of tissue. Since the implant will reflect photons back into the overlying tissue, any dose delivered to the overlying tissue should be reduced. In most cases, this is accomplished simply by delivering only a small amount of the entire laser treatment over the implant.

Microbial Infection

In vitro, some wavelengths of light have been shown to stimulate the growth of cultures of some bacterial species and to inhibit others (Nussbaum *et al.*, 2003).

Reliance on this information would indicate that microbial infection is a contraindication for laser therapy. On the contrary, however, other studies indicate that laser therapy, when applied *in vivo*, has a variety of immune-stimulating responses that help overcome microbial infection.

An animal-model investigation into the PBM effects of 1072 nm light on the immune response involved in antibacterial and wound-healing processes (Lee *et al.*, 2011) demonstrated enhancement of cutaneous immune response and higher vascular endothelial growth factor (VEGF) levels associated with more favorable clinical outcomes.

A study involving human patients showed the positive fungicidal effects of 830 nm laser light on oral stomatitis in a clinical setting (Maver-Biscanin *et al.*, 2004). Following laser irradiation at both 685 and 830 nm, statistically significant effects were observed *in vitro* on the turbidimetric growth kinetics of *Candida albicans* cultures and *in vivo* on the survival rate of infected mice (Seyedmousavi *et al.*, 2014).

In an animal-model study to see whether 780 nm laser light would stimulate host immunity in fighting fungal infection, neutrophils from mice that received laser therapy were more active metabolically and had higher fungicidal activity (Burger *et al.*, 2015).

A study to investigate the effects of laser therapy on a rat model of mastitis demonstrated that the number of polymorphonuclear cells in the mammary alveolus and the myeloperoxidase activity (an indicator of mastitis in dairy cattle) were decreased after therapy. The authors suggested that laser therapy might be beneficial in decreasing the somatic cell count and improving milk nutritional quality in cows with an intramammary infection (Wang *et al.*, 2014).

In vivo, PBM produces a complex, immune-enhancing effect that improves response to microbial infection. Laser therapy is indicated in microbial infections in veterinary patients.

Photosensitizing Medications

Numerous medications, both topical and systemic, are reported as being photosensitizers. A photosensitivity occurs when a chemical in a medication is photoactivated by light and a cutaneous manifestation arises. It has been suggested that photosensitization might be possible with the wavelengths and treatment parameters used in laser therapy, and thus treatment of both human and veterinary patients on these medications has historically been contraindicated.

In 2014, a review of publications for any report of adverse effects from laser therapy in patients on photosensitizing medication was conducted (Kerstein *et al.*, 2014). Only four publications linked the search term "laser therapy" with multiple terms for photosensitive reactions. No adverse effects were reported.

In the absence of any published evidence that laser therapy-induced photosensitization occurs in veterinary patients, this should be considered a false contraindication.

Conclusion

The historical contraindications for laser therapy are inconsistent, inaccurate, and outdated. Knowledge from 5 decades of research and clinical application has rewritten the recommendations against using laser therapy on many conditions and anatomical sites once thought to be contraindicated. Direct eye exposure remains an absolute contraindication for all veterinary providers, patients, and owners. Some historical contraindications now require special consideration before treatment can be indicated, others simply require precaution when treating, and still others have been demonstrated to be false. Practitioners are encouraged to update their use of laser PBM with current knowledge about contraindications, special considerations, and precautions.

References

Anderson, R.R. and Parrish, J.A. (1981) The optics of human skin. *J Invest Dermatol.* **77**(1):13–19.

ANSI. (2011) *American National Standard for Safe Use of Lasers in Health Care Facilities ANSI Z136.3 – 2011.* American National Standards Institute, Washington, DC.

Aoki, A. *et al.* (2015) Periodontal and peri-implant wound healing following laser therapy. *Periodontol 2000.* **68**(1):217–269.

Avila, R. *et al.* (1999) Structural changes induced by He-Ne laser on the chick embryo ovary. *Rev Fac Cien Med Univ Nac Cordoba.* **50**(1):7–10.

Azevedo, L. H. *et al.* (2005) Evaluation of low intensity laser effects on the thyroid gland of male mice. *Photomed Laser Surg.* **23**(6):567–570.

Batista, J.D. *et al* (2015) Low-level laser therapy on bone repair: is there any effect outside the irradiated field? *Lasers Med Sci.* **30**(5):1569–1574.

Burger, E. *et al.* (2015) Low-level laser therapy to the mouse femur enhances the fungicidal response of neutrophils against Paracoccidioides brasiliensis. *PLoS Negl Trop Dis.* **9**(2):e0003541.

Censabella, S. *et al.* (2016) Photobiomodulation for the management of radiation dermatitis: the DERMIS trial, a pilot study of MLS® laser therapy in breast cancer patients. *Support Care Cancer.* **24**(9):3925–3933.

Chung, H. *et al.* (2012) The nuts and bolts of low-level laser (light) therapy. *Ann Biomed Eng.* **40**(2):516–533.

Cialdai, F. *et al.* (2015) In vitro study on the safety of near infrared laser therapy in its potential application as postmastectomy lymphedema treatment. *J Photochem Photobiol B.* **151**:285–296.

Cressoni, M.D. *et al.* (2010) Effect of GaAlAs laser irradiation on the epiphyseal cartilage of rats. *Photomed Laser Surg.* **28**(4):527–532.

Dastanpour, S. *et al.* (2015) The effect of low-level laser therapy on human leukemic cells. *J Lasers Med Sci.* **6**(2):74–79.

de Andrade, A.R. (2012) The effects of low-level laser therapy, 670 nm, on epiphyseal growth in rats. *Scientific WorldJournal.* **2012**:231723.

Dias Schalch, T. *et al.* (2016) Photomodulation of the osteoclastogenic potential of oral squamous carcinoma cells. *J Biophotonics.* doi:10.1002/jbio.2015 00292.

Firestone, R. *et al.* (2012) The effects of low-level laser light exposure on sperm motion characteristics and DNA damage. *J Androl.* **33**(3):469–473.

Gomes, H. *et al.* (2014) Low-level laser therapy promotes proliferation and invasion of oral squamous cell carcinoma cells. *Lasers Med Sci.* **29**(4):1385–1395.

Höfling, D.B. (2010) Low-level laser therapy in chronic autoimmune thyroiditis: a pilot study. *Lasers Surg Med.* **42**(6):589–596.

Höfling, D.B. *et al.* (2013) Low-level laser in the treatment of patients with hypothyroidism induced by chronic autoimmune thyroiditis: a randomized, placebo-controlled clinical trial. *Lasers Med Sci.* **28**(3):743–753.

Houghton, P. *et al.* (2010) Electrophysical agents – contraindications and precautions: an evidence-based approach to clinical decision making in physical therapy. *Physiother Can.* **62**(5):1–80.

IEC. (2014) *Safety of Laser Products – Part 1: Equipment Classification and Requirements*, 3 edn. IEC 60825-1:2014. International Electrotechnical Commission, Geneva.

Jawad, M.M. *et al.* (2013) Effect of 940 nm low-level laser therapy on osteogenesis in vitro. *J Biomed Opt.* **18**(12):12800.

Karu, T. (2010) Mitochondrial mechanisms of photobiomodulation in context of new data about multiple roles of ATP. *Photomed Laser Surg.* **28**(2):159–160.

Kerstein, R.L. *et al.* (2014) Laser therapy and photosensitive medication: a review of the evidence. *Lasers Med Sci.* **29**(4):1449–1452.

Lanzafame R.J. (2011) Photobiomodulation and cancer and other musings. *Photomed Laser Surg.* **29**(1):3–4.

Larkin, K. *et al.* (2012) Limb blood flow after class 4 laser therapy. *J Athl Train.* **47**(2):178–183.

Lee, S.Y. *et al.* (2011) Enhancement of cutaneous immune response to bacterial infection after low-level light therapy with 1072 nm infrared light: a preliminary study. *J Photochem Photobiol B.* **105**(3):175–182.

Liang, W.Z. *et al.* (2015) Selective cytotoxic effects of low-power laser irradiation on human oral cancer cells. *Lasers Surg Med.* **47**(9):756–764.

Maegawa, Y. *et al.* (2000) Effects of near-infrared low-level laser irradiation on microcirculation. *Lasers Surg Med.* **27**(5):427–437.

Maver-Biscanin, M. *et al.* (2004) Fungicidal effect of diode laser irradiation in patients with denture stomatitis. *Lasers Surg Med.* **35**(4):259–262.

Mester, E. *et al.* (1968) The effect of laser beams on the growth of hair in mice. *Radiobiol Radiother (Berl).* **9**(5):621–626.

Navratil, L. and Kymplova, J. (2002) Contraindications in noninvasive laser therapy: truth and fiction. *J Clin Laser Med Surg.* **20**(6):341–343.

Nussbaum, E.L. *et al.* (2003) Effects of low-level laser therapy (LLLT) of 810 nm upon in vitro growth of bacteria: relevance of irradiance and radiant exposure. *J Clin Laser Med Surg.* **21**(5):283–290.

OSHA. (n.d.) Occupational Safety & Health Administration Technical Manual: Laser Hazards. Available from: https://www.osha.gov/dts/osta/otm/otm_iii/otm_iii_6.html#6 (accessed November 30, 2016).

Oliveira, S.P. *et al.* (2012) Low-level laser on femoral growth plate in rats. *Acta Cir Bras.* **27**(2):117–122.

Ottaviani, G. *et al.* (2013) Effect of class IV laser therapy on chemotherapy-induced oral mucositis: a clinical and experimental study. *Am J Pathol.* **183**(6):1747–1757.

Parrado, C. *et al.* (1990) Quantitative study of the morphological changes in the thyroid gland following IR laser radiation. *Lasers Med Sci.* **5**(1):77–80.

Parrado, C. *et al.* (1999) A quantitative investigation of microvascular changes in the thyroid gland after infrared (IR) laser radiation. *Histol Histopathol.* **14**(4):1067–1071.

Salman, Y.R. *et al.* (2014) Effect of 830-nm diode laser irradiation on human sperm motility. *Lasers Med Sci.* **29**(1):97–104.

Santana-Blank, L. *et al.* (2012a) Solid tumors and photobiomodulation: a novel approach to induce physiologically reparative homeostasis/homeokinesis – review. *J Solid Tumors.* **2**(6):623–635.

Santana-Blank, L. *et al.* (2012b) Concurrence of emerging developments in photobiomodulation and cancer. *Photomed Laser Surg.* **30**(11):615–616.

Santana-Blank, L. *et al.* (2016) "Quantum leap" in photobiomodulation therapy ushers in a new generation of light-based treatments for cancer and other complex diseases: perspective and mini-review. *Photomed Laser Surg.* **34**(3):93–101.

Seyedmousavi, S. *et al.* (2014) Effects of low-level laser irradiation on the pathogenicity of *Candida albicans*: in vitro and in vivo study. *Photomed Laser Surg.* **32**(6):322–329.

Son, J. *et al.* (2012) Bone healing effects of diode laser (808 nm) on a rat tibial fracture model. *In Vivo.* **26**(4):703–709.

Standards Australia. (2004) *Guide to the Safe Use of Lasers in Health Care. AS/NZS 4173:2004.* Standards Australia Publications, Sydney.

Taha, M.F. and Valojerdi, M.R. (2004) Quantitative and qualitative changes of the seminiferous epithelium induced by Ga. Al. As. (830 nm) laser radiation. *Lasers Surg Med.* **34**(4):352–359.

Tang, E. and Arany, P. (2013) Photobiomodulation and implants: implications for dentistry. *J Periodontal Implant Sci.* **43**(6):262–268.

Tuner, J. and Hode, L. (2010) Contraindications. In: *The New Laser Therapy Handbook*, pp. 473–481. Prima Books, Coeymans Hollow, NY.

Wang, Y. *et al.* (2014) Low-level laser therapy attenuates LPS-induced rats mastitis by inhibiting polymorphonuclear neutrophil adhesion. *J Vet Med Sci.* **76**(11):1443–1450.

Part IV

Clinical Applications of Laser Therapy in Companion Animals

8

Laser Therapy and Pain Management

Jennifer F. Johnson

Stoney Creek Veterinary Hospital, Morton, PA, USA

Introduction

As veterinarians, we are morally and ethically required to consider the concept of pain in our patients. Upon graduation, we recite the veterinary oath, promising to use our knowledge for "the prevention and relief of animal suffering." Though the actual wording of the oath varies across the world, the commitment we make is universal.

Despite the long history of our oath and of making that commitment, it has only been in the last few decades that veterinarians have taken a more proactive approach to pain management in our patients. Historically, there were few textbooks published before the 1980's exploring the pathophysiology and treatment of pain. Veterinary doctors were reluctant to provide patients with substantial pain relief, fearing the potential re-injuring of newly repaired bones and joints, or the overuse of healing tissues. Our knowledge of pain perception in animals was lacking. There was a general consensus that if an animal was still eating and appeared fine, it must not feel pain the way that humans did. This paralleled the prevailing thought in human neonatology, where until the early 1990's many human neonatal surgeries were performed without anesthesia or analgesia because studies had never shown that babies felt pain (Lee, 2002).

Luckily, medical advancements and the study of pain management in all species have allowed us to enter a new era in the care of our patients. With the establishment of more organizations to study and teach veterinary pain management, the printing of new textbooks on veterinary pain management, and the publication of pain management guidelines by the American Animal Hospital Association (AAHA) (Epstein *et al.*, 2015), there has been a great surge of knowledge regarding effective pain management for veterinary patients.

In 2016, our modern, evolved relationship with animals places great emphasis on recognizing and preserving the human–animal bond. Consequently, we are now acutely aware of the benefit of maintaining and strengthening that bond by improving the health and well-being of our patients. Continued emphasis on pain management in practice is essential when managing patient injury or illness. The exploration of all modalities to alleviate pain is paramount as we strive to provide quality of life for all animal species. The concept that clinicians should combine non-pharmacologic therapies with pharmacotherapy for the management of pain has been well established in human medicine (Chang *et al.*, 2015). The same concept is vital in veterinary medicine.

Photobiomodulation (PBM) through the application of laser therapy can be an important component of the multimodal management of pain. Utilizing laser therapy for its analgesic and anti-inflammatory effects may reduce or eliminate the need for medications and the side effects that can come with their use.

Consequence of Untreated Pain

Studies of pain in humans and animals repeatedly show the significant consequences of unalleviated pain, most notably the increase of mortality in patients suffering from pain. Pain is responsible for a myriad of chemical and neurologic changes that, if untreated, can lead to dire pathophysiologic consequences involving multiple organ systems (Silverstein, 2006). The neurohumoral responses to pain and stress trigger a cascade of events, including changes in cortisol, catecholamines, and other hormones. This stress response to injury and subsequent immune-system stimulation precipitates the release of cytokines, augmenting the systemic inflammatory response syndrome (Davies and Hagen, 1997). Unchecked, the systemic inflammatory response syndrome will lead to multiple-organ dysfunction syndrome (Parke *et al.*, 2003; Wadhwa and Sood, 1997). The cause or extent of the pain and trauma to the body is not the issue. As Aird (2003) so eloquently stated, "it is the host response, rather than the nature of the pathogen, that is the primary determinant of patient outcome." It has been said that stress kills. One could better surmise that unalleviated pain, no matter what the cause, is a prime component of patient mortality.

Examining the Pain Pathway

To better understand where and why photobiomodulation therapy (PBMT) is effective in treating pain, we should first review the basic physiology of pain by following the pain pathway. This includes transduction, transmission, modulation, and perception.

When there is injury to a tissue, damaged cells release a myriad of inflammatory mediators, including prostaglandins, interleukins, arachidonic acid, serotonin, substance P, bradykinin, and glutamate. Specialized sensory nerve fibers, nociceptors, collect this chemical information. Once this "inflammatory soup" of information reaches a specific level (the pain threshold), the nociceptors convert the chemical signal to an electrical impulse. The conversion of these chemicals into a nerve impulse is called *transduction* (Gaynor and Muir, 2015; McMahon *et al.*, 2013).

The second step in the pathway involves sending the electrical signal to the spinal cord. There are three main types of afferent nerve that accomplish *transmission* of the pain signal, A-beta, A-delta, and C fibers. The A-beta fibers are responsible for low-threshold, or non-painful information, such as touch, pressure, vibration, movement, and proprioception. The A-delta fibers are covered in myelin, which helps to transmit the signal quickly. A-delta fiber stimulation is responsible for the withdrawal reflex and for sharp, acute pain. A-delta fibers respond to thermal and mechanical stimulation. C fibers are likewise activated by thermal and mechanical stimulation, but also by chemical stimulation. They are un-myelinated fibers, which causes them to transmit their signals more slowly. They are responsible for slow, burning pain, which can intensify. C fibers have been implicated in the formation of chronic pain. Some C fibers have very high pain thresholds, meaning that they require a very large physical or chemical stimulation to activate a transmission response. These "sleeping" C fibers are found in places such as articular cartilage and tooth pulp canals, where intense, intractable pain can commonly become an issue. Aggressively blocking the awakening of sleeping C fibers holds great value in the pre-emptive treatment of chronic pain (Gaynor and Muir, 2015).

Modulation of the electrical signal carried by the afferent fibers occurs in the spinal cord. The signals from A-delta and C fibers change in the dorsal horn, being either inhibited or amplified. Excitatory and inhibitory neurotransmitters work to transform the signals before they reach the brain. For example, gamma-amino butyric acid (GABA) acts as an inhibitor, while glutamate works to intensify the signal. Other chemicals, such as serotonin, can help stifle glutamate and augment GABA, modifying the signal before it reaches the brain. A-beta fiber impulses that reach the dorsal horn can work as gate controls, to inhibit the modulated signal from reaching the brain. This gate-control theory explains why tissue massage at the site of injury can help decrease the perception of pain. Modulation will also initiate the release of endogenous opioids in response to transmitted pain signals, which work at opioid receptors found in the periphery, spinal cord, and brain to inhibit the release of excitatory neurotransmitters (Gaynor and Muir, 2015).

The last phase of the pain pathway is *perception*, the integration and recognition of the sensory information. Multiple ascending pathways and brain regions are involved in the processing of pain. These brain regions are responsible for several pain components, including sensory, immediate affective, and secondary affective dimensions. They include spinal ascending pathways that directly target limbic and brainstem structures involved in pain-related responses (Price *et al.*, 2006). Multiple areas of the brain are responsible for various tasks as the awareness of pain is processed. They work together to create a coordinated response to the pain stimuli, including fear, anxiety, aggression, motor, autonomic, and endocrine activity. For example, the amygdala controls the fear or anxiety response, the cortex controls perception, and the hippocampus controls memory. The body sends parallel signals from the periphery to ensure the cortex receives adequate information about the insult. The perception centers spearhead the overall autonomic, emotional, and physical (motor) response to pain (Gaynor and Muir, 2015; McMahon *et al.*, 2013).

PBMT and the Pain Pathway

Blocking various biochemical and physiologic responses along the pain pathway is the goal of all pharmacological and adjunct pain relief. Pharmaceuticals have been developed to block specific processes of the pain pathway, with great success. For example, non-steroidal anti-inflammatories can effectively reduce the production of arachidonic acid and inhibit prostaglandin release, while the exogenous opioid morphine works to agonize mu receptors in the brain, spinal cord, and periphery. Local anesthetics, such as lidocaine, stop the flow of sodium ions, decreasing depolarization of nociceptive fibers and thereby interfering with signal transmission. In a like manner, PBMT creates biochemical changes along the pain pathway to produce substantial and effective pain relief. The use of PBMT for pain and the biochemical mechanisms of action has been well established (Cotler *et al.*, 2015).

Increasing Serotonin

Serotonin is an excitatory neurotransmitter peripherally, but also works in the dorsal horn to modulate the pain response. Laser therapy increases serotonin levels (Walker, 1983). Serotonin enhances mood, instilling the feeling of general well-being.

Beta-Endorphin Release

Laser therapy causes an increase in the body's production of endogenous opioids, notably beta-endorphin (Labajos, 1988). Beta-endorphins are produced by the pituitary in response to a pain stimulation that is sent from the hypothalamus. In the periphery, they bind to opioid receptors pre- and post-synaptically and block the release of substance P, an excitatory neurotransmitter. In the spinal cord and central nervous system (CNS), increases in beta-endorphins cause a decrease in the production of GABA, and consequently increase the production of dopamine. Large increases in dopamine signal the pleasure center in the brain.

It is interesting that with acute or surgical pain, measurements of pain intensity correlate with the amount of circulating beta-endorphin. Patients that report more pain have lower levels of circulating beta-endorphins. The use of synthetic opioids (e.g., morphine or fentanyl) will decrease the production of beta-endorphins and, if used chronically, the number of opioid receptors. The negative mechanisms that occur with the use of opioid medications can lead to the issues of drug tolerance, withdrawal, and allodynia associated with chronic narcotic use. Studies continue to measure the serum levels of beta-endorphins in patients experiencing pain and the dynamics between various combinations of non-opioid analgesics in the hope of discovering more effective pain relief that does not involve the risk of giving continued opioid medications. Because of the effect of PBMT on the release of endogenous beta-endorphins, we can expect to have a decreased need for exogenous opioid use (Cramond *et al.*, 1994; Sprouse-Blum *et al.*, 2010).

Increasing Acetylcholine

Acetylcholine is an inhibitory neurotransmitter. PBMT has been shown to increase the activity of acetylcholine receptors in damaged muscle (Nicolau *et al.*, 2004; Rochkind and Shainberg, 2013). Acetylcholine is an important component in both the autonomic pathways in the CNS and peripheral-muscle motor function. Increases in acetylcholine decrease the discharge frequency of excitatory neurons and increase the frequency of inhibitory neurons. Ongoing clinical investigation continues to prove that the use of pharmacologic drugs that increase the concentration of acetylcholine (such as neostigmine) is beneficial in the treatment of pain (Lauretti, 2015;

Zhenghong *et al.*, 2008). Accordingly, with evidence that PBMT increases acetylcholine, we can surmise that the analgesic effects of that increase are the same.

Decreasing Bradykinins

When tissue is injured, a key component of the inflammatory soup that establishes the transduction of nociception is bradykinin. Some of the first *in vitro* work showed that bradykinin stimulation of action potentials in C fibers was blocked by laser irradiation (Jimbo *et al.*, 1998). More recent work suggests that wavelengths that cause photobiostimulation decrease kinin receptor activity at the source of inflammation (Bortone *et al.*, 2008). Blocking bradykinin's effects at the source of the injury can significantly increase the pain threshold required for transmission of the sensory nerve input.

The Importance of Nitric Oxide

Nitric oxide (NO) levels are increased in injured and hypoxic cells. Consequently, it seems counterintuitive to suggest that increasing NO levels can reduce pain; however, NO plays an important role as a neurotransmitter as well as a chemical messenger between cells. The increased levels of intracellular NO at the site of injury will essentially block the mitochondrial production of adenosine triphosphate (ATP) and oxygen by binding to cytochrome c oxidase (CCO). CCO is the key photoreceptor of PBMT induced by near-infrared light (Kim, 2014; Passarella and Karu, 2014). Once laser stimulation of the cell occurs, NO becomes unbound, allowing increased cellular metabolism. Unbound NO, which diffuses easily between cells, works to relax vascular smooth muscle, promoting vasodilation, and thereby oxygenation. A key component of pain relief may stem from the removal of inflammatory mediators from the site of injury by an increase of vascular blood flow. Increased unbound NO levels have been shown to inhibit sensory afferents in the peripheral nervous system and activate endorphin release within the CNS, likely by increasing cyclic guanosine monophosphate (cGMP) production (Hancock and Riegger-Krugh, 2008; Mitchell and Mack, 2013; Poyton and Ball, 2011).

Direct Analgesic Effect on Nerves

Nerve cell action potentials are decreased when there is injury to a nerve cell, causing a decreased pain threshold. Through application of photonic energy to nerve cells, we can increase the resting potential closer to the normal transmission voltage. At the same time, the speed of transmission of the nociceptive signal can be decreased by blocking the depolarization of C fiber afferents (Wakabayashi, 1993). Slowing transmission and increasing the amount of nociception it takes to convert a pain

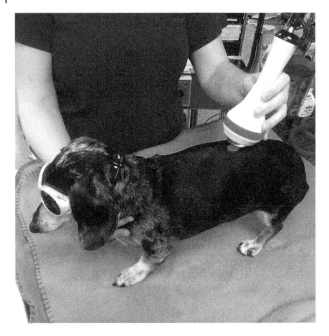

Figure 8.1 Use of therapeutic PBM to increase the speed of nerve cell healing. When treating the acute pain of intervertebral disk disease, apply laser therapy from a dorsal and both lateral directions.

> **Box 8.1 Laser therapy pain management dose recommendations.**
>
> **Acute Superficial Wounds/"Hot" Inflammatory Conditions**
> $1-4\,\text{J/cm}^2$
> **Chronic Superficial Conditions/Chronic Wounds**
> $4-30\,\text{J/cm}^2$
> **Acute Superficial Pain/Injury**
> $2-4\,\text{J/cm}^2$
> **Acute Deep Pain/Injury**
> $4-8\,\text{J/cm}^2$
> **Chronic Deep Pain/Injury**
> $6-20\,\text{J/cm}^2$

signal are more helpful for acute pain. Additionally, multiple studies have shown the remarkable ability of laser therapy to promote nerve cell regeneration by sprouting new axons and repairing nerve cells. Specific power densities and treatment wavelength recommendations are ongoing and continue to be defined. Use of results achieved *in vitro* helps establish parameters *in vivo* (Anders *et al.*, 2004, 2014; Blom *et al.*, 2000; Byrnes *et al.*, 2005). Allodynia and neuropathic pain syndromes are amplified in areas of direct nerve cell injury. Using PBMT to increase the speed of nerve cell healing is a key component of laser therapy's pain relief (Figure 8.1).

Putting Theory into Practice: Incorporating Laser Therapy for Pain

Research continues, and evidence is being compiled on the efficacy of laser therapy for various painful conditions in humans and animals. An investigation of the thousands of published papers on phototherapy shows variable and sometimes unfavorable results. However, published reviews of previous publications continue to support the efficacy of laser therapy for acute and chronic conditions (Bjordal, 2006). Most do so with the caveat that the wavelength, dose, and application technique appear to be key components in the successful outcome of therapy. One seminal review published in the *Lancet* in 2009 showed the success of laser therapy for the management of neck pain once trials were

excluded that showed suboptimal dosing or inappropriate wavelengths (Chow *et al.*, 2009).

The therapeutic dose of energy required for effective pain management is related to the amount of energy that can penetrate into cells to cause the photobiochemical responses previously described. Commercially available veterinary-specific therapy lasers are designed with wavelengths appropriate for depth of penetration that allows cellular stimulation. Power levels vary. Dosing is dependent on the tissue type and depth (Enwemeka, 2009; Weersink, 2007). Current literature recommends doses ranging from 2 to $12\,\text{J/cm}^2$. The range of dose considers both the depth of the tissue requiring stimulation and the incidental scatter and absorption of the beam by pigmented tissues, the hair coat, and the overall body mass (Box 8.1).

Frequency of treatment is dependent on the type of painful condition being treated. Routine surgical incisional pain may only require one treatment immediately after the procedure, and perhaps, if pain persists, a second treatment the next day.

More complex acute pain conditions require an aggressive treatment daily for the initial resolution of pain, and then merit treatments of tapering frequency until the condition is resolved.

Chronic pain conditions require the longest treatment plan for best outcome. One should begin with frequent treatments (three or four times a week) for the initial reduction in pain, and then taper slowly as continued response is measured. Most chronic cases, especially those that include chronic osteoarthritis pain, require continued maintenance therapy, usually once every 4–6 weeks.

Measuring Success in a Clinical Setting

The preceding treatment recommendations may sound vague, which underscores the importance of evaluating the success of treatment in an unbiased and equivalent fashion. In veterinary medicine, we must continue to collect data, we must continue to collect clinical evidence, and we must exercise care to document responses or non-responses to treatment in the most unprejudiced way possible. To this end, it is important to review reasonable ways of documenting pain management protocol results in order to carefully quantify laser therapy protocol results.

Pain Scales

Lord Kelvin stated, "If you cannot measure it, you cannot improve it." Using a practice-specific pain scale for evaluation of patients before, during, and after treatment is critical to measuring treatment success. There are many published references available to help you design and implement a protocol for pain assessment in your hospital, including subjective, objective, and semi-objective tools (Wiese, 2015). It is helpful to consider implementing both a practice-specific pain assessment scale and a validated tool such as the Canine Brief Pain Inventory (Canine BPI) for owner evaluation (Brown, 2008; PennVet, 2016). A recently published Feline Musculoskeletal Pain Index (FMPI) is also available (NC State, 2016). The consistent use of pain scales for all patients with documentation in their medical record is an easy way to evaluate the success of laser therapy. The International Veterinary Association of Pain Management (IVAPM) provides excellent client education handouts to its members (IVAPM, 2016).

Digital Thermal Imaging

Digital thermal imaging technology continues to improve. Digital thermal cameras are now readily available in veterinary medicine to help identify possible areas of pain, as well as to monitor response to treatment. Digital thermography records radiated energy from the body. Software uses that record to construct an image with a thermal gradient: a color image of temperature gradients in the body (Grossbard *et al.*, 2014). The technology is valuable, since it can help identify anatomical areas of increased energy, which are responses to increases in blood flow and inflammation, as well as areas with decreased thermal energy, suggesting chronic muscle or nerve disease. Thermal imaging is a valuable tool to help investigate the physiologic state of the patient. Pain management clinicians can use digital thermal images to locate areas of the body that may have painful conditions, and then monitor treatment response with follow-up imaging (Diakides *et al.*, 2013).

Stance Analyzer

Objective measurement of limb weight bearing can be accomplished using commercially available stance analyzers (Figure 8.2). Measuring weight while a patient

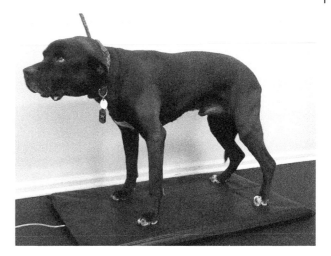

Figure 8.2 Objective measurement of limb weight bearing can be accomplished using commercially available stance analyzers. Have the patient stand squarely on the mat for the best analysis of weight bearing.

is standing can be used first to ascertain likely occult leg pain, then to monitor response to treatment. Response to treatment is measured by comparing weight bearing before it to weight bearing after (Millis and Levine, 2014).

Surgical Pain Multimodal Management

Routine surgeries such as ovariohysterectomy and orchiectomy in small-animal practice create painful stimuli both viscerally and somatically. The somatic pain can be classified as acute and of short duration, caused by inflammation at the surgical site due to tissue trauma. Visceral pain is associated with stretching or tearing of tissue ligaments and, especially in the case of ovariohysterectomy, the manipulation of abdominal viscera. A balanced, multimodal analgesic approach is recommended and might include:

- Preoperative analgesia: Hydromorphone 0.08 mg/kg and dexmedetomidine 10 µg/kg IM.
  - Carprofen 4.4 mg/kg SQ.
- Intraoperative analgesia: Ketamine constant rate infusion, 10 µg/kg/min in surgical fluids.
- Postoperative analgesia: PBM dose 2–4 J/cm^2 immediately postoperatively over and adjacent to incision.
  - Repeat narcotic, hydromorphone 0.08 mg/kg SQ or buprenorphine 0.01 mg/kg SQ.
  - Carprofen 4.4 mg/kg PO × 4 days to go home.

The addition of one therapy laser treatment will reduce post-incisional inflammation, reduce the need for rescue narcotic injection, and reduce the need for oral opioids postoperatively.

More invasive and tissue-disruptive surgeries, such as laparotomies, thoracotomies, or orthopedic surgeries, warrant multiple laser therapy treatments postoperatively. In a double-blind, controlled, randomized clinical trial, human patients who were candidates for tibial fracture surgery were allocated randomly to a control or a laser therapy group (Nesioonpour *et al.*, 2014). Patients were evaluated for pain intensity according to the visual analogue scale and the amount of pharmacological analgesia use during 24 hours after surgery. The laser therapy-treated group experienced less pain intensity and consumed significantly less opioid than the control group. This study demonstrated that laser therapy is a proper method for reducing postoperative pain, because it is painless, safe, and non-invasive, and can reduce the need for pharmacological agents.

Treatment for more tissue-disruptive surgeries should begin immediately after surgery and continue daily for several days, and then perhaps every other day until satisfactory pain and mobility levels are reached.

Ovariohysterectomy Multimodal Pain Management

Signalment
"Amber," 6 months old, Fe, canine Shih Tzu, 5.5 kg.

Client Complaint
Routine ovariohysterectomy.

Medical Pain Management
Preoperatively, Amber received 0.44 mg hydromorphone with 55 µg dexmedetomidine IM, plus carprofen 22 mg SQ. During the surgical procedure, she received IV surgical fluids with ketamine 60 mg/L, at a rate of 10 mL/kg/hr, to achieve a 10 µg/kg/min dose, effectively blocking N-methyl-D-aspartate (NMDA) receptor stimulation (wind-up).

Carprofen 12.5 mg was dispensed for oral administration at home daily for 4 days.

Laser Therapy Treatment
Laser therapy was administered over the abdominal incision site postoperatively using a non-contact delivery with laser settings that delivered 3–4 J/cm^2.

Outcome
Pain was assessed by abdominal palpation hourly until discharge from the hospital 8 hours after the procedure, using a hospital descriptive, semi-objective pain scale. A follow-up owner assessment 30 hours after the procedure noted that Amber was eating normally, leash walking, and displaying no incisional pain or swelling.

Oral Surgery Multimodal Pain Management

Oral pain following dental extractions can be profound and has a higher incidence of developing into intractable pain due to the high-concentration C fibers found in pulp tissue. Clinicians may consider avoiding laser therapy post-extraction for fear of creating more post-extraction bleeding, but published human studies confirm that immediate laser therapy post-extraction has significant benefit when compared with delayed therapy (Abdel-Alim *et al.*, 2015). The medical pain-management protocol is similar to the one cited for surgical pain, with the addition of a local anesthetic dental block prior to extraction.

Signalment
"Griffen," 10 years old, MN, canine mixed breed, 20.5 kg.

Client Complaint
Griffen was presented for dental prophylaxis and extraction of his right upper carnassial tooth with a small crown fracture, pulp exposure, and dental radiographic evidence of maxillary bone loss.

Medical Pain Management
Preoperatively, Griffen received 2 mg hydromorphone IM, 200 µg dexmedetomidine IM, and carprofen 90 mg SQ. An infraorbital nerve block was performed with 3 mL bupivicaine (0.15 mL/kg) 15 minutes prior to extraction. During the procedure, Griffen received IV surgical fluids with ketamine 60 mg/L at 200 mL/hr to achieve a 10 µg/kg/min ketamine dose. Postoperatively, a 1.5 mg dose of hydromorphone was given 4 hours after the procedure. Griffen was discharged after 6 hours. Carprofen 75 mg was dispensed for oral administration at home daily for 4 days.

Laser Therapy Treatment
Laser therapy was administered immediately after the procedure, treating the extraction site as well as all of the gingiva. A non-contact delivery was used, with laser settings that delivered 3–4 J/cm^2.

Acute Pain Multimodal Management

Laser therapy is an invaluable tool for providing rapid and substantial pain relief in acute pain situations.

Otitis Externa Multimodal Management

Signalment
"Pride," 2 years old, MN, canine English bulldog.

Client Complaint
Rubbing the left ear and shaking the head.

Physical Examination

Upon presentation, the left pinna was erythematous, edematous, and painful to the touch. The external ear canal opening was inflamed, and otoscopic examination was difficult and painful. Pride was intolerant during the ear examination. Visualization of the deep, horizontal canal was not possible in the absence of sedation.

Laboratory Data

Cytology using a commercial Romanowsky stain was performed on samples collected from the left ear. Large numbers of budding yeast and squamous epithelial cells were present.

Medical Management

Pride was given an injection of dexamethasone at a dose of 0.2 mg/kg. No topical treatment was initiated on presentation, because of Pride's intolerance of having his ear handled.

Laser Therapy Treatment

Laser therapy was applied to Pride's left ear using non-contact delivery of 3–4 J/cm^2 over the affected areas of the pinna and visible parts of the ear canal and 8.10 J/cm^2 transcutaneously over the more proximal portions of the ear canal.

Outcome

The owner returned Pride 24 hours later. Rapid reduction of edema, swelling, and pain resulted in the owner reporting a decrease in redness and head shaking. Pride was tolerant of a full ear canal otoscopic examination. A second laser therapy treatment was administered and topical treatment was initiated based on cytology results.

Acute Abdominal Pain Multimodal Management

Signalment

"Shultz," 5 years old, MN, canine miniature schnauzer

Client Complaint

Shultz presented with a 12-hour history of anorexia and vomiting bile.

Physical Examination

Examination revealed physical signs of nausea (lip licking and salivating) and pain on palpation of the cranial abdomen.

Laboratory Data

Complete blood count and serum chemistries were unremarkable. A canine-specific pancreatic lipase enzyme-linked immunosorbent assay (ELISA) was positive.

Diagnostic Imaging

Abdominal radiographs showed loss of detail in the cranial right quadrant and a laterally deviated gas-filled duodenum.

Diagnosis

Acute pancreatitis.

Medical Management

The patient was hospitalized and given intravenous fluids and anti-nausea medications.

Laser Therapy Treatment

Laser therapy was administered once every 24 hours over the surface of the abdomen, concentrating on the right cranial quadrant, using a contact delivery of 10 J/cm^2.

Outcome

No further vomiting was noted in the hospital. Shultz's abdominal pain decreased significantly and he began to eat 24 hours after hospitalization.

Acute Neck Pain Multimodal Management

Signalment

"Lady," 5 years old, FS, canine beagle.

Client Complaint

The owner presented Lady with the concern that she did not eat her breakfast. The previous day, Lady had been very active, running in the yard on her tie-out leash and barking at the neighbor.

Physical Examination

A physical examination showed that Lady was walking gingerly with her head down. Palpation revealed muscle spasms and pain in her neck, with a pain score of 7/10.

Diagnosis

Acute pain and muscle spasms in the cervical area.

Medical Management

Carprofen 4.4 mg/kg once a day and tramadol 5 mg/kg were dispensed for oral administration at home.

Laser Therapy Treatment

Laser therapy of the neck using contact delivery was instituted, administering 10 J/cm^2. The application of laser therapy was accomplished perpendicular to the neck dorsally, ventrally, and both right and left laterally. Lady was released with instructions to give her strict rest at home.

Outcome

Lady returned for a second laser therapy treatment 16 hours after initial presentation. Her pain score had reduced to 4/10. She no longer exhibited muscle spasms in her neck and was able to lower her head to eat. A third and final laser treatment was administered 48 hours later and the owner noted that Lady was behaving normally. Long-term recommendations included the use of a harness for walking and discontinuation of the use of a tie-out cable in the yard.

Recurrent Urinary Tract Disease Multimodal Management

Signalment

"Sara," 4 years old, SF, feline domestic short hair, 5 kg.

Client Complaint

Sara had a history of intermittent straining and blood in the urine, extending back for 2 years.

History

The most recent episode of straining and blood in the urine was 4 months prior to presentation. Sara's history included a previous negative urine culture. Previous radiographs and urinary tract ultrasound were normal. Previous therapies had included the use of corticosteroids, antibiotics, non-steroidal anti-inflammatories, a tricyclic antidepressant, and a glucosamine chondroitin supplement. The owner reported that regardless of the treatment, Sara appeared to recover over a course of 2 weeks, but would later relapse. Because oral medication was difficult to administer, Sara was not on any oral medications. A canned commercial diet, formulated to help reduce lower urinary tract disease, was being fed.

Physical Examination

Upon presentation, Sara's bladder was mostly empty, and she was painful on bladder palpation. She was intermittently dribbling small amounts of bloody urine.

Diagnosis

Chronic, recurrent, feline lower urinary tract disease.

Medical Management

Sara was given a subcutaneous injection of 0.24 mg/kg buprenorphine that had a duration of action of 24 hours. She also was given 300 mL of subcutaneous fluids (60 mg/kg/day).

Laser Therapy Treatment

Laser therapy was instituted immediately to reduce pain and muscle spasms of the urinary bladder and urethra (see Figure 8.3). Using a contact delivery over the bladder in the caudal abdomen, the treatment delivered 8–9 J/cm^2.

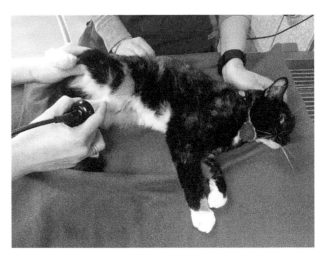

Figure 8.3 Applying laser therapy to a cat with interstitial cystitis. Note the minimal restraint necessary and that the patient is clearly enjoying the treatment!

The management plan included the recommendation that laser therapy be continued long-term as needed to help reduce occurrences of symptoms.

Outcome

The following day, Sara returned for a second laser treatment. The owner reported she was no longer straining and a good volume of urine had been observed in the litter box. Laser therapy was repeated the following day and, based on the positive response, was continued twice a week for two more weeks, then once a week for a month, then twice a month for a month. Sara currently receives maintenance laser therapy treatments every 4–6 weeks and has not had a repeat episode of straining or blood in her urine for over a year.

Chronic Pain Multimodal Management

Chronic pain in animals can be positively improved by the use of deep-tissue laser therapy. The most common causes of chronic pain in veterinary medicine are osteoarthritis and degenerative joint disease. Multiple studies have been published on the results of PBMT in lab animals with experimentally induced arthritis (Assis *et al.*, 2016; Carlos *et al.*, 2014; Peimani and Sardary, 2014). In clinical application, laser therapy is most often added to a full multimodal management protocol for these conditions.

There are three key points that should be addressed with every chronic musculoskeletal case. First, each patient should be completely evaluated for affected joints and areas of pain. It is not unusual to have pain in the elbows and shoulders in dogs with significant osteoarthritis and dysplasia of the hips. Do not assume that the pain is localized to the joints that show radiographic evidence of osteoarthritis. Clinicians should utilize all of the pain-assessment tools at their disposal to establish a treatment pain prior to initiating therapy. In this way, positive outcomes can be objectively evaluated.

Second, it is critical to provide the proper dose of PBMT necessary to stimulate the deep tissues. Delivering the appropriate dose ($8-15 \text{J/cm}^2$) is important in creating an effective cellular response. The cellular response will vary greatly if an inappropriate dose is used or if laser application is not performed on the correct target joints.

Third, chronic pain requires aggressive therapy initially, to establish good cellular response and the initiation of the anti-inflammatory and regenerative healing process stimulated by PBMT. We cannot expect a good response if we do not treat the painful target tissues at least twice a week for a few weeks. The recommendation is to treat two or three times a week for the first 2 weeks, then increase the time between treatments as the patient continues to show a positive response. In the case of chronic osteoarthritis, the underlying cause may always be present (e.g., joint dysplasia, cartilage degradation), so continued laser therapy may be required to maintain pain relief. Once good pain relief has been accomplished, the time between therapy sessions can be slowly increased. The majority of chronic pain cases require therapy every 4–6 weeks to maintain adequate pain relief.

Chronic Multiple-Joint Osteoarthritis Multimodal Management

Signalment

"Major," 12 years old, MN, canine German shepherd retriever mixed breed.

Client Complaint

Over the past 2 months, the clients had noticed that Major was losing weight in his rear legs and was starting to slip on the kitchen floor. He was also having more trouble going up and down the steps.

History

At the first signs of weakness in his rear quarters 6 years ago, radiographs showed that Major had bilateral hip dysplasia with moderate subluxation of his hip joints and degenerative joint changes in his hips and stifles. Osteoarthritis was diagnosed.

Physical Examination

Physical examination showed mild thoracolumbar back pain, bilateral elbow pain, muscle atrophy of both hind legs, bilateral iliopsoas pain, limited extension of both hips, and mild proprioceptive deficits in the rear legs, with increased time to placement of both hind limbs after knuckling.

Current Medications

Major had been on carprofen 3 mg/kg daily. He had also received daily administration of an oral glucosamine, chondroitin, methylsulfonylmethane, and avocado soybean unsaponifiables product.

Multimodal Management Plan

Deep-tissue laser therapy was initiated, and Major received treatment over the hips, stifles, lumbosacral spine, thoracolumbar spine, and both elbows. Each treatment area received a dose of $10-12 \text{J/cm}^2$ using a contact delivery. The hips and knees were manipulated with slow, passive range of motion during the laser application, with delivery from as many different directions as possible.

Major's degree of pain and dysfunction indicated a need for increased medical pain management. Gabapentin, 10 mg/kg twice a day, was dispensed for oral administration at home.

The owners were instructed to continue low-impact exercise with Major, concentrating on muscle-strengthening exercises for the rear quarters.

Major was scheduled to receive 10 induction-phase laser therapy sessions 2–3 days apart.

Outcome

Both client and clinician pain assessment improved after the initial laser therapy treatments. Laser therapy was slowly tapered over 2 months until a maintenance-phase schedule of once-a-month treatment was achieved. Major continued to develop muscle strength in his rear quarters, his proprioception improved, and he had a much easier time getting up and down.

Conclusion

Adding laser therapy to a pain-management protocol provides great additional benefit, complementing the multimodal analgesia program. The synergy with traditional pharmaceuticals and other adjunct therapies that PBMT provides is paramount as we strive to conquer pain in patients that spend most of their life trying to deny that they are indeed in any type of distress. Astute clinicians realize the great importance of evaluating and recognizing pain in animal patients, and the true benefit of alleviating pain by all means possible. It is with great excitement that we continue to document positive responses to PBMT and continue to incorporate PBMT as a key component of patient health and welfare.

References

Abdel-Alim, H.M. *et al.* (2015) A comparative study of the effectiveness of immediate versus delayed photobiomodulation therapy in reducing the severity of postoperative inflammatory complications. *Photomed Laser Surg.* **33**(9):447–451.

Aird, W.C. (2003) The hematologic system as a marker for organ dysfunction in sepsis. *Mayo Clin Proc.* **78**(7):869–881.

Anders, J.J. *et al.* (2004) Phototherapy promotes regeneration and functional recovery of injured peripheral nerve. *Neurol Res.* **26**(2):233–239.

Anders, J.J. *et al.* (2014) In vitro and in vivo optimization of infrared laser treatment for injured peripheral nerves. *Lasers Surg Med.* **46**(1):34–45.

Assis, L. *et al.* (2016) Aerobic exercise training and low-level PBMT modulate inflammatory response and degenerative process in an experimental model of knee osteoarthritis in rats. *Osteoarthritis Cartilage.* **24**(1):169–177.

Bjordal, J.M. *et al.* (2006) Low-level laser therapy in acute pain: a systematic review of mechanisms of action and clinical effects in randomized placebo-controlled trials. *Photomed Laser Surg.* **24**(2):158–168.

Blom, K. *et al.* (2000) The influence of low intensity infrared laser irradiation on conduction characteristics of peripheral nerve: a randomized, controlled, double blind study on the sural nerve. *Lasers Med Sci.* **15**(3):195–200.

Bortone, F. *et al.* (2008) Low level laser therapy modulates kinin receptor expression in the subplantar muscle of rat paw subjected to carrageenan-induced inflammation. *Int Immunopharm.* **8**(2):206–210.

Brown, D.C. *et al.* (2008) Ability of the Canine Brief Pain Inventory to detect response to treatment in dogs with osteoarthritis. *J Am Vet Med Assoc.* **233**(8):1278–1283.

Byrnes, K. *et al.* (2005) Low power laser irradiation alters gene expression of olfactory ensheathing cells in vitro. *Lasers Surg Med.* **13**(1):72–82.

Carlos, F.P. *et al.* (2014) Protective effect of low-level PBMT (LLLT) on acute zymosan-induced arthritis. *Lasers Med Sci.* **29**(2):757–763.

Chang, K.L. et al. (2015) Cronic pain management: pharmacotherapy for chronic pain. *FP Essent.* **432**:27–38.

Chow, R. *et al.* (2009) Efficacy of low-level laser therapy in the management of neck pain: a systematic review and meta-analysis of randomized placebo or active-treatment controlled trials. *Lancet.* **374**(9705):1897–1908.

Cotler, H.B. *et al.* (2015) The use of low level laser therapy (LLLT) for musculoskeletal pain. *MOJ Orthop Rheumatol.* **2**(5):pii:00068.

Cramond, T. *et al.* (1994) ACTH and beta-endorphin levels in response to low level laser therapy for myofascial trigger points. *Laser Ther.* **6**(3):133–142.

Davies, M.G. and Hagen, P.O. (1997) Systemic inflammatory response syndrome. *Br J Surg.* **84**(7):920–935.

Diakides, M. *et al.* (2013) *Medical Infrared Imaging Principles and Practices.* CRC Press, Boca Raton, FL.

Enwemeka, C.S. (2009) Intricacies of dose in laser phototherapy for tissue repair and pain relief. *Photomed Laser Surg.* **3**:387–393.

Epstein, M. *et al.* (2015) 2015 AAHA/AAFP pain management guidelines for dogs and cats. *JAAHA.* **51**(2):67–84.

Gaynor, J.S. and Muir, W.W. (2015) *Handbook of Veterinary Pain Management*, 3 edn. Elsevier, New York.

Grossbard, B.P. *et al.* (2014) Medical infrared imaging (thermography) of type I thoracolumbar disk disease in chondrodystrophic dogs. *Vet Surg.* **43**(7):869–876.

Hancock, C.M. and Riegger-Krugh, C. (2008) Modulation of pain in osteoarthritis: the role of nitric oxide. *Clin J Pain.* **24**(4):353–365.

IVAPM. (2016) Animals and pain. Available from: https://ivapm.org/for-the-public/animals-and-pain-articles/(accessed November 30, 2016).

Jimbo, K. *et al.* (1998) Suppressive effects of low-power laser irradiation on bradykinin evoked action potentials in cultured murine dorsal root ganglion cells. *Neurosci Lett.* **240**(2):93–96.

Kim, H.P. (2014) Lightening up light therapy: activation of retrograde signaling pathway by photobiomodulation. *Biomol Ther (Seoul).* **22**(6):491–496.

Labajos, M. (1988) Beta-endorphin levels modification after GaAs and HeNe laser irradiation on the rabbit. *Comparative study. Invest Clin.* **1–2**:6–8.

Lauretti, G.R. (2015) The evolution of spinal/epidural neostigmine in clinical application: thoughts after two decades. *Saudi J Anaesth.* **9**(1):71–81.

Lee, B.H. (2002) Managing pain in human neonates, applications for animals. *J Am Vet Med Assoc.* **221**(2):233–237.

McMahon, S.B. *et al.* (2013) *Wall and Melzack's Textbook of Pain*, 6 edn. Elsevier, New York.

Millis, D.L. and Levine, D. (2014) *Canine Rehabilitation and Physical Therapy*, 2 edn. Elsevier, New York.

Mitchell, U.H. and Mack, G.L. (2013) Low-level laser treatment with near-infrared light increases venous nitric oxide levels acutely: a single-blind, randomized clinical trial of efficacy. *Am J Phys Med Rehabil.* **92**(2):151–156.

NC State. (2016) Feline Musculoskeletal Pain Index (FMPI). Available from: https://cvm.ncsu.edu/research/

labs/clinical-sciences/comparative-pain-research/ clinical-metrology-instruments/(accessed November 30, 2016).

Nesioonpour, S. *et al.* (2014) The effect of low-level laser on postoperative pain after tibial fracture surgery: a double-blind controlled randomized clinical trial. *Anesth Pain Med.* **4**(3):e17350.

Nicolau, R.A. *et al.* (2004) Neurotransmitter release changes induced by low power 830 nm diode laser irradiation on the neuromuscular junctions of the mouse. *Lasers Surg Med.* **35**(3):236–241.

Parke, A.L. *et al.* (2003) Multiple organ dysfunction syndrome. *InflammoPharmacology.* **11**(1):87–95.

Passarella, S. and Karu, T. (2014) Absorption of monochromatic and narrow band radiation in the visible and near IR by both mitochondrial and non-mitochondrial photoacceptors results in photobiomodulation. *J Photochem Photobiol B.* **140**:344–358.

Peimani, A. and Sardary, F. (2014) Effect of low-level laser on healing of temporomandibular joint osteoarthritis in rats. *J Dent (Tehran).* **11**(3):319–327.

PennVet. (2016) Canine Brief Pain Inventory (Canine BPI). Available from: http://www.vet.upenn.edu/research/ clinical-trials/vcic/pennchart/cbpi-tool (accessed November 30, 2016).

Poyton, R.O. and Ball, K.A. (2011) Therapeutic photobiomodulation: nitric oxide and a novel function of mitochondrial cytochrome c oxidase. *Discov Med.* **11**(57):154–159.

Price, D.D. *et al.* (2006) Plasticity in brain processing and modulation of pain. *Prog Brain Res.* **157**:333–352.

Rochkind, S. and Shainberg, A. (2013) Protective effect of laser phototherapy on acetylcholine receptors and creatine kinase activity in denervated muscle. *Photomed Laser Surg.* **31**(10):499–504.

Silverstein, D. (2006) SIRS, MODS, and sepsis in small animals. Available from: http://www.ivis.org/ proceedings/scivac/2006/silverstein2_en.pdf?LA=1 (accessed November 30, 2016).

Sprouse-Blum, A.S. *et al.* (2010) Understanding endorphins and their importance in pain management. *Hawaii Med J.* **69**(3):70–71.

Wadhwa, J. and Sood, R. (1997) Multiple organ dysfunction syndrome. *Natl Med J India.* **10**(6):277–282.

Wakabayashi, H. (1993) Effect of irradiation by semiconductor laser on responses evoked in trigeminal caudal neurons by tooth pulp stimulation. *Lasers Surg Med.* **13**(6):605–610.

Walker, J. (1983) Relief from chronic pain by low-power laser irradiation. *Neurosci Lett.* **43**(203):339–344.

Weersink, R. (2007) Light dosimetry for low level laser therapy: accounting for difference in tissue and depth. *Proc of SPIE.* **6428**:642803.

Wiese, A.J. (2015) Assessing pain. In: *Handbook of Veterinary Pain Management*, 3 edn. Elsevier, New York.

Zhenghong, Z. *et al.* (2008) Morphine increases acetylcholine release in the trigeminal nuclear complex. *Sleep.* **31**(12):1629–1637.

9

Intra- and Postoperative Laser Therapy

Steven Buijs[1] and John C. Godbold, Jr.[2]

[1] *Dierenhospitaal Visdonk, Roosendaal, Netherlands*
[2] *Stonehaven Veterinary Consulting, Jackson, TN, USA*

Introduction

For the past 15 years, my colleagues and I have been performing basic and advanced surgical procedures at our hospital, Dierenhospitaal Visdonk, in Roosendaal, Netherlands. Our surgeries range from standard ovariectomies and ovariohysterectomies to complicated corrective osteotomies. During the postoperative phase of these surgeries, we have historically expected to encounter predictable, minor surgical complications such as edema, pain, inflammation, time required for return of function, and occasional wound problems.

For the past 3 years, we have been incorporating laser therapy into our surgical protocols. My colleagues and I have been astonished to see the results when we incorporate laser therapy during and after surgery. The addition of laser therapy does not significantly increase the overall time required for surgeries (as most laser therapy sessions are only minutes in duration) and significantly decreases complications. The use of laser therapy and photobiomodulation (PBM) in conjunction with surgery has been previously reported for both human and veterinary patients (Draper *et al.*, 2012; Karlekar *et al.*, 2015; Nesioonpour *et al.*, 2014). The therapeutic use of PBM, which is aimed at alleviating pain and inflammation, modulating immune responses, and promoting wound healing and tissue regeneration, continues to be reviewed (Arany, 2016; Pryor and Millis, 2015).

While treating a high percentage of our surgery patients with laser therapy, we get the chance to observe those patients when they are hospitalized, witness their improvement, and appreciate how laser PBM is helping them. Laser therapy leads to increased comfort in our patients and to more satisfied owners. Owners have readily accepted the technology, despite higher costs for them from laser therapy fees. After 3 years, we can't imagine going into our surgery theater for a procedure without the possibility of using laser therapy for our patients.

This chapter reflects the success we have had with laser therapy and PBM at Dierenhospitaal Visdonk. As the lead author of this chapter, I am indebted to the second author, my colleague from the United States, John C. Godbold, Jr., DVM, for contributing literature searches and references.

Overview

Surgical interventions are selected to give expected outcomes for our patients. If, for example, we want to treat a ruptured cruciate ligament, we must select a procedure that will stabilize the stifle joint and provide a return of function of the stifle. But, during any type of surgery, there will be tissue handling, which results in unwanted responses from the body. The more invasive the procedure, the more tissue is disrupted, and the greater the response that follows. These responses cause most of the unwanted side effects of surgery. Inflammation will occur, swelling will develop, changes in vasculature are unavoidable, and suture materials will cause enzymatic processes, which will absorb the materials. All of these processes result in pain, inflammation, and discomfort, and affect the speed of healing. Our goals for the successful use of a therapeutic laser are to minimize the responses of the body that we do not want, increase those we do want, increase patient comfort, and decrease healing time.

The first patients we treated perioperatively with laser therapy were dogs with cruciate ligament ruptures. Our surgical procedure for these patients before that point was usually tibial tuberosity advancement (TTA), by KYON (n.d. c). Due to swelling and inflammation at the surgical site, we routinely saw the development of edema in the distal part of the hind limb. This occurred in all patients within 2 days following surgery, causing discomfort and delaying use of the leg. Sometimes, the swelling

Table 9.1 Examples of procedures in which intraoperative or postoperative treatment is indicated.

Procedure	Intraoperative laser therapy	Postoperative laser therapy
Amputation (leg, tail, claws, etc.)		×
Arythenoid lateralization	×	×
Arthroscopy		×
Arthrotomy	×	×
Aural hematoma (othematoma)		×
Brachycephalic obstructive syndrome	×	×
Caudectomy		×
Coeliotomy (laparotomy)		×
Corrective osteotomy (TTA, TPLO, TPO, etc.)	×	×
Cystotomy	×	×
Dorsal hemilaminectomy	×	×
Enterectomy	×	×
Enterotomy	×	×
Enucleation of the eye		×
Episioplasty		×
Femoral head excision	×	×
Gastric dilation and volvulus	×	×
Gastrotomy	×	×
Laparoscopy		×
Orchiectomy		×
Osteosynthesis (fracture stabilization)	×	×
Ovario(hyster)ectomy		×
Promotion of secondary healing	×	×
Thoracoscopy		×
Thoracotomy	×	×
Total ear canal ablation	×	×
Total hip prosthesis	×	×
Urethrostomy (perineal or scrotal)	×	×
Ventral slot	×	×

was massive and needed additional treatment, including diuretic medication, massage, and pressure bandaging. We started to use a therapeutic laser immediately after these surgeries 3 years ago and noticed that in the majority of patients there was hardly any edema formation, and that most patients returned to weight-bearing use of the hind limb within 2 days.

We recognized that an important part of patients assuming more rapid weight bearing was better pain control as a result of laser therapy. Treating them with the laser every other day for the first 10 days has significantly improved the speed of their return to function. Monitoring and comparing their pain scores has verified that laser-treated patients are more comfortable than we had expected them to be. We also note that these patients show less interest in the wound, and we have fewer cases of wound complications due to licking. Our observations of reduced pain in postoperative patients after laser therapy mirror what has been reported in benchtop studies and in animal-model and human studies (Bjordal *et al.*, 2006; Enwemeka *et al.*, 2004; Fulop *et al.*, 2010; Hawkins and Abrahamse, 2006; Sprouse-Blum *et al.*, 2010).

We have now started using laser therapy intraoperatively during ruptured cranial cruciate stabilization, as well as postoperatively. We can effectively apply laser therapy without touching the tissue during surgery, maintaining asepsis. We now apply laser therapy to our closed arthrotomy wounds, before we close the subcutis and skin. This technique is much more efficient, since we are delivering the laser light directly to the surgical site, without any absorption of photons by the skin.

Because of the success we have had with this group of patients, we have expanded our perioperative use of laser therapy to all of our surgical procedures (Table 9.1).

Intraoperative Laser Therapy

There are multiple advantages of the intraoperative use of a therapeutic laser. The laser light can be delivered much earlier in the process. A 2015 study of human dental patients reported the effectiveness of immediate versus delayed photobiomodulation therapy (PBMT) in reducing the severity of postoperative inflammatoion (Abdel-Alim *et al.*, 2015). When applying laser therapy almost immediately after tissue trauma, PBMT will result in a decrease in the release of cytokines and a reduction in inflammatory cell activity. Healing will be stimulated very quickly. The therapy laser beam can be pinpointed to localized areas we want to treat, such as an arthrotomy wound, or an enterotomy or cystotomy wound. Since this technique allows treatment directly in the deeper tissues, photon absorption by more superficial tissue is avoided.

During surgery, we have to be sure not to interfere with the aseptic environment and technique. We can easily deliver laser therapy intraoperatively without touching the tissue. When treating intraoperatively, the tissues being targeted are in clear sight and do not require a deep-tissue dose and technique; contact with the tissue is not necessary. To maintain asepsis, the laser therapist

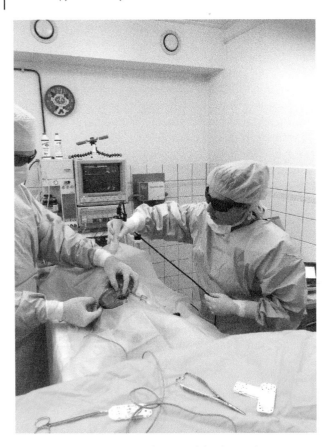

Figure 9.1 Intraoperative application of the therapy laser, maintaining aseptic technique.

must be a well-trained member of the surgery team. There has to be good coordination between the therapist and the surgeon so there is no unwanted touching of tissue with the laser handpiece.

Before surgery, the handpiece and cable should be thoroughly cleaned, as we don't want any particles or dust falling into the surgical field. The laser therapist should wear sterile surgical gloves for the same purpose. The therapist must make sure that the handpiece and the cable remain clear of the surgical field and do not touch any part of the patient (Figure 9.1).

The surgeon should present the organ or surgical wound to the therapist, so a maximal exposure can be achieved. Whenever the surgeon is going to move the patient or tissue, this should be communicated so that the therapist can avoid accidental touching. When treating intraoperatively and the target tissue can be visualized, the laser settings should deliver a dose of $3–4\,J/cm^2$. The tissue being targeted is often sensitive and traumatized, so we recommend not exceeding 4 W power. Since the tissue areas being treated are relatively small, and the dose being delivered is relatively low, using a lower power setting does not increase the treatment time significantly.

Postoperative Laser Therapy

As soon as the surgery wounds are closed, it is an ideal time to treat the wound and the surrounding tissues with the therapy laser without interfering with sterility. A member of the surgical team should treat the wounds and tissues as soon as surgery has finished. The tissue can be touched with the laser handpiece, using a contact delivery. Since, in this application, we are treating the skin, subcutis, and deeper tissues, the laser settings should deliver $8–10\,J/cm^2$. A well-trained laser therapist will apply a gentle massage with the handpiece and will treat from all directions to facilitate photon permeation of the tissue. When treating a wound where the skin and more superficial tissues have been affected, like a coeliotomy wound, the treatment area should include the immediate wound area, including the skin, subcutis, and underlying musculature, as well as a margin of normal tissue around the wound. Following a surgery that results in a greater degree of tissue damage and disruption, a larger area should be treated. For example, following a stifle surgery, the tissue being treated should include the surgical wound, the entire stifle, the musculature associated with the stifle, and the vasculature caudal to the stifle.

Patients that have had invasive procedures should be scheduled to return to the hospital daily or every other day to repeat the laser therapy. The main goals are to reduce pain, reduce edema by improving blood flow and reducing swelling, reduce inflammation, promote healing, and promote quicker return of function. When patients have reached a point of expected healing and return to function, laser therapy can be discontinued. The effects of PBMT on wound healing are outlined in Chapter 10 and are well established in current publications (Avci *et al.*, 2013; Hawkins and Abrahamse, 2006; Medrado *et al.*, 2003; Silveira *et al.*, 2007). Other studies and literature reviews verify the effective pain-reduction mechanisms of PBMT (Chow *et al.*, 2007, 2011; Fulop *et al.*, 2010).

Clinical Examples of Intra- and Postoperative Laser Therapy Application

The following procedures are examples of how laser therapy can be used intra- and postoperatively to effectively impact overall patient care.

Ruptured Cruciate Ligament

The majority of canine patients with a ruptured cranial cruciate ligament seen at Dierenhospitaal Visdonk are treated with a correctional osteotomy to neutralize the forces associated with the ligament dysfunction. Our goals with this type of surgery are to regain comfortable function as soon as possible and to have a very low complication rate. Laser therapy is a very useful adjunct to surgery in accomplishing these goals. Neither surgery nor laser therapy can replace the other; but, when used together properly, they can enhance the outcome.

The first step in surgery is an arthrotomy or arthroscopy to confirm the diagnosis, examine for possible meniscal injury, remove the remnants of the ruptured cruciate ligament, and, if a meniscal tear is present, remove the loose border or body of the meniscus. In addition to confirming the diagnosis, the purpose of this part of the surgery is to reduce the inflammatory response of the body. If remnants of the cruciate ligament are left in the joint, the body will attempt to absorb them. The accompanying joint inflammation will be an onset for the development of osteoarthritis and an increased effusion of synovial fluid, which will distend the joint capsule and cause more discomfort and pain. After inspection of the joint, removal of cruciate ligament remnants, and possible meniscectomy, we close the joint capsule in two layers, incorporating the patellofemoral ligament if it was severed with an open approach.

Due to the tissue damage when opening the joint, the handling of instruments in the joint, and suture placements in the joint capsule, we induce significant tissue disruption, which will in turn induce an inflammatory response. We can temper the inflammatory response with laser therapy. In 2014, a study demonstrated that laser therapy, using an 808 nm laser and doses of 10 and 50 J/cm^2, prevented features related to the articular degenerative process, such as increased release of inflammatory mediators, in the knees of rats after anterior cruciate ligament transection (Bublitz *et al.*, 2014).

After closure of the joint capsule, the nurse serving as laser therapist will take the prepared laser handpiece. Her hands become non-sterile at this point. Using a non-contact delivery, she will focus the laser beam on the joint only, with emphasis on the surgical wound (Figure 9.2).

A correct laser therapy dose is delivered by estimating the surface area to be treated and setting the laser to deliver 3–4 J/cm^2. We recommend not exceeding a laser power setting of 4 W, to minimize any potential of heating in the tissues. The time required for laser therapy treatment of this area is no more than 1–2 minutes. The benefits of administering laser therapy at this point are that PBMT can be started as soon as possible in order to reduce the inflammation and that the target tissues can be exactly located, without any overlying skin.

The nurse will then change gloves and re-join the surgery aseptically to continue with the procedure. We approach the medial side of the proximal tibia to

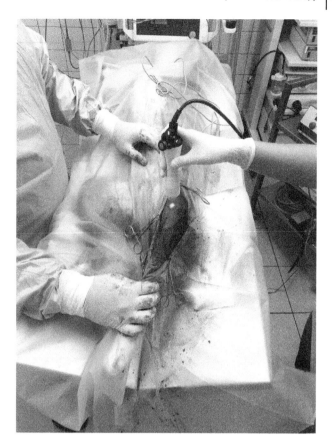

Figure 9.2 Intraoperative treatment during a stifle surgery, after closure of the arthrotomy wound, maintaining aseptic technique.

perform a tibial plateau leveling osteotomy (TPLO) (KYON, n.d. b), TTA, or other correctional techniques. At Dierenhospitaal Visdonk, we have performed mostly TTA (KYON, n.d. c), but more recently we have added TTA-2 (KYON, n.d. c) to our possibilities for treating this condition. In performing these surgeries, we cause a lot of tissue damage. All techniques involve performing an osteotomy, which means that in addition to cutting bone, we cut through soft tissues on the medial side of the tibia. The osteotomy is either circular with a TPLO, or curved with a TTA. Securing the implants requires bone screws (except in TTA-2). Drilling screw holes and placing screws also inflicts tissue damage. Closing and restoring the medial soft tissue is important, in order to fully cover the implants and provide added support in reducing cranial thrust of the tibia. Due to the extensive damage to these tissues during surgery, we expect to see swelling in the entire stifle area. The swelling puts pressure on the saphenous vein, reducing venous return, and promotes accumulation of fluid and edema in the distal area of the limb.

To help reduce postoperative swelling and edema after medial closure of the subcutis and skin, we administer laser therapy again. Since this is a postoperative application, maintaining asepsis is no longer required. Delivery in contact with the tissue is recommended, with gentle massage and laser settings that will deliver 3–4 J/cm^2 to the superficial soft tissues. Addressing all of the affected superficial soft tissue, the nurse serving as laser therapist should treat the entire stifle area from all directions. Treatment should extend distal and medial to the stifle to include all soft tissues over the osteotomy site.

To facilitate continued applications of laser therapy, we recommend not applying a bandage after surgery. When required, the surgical site can be protected with wound-protection sleeves or an Elizabethan collar. Patients are scheduled for their next postoperative laser therapy treatment 24 hours after surgery.

Patients we have treated with laser therapy intra- and postoperatively are weight bearing either at release the day of surgery or within 24 hours. Occasionally, we will see a moderate amount of edema appear at the distal tibia and hock region. When this occurs, we administer laser therapy using contact delivery and gentle massage, starting in the stifle area in order to enhance blood flow in venous return. Gentle handpiece massage is accompanied by the therapist massaging the hock and distal tibia with the other hand. Halfway through the treatment, the therapist will move to the distal part of the leg and treat over the edematous area. During the treatment, the edema will visibly reduce, and rapid pain reduction results in an immediate improvement in weight bearing (Figure 9.3).

In our postoperative laser therapy management plan, the patient will return every other day for the first 10 days. At each return visit, we treat the stifle and proximal tibia and the associated soft tissues with contact delivery, gentle massage, movement of the stifle through passive range of motion, and laser settings that deliver 8–10 J/cm^2. Normally, beginning at the second visit, we do not see any edema in the distal parts of the limb. At 10 days after surgery, we discontinue the laser therapy treatments, unless we are not satisfied with the results, in which case we continue with twice-weekly treatments until better function is noted.

Using this combination of surgery and intense laser therapy treatment, canine cranial cruciate ligament rupture patients can have a 99% chance of having a successful outcome, without any minor or major complications, and a much quicker return to full function.

Medial-Compartment Disease in the Elbow Joint

At Dierenhospitaal Visdonk, medial-compartment disease in the elbow joint is treated with the gold standard: arthroscopy. This developmental condition most often affects the medial coronoid process of young to middle-aged patients and is a result of an overload of pressure on the medial aspect of the elbow joint. In many cases, it will be the result of a limb malalignment that develops during bone growth. If treatment is focused only on the intra-articular fragment and the underlying cause is not treated, symptoms may reoccur, with joint distention, osteoarthritis, and reduced range of motion of the elbow joint. Two different approaches are required to properly manage these patients: arthroscopy alone or limb-realignment osteotomy to correct the predisposing cause of the condition.

Arthroscopy is very useful in verifying the diagnosis and can be helpful in providing treatment at the same time. It allows visual inspection of the joint, an evaluation of the degree of inflammation, and visualization of collateral damage caused by the fragment in kissing lesions on the medial humeral condyle. In an affected joint, the medial coronoid process may have a fissure,

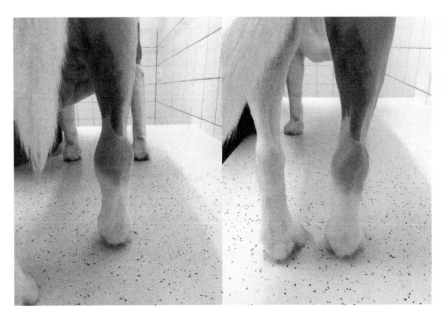

Figure 9.3 Left: Marked swelling of the hock 2 days after TTA, with patient placement of the leg more cranially to avoid weight bearing. Right: Reduced edema and normal weight bearing immediately after laser therapy treatment.

a non-displaced fragment, or a displaced fragment, or worn cartilage in complete medial-compartment disease.

Whenever applicable, loose fragments should be removed during arthroscopy to minimize iatrogenic damage to the joint and surrounding soft tissue. If successful, the only wounds will be 3–4 mm arthroscopy puncture wounds, which can be closed with a simple suture. Immediately after the arthroscopy, we administer a laser therapy treatment. We treat the elbow joint using a contact delivery and laser settings that deliver 8–10 J/cm^2. The laser therapist will treat the joint from all directions and through a full passive range of motion. This first postoperative treatment helps reduce the pain and inflammation caused by the arthroscopy, and begins to address any chronic arthritic caused by the condition.

In order to reduce joint inflammation, reduce pain, improve function, and promote healing of the cartilage defects, we recommend continuing laser therapy every other day (Assis *et al.*, 2016). The treatment protocol is the same as that used immediately after surgery, so a deep-tissue target dose of 8–10 J/cm^2 is delivered.

For most patients, a limb-correction alignment surgery is recommended following arthroscopy. When owners decline this option, we begin conservative management to slow degenerative joint disease and improve function.

After an induction phase of five or six every-other-day laser therapy treatments following the arthroscopy, we go through a transition phase of treatments, tapering the frequency by treating twice a week for 2 weeks and then once a week for 2 weeks. Long-term maintenance-phase treatments are prescribed every 2–4 weeks and continued lifelong. In these conservatively managed patients, progressive degenerative joint disease is expected; however, with continued laser therapy, the progression occurs at a slower pace (Wang *et al.*, 2014).

When patients require limb alignment correction and the owners accept the recommendation, the surgery is scheduled 1–2 weeks after the arthroscopy. Laser therapy is continued between the arthroscopy and the alignment correction. We perform a proximal abducting ulnotomy (PAUL) (KYON, n.d. a) and continue laser therapy as part of overall patient management, as with any osteosynthesis.

Osteosynthesis

Every patient that is subject to a fracture is confronted with hematoma, edema, pain, and dysfunction. The majority of patients will be treated with some form of osteosynthesis, in order to repair the damage to the bones (and the soft tissue, if necessary). There is a definite indication to treat these patients with a therapeutic laser, before and after surgery. In addition to its important effects on soft tissue, PBMT plays an important role in activating osteogenic factors, stimulating osteoblastic cells, and accelerating bone healing (Barbosa *et al.*, 2014; Chang *et al.*, 2014; Ebrahimi *et al.*, 2012; Jawad *et al.*, 2013; Mota *et al.*, 2013; Son *et al.*, 2012; Tim *et al.*, 2014).

The way laser therapy is used in managing fractures is the same whether in treatment of traumatic fractures or in elective surgeries such as corrective osteotomies. Examples of elective, corrective osteotomies are distal femoral osteotomy, proximal tibial osteotomy, PAUL, and proximal sliding ulnotomy.

In patients with traumatic fractures, we are presented with an instability, which will be accompanied with a hematoma, profuse swelling, and skin wounds. If fracture fixation is delayed by the presence of other injuries and the need to stabilize the patient, the surgeon is often confronted with massive soft-tissue swelling. To help prevent and control swelling before surgery, the application of a splint or bandaging is recommended. Laser therapy is administered before bandage or splint application and during each change of the bandage or splint. Note that laser therapy cannot be administered through bandage or splint material. Even very thin layers of bandage material produce massive scattering of the coherent laser beam and significant reduction of the percentage of photons reaching the target tissue. Repeat laser therapy as often as twice a day until surgery for osteosynthesis is performed. A combination of bandaging, support, and laser therapy will result in a markedly decreased amount of swelling and edema, and improved visualization for the surgeon during surgery.

After osteosynthesis, regardless of the indication or location, we start laser therapy immediately after closure of the wounds with a contact delivery and laser settings that will deliver 8–10 J/cm^2. This deep-tissue target dose is appropriate for osteosynthesis sites and will also treat the more superficially damaged soft tissue. During this treatment, the laser is applied to the fracture site, circumferentially around the fractured bone, moving from proximal to distal. This laser therapy treatment will help reduce swelling and pain, and at the same time promote soft-tissue healing and ostoegenesis.

Laser therapy will then be repeated every day for the first 3–5 days, then every other day until 10–14 days after surgery. Depending on the functional result, the degree of swelling, and the progression of wound healing, we will discontinue laser therapy at that time; alternatively, when necessary, we may continue with twice a week treatments for as long as needed. If a patient has any risk of a delayed healing, as for example with a fracture of the proximal ulna, we will continue laser therapy twice weekly until the fracture is stable.

Femoral Head Excision

Femoral head excision is primarily indicated in cats with trauma to the acetabulum, femoral head, or femoral neck. In dogs, excision is most often required in toy breeds with similar trauma or with hereditary diseases of the femoral head, such as avascular femoral head necrosis. After femoral head excision, patients are dependent on the development of a neoarthrosis to regain a full functional hind limb with a normal range of motion. Managing postoperative pain in these patients is critical, since they should begin using their leg as soon as possible after surgery to facilitate a return to function. If the surgical area is painful, the patient will be reluctant to use the leg, leading to a lengthening of functional healing time.

We recommend starting laser therapy as soon as the femoral head excision is completed and the surgical wound has been closed. While still in the surgical theater, deliver a laser therapy treatment, using a contact delivery, with laser settings that deliver a deep-tissue target dose of 8–10 J/cm^2. Direct the laser beam toward the acetabulum, circling around the major trochanter, and into the surgical site from the medial aspect of the proximal femur. Move the femur through passive range of motion, through flexion and extension, as the treatment is delivered.

Continue daily laser therapy until weight bearing is comfortable for the patient. Use the same laser settings and delivery as used immediately after the surgery. At Dierenhospitaal Visdonk, we see much better and quicker results when we incorporate laser therapy in the rehabilitation of femoral head excision patients compared to similar patients in which laser therapy is not used. A return to full function is expected in 2–3 weeks after surgery when incorporating laser therapy. We continue laser therapy twice a week for 6 weeks after surgery to facilitate healing and increased formation of connective tissue between the acetabulum and proximal femur.

Coeliotomy (Laparotomy)

Laser therapy is indicated for every abdominal surgery that does not involve a malignancy. In our practice, when we began applying laser therapy to the abdominal wall and surgical wounds following coeliotomy, we noted that the reduction in pain and swelling resulted in patients showing less interest in their wounds and engaging in less licking of and biting at the wounds. The application of laser therapy after an abdominal surgery is quick, easy, and efficacious (Figure 9.4). Use either a contact or a non-contact delivery with laser settings that delivery 3–4 J/cm^2.

Regardless of the reason for the surgery, with a normal approach into the abdomen, through healthy tissue, we prescribe laser therapy a single time for these patients.

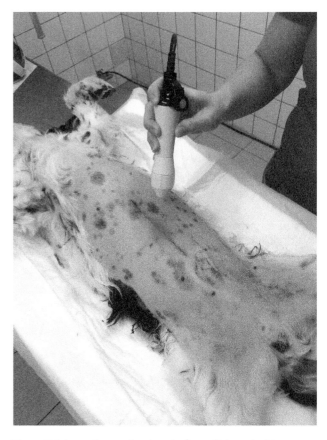

Figure 9.4 Laser therapy treatment of a coeliotomy incision immediately after closure.

If conditions within the abdomen warrant continued treatment, as, for example, when enteritis, cystitis, or peritonitis is present, we will treat immediately after surgery using a contact delivery and laser settings that deliver 8–10 J/cm^2, and will then continue daily or twice-daily treatments until the intra-abdominal condition has resolved.

Enterotomy and Enterectomy

The most common indication for an enterotomy or enterectomy (resection and anastomosis) is a foreign object in the small intestines that is just too large to pass through the lumen with normal peristaltic movements. If the foreign object can't move, the damage to the intestinal wall may be minor, or it may result in significant pressure necrosis, vascular impairment, and perforation. Similarly vascular compromise, necrosis, and perforation are also seen with an intussusception.

If vascular supply has not been compromised, a foreign object can be removed with an enterotomy. If there is doubt about the vascular integrity, or if tissue changes show the vascular supply is compromised, an enterectomy is indicated. Regardless of the procedure, laser therapy is indicated immediately after closure of the

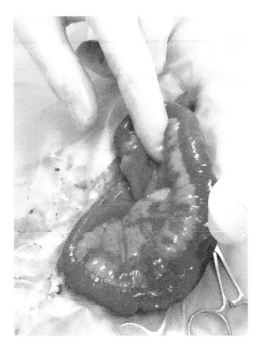

Figure 9.5 Intraoperative treatment of an enterotomy wound. The surgeon is presenting the jejunum, and the nurse is aiming the handpiece, making sure to maintain aseptic technique.

small intestines with suturing or stapling. The sterile-gloved nurse serving as laser therapist will take the cleaned, prepared laser handpiece. The nurse's hands become non-sterile at this point. The size of the intestinal tract to be treated will be estimated and the laser will be set to deliver a dose of $3–4 J/cm^2$. It is helpful for the surgeon to "present" and move the intestines during treatment to maximize photon penetration from as many different directions as possible (Figure 9.5). Communication between the surgeon and the nurse is important in order that unpredictable movements and inadvertent contamination of the tissue do not occur. In this application, it is not unusual to be able to actually visualize the effect of PBMT on the tissues. Visible improvement in tissue color and motility can frequently be seen within a few minutes as tissue perfusion improves. Laser therapy has been demonstrated to cause potent dilation in rat mesenteric arterioles *in vivo*, which leads to a marked increase in the arteriolar blood flow (Maegawa *et al.*, 2000). If ischemia and reperfusion injury are present, laser therapy will reduce their impact on distant organs (Kirkby *et al.*, 2012).

After direct laser therapy of the intestinal wound, closure of the coeliotomy is performed in the routine manner. Then, as already described for coeliotomies, the abdominal incision and abdominal wall are treated with laser therapy, with a laser setting that will deliver $3–4 J/cm^2$.

If the surgery encounters focal or generalized peritonitis, laser therapy treatment through the body wall is repeated after 24 hours, using a contact delivery and with the laser set to deliver $8–10 J/cm^2$. Daily treatments should be continued until the problem has been resolved.

Since we began adding laser therapy to gastrointestinal surgeries, we have seen improved patient comfort after surgery, much quicker healing, and reduced frequency of leakage and dehiscence of enterotomy and enterectomy wounds.

Cystotomy

The technique of administering laser therapy intraoperatively, directly to the target tissue, has been very beneficial in cystotomy patients. When performing a cystotomy to remove bladder stones or polyps from the urinary bladder, we treat the cystotomy wound immediately after closure, prior to returning the bladder to the abdomen. As with other intraoperative applications, a cleaned, prepared handpiece is used by a nurse wearing sterile gloves. The surface area of the bladder to be treated is estimated and the laser is set to deliver $3–4 J/cm^2$. As seen in intestinal tissue during the treatment of enterotomy and enterectomy surgery sites, the bladder wall and serosa show immediate response to therapy laser treatment, with improved perfusion. Closure of the abdominal wall is done routinely, and the incisional area is treated immediately after surgery, as previously described.

Since virtually all cystotomy patients have some degree of cystitis, the bladder is treated with laser therapy administered through the abdominal wall daily for 3–5 days following surgery. A contact delivery is used, with laser settings that deliver $8–10 J/cm^2$. Since the bladder is in a predictable position in the caudal abdomen, treatment can be delivered from the ventral and both lateral directions. Cystotomy patients appear to be more comfortable when laser therapy is added to their management, and most display a return to normal frequency of urinations within 24 hours.

Urethrostomy

Though the combination of medical and dietary management can reduce the incidence of urinary calculi, male cats continue to be susceptible to blockage of the distal urethra, and male dogs can have calculi lodge in the distal urethra caudal to the bone of the penis (baculum).

In both cats and dogs, the success rate of displacing the urethral blockage or calculi with retrograde flushing will be higher if laser therapy is administered before passing a catheter. Using a contact delivery and a laser setting that delivers $6–8 J/m^2$, the suspected location of the obstruction and the surrounding tissue are treated to decrease edema and swelling, and to help relax muscle spasms in the urethra. In most cases, subsequent passage of a urinary catheter and retrograde flushing of urethral contents will then be easier.

If it is impossible to dislodge the obstruction, surgery is required. If frequent recurrence of a blockage occurs, surgery to reroute the urethra is indicated. The mucosal lining of the urethra is sensitive tissue and develops inflammation rapidly. Performing a urethrotomy to remove calculi or a urethrostomy to reroute the urine passage requires delicate handling of tissue. In addition to pre-existing and intraoperative tissue damage, the urethral mucosa will be damaged during the suturing process. The responses to tissue damage and the presence of sutures will be pain, swelling, and inflammation, all of which can cause urinary straining and patient self-trauma.

Important to this procedure is the delicate handling of the urethral mucosa to minimize trauma. In both perennial urethrostomy in the cat and scrotal urethrostomy in the dog, the diameter of the stoma is of great importance. Prevention of licking of the urethral surgical wounds is critical to a successful result. Laser therapy is indicated to reduce swelling, inflammation, and pain immediately after creating the stoma and placing sutures. For this treatment, a non-contact delivery is recommended, along with laser settings that deliver $3-4\,\text{J/cm}^2$. Laser therapy is repeated daily for 5–10 days. Laser therapy markedly decreases swelling at the stoma, and patients seem to be more comfortable and less tempted to lick the site.

Thoracotomy

Because of the invasiveness of thoracotomies, and the level of patient discomfort postoperatively, laser therapy can play an important role in a patient's return to function following this surgery. Whether the approach is intercostal or sternal, there simply is a lot of postoperative pain. Respirations produce more motion of the cut tissues and increased pain compared to other surgeries. Use of the therapy laser intra- and postoperatively is an important adjunct to other pain-management modalities.

At Dierenhospitaal Visdonk, the most common reasons for performing thoracotomies are lung lobe removal, pericardiectomy, vascular ring anomaly, persistent ductus arteriosus (duct of Botalli), thymoma removal, and biopsy. All of these thoracotomy patients will benefit from laser therapy. After closure of the ribs or sternum, and after re-establishing negative pressure in the thorax, laser therapy is administered prior to skin closure. Using non-contact delivery, and maintaining aseptic technique as in other intraoperative applications, the laser therapy treatment is delivered to the closed entrance to the thorax. We estimate the size of the area and deliver a dose of $3-4\,\text{J/cm}^2$. After this treatment, we routinely close the overlying muscle, subcutis, and skin. When all of the soft tissues have been closed, we treat the closed incision using a contact delivery with laser settings that deliver a dose of $3-4\,\text{J/cm}^2$. Laser therapy is repeated every day for 3–5 days. The result of incorporating laser therapy for these patients is much less postoperative discomfort and less frequent seroma formation.

Stimulation of Secondary Healing

When trauma or surgical intervention results in a large area of skin loss, laser therapy is certainly indicated (Peplow *et al.*, 2010; Skopin and Molitor, 2009; Takashi, 1988).

Addressing the wound surgically is the first step, to remove all devitalized tissue, clean the remaining tissue as well as possible, and begin to prevent movement of loose skin by suturing it to underlying tissues. Regardless of whether open healing by second intention or support and healing of skin grafts is the goal, laser therapy will contribute to faster healing (Calisto *et al.*, 2015; Hodjati *et al.*, 2014; Hopkins *et al.*, 2004; Kovacs, 2015; Kuffler, 2016).

An excellent example is a Belgian shepherd that presented with a large area of necrosis, which was caused by a wound inflicted by a cat. There was a small, extremely painful area of necrosis visible through the fur 5 days after the incident. Under full anesthesia, we clipped the area, and a much larger area of involvement became visible (Figure 9.6a). This kind of wound is not a candidate for closure or grafting, and needs to be treated, at least initially, in a conservatively manner to encourage granulation formation.

We debrided to remove necrotic tissue, cleaned with sterile physiologic fluids, and placed simple interrupted sutures to fix the skin edge to the underlying tissue. Suturing is necessary to limit the exposed area and prevent movement of skin in relation to the underlying tissue, as movement will delay healing (Figure 9.6b).

Applying bandages or dressings was impossible with this patient. It removed any dressing within hours after placement, and it was very difficult to prevent licking of the wounds. After 5 days, we decided to leave the wounds open and uncovered, without any bandage or dressing, and began laser therapy treatment. We used a laser setting that delivered $3-4\,\text{J/cm}^2$ to the affected area via a non-contact delivery. Immediately after the first treatment, the patient showed decreased interest in the wounds. We treated the wounds with laser therapy twice a day for the first week, then every day for the next week. After the initial 2 weeks of laser therapy, the wounds were fully granulated and an epithelial margin was noted around all wound edges.

Since the patient was not showing interest in the wounds, we decided to continue conservative treatment and wait for secondary healing. At this point, we could have decided to perform surgery again and use skin grafts to cover the wounds, but the owner saw the rapid

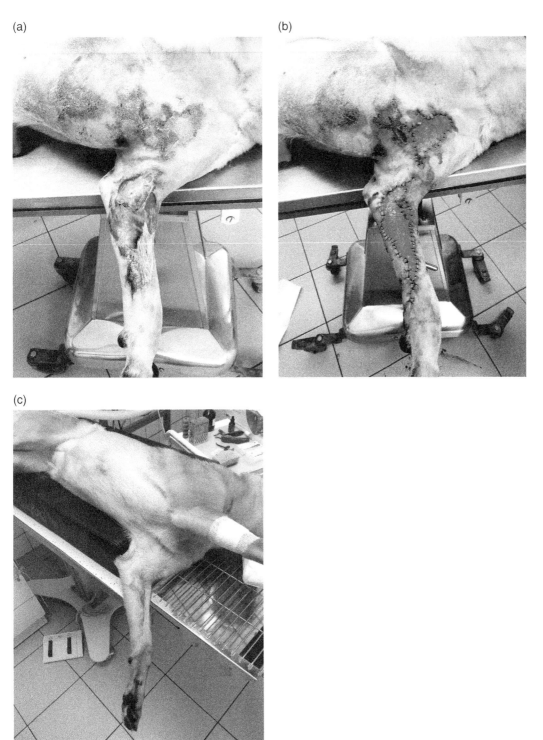

Figure 9.6 (a) Necrotic wound at initial presentation. (b) Necrotic wound after cleaning and suturing at the starting point of secondary healing. (c) Necrotic wound 45 days after starting laser therapy treatment. Note the complete healing, hair regrowth, and relatively small scars.

closure of the wounds and elected to continue with secondary healing.

We tapered the frequency of laser therapy treatments down to every other day until complete healing was noted 45 days after starting the laser therapy treatments (Figure 9.6c).

Measurements of the rate of wound healing indicated a closure rate of approximately 1.4 mm/day, which is significantly faster than expected without laser therapy. In this case, in addition to an accelerated rate of healing, laser therapy provided the important benefit of creating non-interest in the wounds for the dog. We observed that scar formation was very limited and that the scars that did form were flexible and did not limit motion of the foreleg.

Conclusion

In 3 years of using laser therapy during and after surgery, my colleagues and I have seen a significant improvement in the comfort level of our patients, and in their speed of healing and return to function after surgery. We find no disadvantages in using the therapy laser in our surgical theater. The procedures described in this chapter are examples of how laser therapy and PBM can be used as a valuable adjunct to other modalities in generating better surgical outcomes. By adopting the laser therapy application techniques described here, administering appropriate laser therapy doses, and prescribing an appropriate schedule of treatments intra- and postoperatively, laser therapy can be made a successful part of virtually all veterinary surgeries.

References

Abdel-Alim, H.M. *et al.* (2015) A comparative study of the effectiveness of immediate versus delayed photobiomodulation therapy in reducing the severity of postoperative inflammatory complications. *Photomed Laser Surg.* **33**(9):447–451.

Arany, P.R. (2016) Craniofacial wound healing with photobiomodulation therapy: new insights and current challenges. *J Dent Res.* **95**(9):977–984.

Assis, L. *et al.* (2016). Aerobic exercise training and low-level laser therapy modulate inflammatory response and degenerative process in an experimental model of knee osteoarthriti in rats. *Osteoarthritis Cartilage.* **24**(1):169–177.

Avci, P. *et al.* (2013) Low-level laser (light) therapy (LLLT) in skin: stimulating, healing, restoring. *Semin Cutan Med Surg.* **32**(1):41–52.

Barbosa, D. *et al.* (2014) Laser therapy in bone repair in rats: analysis of bone optical density. *Acta Ortop Bras.* **22**(2):71–74.

Bjordal, J.M. *et al.* (2006) Low-level laser therapy in acute pain: a systematic review of mechanisms of action and clinical effects in randomized placebo-controlled trials. *Photomed Laser Surg.* **24**(2):158–168.

Bublitz, C. *et al.* (2014) Low-level laser therapy prevents degenerative morphological changes in an experimental model of anterior cruciate ligament transection in rats. *Lasers Med Sci.* **29**(5):1669–1678.

Calisto, F.C. *et al.* (2015) Use of low-power laser to assist the healing of traumatic wounds. *Acta Cir Bras.* **30**(3):204–208.

Chang W. et al (2014) Therapeutic outcomes of low-level laser therapy for closed bone fracture in the human wrist and hand. *Photomed Laser Surg.* **32**(4):212–218.

Chow, R.T. *et al.* (2007) 830 nm laser irradiation induces varicosity formation, reduces mitochondrial membrane potential and blocks fast axonal flow in small and medium diameter rat dorsal root ganglion neurons: implications for the analgesic effects of 830 nm laser. *J Peripher Nerv Syst.* **12**(1):28–39.

Chow, R. *et al.* (2011) Inhibitory effects of laser irradiation on peripheral mammalian nerves and relevance to analgesic effects: a systematic review. *Photomed Laser Surg.* **29**(6):365–381.

Draper, W. *et al.* (2012) Laser therapy reduces time to ambulation in dogs after hemilaminectomy. *J Small Anim Pract.* **53**(8):465–469.

Ebrahimi, T. *et al.* (2012) The influence of low-intensity laser therapy on bone healing. *J Dent (Tehran).* **9**(4):238–248.

Enwemeka, C.S. *et al.* (2004) The efficacy of low-power lasers in tissue repair and pain control: a meta-analysis study. *Photomed Laser Surg.* **22**(4):323–329.

Fulop, A. *et al.* (2010) A meta-analysis of the efficacy of laser phototherapy on pain relief. *Clin J Pain.* **26**(8):729–736.

Hawkins, D. and Abrahamse, H. (2006) The role of laser fluence in cell viability, proliferation, and membrane integrity of wounded human skin fibroblasts. *Lasers Surg Med.* **38**(1):74–83.

Hodjati, H. *et al.* (2014) Low-level laser therapy: an experimental design for wound management: a case-controlled study in rabbit model. *J Cutan Aesthet Surg.* **7**(1):14–17.

Hopkins, T. J. *et al.* (2004) Low-level laser therapy facilitates superficial wound healing in humans: a triple-blind, sham-controlled study. *J Ath Train.* **39**(3):223–229.

Jawad, M.M. *et al.* (2013) Effect of 940 nm low-level laser therapy on osteogenesis in vitro. *J Biomed Opt.* **18**(12):128001.

Karlekar, A. *et al.* (2015) Assessment of feasibility and efficacy of class IV laser therapy for postoperative pain relief in off-pump coronary artery bypass surgery patients: a pilot study. *Ann Card Anaesth.* **18**(3):317–322.

Kirkby, K. *et al.* (2012) The effects of low-level laser therapy in a rat model of intestinal ischemia-reperfusion injury. *Lasers Surg Med.* **44**(7):580–587.

Kovacs, K. (2015) Low Level Laser Therapy of Serious Wounds of Dogs. Poster presentation. ASLMS Annual Meeting, April 24–26. Orlando, FL.

Kuffler, D.P. (2016) Photobiomodulation in promoting wound healing: a review. *Regen Med.* **11**(1):107–122.

KYON. (n.d. a) Proximal Abducting ULnar Osteotomy (PAUL). Available from: http://www.kyon.ch/current-products/proximal-abducting-ulnar-osteotomy-paul (accessed November 30, 2016).

KYON. (n.d. b) Tibial Plateau Leveling Osteotomy (TPLO). Available from: http://www.kyon.ch/current-products/tibial-plateau-leveling-osteotomy-tplo (accessed November 30, 2016).

KYON. (n.d. c) TTA surgery. Available from: http://www.kyon.ch/current-products/tibial-tuberosity-advancement-tta (accessed November 30, 2016).

Medrado, A.R. *et al.* (2003) Influence of low level laser therapy on wound healing and its biological action upon myofibroblasts. *Lasers Surg Med.* **32**(3):239–244.

Maegawa, Y. *et al.* (2000) Effects of near-infrared low-level laser irradiation on microcirculation. *Lasers Surg Med.* **27**(5):427–437.

Mota, F.C. *et al.* (2013) Low-power laser therapy for repairing acute and chronic-phase bone lesions. *Res Vet Sci.* **94**(1):105–110.

Nesioonpour, S. *et al.* (2014) The effect of low-level laser on postoperative pain after tibial fracture surgery: a double-blind controlled randomized clinical trial. *Anesth Pain Med.* **4**(3):e17350.

Peplow, P.V. *et al.* (2010) Laser photobiomodulation of wound healing: a review of experimental studies in mouse and rat animal models. *Photomed Laser Surg.* **28**(3):291–325.

Pryor, B. and Millis, D.L. (2015) Therapeutic laser in veterinary medicine. *Vet Clin North Am Small Anim Pract.* **45**(1):45–56.

Silveira, P.C. *et al.* (2007) Evaluation of mitochondrial respiratory chain activity in wound healing by low-level laser therapy. *J Photochem Photobiol B.* **86**(3):279–282.

Skopin, M.D. and Molitor, S.C. (2009) Effects of near-infrared laser exposure in a cellular model of wound healing. *Photodermatol Photoimmunol Photomed.* **25**(2):75–80.

Sprouse-Blum, A.S. *et al.* (2010) Understanding endorphins and their importance in pain management. *Hawaii Med J.* **69**(3):70–71.

Son, J. *et al.* (2012) Bone healing effects of diode laser (808 nm) on a rat tibial fracture model. *In Vivo.* **26**(4):703–709.

Takashi, K. (1988) Low level diode laser treatment for hematomas under grafted skin and its photobiological mechanisms. *Keio J Med.* **37**(4):415–428.

Tim, C.R. et al. (2014) Low-level laser therapy enhances the expression of osteogenic factors during bone repair in rats. *Lasers Med Sci.* **29**(1):147–156.

Wang, P. *et al.* (2014) Effects of low-level laser therapy on joint pain, synovitis, anabolic, and catabolic factors in a progressive osteoarthritis rabbit model. *Lasers Med Sci.* **29**(6):1875–1885.

10

Wounds

David S. Bradley

K-Laser USA, Oakdale, CA, USA

Introduction

Laser therapy for improved wound healing and other dermatologic conditions is one of the most studied and widely used applications of the technology. It was actually described as the founding concept behind laser therapy back in 1968, when Dr. Endre Mester was first experimenting with the laser's effect on recalcitrant cells that he implanted in rats. Though the proposed experiment was a failure, he observed that the implantation sites healed faster, and the hair grew back faster, on those rats that received laser exposure (Mester *et al.*, 1968).

Wound applications integrate all available laser parameters for optimal results. These include wavelength, delivery mode, and dosage. We will look at these factors and how to adjust them in order to obtain the best, most efficient, and safest clinical results. First, we need to briefly review the process of wound healing. Though a complete discussion of wound healing is not the subject of this text, some important points need to be highlighted.

Wound Healing

Wound healing is a multi-stage process. For optimal results, a well-orchestrated series of events needs to unfold, including clotting, inflammation, granulation tissue formation, collagen synthesis, epithelialization, and tissue remodeling. An inappropriate inflammatory response, poor angiogenesis, or defects in collagen production and differentiation can lead to delayed healing and an increased risk of infection (Meireles *et al.*, 2008).

Laser therapy aims to restore the normal biological function of injured or stressed cells. "Normalization" is the key word when it comes to laser therapy (Tuner and Hode, 2002). The cellular effects of photobiomodulation therapy (PBMT) can be classified as either primary effects, which are light-induced, or secondary effects,

which occur in response to the primary effects (Hawkins and Abrahamse, 2007).

In primary effects, a direct photochemical reaction occurs when photons emitted by the laser reach the mitochondria and membranes of cells (e.g., fibroblasts, keratinocytes, and endothelial cells) and the photonic energy is absorbed by endogenous chromophores (mitochondrial cytochromes, porphyrins, and flavoproteins) and converted into a chemical kinetic energy within the cells. This causes an improved efficiency of the respiratory chain within the mitochondria, due to changes in membrane permeability, improved signaling between mitochondria, nucleus, and cytosol, and increased oxidative metabolism, which enables more adenosine triphosphate (ATP) to be produced (Karu, 1989). In addition, reactive oxygen species (ROS) such as nitric oxide (NO) and superoxide dismutase (SOD) are produced, and there is a shift in the redox state.

Secondary effects lead to the amplification of the previously mentioned primary photoreactions. Calcium is released from the mitochondria into the cytoplasm with changes in intracellular calcium levels (Tuner and Hode, 2002), which stimulates cell metabolism and the regulation of the signaling pathways responsible for the events required for wound repair, such as cell migration, DNA and RNA synthesis, cell mitosis, protein secretion, and cell proliferation. A cascade of metabolic effects results in various physiological changes at the cellular level, such as activation of fibroblasts, macrophages, and lymphocytes, growth factor release, neurotransmitter release, vasodilation, collagen synthesis, and improvement of cell membrane permeability and the function of the Na^+/K^+ pump. Laser therapy has a positive effect on prostaglandin production, mediating neutrophil activation, lymphocyte accumulation, and other inflammatory effects. Increased metabolic activity increases oxygen and nutrient availability, leading to enhanced protein and enzyme production. These factors ultimately lead to normalization of cell function. They stimulate and

Laser Therapy in Veterinary Medicine: Photobiomodulation, First Edition. Edited by Ronald J. Riegel and John C. Godbold, Jr.
© 2017 John Wiley & Sons, Inc. Published 2017 by John Wiley & Sons, Inc.

accelerate cell reproduction and growth, leading to faster repair of damaged tissues and moderation of the inflammatory response. Concurrently, a sequence of cellular events provides analgesia (Hamblin and Demidova, 2006; Karu, 1989, 1999; Karu and Kolyakov, 2005; Martin, 2003; Peavy, 2002; Wray *et al.*, 1988).

In laboratory animals, biostimulation of the wound-healing process, as reported by several investigators, results in the stimulation of fibroblast proliferation, significant increases in re-epithelialization, increased collagen synthesis and granulation tissue formation, acceleration of wound closure, improved tensile strength of scars, and faster healing of burns (Calisto *et al.*, 2015; Gal *et al.*, 2006; Hodjati *et al.*, 2014). In rodent skin-wound models, laser therapy leads to earlier regression of the inflammatory phase, faster re-epithelization, and acceleration of the maturation phase. Production of growth factors increases, including vascular endothelial growth factor (VEGF), keratinocyte growth factor (KGF), transforming growth factor (TGF), and platelet-derived growth factor (PDGF) (Stadler *et al.*, 2001). The photochemical effects of near-infrared exposure on human fibroblast growth rates in an *in vitro* model of wound healing demonstrate that photobiomodulation (PBM), at appropriate exposure levels, accelerates cell growth (Skopin and Molitor, 2009).

There are a variety of cells integral to proper wound healing. Mast cells release histamine, which reacts with collagen and interleukin 4 (IL4) to stimulate fibroblasts to proliferate and migrate. New investigations show that skin mast cells modulate the inflammatory response in healing wounds, play a role in angiogenesis, and may participate in tissue remodeling in the late phase of wound healing. Recent evidence has shown that skin mast cells are important for the formation of granulation tissue and for the synthesis of collagen fibers at the edge of a wound (Vasheghani *et al.*, 2008).

Important processes that occur in wound healing are:

- Formation of a platelet- and fibrin-containing plug at the wound site.
- Invasion of the wound by neutrophils, monocytes, and macrophages.
- Proliferation and migration of keratinocytes from the wound edge to begin re-epithelization of the wound.
- Proliferation of fibroblasts at the dermal edge.
- Formation of granulation tissue, comprising fibroblasts, macrophages, lymphocytes, plasma cells, and an extracellular matrix (ECM) containing collagen fibers and macromolecular components such as glycoproteins, as well as the formation of new blood vessels.
- Maturation of granulation tissue and collagen fibers and vascularization of wound tissue.

The processes involved in inflammation, re-epithelization, granulation tissue, ECM formation, angiogenesis, and tissue remodeling are controlled by growth factors and cytokines produced by the cellular elements present in the wounds and in blood. Cytokines regulate inflammatory cells during the early stages of wound healing, and influence the gene expression and release of growth factors important in the proliferation and differentiation of cells and the synthesis of ECM. The presence of receptors or binding proteins for specific growth factors on cells is also important in determining cellular responses (Pavletic, 2010; Stadelman *et al.*, 1998).

Effects of Laser Therapy on Wound Healing

It is important to emphasize again that laser therapy normalizes cell function. It enables the cell to do its job better. This does not mean it makes normal cells super cells. It does not just ramp everything up or turn everything down. It allows the cell to do its job, which sometimes means doing nothing! *In vitro* studies demonstrate that part of a cell's normal function is to recognize normal cell-to-cell contact inhibition once cell cultures approach confluence (Martz and Steinberg, 1972). This is analogous, *in vivo*, to a healthy organism, which will regenerate healing tissue, but stop further growth when healing is complete. It is important to note that laser treatment accelerates normal healing and tissue regeneration without producing overgrowth or neoplastic transformation.

Laser therapy stimulates a better alignment and organization of collagen fibers. Collagen organization is important to the strength and elasticity of healing wounds (Doillon *et al.*, 1988). Similarly, there is a linear relationship between the tensile strength of a tendon and both the content and the arrangement of collagen fibers. In a study analyzing cutaneous wounds in the dorsum of Wistar rats, irradiated subjects showed increased collagen production and organization when compared to non-irradiated controls (Mendez *et al.*, 2004). PBM stimulates a more normal distribution of type I and III collagen during healing in wounds, as well as in tendons (Paraguassu *et al.*, 2014; Wood *et al.*, 2010).

As a general mechanism, enhancing blood flow and oxygenation to a diseased area will help tissue healing (Larkin *et al.*, 2012). The effect of laser light on blood flow is extended after the exposure to the light has finished. It is supported by an increased angiogenesis promoted by basic fibroblastic growth factor (FGF) and VEGF. These benefits in wound healing apply to clean surgical wounds, second-intention healing, graft and flap survival, and contaminated and infected wounds (Kubota 2002).

The increased oxygenation also helps with infections, since many pathogenic microorganisms grow poorly in an oxygen-rich environment. Laser therapy has other indirect effects that can help treat infection: it enhances macrophage function and modulates immune response and ROS production (Burger *et al.*, 2015).

There is also a potential direct effect on microorganisms. *In vitro* studies have not fully elucidated the underlying mechanisms of the antimicrobial effect and have provided different results. Most experiments seem to show a decreased microbial growth after exposure to laser light, including common pathogenic and opportunistic species such as *Staphylococcus aureus*, *Escherichia coli*, *Pseudomonas aeruginosa*, and *Candida albicans* (Redondo, 2015). It is important to realize that some bacteria show no effect, or even experience increased growth, from exposure to laser light. However, decreased microbial growth after laser therapy *in vivo* is almost universally accepted, and *in vivo* experiments (as well as case reports) have provided consistent and encouraging results to support laser use in infected tissues (Nussbaum *et al.*, 2003). In addition, these results seem to be consistent despite the different technical parameters encountered when comparing *in vivo* studies.

Due to the problem of increasing antibiotic resistance worldwide, focus has been directed on PBMT as a non-pharmacological antimicrobial tool. Laser therapy, using a dose of 5 J/cm^2 in both intact skin and wounds of rats infected with methicillin-resistant *S. aureus* (MRSA), has been shown to reduce bacterial proliferation (Silva *et al.*, 2013). In another animal study using rats, laser therapy showed promise as an adjunct or alternative to pharmacological agents in the treatment of osteomyelitis experimentally induced by MRSA (Kaya *et al.*, 2011).

Optimal Parameters for Laser Therapy

The variety of mechanisms behind the physiologic effects of laser therapy is becoming better understood every day. Certainly, there is still more to learn, but the question, "Does laser therapy work?" is no longer relevant. The more pertinent questions today, and where most laser research is now being focused, are how to optimize laser therapy and expand the applications of this remarkable modality. Let us review the parameters found in today's therapy lasers and their software, and discuss how they can be modified to enhance the clinical response. These parameters include wavelength, delivery mode, and dosage.

Wavelength

Wavelength is what actually determines the best function of any particular laser. Laser therapy works by a wavelength-specific form of PBM. Cellular chromophores within blood and tissue mitochondria absorb the

laser energy and a series of direct biochemical processes are stimulated or enhanced, along with a broad cascade of secondary and tertiary effects. The reason most therapy lasers now have the capability to produce more than one wavelength is because of our improved understanding of the direct photochemical effects that are produced when a photon of light is absorbed by specific chromophores within the body (Assis *et al.*, 2012; Emanet *et al.*, 2010; Joensen *et al.*, 2012; Longo *et al.*, 1987; Moriyama *et al.*, 2009).

The most important target chromophores are: melanin and other superficial chromophores, which absorb wavelengths in the visible red range (630–660 nm); water, which has a nice peak of absorption in the 970–980 nm range; hemoglobin, which has a broad absorption peak at 890–990 nm; and cytochrome c oxidase (CCO), which has a peak absorption at 790–830 nm (Anderson and Parrish, 1981).

The shorter wavelengths (630–660 nm) are absorbed more superficially and therefore do not have the ability to penetrate as readily as the longer wavelengths. These are very beneficial in wound healing (Al-Watban *et al.*, 2007). The wavelengths near the 970–980 nm range have a moderately increased absorption by water. This produces a mild warming effect in local tissues when higher-powered therapy lasers are used, and therefore creates a thermal gradient. Blood will tend to flow along thermal gradients from warm to cool or from higher pressure to lower pressure. This increases circulation in these areas. An important discovery is related to wavelengths in a range near 800 nm (750–830 nm). These are at the peak of absorption for the CCO enzyme. As a rate-limiting step in the conversion of oxygen to ATP within the electron transport cycle, CCO that has absorbed energy from a photon of light can accelerate the step to improve ATP production, along with production of NO.

As our understanding of basic photochemistry has expanded, therapy laser manufacturers have begun including more than one wavelength within a single device. Simultaneously delivering multiple wavelengths can give a synergistic effect and a wider range of treatment options, resulting in better clinical outcomes.

Delivery Mode

How laser light is delivered to the tissue has clinical significance. The delivery modes used in laser applications can be modified and tailored to optimize laser therapy across a broad range of applications and patient parameters. Laser light can be delivered in continuous-wave (CW), pulsed, or superpulsed modes.

If being pulsed, the pulse rate with which laser light is delivered can have differing physiologic effects on cell-tissue structures (Cheida *et al.*, 2002). Different tissue culture types respond differently to different pulse rates

(Karu *et al.*, 1997). In cell cultures, lower pulse rates and CW impart a better effect on pain-modulation processes, while higher frequencies have more anti-inflammatory and biostimulatory effects (Tuner and Hode, 2004). These *in vitro* effects in tissue cultures may not be as simple as the rate of pulsing: they might also include the time for which the laser is on versus off (Karu *et al.*, 1999).

The literature continues to show that adding pulse frequencies to treatment protocols may have an effect on overall long-term results. For example, pulsing may improve outcomes by mitigating the filtration effects of cutaneous melanin (Brondon, 2009). Another example is a 2009 study in a transgenic murine model, which demonstrated that different wavelengths and CW versus pulsed delivery mode resulted in different effects in an induced inflammatory process (Moriyama *et al.*, 2009). The importance of evaluating the effects of pulsing was addressed in a 2014 guest editorial in *Photomedicine and Laser Surgery*, in which it was noted, "The PW [pulsed] LLLT [low-level laser therapy] device has more laser (illumination) parameters, such as peak and average power outputs, pulse frequency, and pulse duration, than CW LLLT, all of which add to the medical applicability of this technique. It is assumed that by investigating different values of these parameters, researchers can select better protocols and achieve more satisfactory outcomes with PW LLLT devices than with CW LLLT devices" (Bayat, 2014).

A 2010 review analyzed relevant laser literature from 1970–2010 regarding the effects of pulsing versus CW in laser therapy. This review suggested that though CW light has been the gold standard, and has been used for all types of laser therapy application, pulsed light may be superior, particularly for wound healing and post-stroke management. As noted in the review, there is unfortunately no consensus on the very best pulsing parameters for specific diseases or pathologies, due to inconsistent reporting of parameters in studies. It is suggested that future researchers record all laser parameters in order to help determine optimal protocols for a wider variety of conditions (Hashmi *et al.*, 2010).

A recent unpublished study conducted by the International Centre for Genetic Engineering and Biotechnology (ICGEB) in Trieste, Italy showed a more consistent and prolonged stimulation of cellular ATP production using pulsed versus CW delivery modes (Ottaviani *et al.*, 2015). This study was done subsequent to several other studies from the University of Trieste illustrating the profound beneficial effects of laser therapy in resolving oral mucositis secondary to chemotherapy and radiation therapy in human patients with head and neck cancer (Chermetz *et al.*, 2014; Gobbo *et al.*, 2014; Ottaviani *et al.*, 2013).

Superpulse is another laser delivery mode that is available for some lasers, including some surgical, therapeutic,

and industrial lasers. Superpulsing in therapeutic lasers can mitigate the thermal and absorption effects of pigmented tissue. In theory, it may therefore improve penetration, and with proper parameters increase the number of photons that reach the target tissue. Data on depth of penetration using superpulsing with different wavelengths vary considerably, and more recent work challenges the notion (Anders and Wu, 2015; Joensen *et al.*, 2012).

It is very important to keep in mind the average power and the total joules per minute being delivered for effective results. Don't be misled by statements that suggest the peak power capability of a pulsing or superpulsing laser device results in an increased average power.

Another concept related to delivery mode is administering therapy in a contact or non-contact mode. Though in wound healing almost all treatments will be performed while not touching the tissue (non-contact mode), this is still an important concept to discuss (Enwemeka, 2009). Just to clarify, unless you are using a laser for surgical applications, no laser fiber directly touches the patient during laser therapy. All lasers transmit their energy through some configuration of a delivery handpiece. This is especially important in veterinary patients, because with many of the conditions that we treat (other than wounds), the laser energy is administered through the hair coat. In human treatments, clothing is removed. Hair can be just as big a barrier to laser energy as clothing, but if we had to shave all of our patients for every treatment it would greatly decrease client compliance. By using a delivery handpiece (and proper dosage), the hair can be displaced adequately to allow enough photons to reach our target tissue.

No study shows any delivery system or handpiece design is superior to any other. The most pertinent features of the delivery handpiece, therefore, are related to ease of use, cleaning and sanitization, durability, and adjustability. Since most wounds will probably have lost hair due to the inciting trauma, or be shaved as some part of the treatment process, the delivery handpiece just needs to be close to the area to be treated, and directed perpendicular to the tissue.

Dosage

The last parameter to discuss is dosage, and how it relates to the average power delivered by specific laser products. Dosage is one of the primary factors that will determine the success of laser therapy. It also seems to be one of the more confusing issues among those with whom I consult.

Let's start with some basic laser terminology:

- Power is the rate of delivery of energy and is measured in watts (W), where $1\,W = 1\,J/sec$.
- Energy is the total number of joules (J) delivered and is simply calculated by multiplying power (W) by time (sec).

- Irradiance (W/cm^2) is the amount of power (W) delivered to a specific area (cm^2).
- Fluence (J/cm^2) is the total amount of energy (J) delivered to a given area (cm^2).

Using simple math, it is always possible to accurately calculate the dosage (fluence) delivered to an area, whether you are holding the handpiece stationary or using a scanning technique. Most of the confusion in varying dosage recommendations does not come from the physics of laser energy delivery, but rather from ignoring the principles related to the optics of human tissue. The photons of laser light (or any light) are constantly scattered, reflected, and absorbed. The "decay" of the laser beam as it travels through tissue, which has a turbidity that can be calculated, must be considered when calculating the number of photons needed to elicit a direct photochemical effect on a structure that is not on the surface. The math behind this is too complicated to be described here, but it takes into account Beer's law and the Kubelka–Munk theory, which incorporates scatter coefficients, the absorption coefficients found in Boltzmann's equation, and other diffusion constants (Anderson and Parrish, 1981).

Power dictates the rate of delivery and is an important component when determining efficiency, efficacy, and safety. Being able to adjust the power should be one of the critical features looked for when deciding which therapy laser is best for you. If power is too high, with too many photons delivered too rapidly, especially to a very small area (high irradiance), then superficial tissue heating may occur. If power is too low, with too few photons delivered too slowly (very low irradiance), there will be too much absorption and scatter to allow the photons to saturate large volumes of deep tissue. If delivered at an appropriate irradiance, all the positive effects will be experienced safely. This can be tailored to properly stimulate small or superficial conditions, or for direct tissue stimulation of a large volume of tissue. The total energy (fluence) delivered to a tissue or body part will be a direct measure of the irradiance (power delivered per unit area) times the time of exposure.

Dosages listed and recommended in the literature range from 1 to $10 J/cm^2$ (or higher), depending on the size and depth of the lesion, the severity, and the chronicity (Al-Watban *et al.*, 2007; Hawkins and Abrahamse, 2007; Peplow *et al.*, 2010; Tuner and Hode, 2002). You will no longer see credible studies in the literature that do not list the dosage used.

A simple wound of 3×3 cm has an area of roughly $10 cm^2$. To deliver $1 J/cm^2$ requires delivery of $10 J$. With a 1 W laser, that takes 10 seconds. With a 500 mW laser, it takes 20 seconds. With a 5 mW laser, it takes 2000 seconds, or over 30 minutes.

The classification of lasers is dictated by ANSI Standards and relates to the maximum *average* laser output (ANSI, 2014). Maximum laser output is calculated by the total average power (J/sec), not a single burst or peak power. If you want to administer laser therapy to small patients and superficial wounds, as well as to larger patients and deep musculoskeletal or neurologic conditions, then a laser that has a broad range of power adjustability will give the best results on the widest range of conditions. Most high-power lasers can be turned down to 500 mW or less when needed for small patients, delicate tissue, or very superficial lesions.

Understanding the science and physics of laser–tissue interactions is just as important as understanding the physiology and biochemistry. As we increase our understanding, we can more accurately quantify minimum desired dosages, and lasers can then be preset to deliver these dosages safely and accurately in order to simplify treatments. Realize, though, that there is no perfect dosage. There are many patient variables that affect dose: coat length and color, skin color, hydration, vascularity, chronicity, severity, and even individual patient response. Minimum dosages can be calculated and preset for ease of use (see Boxes 10.1 and 10.2), but keep in mind two principles: (i) the only thing we can say for sure is that if

---

Box 10.1 Laser therapy dosage recommendations. Adapted from Hawkins and Abrahamse (2007) and Peplow *et al.* (2010).

Acute Superficial Wounds or "Hot" Inflammatory Conditions
$1–4 J/cm^2$
Chronic Superficial Conditions or Chronic Wounds
$4–30 J/cm^2$
Acute Superficial Pain or Injury
$2–4 J/cm^2$
Acute Deep Pain or Injury
$4–8 J/cm^2$
Chronic Deep Pain or Injury
$6–20 J/cm^2$

Box 10.2 Pulse frequency recommendations based on *in vitro* cell studies (Tuner Hode, 2002).

Pain/Neuralgia
2–20 Hz or CW
Edema/Swelling
1000 Hz
General Stimulation
500 Hz
Inflammation
5000 Hz
Infection
10 000 Hz

you give too little a dosage, you will produce little to no response; and (ii) there is a very wide margin of safety.

Basic Principles of Laser Wound Therapy

Laser therapy may seem a very complicated proposition. Though the principles behind it can be very intricate, they are well understood. More important is that all this information is being used to produce very user-friendly laser products. The software protocols already set up in most therapeutic lasers simplify all parameters in an easy-to-use "point-and-shoot" technique. Because of the wide margin of safety, laser therapy can be instituted quickly and easily. It can and should be delegated to the veterinary staff for the most efficient and economic benefits. Initial training is essential, and continuing education is necessary to fully realize the benefits of laser therapy.

Treatment Techniques

There are two basic delivery methods for laser therapy: direct contact of the delivery handpiece with the tissue, and delivery with the handpiece not in contact with the tissue. Direct contact is rarely used for wound therapy, but is the technique of choice when treating most non-wound conditions. It can be done on light-coated, short-haired, or shaved patients (Enwemeka, 2009). It is especially important to help separate hairs on long-coated animals. You can use your other hand to do this, while monitoring for superficial warmth.

Whether in contact with the tissue or not, treat in a grid pattern or use a scanning technique. Treat the area of interest, as well as a border of surrounding healthy tissue. Treatment can be administered in conjunction with stretching or range-of-motion movement.

A scanning delivery technique in contact or non-contact mode employs a slow, steady movement of the laser handpiece in a pattern that uniformly covers the desired treatment area. This could be large, even, parallel strokes, small expanding circles, large concentric circles, or any pattern that thoroughly covers the area. The area can be treated in a methodical process with repeat passages until the total calculated dosage is delivered. Move at a rate that is not too slow or too fast, and is comfortable for the patient. About 3 cm/sec is adequate.

The thermal effect of laser therapy varies with coat color and skin pigmentation. Darker colors absorb more. If, due to heavy pigmentation and unexpected tissue warming, you notice patient sensitivity, as evidenced by

a withdrawal response or aversion reactions, try using the following techniques:

- Increase hand speed.
- Increase distance between the laser handpiece and the patient.
- Use a larger-diameter spot size (decrease the power density).
- Decrease the power (the time must be increased to maintain proper dosage).

A grid-pattern delivery technique involves holding the handpiece in a fixed spot for 1–3 seconds then moving it in a uniform pattern every 1–3 seconds to cover the entire area. It is important to try not to immediately overlap with this technique.

Non-contact delivery is how most wounds will be treated. This is usually done using a scanning technique. Scan 1–2 cm from the surface with slow passage over the affected area. This delivery is used for open wounds or any area with discharge or exudates. It is also used on very painful or sensitive areas. Use the other hand to separate hair to aid in penetration, if needed.

Always apply the laser to a 2–5 cm border of healthy tissue surrounding the area of greatest concern. Include any other structures that may be injured or are adding stress to the injured area. If treating for edema, swelling, ischemia, or large and severe wounds, start treating proximal and work distal. Laser the major draining lymph nodes in the axilla or groin and associated lymphatic and blood supply.

Some wounds will only need one to three treatments to help stimulate faster, better healing. Most will need an initial phase of at least six. It is always warranted to begin laser therapy as soon as possible after the initial injury. Acute injuries and wounds should be treated daily for 2–5 days, then every other day for three to five treatments. In very severe trauma or compromised tissues, treating twice daily for the first 1–2 days may be beneficial. If further treatment is needed, continue twice weekly (or at least weekly) until the condition is resolved or plateaus.

Chronic conditions and wounds can initially be treated on an every-other-day basis for the first three to five treatments. Then continue twice weekly (or at least weekly) until the condition is healed, has resolved, or plateaus. Some conditions with underlying factors (allergies, autoimmune disorders, immunocompromised patients, or repetitive stress or trauma) will need ongoing maintenance treatments at least monthly. Shorter intervals may be warranted and are perfectly safe if owner compliance allows.

Laser therapy effects are cumulative. Observable response, or the duration of response, should increase with each treatment until the condition is healed or plateaus. Laser therapy has a wide margin of safety. It is prudent to start with a more conservative dosage with acute or "hot" lesions. Injured tissue is very responsive to laser therapy. Most patients will show at least a mild positive response within the first couple treatments. If a positive response is not noted within three or four treatments with a standard protocol, re-evaluate the condition, diagnosis, or treatment protocol. If the diagnosis is correct and other underlying contributing factors are being addressed, make sure you are delivering at least the minimum recommended dose. You can then begin to increase the delivered dosage by 25–50% per treatment until a positive response is being noted. Do this by adjusting the time first and the power second, if the time is becoming too prolonged (Lanzafame *et al.*, 2007).

Wound Classification and Treatment

The types of wound to be discussed will start with the simplest acute clean wounds and progress to the more extensive, infected, and chronic wounds. This discussion will encompass postoperative wounds, minor abrasions, pressure sores and ulcers, burns, degloving injuries, grafts, and flaps. The same principles apply whether the wound was caused by surgical intervention, external trauma, self-trauma, thermal injury, ischemic injury, tissue toxins, or envenomation. Any underlying or predisposing pathology or repetitive trauma needs to be addressed. Laser therapy will almost always be an adjunct treatment, with other standard protocols being implemented simultaneously. These will include: proper cleaning, debriding, lavage, topical treatments, dressing, systemic therapies, Elizabethan collars or other preventive mechanisms, wraps, and bandages. It is important to note that laser therapy will not penetrate wraps or bandage material of any kind. If laser therapy is warranted more frequently than a bandage will be changed, consideration must be made when applying the bandage. A window that can be easily unwrapped and re-wrapped without disrupting the integrity of the bandage or support should be included over the area to be treated. When treating large wounds or extremely compromised or infected tissue, it is recommend to always start by treating the vasculature and lymphatic vessels proximal or central to the area and then progress distally.

Surgical Incisions and Clean Wounds

Simple, clean wounds and postoperative incisions in healthy patients will benefit from a single laser therapy treatment administered during recovery. If the patient is staying overnight, a second treatment may be administered the following day. Larger incisions, incisions with undue tension or stress on them, incisions near or involving compromised tissue, and incisions in older or

debilitated patients should all receive a minimum of three treatments. Keep in mind the general principles of wound treatment and be sure to include a margin of healthy tissue surrounding the incision as part of the treatment area. Though cases of acute pyotraumatic dermatitis (hot spots) are usually infected, they can be included in this category and treated in a similar fashion.

Measure the incision or wound area and the surrounding margin of healthy tissue. This margin may be as small as 1 cm for wounds on very small animals or 3 cm or more for large or severe wounds. Deliver a starting dosage of $2-4 \, \text{J/cm}^2$. Treat daily for 2–3 days if possible, then every other day.

Figure 10.1 shows sibling patients. These two dogs were from the same breeder, owned by the same person, and both had an ovariohysterectomy on the same day, performed by the same surgeon. The patient on the left did not receive laser therapy postoperatively. The patient on the right received one laser therapy treatment immediately postoperatively. The patients were otherwise not managed differently. There is an observable reduction in the tissue swelling and reaction to the sutures in the laser-treated incision. There also appears to be less papular and macular reaction in the surrounding skin. Using laser therapy will not guarantee that your patients never experience postoperative incisional complications or reactions, but it will decrease the incidence and severity of these reactions.

Chronic, Granulomatous, and Infected Wounds

Chronic, granulomatous, and infected wounds will often require a prolonged and aggressive treatment regimen (Figure 10.2). It is recommended to start with daily treatments, along with standard adjunct therapies. Often, very high dosages of laser therapy will be needed to resolve these lesions. If the wound is not progressing or stalls, do not hesitate to increase the dosage significantly based on the guidelines in Box 10.1. With consistent treatment, a high number of these problems can be cured. It is important to persevere and continue all measures until complete resolution.

Measure the incision or wound area and the surrounding margin of healthy tissue. This margin may be as small as 1 cm for wounds on very small animals or 3 cm or more on large or severe wounds. Deliver a starting dosage of $4-6 \, \text{J/cm}^2$. Treat daily for 2–5 days if possible, then every other day. If no improvement is noted within the first two to four treatments, start increasing the dosage (joules) by 25–50% per treatment until a positive response is being noted. Do this by first adjusting the treatment time, then, if the treatment time is becoming too long, adjusting the power up. In very large wounds such as degloving injuries or lick granulomas, you can

Figure 10.1 Postoperative ovariohysterectomy incisions. The patient on the left did not receive laser therapy postoperatively. The patient on the right did receive laser therapy immediately postoperatively. Images courtesy of Dr. Susan Kelleher.

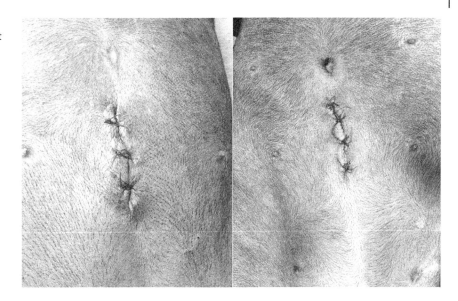

Figure 10.2 Chronic granulomatous lesion on the front paw of a leopard at a rescue sanctuary. Multiple other therapies, along with environmental enrichment, had been attempted, with no success at reducing continued self-trauma. Laser therapy was instituted (left) and improvement was noted (right).

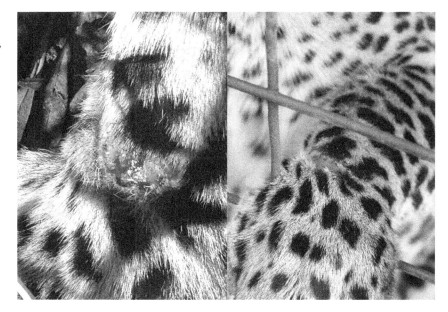

decrease treatment intervals to twice weekly once the wound is showing strong positive clinical response, usually after 10–20 days.

Traumatic Wounds and Burns

Traumatic wounds encompass a wide range of potential complicating factors. Many traumatic wounds will appear worse several days after the incident. This is due to the unseen damage from crushing and pressure injuries or from thermal insults. It can also be a result of disruption to the integrity of the blood supply. Ongoing damage due to a tissue toxin such as snake or insect envenomation will also result in delayed onset of the full extent of tissue damage. To improve results, these possibilities should be anticipated during initial evaluation. Proper laser therapy protocols should be utilized to treat the wider margin of potential injury, as well as the vasculature supplying or draining the injured area (Kovacs, 2015).

Measure the wound area and the surrounding margin of healthy tissue. As with other types of wound, this margin may be as small as 1 cm for wounds on very small animals or 3 cm or more on large or severe wounds. For burns, it is recommended to start with low power initially, and only about 2 J/cm^2. For all other traumatic wounds, plan on delivering a starting dosage of 4–6 J/cm^2. Treat daily for 2–3 days if possible, then every other day. If no improvement is noted within the first two to four treatments, start increasing the dosage (joules) by 25–50% per treatment until a positive response is being noted. Do this by first adjusting the treatment time, then,

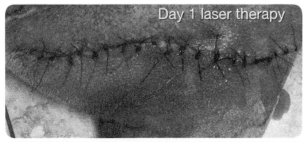

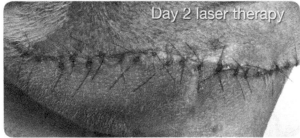

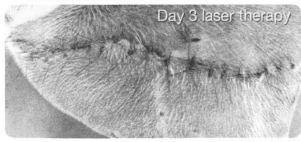

Figure 10.3 Soft-tissue wound prior to laser therapy (top), and 1 (middle) and 2 (bottom) days after starting laser therapy. Images courtesy of Dr. Boaz Man.

if the treatment time is becoming too long, start adjusting the power upwards. In very large or severe wounds, you can decrease treatment intervals to twice weekly once the wound is showing strong positive clinical response, usually after 10–20 days.

Figure 10.3 shows a patient that had been attacked by another dog with severe bite wounds. It had initial treatment and repair at an emergency facility 4 days earlier. The picture on top shows the wounds with severe swelling, bruising, and copious drainage of serosanguinous fluid. Laser therapy treatment was instituted daily for 3 days. Antibiotics were continued, but no other therapy was used. The swelling, bruising, and discharge improved measurably over the next 2 days.

Figure 10.4 shows a patient with a substantial sloughing of tissue 7 days after sustaining fight wounds over the left hip region. Laser therapy was initiated along with standard management appropriate for an open wound healing by second intention. Figure 10.5 shows the healing at 28 and 56 days.

Degloving Injuries

Degloving injuries often require weeks of therapy to heal. PBMT will improve the granulation bed, help prevent infection, and improve the rate and quality of epithelialization. Regular laser therapy treatments, along with proper bandaging and other management protocols, will greatly improve the success of full coverage, with minimal scarring. If tissue grafts or flaps are employed, laser therapy will enhance the survival and proliferation of the grafted tissue and heal the donor sites. Treat the entire area, as well as a generous margin of healthy tissue surrounding the denuded area. Stimulation of the contributing vasculature will

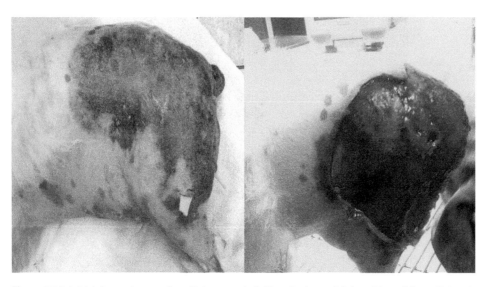

Figure 10.4 Initial tissue changes from fight wounds (left) and substantial sloughing of tissue 7 days later (right). Images courtesy of Dr. Daniel M. Core.

Figure 10.5 Progression of healing of the wound in Figure 10.4 at days 28 (left) and 56 (right) following standard open-wound management and laser therapy. Images courtesy of Dr. Daniel M. Core.

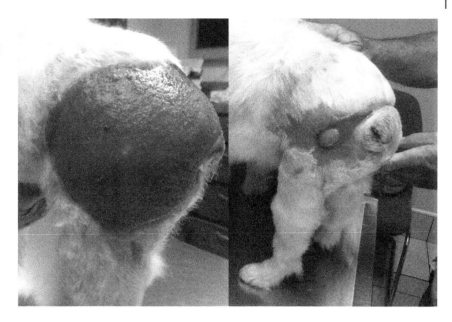

Figure 10.6 Degloving injury to the medial aspect of the distal foreleg at presentation (left), at 7 days (middle), and at 14 days (right). Images courtesy of Dr. Azeddine Menighed and Sandy Skouras, RVT.

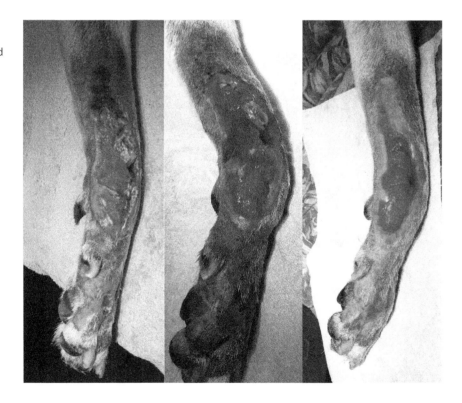

be beneficial to tissue proliferation and graft survival. This can be accomplished by applying laser energy to the proximal or central blood supply. Start at the axilla or groin, or at least one joint above the area of injury.

Deliver a starting dosage of 4–6 J/cm^2. Treat daily for 2–3 days if possible, then every other day. If no improvement is noted within the first two to four treatments, start increasing the dose by 25–50% per treatment until a positive response is being noted. Do this by first adjusting the treatment time, then, if the treatment time is becoming too long, start adjusting the power upwards. In very large or severe wounds, you can decrease treatment intervals to twice weekly once the wound is showing strong positive clinical response, usually after 10–20 days.

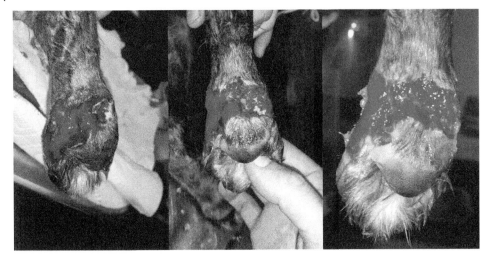

Figure 10.7 Traumatic wound that has been closed and dehisced (left). Traditional open-wound management and laser therapy were instituted. Rapid improvement was noted 1 (center) and 4 (right) days later, with the formation of a healthy granulation bed and significant epithelial migration. Images courtesy of Dr. Seth Narwold.

Figure 10.6 shows a degloving injury to the distal medial aspect of the left front limb of a canine patient. There was also rupture and avulsion of the extensor carpi radialis tendon. Laser therapy was instituted after proper cleaning. Topical dressing with bandaging and a splint were applied. The progression of a healthy wound bed and rapid epithelial migration in the early stages are evident in the images. This wound healed completely within 6 weeks. The carpal joint also regained full strength and integrity.

Vasculitis and Ischemia

Some wounds and tissue damage result from vasculitis or vascular damage and lead to tissue ischemia. This may have a number of different etiologies, including infections, autoimmune disease, trauma, vascular occlusion, clotting disorders, and cardiovascular disease (CVD). Alternatively, the etiology may be idiopathic. Of course, the underlying pathology and contributing factors must be addressed with proper medications. Laser therapy is indicated, since it improves blood flow and circulation via the mechanisms discussed earlier: thermal gradients, vasodilation, and angiogenesis (Kubota, 2002). Laser therapy will also help to modulate the inflammatory response and will have a positive immunomodulating effect. Treat the affected area and the entire vascular branch involved. It is always recommended to start centrally and work peripherally.

Measure the wound area and the surrounding margin of healthy tissue. Deliver a starting dosage of $4–6\,\mathrm{J/cm^2}$. Treat daily for 2–3 days if possible, then every other day. If no improvement is noted within the first

two to four treatments, start increasing the dose (joules) by 25–50% per treatment until a positive response is being noted. In very large or severe wounds, you can decrease treatment intervals to twice weekly once the wound is showing strong positive clinical response, usually after 10–20 days.

Figure 10.7 shows the early stages of healing in a fence trauma wound that devitalized and dehisced due to ischemia. The wound was initially debrided and sutured upon presentation. Due to the initial trauma and vascular compromise, the wound dehisced 5 days later. After cleaning and further debriding, laser therapy was instituted. The figure shows a rapid improvement, with the formation of a healthy granulation bed and improved epithelial margins. The wound progressed satisfactorily and was completely healed in 3 weeks.

Autoimmune and Allergic Conditions

Many autoimmune diseases have a dermatologic component as their primary clinical complaint, or as part of the disease complex. Allergic reactions often manifest as a dermatologic problem. Systemic therapy is always warranted to help regulate the immune system, and laser therapy can be used to mitigate the local dermatologic effects. Other topical and immunomodulating treatments should be used in conjunction with laser therapy (Gobbo *et al.*, 2012).

Deliver a starting dosage of $4–6\,\mathrm{J/cm^2}$. These conditions can improve or resolve completely, but when a response is noted, the underlying allergy or immune system dysfunction has not been corrected. Therefore, two options for ongoing treatment are recommended: a

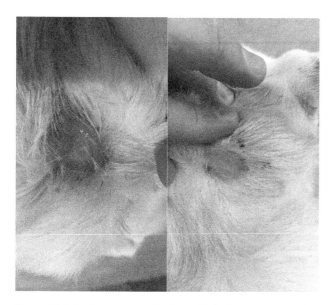

Figure 10.8 Acute pyotraumatic dermatitis lesion on presentation (left) and after therapy laser treatment (right). Images courtesy of Claus Walther.

routine prophylactic treatment can be performed every 2–4 weeks, depending on patient response; or the owner can be counseled to be vigilant in monitoring for any signs of recurrence – at the first sign of a flare-up, start medications and laser therapy to suppress the reaction and minimize the length and severity of outbreak.

Figure 10.8 shows the immediate anti-inflammatory effects that a laser can provide to an acute pyotraumatic dermatitis lesion.

Conclusion

Laser therapy can be a tremendous adjunct to your armamentarium for wound therapy (Hopkins *et al.*, 2004). When used appropriately, it can help both acute and chronic wounds heal more efficiently, with fewer complications. Keep in mind all the parameters and principles needed for optimal results, and your success rate will continue to grow.

References

Al-Watban, F.A.H. *et al.* (2007) Low-level laser therapy enhances wound healing in diabetic rats: a comparison of different lasers. *Photmed Laser Surg.* **25**(2):72–77.

Anders, J.J. and Wu, X. (2015) Comparison of light penetration of 810 nm and 904 nm wavelength light in anesthetized rats. *Lasers Med Sci.* **30**(8):2041.

Anderson, R.R. and Parrish, J.A. (1981) The optics of human skin. *J Invest Dermatol.* **77**(1):13–19.

ANSI. (2014) *American National Standard for Safe Use of Lasers. ANSI Z136.1 – 2014.* American National Standards Institute, Washington, DC.

Assis, L. *et al.* (2012) Low-level laser therapy (808 nm) reduces inflammatory response and oxidative stress in rat tibialis anterior muscle after cryolesion. *Lasers Surg Med.* **44**(9):726–735.

Bayat, M. (2014) The necessity for increased attention to pulsed low-level laser therapy. *Photomed Laser Surg.* **32**(8):1–2.

Brondon, P. (2009) Pulsing influences photoradiation outcomes in cell culture. *Lasers Surg Med.* **41**(3):222–226.

Burger, E. *et al.* (2015) Low-level laser therapy to the mouse femur enhances the fungicidal response of neutrophils against *Paracoccidioides brasiliensis. PLoS Negl Trop Dis.* **9**(2):e0003541.

Calisto, F.C. *et al.* (2015) Use of low-power laser to assist the healing of traumatic wounds. *Acta Cir Bras.* **30**(3):204–208.

Cheida, A.A. *et al.* (2002) Resonance response of cell tissue structures to impulse frequency of infrared laser radiation of low intensity. *Vopr Kurortol Fizioter Lech Fiz Kult.* **6**:33–35.

Chermetz M. *et al.* (2014) Class IV laser therapy as treatment for chemotherapy-induced oral mucositis in onco-haematological paediatric patients: a prospective study. *Int J Paediatr Dent.* **6**:441–449.

Doillon, C.J. *et al.* (1988) Relationship between mechanical properties and collagen structure of closed and open wounds. *J Biomech Eng.* **110**(4):352–356.

Emanet, S. K. *et al.* (2010) Investigation of the effect of GaAs laser therapy on lateral epicondylitis. *Photomed Laser Surg.* **28**(3):397–403.

Enwemeka, C.S. (2009) Intricacies of dose in laser phototherapy for tissue repair and pain relief. *Photomed Laser Surg.* **3**:387–393.

Gal, P. *et al.* (2006) Histological assessment of the effect of laser irradiation on skin wound healing in rats. *Photomed Laser Surg.* **24**(4):480–488.

Gobbo, M. *et al.* (2012) Acneifrom rash due to epidermal growth factor receptor inhibitors: high-level laser therapy as an innovative approach. *Lasers Med Sci.* **27**(5):1085–1090.

Gobbo M. *et al.* (2014) Evaluation of nutritional status in head and neck radio-treated patients affected by oral mucositis: efficacy of class IV laser therapy. *Support Care Cancer.* **7**:1851–1856.

Hamblin, M.R. and Demidova, T.N. (2006) Mechanisms of low level light therapy. *Proc of SPIE.* **6140**(612001):1–12.

Hashmi, J. *et al.* (2010) Effect of pulsing in low-level light therapy. *Lasers Surg Med.* **42**(6):450–466.

Hawkins, D. and Abrahamse, H. (2007) Phototherapy – a treatment modality for wound healing and pain relief. *African J Biomed Res.* **10**:99–109.

Hodjati, H. *et al.* (2014) Low-level laser therapy: an experimental design for wound management: a case-controlled study in rabbit model. *J Cutan Aesthet Surg.* **7**(1):14–17.

Hopkins, T. J. *et al.* (2004) Low-level laser therapy facilitates superficial wound healing in humans: a triple-blind, sham-controlled study. *J Ath Train.* **39**(3):223–229.

Joensen, J. *et al.* (2012) Skin penetration and time-profiles for continuous 810nm and superpulsed 904nm lasers in a rat model. *Photomed Laser Surg.* **30**(12):688–694.

Karu, T. (1989) *Photobiology of Low Power Laser Therapy.* Harwood Academic Publishers, London.

Karu, T. (1999) Primary and secondary mechanisms of action of visible to near-IR radiation on cells. *J Photochem Photobiol B.* **49**(1):1–17.

Karu, T. and Kolyakov S.F. (2005) Exact action spectra for cellular responses relevant to phototherapy. *Photomed Laser Surg.* **23**(4):355–361.

Karu, T. *et al.* (1997) Nonmonotomic behavior of the dose dependence of the radiation effect on cells in vitro exposed to pulsed laser radiation at 820 nm. *Lasers Surg Med.* **21**(5):485–492.

Karu, T. *et al.* (1999) Studies into the action specifics of a pulsed GaAlAS laser (820 nm) on a cell culture. *Lasers Life Sci.* **9**:211–219.

Kaya, G.Ş. *et al.* (2011) The use of 808-nm light therapy to treat experimental chronic osteomyelitis induced in rats by methicillin-resistant *Staphylococcus aureus.* *Photomed Laser Surg.* **29**(6):405–412.

Kovacs, K. (2015) Low Level Laser Therapy of Serious Wounds of Dogs. Poster presentation. ASLMS Annual Meeting. April 24–26, 2015. Orlando, FL.

Kubota, J. (2002) Effects of diode laser therapy on blood flow in axial pattern flaps in the rat model. *Lasers Med Sci.* **17**(3):146–153.

Lanzafame, R.J. *et al.* (2007) Reciprocity of exposure time and irradiance on energy density during photoradiation on wound healing in a murine pressure ulcer model. *Lasers in Surg Med.* **39**(6):534–542.

Larkin, K.A. *et al.* (2012) Limb blood flow after class 4 laser therapy. *J Ath Train.* **47**(2):178–183.

Longo, L. *et al.* (1987) Effects of diode-laser silver arsenide-aluminum (Ga-Al-As) 904 nm on healing of experimental wounds. *Lasers Surg Med.* **7**(5):444–447.

Martin, R. (2003) Laser accelerated inflammation/pain reduction and healing. *Practical Pain Management.* **3**(6):20–25.

Martz, E. and Steinberg, M.S. (1972) The role of cell-cell contact in "contact" inhibition of cell division: a review and new evidence. *J Cell Physio.* **79**(2):189–210.

Meireles, G.C. *et al.* (2008) Effectiveness of laser photobiomodulation at 660 or 780 nanometers on the repair of third-degree burns in diabetic rats. *Photomed Laser Surg.* **26**(1):47–54.

Mendez, T.M. *et al.* (2004) Dose and wavelength of laser light have influence on the repair of cutaneous wounds. *J Clin Laser Med Surg.* **22**(1):19–25.

Mester, E. *et al.* (1968) The effect of laser beams on the growth of hair in mice. *Radiobiol Radiother (Berl).* **9**(5):621–626.

Moriyama, Y. *et al.* (2009) In vivo effects of low level laser therapy on inducible nitric oxide synthase. *Lasers Surg Med.* **41**(3):227–231.

Nussbaum, E.L. *et al.* (2003) Effects of low-level laser therapy (LLLT) of 810 nm upon in vitro growth of bacteria: relevance of irradiance and radiant exposure. *J Clin Laser Med Surg.* **21**(5):283–290.

Ottaviani G. *et al.* (2013) Effect of class IV laser therapy on chemotherapy-induced oral mucositis: a clinical and experimental study. *Am J Pathol.* **183**(6): 1747–1757.

Ottaviani, G. *et al.* (2015) Study on Human Skin Fibroblasts and Data Related to ATP Content after Laser Exposure Compared to a Control Group. International Centre for Genetic Engineering and Biotechnology and the University of Trieste. Unpublished.

Paraguassu, G. *et al.* (2014) Effect of laser phototherapy (660nm) on type I and III collagen expression during wound healing in hypothyroid rats: an immunohistochemical study in a rodent model. *Photomed Laser Surg.* **32**(5):281–288.

Pavletic, M.M. (2010) *Basic Principles of Wound Healing. Atlas of Small Animal Wound Management and Reconstructive Surgery*, 3 edn., pp. 18–28. Wiley-Blackwell, Hoboken, NJ.

Peavy G.M. (2002) Lasers and laser-tissue interaction. *Vet Clin Small Anim.* **32**(3):517–534.

Peplow, P.V. *et al.* (2010) Laser photobiomodulation of wound healing: a review of experimental studies in mouse and rat animal models. *Photomed Laser Surg.* **28**(3):291–325.

Redondo, M.S. (2015) Laser therapy approach to wound healing in dogs. Available from: http://www.vettimes. co.uk/article/laser-therapy-approach-to-wound-healing-in-dogs/(accessed November 30, 2016).

Silva, D.C. *et al.* (2013) Low level laser therapy (AlGaInP) applied at 5J/cm2 reduces the proliferation of *Staphylococcus aureus* MRSA in infected wounds and intact skin of rats. *An Bras Dermatol.* **88**(1): 50–55.

Skopin, M.D. and Molitor, S.C. (2009) Effects of near-infrared laser exposure in a cellular model of wound healing. *Photodermatol Photoimmunol Photomed.* **25**(2):75–80.

Stadelman, W.K. *et al.* (1998) Physiology and healing dynamics of chronic cutaneous wounds. *Am J Surg.* **176**(2A Suppl.):26S–38S.

Stadler, I. *et al.* (2001) 830-nm irradiation increases the wound tensile strength in a diabetic murine model. *Lasers Surg Med.* **28**(3):220–226.

Tuner J. and Hode L. (2002) Some basic laser physics. In: *Laser Therapy – Clinical Practice and Scientific Background*, pp. 12, 21–22. Prima Books AB, Grängesberg.

Tuner J. and Hode L. (2004) *The Laser Therapy Handbook*, pp. 78–80. Prima Books AB, New York.

Vasheghani, M.M. *et al.* (2008) Effect of low-level light therapy on mast cells in second-degree burns in rats. *Photomed Laser Surg.* **26**(1):1–5.

Wood, V.T. *et al.* (2010) Collagen changes and realignment induced by low-level laser therapy and low-intensity ultrasound in the calcaneal tendon. *Lasers Med Surg.* **42**(6):559–565.

Wray, S. *et al.* (1988) Characterization of the near infrared absorption spectra of cytochrome aa3 and haemoglobin for the non-invasive monitoring of cerebral oxygenation. *Biochimica et Biophysica Acta.* **933**(1):184–192.

11

Dermatological and Non-musculoskeletal Soft-Tissue Conditions

Daniel M. Core[1] and John C. Godbold, Jr.[2]

[1] Airline Animal Health and Surgery Center, Bossier City, LA, USA
[2] Stonehaven Veterinary Consulting, Jackson, TN, USA

Introduction

Early use of therapy lasers in veterinary medicine focused on the treatment of musculoskeletal disorders. The clinical success of veterinary practitioners treating musculoskeletal disorders with laser therapy (photobiomodulation therapy, PBMT) mirrors the evidence-based data being published about similar responses in animal-model studies and clinical trials with human patients (Assis *et al.*, 2016; Bjordal *et al.*, 2008; Chow *et al.*, 2009; de Carvalho *et al.*, 2016; Jang and Lee 2012). As veterinarians have grown confident in the successful application of PBMT to the musculoskeletal system, they have begun to treat conditions involving other organ systems. Wounds and other skin and soft-tissue conditions are commonly-used experimental models for ongoing research into the effects of photobiomodulation (PBM) (Calisto *et al.*, 2015; Hodjati *et al.*, 2014; Kovacs, 2015; Kuffler, 2016). Laser therapy has now become a standard of care for many practices in the treatment of many conditions involving the skin and other non-musculoskeletal soft tissues. Not surprisingly, the current experience of practitioners treating these disorders mirrors evidence being published (Avci *et al.*, 2013; Peplow *et al.*, 2010).

Skin makes up 12–24% of the total body weight and is the largest organ of the body. Dermatological complaints are the number one reason patients are presented for small-animal consultations (Hill *et al.*, 2006). Skin disorders, including ear problems, skin allergies, and pyoderma, are the top reasons for insurance claims in dogs, and number five in cats (PRNewswire, 2015). Patients with disorders of the skin and other non-musculoskeletal soft tissues thus make up a significant number of those that are candidates for laser therapy. In practices that are fully utilizing the capabilities of a therapeutic laser, they should represent a significant percentage of the overall number of cases treated with PBMT.

This chapter will focus on the most common conditions involving dermatological and non-musculoskeletal soft-tissue conditions for which laser therapy is indicated, with the exclusion of traumatic wounds. Chapter 10 addresses wounds, wound healing, and the important role laser therapy plays in managing wounds of all types.

Laser therapy is indicated for virtually any condition that requires healing, reduction of pain, modulation of inflammation, acceleration of healing, and restoration of function (Chung *et al.*, 2012). It is compatible with traditional protocols for the treatment of skin and soft-tissue disorders, is non-invasive, and has minimal side effects if used properly. The complex mechanisms by which PBMT exerts these effects are discussed in detail in Chapter 5. This chapter will focus on the practical clinical application of PBMT in common, everyday conditions affecting dermatological and non-musculoskeletal soft tissues.

Acral Lick Dermatitis

Acral lick dermatitis, also known as lick granuloma, acral pruritic nodule, or canine neurodermatitis, is a common skin disorder in dogs. The lesions are the result of obsessive self-licking. The licking is a stereotypic behavior, a pattern of repetitive licking, repeated without variation, without any apparent purpose (Knol and Wisselink, 1996).

Acral lick dermatitis usually begins as an area of inflamed alopecia. As the licking continues, the lesion increases in size and becomes thickened, and secondary bacterial infections are common. Acral lick dermatitis lesions can become deeply ulcerated and can range in size from small lesions a few centimeters in diameter to large masses. Lesions most commonly occur in the distal, dorsal surface of the fore and hind legs, but can occasionally occur on the flank and near the tail base (Ackerman, 2008a).

The etiology of acral lick dermatitis is not completely understood but is thought to be multifactorial. Potential causes include atopy, food allergy, bacterial folliculitis, behavior disorders, boredom, foreign-body penetration, local trauma, underlying musculoskeletal disorder, and peripheral neuropathy (Ackerman, 2008a; Rosychuk, 2011). Those individuals with behavioral- or psychogenic-induced acral lick dermatitis may have other accompanying behavioral disorders, such as separation anxiety or storm anxiety. Canine acral lick dermatitis has served as an animal model of obsessive–compulsive disorder (OCD) (Rapoport *et al.*, 1992). Secondary bacterial infections are common, with a 50% incidence of multi-drug-resistant organisms (Shumaker *et al.*, 2008).

Acral lick dermatitis is best managed with a multimodal therapeutic protocol. Treatment should be preceded by detailed diagnostics, including radiography, to try to determine the etiology. Extended use of an appropriate antibiotic based on culture and sensitivity is required, since lesions usually develop a deep pyoderma component with micro-abscesses and fistulas. Allergy testing and treatment with hyposensitization, avoidance, and anti-inflammatory drugs such as corticosteroids are often warranted. Bandages, Elizabethan collars, and leggings can be beneficial in limiting patient access to the lesions. Behavioral modification with medications, therapy, and change of environment can be helpful in those individuals suspected of having a behavioral etiology.

Laser therapy for acral lick dermatitis is most appropriately added to other forms of therapy. Practitioner experience indicates these dense, complex lesions require higher doses of laser therapy than are used for most conditions, and that treatment is required over an extended period of time. Laser settings that deliver $30–40\,J/cm^2$ are recommended. Treatment with the delivery handpiece in contact with the lesion will increase photon penetration into the tissue (Enwemeka, 2009).

Lesions should be treated through an induction phase, every other day or twice a week, with treatments coinciding with bandage changes. Note that laser therapy cannot be administered through a bandage: photons are absorbed and scattered by bandaging materials, resulting in an unpredictable dose reaching the target tissue.

Once a clinical response has been noted, treatment frequency can be reduced, through a transition phase. A complete resolution of acral lick dermatitis is not always possible. Lesions that persist should continue to be treated indefinitely, with maintenance-phase treatments every 3–4 weeks.

Acute Moist Dermatitis, Hot Spots, and Pyotraumatic Dermatitis

Lesions of acute moist dermatitis, also known as pyotraumatic dermatitis or hot spots, result from self-trauma and are characterized by focal, moist, erythematous wounds with partial alopecia. There are multiple causes, including hypersensitivity due to flea allergy or atopy, trauma in the form of abrasions, foreign bodies, and in some cases behavior disorders. Heat and moisture act to exacerbate this condition. Progressive self-trauma often leads to rapidly enlarging lesions (Ackerman, 2008b).

Acute moist dermatitis can occur on any part of the body. In one study in 2004, males were over-represented and 25 of 27 cases cultured grew *Staphylococcus intermedius* (Holm *et al.*, 2004). Traditional treatment includes clipping hair from the lesions and a border of normal skin around the lesion, local cleansing with a topical antimicrobial solution or shampoo, systemic corticosteroids, appropriate systemic antibiotics, and topical anti-inflammatory and antibiotic medications. The efficacy of a topical preparation containing a bacteriostatic antibiotic and a corticosteroid was compared to systemic therapy (comprising a combination of parenteral corticosteroid and an oral antibiotic) in the treatment of 104 dogs with acute moist dermatitis. Significant improvement was evident after 7 days in both treatment groups, and there was no significant difference in the overall response between the two groups (Cobb *et al.*, 2005).

Laser therapy can be a valuable adjunct to traditional topical or systemic therapeutics for acute moist dermatitis. In the authors' experience, when PBMT is used as an adjunct to topical or systemic therapy, or a combination of both, the lesions appear to resolve more quickly than with traditional therapy alone. Laser therapy rapidly reduces how painful these lesions are, and thus reduces patient obsession with the lesions and self-trauma. Edema, swelling, and inflammation are reduced. Complex photobiomodulatory mechanisms may also result in enhanced macrophage and neutrophil response against any microorganisms present (Burger, 2015).

Acute moist dermatitis is normally treated, as its name implies, as an acute condition. Laser treatment normally follows clipping and cleaning during the initial patient presentation (Figure 11.1). Laser settings that deliver $3–4\,J/cm^2$ are recommended. The treatment should be delivered in a non-contact manner, with the delivery handpiece not touching the inflamed and contaminated tissue. Since the lesion is superficial, contact delivery, preferred for best photon penetration when treating deep-tissue conditions, is not necessary.

In most cases, clipping, cleaning, laser therapy, and an appropriate medical protocol result in rapid resolution.

(a)

(b)

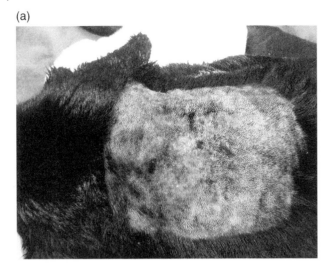
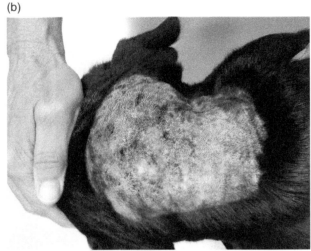

Figure 11.1 (a) Acute moist dermatitis after clipping and rinsing with sterile saline solution. (b) Reduced inflammation and dryness 3 hours after clipping, rinsing with sterile saline solution, and treating with laser therapy at 4 J/cm². Traditional pharmacological agents were withheld for 3 hours for observation of the effects of laser therapy.

If the patient continues to self-traumatize, repeat laser therapy treatments are recommended every 24 hours until resolution. If areas of deeper pyoderma or cellulitis are noted, two to four additional every-other-day treatments are indicated.

Though laser therapy is recommended as an addition to traditional therapeutics for acute moist dermatitis, many practitioners find that its addition eliminates or reduces the need for systemic and topical corticosteroids. Practitioners are encouraged to monitor the effects of adding laser therapy to their traditional protocol and to adjust the protocol accordingly.

Anal Sacculitis and Anal Sac Abscess

The anal sacs, sometimes erroneously referred to as "anal glands," are a pair of sacs lined with sebaceous glands located between the internal and external anal sphincter muscles at the 4 and 8 o'clock positions. They are connected to the exterior via the anal sac ducts, which empty at the 3 and 9 o'clock positions near the anal mucocutaneous junction.

The exact function of the anal sacs is not completely understood. Normal anal sac secretions are liquid, clear to translucent, and often pale yellow in color. Abnormal secretions are thicker in consistency, dark brown in color when impaction has occurred, and pus-colored when infection is present (Halnan, 1976a). The secretions are thought to be involved in territory marking, serving as a form of communication.

Anal sacs are normally emptied by compression of the anal sphincter muscles during a bowel movement, depositing a small amount of anal sac secretion on the feces. Clinical problems usually occur when there is incomplete emptying of the sacs during bowel movement. This results in anal sac impaction and discomfort. A survey of over 3000 dogs presented to two practices, one in England and one in Australia, indicated that 12.5% were affected with some degree of anal sac disease (Halnan, 1976b).

Possible causes of anal sac impaction are hypersecretion of sebaceous glands, constipation, chronic diarrhea, laxity of anal sphincters, narrowing of the anal sac ducts, imperforate ducts, and food allergy (van Duijkeren, 1995). Untreated anal sac impaction can lead to pain, constipation, and self-trauma in the form of licking and rubbing or dragging the perineum. Diagnosis of anal sacculitis is based on history and physical examination. Physical examination should include a rectal examination, with expression of the anal sacs and examination of their contents, as well as careful palpation for masses (Culp, 2012). Findings from analysis of anal sac secretions show no statistically significant cytological differences between secretions from normal dogs and those with anal sac disease. Thus, cytology appears to be an ineffective tool for diagnosing anal sac disease (James *et al.*, 2011).

Acute anal sacculitis, usually a result of short-term impaction, often responds to simple expression of the affected sac. In addition to the discomfort and inflammation present in the anal sac area, patients presenting with acute anal sacculitis may have superficial perianal abrasions from scooting and self-trauma, and may have localized areas of skin irritation around the tail base from licking and chewing. Manual expression of the sacs during rectal palpation may induce increased discomfort and inflammation.

(a) (b)

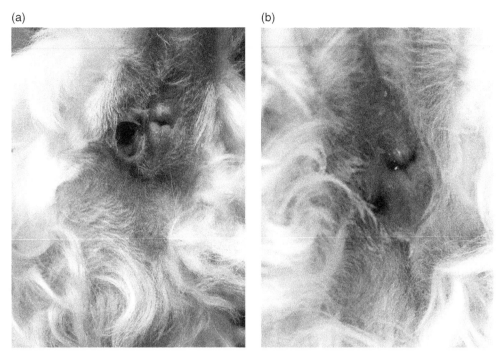

Figure 11.2 (a) Anal sac abscess on initial presentation. In addition to traditional therapeutics, anal sac abscesses should be treated with laser therapy daily for 2–3 days, with laser settings that deliver 8–10 J/cm^2. (b) Anal sac abscess 7 days after initial laser therapy treatment.

Laser therapy can significantly reduce the pain and inflammation of acute anal sacculitis, and is an excellent alternative to corticosteroids in preventing continued symptoms. Laser settings that deliver 6–8 J/cm^2 are recommended, using either contact or non-contact delivery. This dose is appropriate for secondary, superficial lesions, as well as for somewhat deeper anal sacs and the tissue that surrounds them. Most acute anal sac impactions resolve quickly after expression and treatment, and require no further treatment. Anecdotal information from practitioners indicates that performing laser therapy prior to anal sac expression may reduce patient discomfort and resistance, facilitating easier expression.

Chronic anal sacculitis presents a far more difficult therapeutic challenge. Cases often present intermittently with impaction, marked inflammation, bacterial infection of the sacs, and large amounts of noxious, purulent secretions. Systemic antibiotics, anti-inflammatories, and pain medications are indicated, along with repeated manual expression, flushing, and packing of the sacs. Laser therapy should be added to recommended medical protocols for chronic anal sacculitis. As with acute anal sacculitis, laser settings that deliver 6–8 J/cm^2 are recommended, using either contact or non-contact delivery.

Chronic cases should be treated through an induction phase, every other day or twice a week, with treatments coinciding with expression of the sacs. Once a clinical response has been noted, treatment frequency can be reduced through a transition phase, gradually extending the time between treatments. A complete resolution of anal sacculitis is not always possible. Patients with symptoms that persist or reoccur frequently should continue to be treated indefinitely, with maintenance-phase treatments every 3–4 weeks. Administration of maintenance-phase PBMT treatments long-term can, in some cases, control symptoms and flare-ups sufficiently to avoid surgical excision of the sacs.

If anal sac impaction is not resolved, abscess formation can result, accompanied by cellulitis and fistulous tracts. Anal sac abscesses should be managed with traditional incision and drainage, debridement and flushing, and systemic and topical medications (Figure 11.2). Additionally, as with any abscess or deep-tissue infection, treatment with laser therapy is recommended. Because deeper and more extensive tissues are usually affected when anal sacs abscess, laser settings that deliver 8–10 J/cm^2 are recommended. Treatment should be administered daily for 2–3 days, then on alternate days for three or four more sessions, or until the cellulitis and fistulous tracts have healed.

Aural Hematoma

Aural hematoma is a collection of blood between the cartilage of the pinna and the skin. The exact cause of this condition is unknown, however it is often observed in conjunction with acute or chronic otitis. Excessive head shaking and scratching accompanying otitis can result in an aural hematoma, as can direct trauma to the pinna.

Predisposing otitis must be addressed when treating aural hematomas. Untreated, aural hematomas undergo a slow healing process in which the hematoma clot is absorbed and fibroses and the pinna heals with a classical cauliflower appearance (MacPhail, 2016).

The list of therapeutic options for treating aural hematomas reflects the ingenuity of veterinary practitioners. Historically, these hematomas have been treated by incision and drainage, with an incision from proximal to distal along the full length of the hematoma, followed by multiple suture placements through the full thickness of the ear and over-the-head bandaging for 2–3 weeks (Brown, 2010). This technique is successful, but the slow healing and extended bandaging time are uncomfortable for both the patient and the owner, and make addressing predisposing otitis difficult. Partial-thickness suture placement has been suggested as an alternative closure (Győrffy and Szijártó, 2014).

Other therapeutic approaches have resulted in varying degrees of success. The application of fibrin sealant between the cartilage layers has been successful in humans, but proved unsuccessful in a reported canine case (Blättler *et al.*, 2007). Use of the CO_2 laser to produce a drain hole, followed by multiple punctate incisions over the hematoma surface to stimulate adhesions, has been reported (Dye *et al.*, 2002). Incision and laterally placed vacuum drains resulted in excellent cosmetic results in four of five patients (Pavletic, 2015). Treatment with parenteral drainage and intralesion injection of corticosteroids is sometimes attempted with variable success.

The reported effect of laser therapy on other types of hematomas suggests that it can be a valuable tool in managing aural hematomas. Laser therapy improves circulation, enhances hematoma absorption, and accelerates degradation of fibrin in post-surgical hematomas (Takashi, 1988). Anecdotal reports from practitioners indicate that laser therapy appears to be efficacious when added to a number of different aural hematoma management protocols. Laser therapy can be combined with traditional drainage and surgical tacking with or without bandaging. If a bandage is employed, it must be removed prior to laser treatment.

One of the authors (Core) combines laser therapy with surgical placement of a drain at the most dependent portion of the hematoma. A small, round incision, 3–5 mm in diameter, is created with a CO_2 laser at the most dependent portion of the hematoma. The contents are drained and the hematoma is flushed with sterile saline. A small tube, such as a 16–18-gauge polypropylene catheter or teat tube, is inserted in the drain hole and secured with stay sutures. The pinna is treated with laser therapy at a dose of $3–6 J/cm^2$ immediately after surgery, and then every third day until healing is complete. Patients seldom require a bandage. The drain tube is usually removed 10 days post-surgically. Healing with minimal fibrosis and a pleasant cosmetic appearance is expected.

The other author (Godbold) recommends a similar technique in lieu of drain tube placement. In this technique, drainage is accomplished by aspiration with a 16–18-gauge needle, a 5–7 mm biopsy punch, or a 5–7 mm CO_2 laser incision at the most dependent portion of the hematoma, followed by laser therapy ($3–6 J/cm^2$) and a light pressure bandage. The bandage is changed every 2–3 days, with repeated aspiration as required, and laser therapy while the bandage is off. With this technique, healing is expected in 10–14 days.

Bacterial Folliculitis

Bacterial folliculitis is the most frequently encountered form of pyoderma in dogs (Lloyd, 2012). It is more common in dogs than any other mammalian species. The etiology in the majority of cases is *Staphylococcus pseudoepidermititis*. Infection is a result of disruption of the skin barrier. Located within the hair follicle, this bacterial infection causes inflammation in and around the follicle, and appears as multifocal areas of alopecia, follicular papules or pustules, epidermal collarettes, and serous crusts. Pruritus is frequently present. There are a multitude of underlying conditions that lower the skin's defense to bacterial infection. Cushing's disease, diabetes mellitus, hypothyroidism, anatomical disorders such as skin folds, immune deficiencies, allergies, and parasites such as *Demodex canis* and *Sarcoptes scabiei* can adversely predispose individuals to bacterial folliculitis.

Historically, the first-line response to bacterial folliculitis has been systemic administration of a potentiated amoxicillin, a first-generation cephalosporin, or a potentiated sulfonamide. Currently, methicillin-resistant *Staphylococcus pseudintermedius* and *Staphylococcus aureus* (MRSA) are becoming more prevalent in canine bacterial folliculitis (Sousa, 2013). Regrettably, the emergence of these multi-resistant bacteria means that multimodal management of bacterial folliculitis is indicated (Bloom, 2014). Recent updated guidelines have been published for the diagnosis and antimicrobial therapy of canine bacterial folliculitis (Hillier *et al.*, 2014).

As practitioners adopt more comprehensive, multimodal protocols to treat bacterial folliculitis, PBMT should be included. Laser treatment will reduce inflammation and pruritus, reducing self-trauma. Additionally, multiple studies, using multiple laser wavelengths, suggest laser therapy application is indicated for bacterial infections (Nussbaum *et al.*, 2002, 2003; Silva *et al.*, 2013). In a 2009 study, a near-infrared (870 and 930 nm) laser was demonstrated to produce photoinactivation of *S. aureus*, *Escherichia coli*, *Candida albicans*, and *Trichophyton rubrum* at physiologic temperatures

(Bornstein *et al.*, 2009). Equally promising, though not yet available clinically, is the use of lasers with photosensitizers to photodeactivate bacteria (Alves *et al.*, 2014; St. Denis *et al.*, 2011)

Research has also shown that laser therapy enhances healing. A 2016 review indicated that wound healing is stimulated by many different wavelengths and powers, but that optimal parameters are still being identified (Kuffler, 2016). In patients with an endocrinopathy (diabetes mellitus), laser therapy has been shown to increase the rate of healing (Al-Watban *et al.*, 2007; Minatel *et al.*, 2009). As practitioners turn to multimodal management of bacterial folliculitis, any possible laser therapy effect is welcome.

Multimodal therapy for bacterial folliculitis includes culture and sensitivity, treatment with an appropriate systemic antibiotic, topical therapeutics, identification and management of any underlying disorders, and laser therapy. Laser settings that deliver $3–4 J/cm^2$ are recommended, using a non-contact delivery to reduce the possibility of contamination of the handpiece and subsequent nosocomial infections. Since large areas of skin may be involved, treatment times can become prolonged. The laser power may be increased to reduce treatment time as long as the speed of movement of the handpiece and laser beam increases. Likewise, to reduce treatment time, pulsed delivery can be turned off by setting the laser in a continuous delivery mode. Initial treatment daily or every other day for three to five treatments should be followed by twice-weekly treatments until the folliculitis is resolved.

Canine Non-Inflammatory Alopecia

Canine non-inflammatory alopecia is a heterogeneous group of skin disorders with different underlying pathogeneses. In a significant deviation from normal canine hair follicle physiology, the basis of non-inflammatory alopecia is a defect in the formation of the hair follicle or a failure of the follicle to continually cycle (Welle *et al.*, 2016). The alopecia results as hair is gradually lost, follicles remain inactive, and no new hair grows. The common and distinguishing histological characteristic is a marked increase in kenogen follicles, indicating that the induction of the new anagen phase is impaired (Müntener *et al.*, 2012). Seasonal flank alopecia, alopecia X, color-mutant alopecia, and other causes of follicular dysplasia are examples of canine non-inflammatory alopecia. The therapeutic approach is challenging, and new treatment options are desirable.

As is noted elsewhere in this book, the first report of what we now know as PBM was in 1968, when Endre Mester and his colleagues reported their observations of the effect of laser beams on the growth of hair in mice (Mester *et al.*, 1968). More-rapid-than-expected hair growth is often reported by veterinarians after treating patients in which hair has been clipped and the area treated with laser therapy.

Current publications support these anecdotal observations by veterinarians, as well as the observations published by Mester and his colleagues nearly 50 years ago, that laser light stimulates hair growth. Laser therapy treatment accelerated hair regrowth in a rat model of chemotherapy-induced alopecia (Wikramanayake *et al.*, 2013). A 2016 evidence-based review analyzed studies reporting the effects of laser therapy on hair regrowth, finding positive responses (Zarei *et al.*, 2016). A 2015 pilot study reported promising results of laser therapy on hair regrowth in canine non-inflammatory alopecia (Olivieri *et al.*, 2015). Patients were treated twice a week for a maximum of 2 months with a combination of 470, 685, and 830nm laser light at a dose of $3 J/cm^2$. At the end of the study, hair regrowth was significantly improved in six of seven animals and showed some improvement in the remaining one.

Enough evidence exists to warrant clinical treatment of canine non-inflammatory alopecia by practitioners. A suggested protocol is twice-weekly treatment at a dose of $3 J/cm^2$, with treatments continued until hair growth is noted. Since deep-photon penetration is not required, treatment using a non-contact delivery, with the laser beam spread out over a larger area, is appropriate.

Deep-Tissue Infections, Abscesses, and Cellulitis

Skin and soft-tissue infections are common, with complicated, deep-tissue infections being the most extreme and presenting the greatest challenge. Deep-tissue infections, abscesses, and cellulitis frequently begin with some degree of dermatological involvement or penetration, followed by extension of the infection into the deeper tissues. A variety of bacterial and fungal agents may be involved.

As an abscess develops, the abscess wall that is formed by adjacent healthy cells in an attempt to keep pus from infecting neighboring structures creates an encapsulation. If not contained to a focal area and encapsulated, infection spreads between tissue planes, producing cellulitis. Draining fistulous tracts may or may not develop.

Pain, erythema, swelling, and edema increase as the infection spreads.

Successful management involves prompt recognition, timely surgical drainage, appropriate antimicrobial therapy, and pain management. In addition to this traditional management protocol, laser therapy is indicated to help reduce the pain, swelling, and edema, to stimulate host response to the microbial infection, and to accelerate the healing process. The mechanisms by which laser therapy exert PBM effects are similar in deep-tissue infections to those in more superficial infections. These mechanisms have been mentioned previously in this chapter.

Deep-tissue infections generally require a higher laser therapy dose and a longer course of therapy, due to the depth of the involved tissue and the degree of inflammatory changes present. While more superficial infections require laser settings that deliver $3–5\,J/cm^2$, infections involving the subcutaneous tissue require a higher dose of $6–8\,J/cm^2$, and infections extending even deeper into tissue require $8–10\,J/cm^2$ (Box 11.1). Treatment should be administered daily for 2–3 days, and then on alternate days until the infection is resolved. If bandages are being used, treatment should coincide with bandage removal. If the infection is open and draining, use a non-contact delivery to reduce the possibility of contamination of the handpiece and subsequent nosocomial infections. Use a contact delivery if drainage is not present, contamination of the handpiece is not a concern, and patient sensitivity allows touching of the affected area.

Though not a result of microbial infection, juvenile cellulitis is a candidate for the immune-modulating effects of PBM (Figure 11.3). This uncommon granulomatous and pustular disorder of the face, pinnae, and submandibular lymph nodes is most often seen in puppies (White *et al.*, 1989). Aspirates of lesions usually reveal pyogranulomatous inflammation with no microorganisms (Reimann *et al.*, 1989). Cultures are negative. Since the condition responds to high, short-term doses of corticosteroids, an immune etiology is suspected (Hutchings, 2003). Treat affected areas of the skin with laser therapy doses of $6–8\,J/cm^2$, as the lesions frequently coalesce and become deep. Treat the affected regional lymph nodes with deep-tissue doses of $8–10\,J/cm^2$ (see Box 11.1). Early treatment is important, to reduce long-term scarring. Daily treatments should be administered until the lesions and lymphadenopathy resolve.

Elbow Hygroma

A hygroma is a fluid-filled cavity surrounded by a connective-tissue capsule over a bony prominence or pressure point. The elbow is the most common location, but hygromas can occur over any bony prominence. In younger individuals, elbow hygromas are thought to be a response to trauma. In older patients, hygromas tend to occur with impaired ambulation and excessive time spent in recumbency on hard surfaces. A soft, fluctuant, fluid-filled swelling develops, which, with continued trauma, can develop ulceration, infection, abscess formation, fistulous tracts, and proliferative granulomatous tissue.

The pathogenesis of elbow hygroma formation and a number of management protocols have been well reported. Aspiration, injection with anti-inflammatory medications, surgical drainage, excision, and a variety of protective bandaging options have been recommended (Canapp *et al.*, 2012; Johnston, 1975; Newton *et al.*, 1974). Treatment is often frustrating, and surgical options are usually avoided as they result in frequent complications. Recently, closed suction drain management was reported to be a simple, economical, and successful method of collapsing an elbow hygroma (Pavletic and Braum, 2015).

Laser therapy can aid in the management of elbow hygroma. Lasers reduce inflammation and edema and stimulate healing processes. As in laser therapy treatment of hematomas, increased circulation, and fibrin degradation should contribute to improvement (Takashi, 1988).

Laser therapy for elbow hygromas is most appropriately added to other forms of therapy. The use of padded bandages and laser therapy is indicated well before surgical intervention is considered. Practitioner experience indicates these dense, complex lesions require higher doses of laser therapy than are used for most conditions,

---

Box 11.1 Dermatological and non-musculoskeletal soft-tissue-condition treatment doses.

Acral Lick Dermatitis
$30–40\,J/cm^2$

Acute Moist Dermatitis
$3–4\,J/cm^2$

Anal Sacculitis
$6–8\,J/cm^2$

Anal Sac Abscess
$8–10\,J/cm^2$

Aural Hematoma
$3–6\,J/cm^2$

Bacterial Folliculitis
$3–4\,J/cm^2$

Canine Non-Inflammatory Alopecia
$3\,J/cm^2$

Deep-Tissue Infections, Abscesses, and Cellulitis
Superficial: $3–5\,J/cm^2$
Subcutaneous: $6–8\,J/cm^2$
Deep tissue: $8–10\,J/cm^2$

Elbow hygroma
$30–40\,J/cm^2$

Otitis Externa
Superficial component: $3–4\,J/cm^2$
Deep component: $8–10\,J/cm^2$
Deep component with severe hyperplasia: $10–20\,J/cm^2$

Perianal fistulas
$12–14\,J/cm^2$

Pododermatitis
$6–8\,J/cm^2$

(a)

(b)

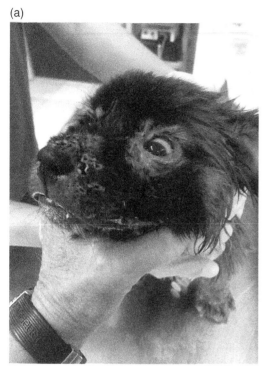
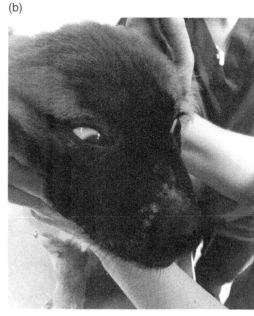

Figure 11.3 (a) Juvenile cellulitis, a candidate for the immune-modulating effects of PBM (affected areas of the skin are treated with laser therapy doses of 6–8 J/cm^2, and the affected regional lymph nodes with doses of 8–10 J/cm^2). (b) Resolution of juvenile cellulitis after 12 days of prednisone (2.2 mg/kg/day) and the immune-modulating effect of PBM. Early resolution of lesions helps reduce scarring.

and that treatment is required over an extended period of time. Laser settings that deliver 30–40 J/cm^2 are recommended. Treatment with the delivery handpiece in contact with the hygroma will increase photon penetration into the tissue.

Hygroma should be treated through an induction phase, every other day or twice a week, with treatments coinciding with removal and change of the padded bandage. Once a clinical response has been noted, treatment frequency can be reduced, through a transition phase, gradually extending the time between treatments. A complete resolution of an elbow hygroma is not always possible. Lesions that persist should continue to be treated indefinitely, with maintenance-phase treatments administered every 3–4 weeks, along with continued protection of the elbow.

Otitis Externa

Otitis is one of the most common reasons for small-animal veterinary consultations. Though acute otitis is often treated successfully with quick results, chronic otitis can be very difficult to manage successfully. Laser therapy can be an important adjunct in the management of both acute and chronic otitis.

Otitis has multiple factors that can contribute to, promote, and predispose individuals to ear infection. In dogs, the ear anatomy, with a long external ear canal and an "L" shape, makes them prone to otitis. The primary and secondary causes of otitis have been well identified in ear-disease texts (Gotthelf, 2004), as well as general dermatology texts.

In virtually all cases of acute otitis, the inflammatory changes produce edema and swelling of the epithelium of the ear canal. The canal narrows, moisture and debris are retained, and infections by bacteria, yeast, and fungi quickly follow. Chronic otitis causes hyperplastic changes within and around the ear canal that result in a permanently narrowed meatus. Traditional diagnostics include identification of primary and secondary causes, physical examination, otoscopy, and cytology.

Often, the ear canal is occluded with wax, hair, and inflammatory debris. The narrowed meatus and debris can make otoscopy and sample collection for cytology painful and difficult. Using laser therapy to reduce pain and swelling in the canal can facilitate otoscopic procedures that visualize, flush, and clean the ear in anesthetized patients. This allows better visualization of the tympanic membrane, to rule out middle- or inner-ear infection or a space-occupying mass. Laser therapy, along with improved otoscopic instrumentation and advanced imaging with radiographs and computed tomography (CT) scans, can contribute to a more accurate diagnosis.

Following a complete diagnostic workup, a multimodal management is recommended for otitis. A number of topical and systemic medications have been recommended that address the pain, swelling, and microbial infections normally present. Laser therapy can be a valuable adjunct to available medical protocols. The rapid reduction of pain from laser therapy increases patient tolerance of topical treatment, and the reduction of epithelial swelling allows more effective penetration of topical medication to the target tissue.

When treating otitis with a therapy laser, two components – or anatomical areas – must be addressed. The first is the affected portion of the pinna and the visible, more distal portion of the ear canal. These tissues should be treated with a laser setting that delivers $3-4\,\text{J/cm}^2$ and are most commonly treated with a non-contact delivery. The second component is the more proximal portion of the ear canal, including most of the vertical and the entire horizontal canal. This deeper tissue component requires a higher target dose of $8-10\,\text{J/cm}^2$ and is most commonly treated with a contact delivery (see Box 11.1).

With acute presentations of otitis externa, laser therapy can be incorporated into the initial visit, facilitating diagnostics and enhancing the overall management protocol. Laser therapy treatments are short enough (8–10 minutes) that treatment can be included during an outpatient consultation. Response to initial treatment is often sufficient that further treatment is not required. If pain and swelling persist, continue laser therapy treatments daily until resolved.

With chronic otitis, thickening of the ear canal epithelium and hyperplastic changes in the cartilage dictate a more prolonged management and a much poorer prognosis. Laser therapy is indicated in these cases, but the long-term goal becomes one of pain reduction and improved quality of life, rather than complete resolution. In these cases, because of the dense and chronic tissue changes, treatment of the deep-tissue component requires a laser setting that delivers $10-20\,\text{J/cm}^2$.

Chronic otitis should be treated through an induction phase, every other day or twice a week, until a reduction in pain and an improvement of quality of life are noted. Once a clinical response is noted, treatment frequency can be reduced, through a transition phase, gradually extending the time between treatments. Long-term maintenance-phase treatments are recommended every 3–4 weeks.

Pemphigus

Pemphigus is an autoimmune disease that results in the formation of bullous lesions of the skin or mucous membranes, or both (Figure 11.4). Patients form autoantibodies against desmogleins that are transmembrane glycoproteins. The breakdown of desmogleins disrupts the adhesion between keratinocytes and results in the formation of detached keratinocytes called "acanthylotic cells." This disruption of the normal connections between the squamous cells of the epidermis causes fragile, superficial, intraepidermal bullae.

Pemphigus foliaceous is the most common form of the disease in dogs and cats. It causes crusts and large pustules, primarily on the face, ears, and feet. The lesions are usually bilaterally symmetrical. Pemphigus vulgaris is much less common in dogs, and has only rarely been reported in cats. It differs from pemphigus foliaceous in that the lesions involve mucous membranes and mucocutaneous junctions. Pemphigus vulgaris is usually more difficult to treat (Blair *et al.*, 2015; Olivry and Linder, 2009).

Treatment of pemphigus requires immune suppression, which normally begins with high doses of glucorticosteroids (Bizikova and Olivry, 2015). Multimodal pharmacological therapy is recommended for long-term maintenance, to help reduce the reliance on glucorticosteroids. The analgesic and immune-modulating effects of PBM suggest that laser therapy should be part of the multimodal management of pemphigus patients. Prompt analgesia and accelerated healing of oral and cutaneous lesions have been reported in humans with pemphigus vulgaris when laser therapy has been added to treatment with systemic glucorticosteroids (Minicucci *et al.*, 2012; Pavli *et al.*, 2014).

The successful response in human patients suggests that laser therapy should be added to other management modalities for pemphigus in dogs and cats. Laser settings that deliver $3-4\,\text{J/cm}^2$ are recommended, using a non-contact delivery to reduce the possibility of contamination of the handpiece and subsequent nosocomial infections. Lesions should be treated through an induction phase, every other day or twice a week. Once a clinical response has been noted, treatment frequency can be reduced, through a transition phase, gradually extending the time between treatments. Patients with symptoms that persist or reoccur frequently should continue to be treated indefinitely, with maintenance-phase treatments every 3–4 weeks.

Perianal Fistulas

Perianal fistulas are a chronic, debilitating, inflammatory condition that results in fistulous tracts in the perianal and perirectal tissues and the surrounding perineum (Figure 11.5). They are rare in cats, more common in dogs, and most commonly seen in German shepherds, as well as in Irish setters and Labrador retrievers. The etiology was once thought to be related to the tail confirmation of German shepherds, but it is now believed to be immune-mediated (Craven, 2010). Comparisons have been made to Crohn's disease in humans.

(a)

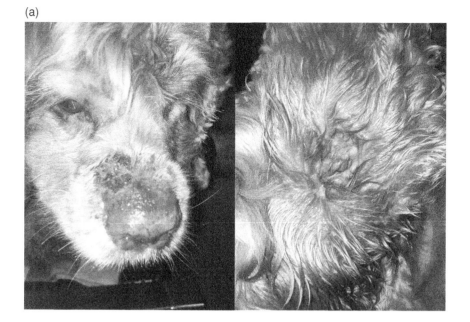

(b)

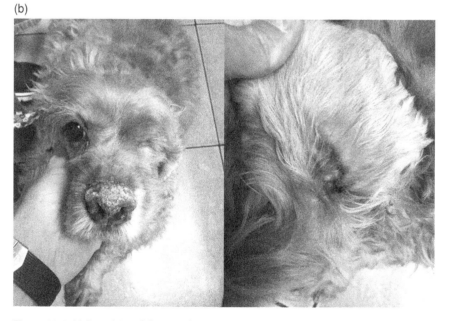

Figure 11.4 (a) Pemphigus foliaceous lesions on the face and pinna prior to laser therapy as an adjunct to immunomodulating pharmacological agents and antibiotics for a resistant bacterial infection. (b) Improvement in pemphigus foliaceous lesions 10 weeks after beginning prednisone, azathioprine, chloramphenicol, and laser therapy.

Patients present with a history of excessive grooming of the perianal area, tenesmus, hematochezia, and dyschezia. As the condition worsens, malodorous, mucopurulent discharge is often present around the anus and elevation of the tail is extremely painful. Inappetence, lethargy, and weight loss may occur in severe cases.

Though surgical excision was once thought to present the best option for resolution, medical management, using different combinations of immunomodulating drugs such as cyclosporine, prednisone, azathioprine, and topical tacrolimus, is now recommended (Craven, 2010; House, 2006; Patricelli *et al.*, 2002; Pieper and McKay, 2011; Stanley and Hauptman, 2009).

Laser therapy is recommended as an adjunct to medical protocols. The reduction of pain and inflammation that laser therapy gives can have a significant effect on patient quality of life. Higher doses of laser therapy are required to successfully target the depth of the fistulas and the extensive secondary inflammatory changes. Laser settings that deliver $12–14\,\mathrm{J/cm^2}$ are recommended, using a non-contact delivery.

(a)

(b)

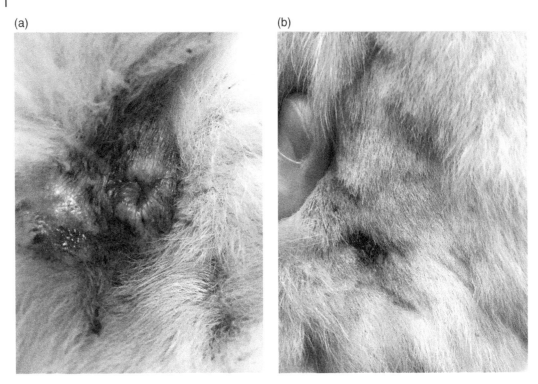

Figure 11.5 (a) Perianal fistula with dorsally draining tract prior to therapy. (b) Reduction in inflammation and swelling 7 days after laser therapy, with the laser set to deliver 12–14 J/cm^2.

Patients should be treated through an induction phase, every other day or twice a week. Initially, patients may be resistant to elevation of the tail for treatment, but as discomfort is reduced through successive treatments, tail elevation normally becomes better tolerated. Once a clinical response has been noted, treatment frequency can be reduced, through a transition phase, gradually extending the time between treatments. Prognosis is guarded, complete resolution of perianal fistulas is often not possible, and reoccurrence is common. Patients with symptoms that persist or reoccur frequently should continue to be treated indefinitely, with maintenance-phase treatments every 3–4 weeks.

Pododermatitis

Pododermatitis, by definition, and as the term is commonly used by veterinary practitioners, refers to any inflammation of the skin of the foot (Figure 11.6). Affected tissues may include interdigital spaces, foot pads, nail folds (paronychia), claws, or other tissues of the foot. There are many potential causes, and therefore many presentations of inflammatory foot disease.

Some veterinary texts use the term "pododermatitis" to refer to pedal folliculitis and furunculosis (Miller *et al.*, 2012), while others use it to refer to the group of as many as a dozen of the most common skin diseases that

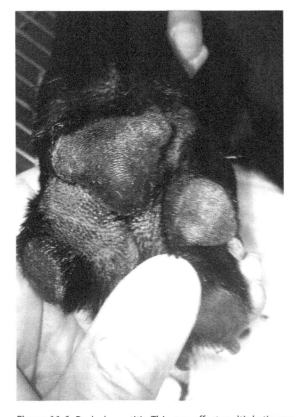

Figure 11.6 Pododermatitis. This may affect multiple tissues, including interdigital spaces, foot pads, nail folds (paronychia), claws, and other tissues of the foot.

cause lesions on the canine paw (Duclos, 2013). The etiology of the various presentations of pododermatitis includes trauma, irritants, allergies (food allergy, atopy, contact dermatitis), infections (bacterial, fungal, and viral), parasites (demodectic mange), and osteomyelitis, as well as immune-mediated (pemphigus), nutritional (zinc deficiency), neoplasia, behavioral, metabolic (hepatic cutaneous syndrome), and inherited and congenital factors (Rosychuk 2002). Some cases have been classified as idiopathic and are now identified as immunomodulatory-responsive lymphotic-plasmocytic pododermatitis (Breathnach et al., 2008).

Pododermatitis, regardless of etiology, is often chronic and painful. Management includes identifying and treating the primary etiology and contributing causes. Therapy includes an appropriate antimicrobial agent, elimination or hyposensitization allergy therapy, immune-modulating medications, pain control, topical therapy, and bandages.

Regardless of the etiology or the management plan, when added as an adjunct, laser therapy can facilitate a reduction in pain, edema, swelling, and inflammation in affected feet.

Though both superficial and deeper tissues may be affected in pododermatitis, because of the anatomy of the foot, the depths of all of the target tissues are relatively shallow. Laser settings that deliver $6-8\,J/cm^2$ are recommended. The complex anatomy and limited surface area of the foot usually require a non-contact delivery. Treatment of the foot should be administered from all directions (360°).

Acute, superficial inflammations of the tissues of the feet may be treated a single time with laser therapy, during the initial outpatient consultation. If inflammation does not respond to medical and laser therapy, treatments can be repeated daily or every other day.

Chronic and deeper involvement of the tissues of the feet should be treated through an induction phase, every other day or twice a week. Once a clinical response has been noted, treatment frequency can be reduced, through a transition phase, gradually extending the time between treatments. Patients with symptoms that persist or reoccur frequently should continue to be treated indefinitely, with maintenance-phase treatments every 3–4 weeks.

Conclusion

As the various conditions summarized in this chapter indicate, laser therapy can be an important tool in the management of dermatological and non-musculoskeletal soft-tissue conditions. In almost all cases, the effects of PBM will be added to an overall, multimodal management plan for these conditions.

The conditions discussed in this chapter are examples of dermatological and non-musculoskeletal conditions for which laser therapy is indicated. Many other conditions affecting the same tissues will also be candidates for laser therapy treatment. Practitioners are encouraged to extrapolate the principles detailed in this chapter and apply them to the diversity of other conditions seen every day in practice.

References

Ackerman, L. (2008a) Acral lick dermatitis. In: *Atlas of Small Animal Dermatology*, pp. 322–326. Inter-Médica, Buenos Aires.

Ackerman, L. (2008b) Pyotraumatic dermatitis (hot spots). In: *Atlas of Small Animal Dermatology*, pp. 8–14. Inter-Médica, Buenos Aires.

Alves, E. *et al.* (2014) An insight on bacterial targets of photodynamic inactivation. *Future Med Chem.* **6**(2):141–164.

Al-Watban, F.A. *et al.* (2007) Low-level laser therapy enhances wound healing in diabetic rats: a comparison of different lasers. *Photomed Laser Surg.* **25**(2):72–77.

Assis, L. *et al.* (2016). Aerobic exercise training and low-level laser therapy modulate inflammatory response and degenerative process in an experimental model of knee osteoarthriti in rats. *Osteoarthritis Cartilage.* **24**(1):169–177.

Avci, P. *et al.* (2013) Low-level laser (light) therapy (LLLT) in skin: stimulating, healing, restoring. *Semin Cutan Med Surg.* **32**(1):41–52.

Bizikova, P. and Olivry, T. (2015) Oral glucocorticoid pulse therapy for induction of treatment of canine pemphigus foliaceus – a comparative study. *Vet Dermatol.* **26**(5):354–358.

Bjordal, J.M. *et al.* (2008) A systematic review with procedural assessments and meta-analysis of low level laser therapy in lateral elbow tendonopathy (tennis elbow). *BMC Musculoskeletal Disord.* **9**:75.

Blair, R.V. *et al.* (2015) Pathology in practice. *Pemphigus vulgaris. J Am Vet Med Assoc.* **246**(4):419–421.

Blättler, U. (2007) Fibrin sealant as a treatment for canine aural haematoma: a case history. *Vet J.* **173**(3):697–700.

Bloom, P. (2014) Canine superficial bacterial folliculitis: current understanding of its etiology, diagnosis and treatment. *Vet J.* **199**(2):217–222.

Bornstein, E. *et al.* (2009) Near-infared photoinactivation of bacteria and fungi at physiologic temperatures. *Photochem Photobiol.* **85**(6):1364–1374.

Breathnach, R.M. *et al.* (2008) Canine pododermatitis and idiopathic disease. *Vet J.* **176**(2):146–157.

Brown, C. (2010) Surgical management of canine aural hematoma. *Lab Anim (NY)*. **39**(4):104–105.

Burger, E. *et al.* (2015) Low-level laser therapy to the mouse femur enhances the fungicidal response of neutrophils against *Paracoccidioides brasiliensis*. *PLoS Negl Trop Dis*. **9**(2):e0003541.

Calisto, F.C. *et al.* (2015) Use of low-power laser to assist the healing of traumatic wounds. *Acta Cir Bras*. **30**(3):204–208.

Canapp, S. *et al.* (2012) Orthopedic coaptation devices and small-animal prosthetics: elbow hygroma. In *Veterinary Surgery: Small Animal*, pp. 638–639. Saunders, St. Louis, MO.

Chow, R. *et al.* (2009) Efficacy of low-level laser therapy in the management of neck pain: a systematic review and meta-analysis of randomized placebo or active-treatment controlled trials. *Lancet*. **374**(9705):1897–1908.

Chung, H. *et al.* (2012) The nuts and bolts of low-level laser (light) therapy. *Ann Biomed Eng*. **40**(2):516–533.

Cobb, M.A. *et al.* (2005) Topical fusidic acid/betamethasone-containing gel compared to systemic therapy in the treatment of canine acute moist dermatitis. *Vet J*. **169**(2):276–280.

Craven, M. (2010) Rectoanal disease: perianal fistula. In: *Textbook of Veterinary Internal Medicine*, 7 edn., pp. 1602–1604. Saunders, St. Louis, MO.

Culp, W.T.N. (2012) Anal sac disease. In: *Small Animal Soft Tissue Surgery*, pp. 399–405. John Wiley & Sons, Chichester.

de Carvalho, P.K. *et al.* (2016) Analysis of experimental tendinitis in rats treated with laser and platelet-rich plasma therapies by Raman spectroscopy and histometry. *Lasers Med Sci*. **31**(1):19–26.

Duclos, D. (2013) Canine pododermatitis. *Vet Clin North Am Small Anim Pract*. **43**(1):57–87.

Dye, T.L. *et al.* (2002) Evaluation of a technique using the carbon dioxide laser for the treatment of aural hematomas. *J Am Anim Hosp Assoc*. **38**(4):385–390.

Enwemeka, C.S. (2009) Intricacies of dose in laser phototherapy for tissue repair and pain relief. *Photomed Laser Surg*. **3**:387–393.

Hodjati, H. *et al.* (2014) Low-level laser therapy: an experimental design for wound management: a case-controlled study in rabbit model. *J Cutan Aesthet Surg*. **7**(1):14–17.

Gotthelf, L. (2004) *Small Animal Ear Diseases: An Illustrated Guide*, 2 edn. Saunders, Philadelphia, PA.

Győrffy, A. and Szijártó, A. (2014) A new operative technique for aural haematoma in dogs: a retrospective clinical study. *Acta Vet Hung*. **62**(3):340–347.

Halnan, C.R.E. (1976a) The diagnosis of anal sacculitis in the dog. *J Small Anim Pract*. **17**(8):527–535.

Halnan, C.R.E. (1976b) The frequency of occurrence of anal sacculitis in the dog. *J Small Anim Pract*. **17**(8):537–541.

Hill, P.B. *et al.* (2006) Survey of the prevalence, diagnosis and treatment of dermatological conditions in small animals in general practice. *Vet Rec*. **158**(16):533–539.

Hillier, A. *et al.* (2014) Guidelines for the diagnosis and antimicrobial therapy of canine superficial bacterial folliculitis (Antimicrobial Guidelines Working Group of the International Society for Companion Animal Infectious Diseases). *Vet Dermatol*. **25**(3):163–175.

Holm, B.R. *et al.* (2004) A prospective study of the clinical findings, treatment and histopathology of 44 cases of pyotraumatic dermatitis. *Vet Dermatol*. **15**(6):369–376.

House, A.K. (2006) Evaluation of the effect of two dose rates of cyclosporine on the severity of perianal fistulae lesions and associated clinical signs in dogs. *Vet Surg*. **35**(6):543–549.

Hutchings, S.M. (2003) Juvenile cellulitis in a puppy. *Can Vet J*. **44**(5):418–419.

James D.J. *et al.* (2011) Comparison of anal sac cytological findings and behaviour in clinically normal dogs and those affected with anal sac disease. *Vet Dermatol*. **22**(1):80–87.

Jang, H. and Lee, H. (2012) Meta-analysis of pain relief effects by laser irradiation on joint areas. *Photomed Laser Surg*. **30**(8):405–417.

Johnston, D.E. (1975) Hygroma of the elbow in dogs. *J Am Vet Med Assoc*. **167**(3):213–219.

Knol, B.W. and Wisselink, M.A. (1996) Lick granuloma in dogs; an obsession for dogs, owners and veterinarians. *Tijdschr Diergeneeskd*. **121**(1):21–23.

Kovacs, K. (2015) Low Level Laser Therapy of Serious Wounds of Dogs. Poster presentation. ASLMS Annual Meeting. April 24–26. Orlando, FL.

Kuffler, D.P. (2016) Photobiomodulation in promoting wound healing: a review. *Regen Med*. **11**(1):107–122.

Lloyd, D.H. (2012) Antimicrobial therapy of bacterial folliculitis in dogs. *Proc Am College Vet Int Med Forum*. May 30–June 1. New Orleans, LA.

MacPhail, C. (2016) Current treatment options for auricular hematomas. *Vet Clin North Am Small Anim Pract*. **46**(4):635–641.

Mester, E. *et al.* (1968) The effect of laser beams on the growth of hair in mice. *Radiobiol Radiother (Berl)*. **9**(5):621–626.

Miller, W. *et al.* (2012) Bacterial skin diseases: pedal folliculitis and furunculosis. In: *Muller and Kirk's Small Animal Dermatology*, 7 edn., p. 201. Saunders, St. Louis, MO.

Minatel, D.G. *et al.* (2009) Phototherapy promotes healing of chronic diabetic leg ulcers that failed to respond to other therapies. *Lasers Surg Med*. **41**(6):433–441

Minicucci, E.M. *et al.* (2012) Low-level laser therapy on the treatment of oral and cutaneous pemphigus vulgaris: case report. *Lasers Med Sci*. **27**(5):1103–1106.

Müntener, T. *et al.* (2012) Canine noninflammatory alopecia: a comprehensive evaluation of common and distinguishing histological characteristics. *Vet Dermatol.* **23**(3):206–e44.

Newton, C.D. *et al.* (1974) Surgical closure of elbow hygroma in the dog. *J Am Vet Med Assoc.* **164**(2):147–149.

Nussbaum, E. L. *et al.* (2002) Effects of 630-, 660-, 810-, and 905-nm laser irradiation delivering radiant exposure of 1–50 J/cm^2 on three species of bacteria in vitro. *J Clin Laser Med Surg.* **20**(6):325–333.

Nussbaum, E.L. *et al.* (2003) Effects of low-level laser therapy (LLLT) of 810 nm upon in vitro growth of bacteria: relevance of irradiance and radiant exposure. *J Clin Laser Med Surg.* **21**(5):283–290.

Olivieri, L. *et al.* (2015) Efficacy of low-level laser therapy on hair regrowth in dogs with noninflammatory alopecia: a pilot study. *Vet Dermatol.* **26**(1):35–39.

Olivry, T. and Linder, K.E. (2009) Dermatoses affecting desmosomes in animals: a mechanistic review of acantholytic blistering skin diseases. *Vet Dermatol.* **20**(5–6):313–326.

Patricelli, A.J. *et al.* (2002) Cyclosporine and ketoconazole for the treatment of perianal fistulas in dogs. *J Am Vet Med Assoc.* **220**(7):1009–1016.

Pavletic, M.M. (2015) Use of laterally placed vacuum drains for management of aural hematomas in five dogs. *J Am Vet Med Assoc.* **246**(1):112–117.

Paveletic, M.M. and Braum, D.E. (2015) Successful closed suction management of canine elbow hygroma. *J Small Anim Pract.* **56**(7):476–479.

Pavli, V. *et al.* (2014) *Pemphigus vulgaris* and laser therapy: crucial role of dentists. *Med Pregl.* **67**(1–2):38–42.

Peplow, P.V. *et al.* (2010) Laser photobiomodulation of wound healing: a review of experimental studies in mouse and rat animal models. *Photomed Laser Surg.* **28**(3):291–325.

Pieper, J and McKay, L. (2011) Perianal fistulas. *Compend Contin Educ Vet.* **33**(9):E4.

PRNewswire. (2015) Top 10 most common medical conditions for dogs and cats. Available from: http://www.prnewswire.com/news-releases/top-10-most-common-medical-conditions-for-dogs-and-cats-300065935.html (accessed November 30, 2016).

Rapoport, J.L. *et al.* (1992) Drug treatment of canine acral lick. An animal model of obsessive-compulsive disorder. *Arch Gen Psychiatry.* **49**(7):517–521.

Reimann, K.A. *et al.* (1989) Clinicopathologic characterization of canine juvenile cellulitis. *Vet Pathol.* **26**(6):499–504.

Rosychuk, R. (2002) Pododermatitis in dogs and cats. *Proc Am College Vet Int Med Forum.* May 29–June 1. Dallas, TX.

Rosychuk, R. (2011) Canine lick granuloma. *World Small Animal Veterinary Association World Congress Proceedings.* October 14–17. Jeju.

St. Denis, T.G. *et al.* (2011) All you need is light: antimicrobial inactivation as an evolving and emerging discovery strategy against infectious disease. *Virulence.* **2**(6):509–520.

Shumaker, A.K. *et al.* (2008) Microbiological and histological features of acral lick dermatitis. *Vet Dermotol.* **19**(5):288–298.

Silva, DC. *et al.* (2013) Low level laser therapy (AlGaInP) applied at 5J/cm^2 reduces the proliferation of *Staphylococcus aureus* MRSA in infected wounds and intact skin of rats. *An Bras Dermatol.* **88**(1):50–55.

Sousa, C.A. (2013) *Staphylococcal pyoderma* in the world of methicillin resistance. *Proc Atlantic Coast Veterinary Conference.* October 14–17. Atlantic City, NJ.

Stanley, B.J. and Hauptman, J.G. (2009) Long-term prospective evaluation of topically applied 0.1% tacrolimus ointment for treatment of perianal sinuses in dogs. *J Am Vet Med Assoc.* **235**(4):397–404.

Takashi, K. (1988) Low level diode laser treatment for hematomas under grafted skin and its photobiological mechanisms. *Keio J Med.* **37**:415–428.

van Duijkeren, E. (1995) Disease conditions of canine anal sacs. *J Small Anim Pract.* **36**(1):12–16.

Welle, M.M. *et al.* (2016) A comparative review of canine hair follicle anatomy and physiology. *Toxicol Pathol.* **44**(4):564–574.

White, S.D. *et al.* (1989) Juvenile cellulitis in dogs: 15 cases (1979–1988). *J Am Vet Med Assoc.* **195**(11):1609–1611.

Wikramanayake, T.C. *et al.* (2013) Low-level laser treatment accelerated hair regrowth in a rat model of chemotherapy-induced alopecia (CIA). *Lasers Med Sci.* **28**(3):701–706.

Zarei, M. *et al.* (2016) Low level laser therapy and hair regrowth: an evidence-based review. *Lasers Med Sci.* **31**(2):363–367.

12

Snake Bites

Barbara R. Gores

Veterinary Specialty Center of Tucson, Tucson, AZ, USA

Introduction

Pit vipers (Crotalinae) form the largest group of venomous snakes in the United States and are involved in an estimated 150 000 bites of dogs and cats annually (Armentano and Schaer, 2011; Peterson, 2006). Rattlesnakes, copperheads, and cottonmouth water moccasins are all pit vipers. At our large multi-specialty 24-hour veterinary emergency and critical care hospital in Tucson, Arizona, we treat an average of 395 rattlesnake envenomation cases each year.

The toxicity of rattlesnake venom varies widely, and envenomation is diagnosed primarily as a focal site with a rapid onset of severe swelling, hemorrhage, pain, and local tissue necrosis. Crotalid venom consists of 90% water and has a minimum of 10 enzymes and 3–12 non-enzymatic proteins and peptides. Envenomation results in potentially severe soft-tissue damage and necrosis, vasculotoxicity, cytotoxicity, and coagulopathy (Armentano and Schaer, 2011; Peterson, 2006). Specifically, hyaluronidase and collagenase work to break down connective tissues, while proteases contribute to coagulopathy and cellular necrosis. Phospholipases are likely the cause of cell-membrane damage and the resultant echinocytosis observed with rattlesnake envenomation. The venom also contains anticoagulants, which contribute to platelet dysfunction and margination of platelets along the vessel wall. Clinically, these patients often have significant prolongation of coagulation times (prothrombin and activated partial thromboplastin times), so hemorrhage is common (Wells, 2012; Witsil *et al.*, 2015).

The clinical manifestations of rattlesnake envenomation depend on the type of snake, anatomical location of the bite, amount of venom injected, age of the snake, and size of the patient. The common presenting signs in dogs and cats include pain, swelling, petechiation or ecchymosis (or both), weakness, hypotension, and local tissue necrosis. In the Mojave rattlesnake, neuromuscular signs such as ataxia, seizures, and respiratory muscle paralysis predominate. The majority of bites occur on the nose and facial region in dogs (Figure 12.1), and secondarily on the extremities in dogs and cats. Cats are more resistant to the effects of rattlesnake venom on a weight basis, but they typically present with more severe clinical signs, due to their smaller body size resulting in a larger relative dose of venom (Wells, 2012; Witsil *et al.*, 2015).

The patient should be hospitalized and monitored closely post-snake bite to determine the degree of envenomation, and to monitor for neuromuscular signs if in a location where Mojave rattlesnakes are present. The only proven, specific therapy against pit viper envenomation is the administration of antivenin, with most dogs and cats requiring one to three vials over 24–36 hours, in our experience. The mainstay of treatment includes antivenin, intravenous crystalloid fluid therapy, and analgesic medications. Antimicrobial therapy and blood products are used if clinically indicated (Armentano and Schaer, 2011). Labwork should initially be run and then monitored closely throughout hospitalization to determine the response to systemic therapies. However, antivenin and other systemic therapies are ineffective in neutralizing the severe, rapid, local tissue damage following snake-bite envenomation.

In 2006, our hospital began implementing photobiomodulation (PBM) as an adjuvant therapy in conjunction with the standard accepted systemic treatment (including antivenin) just described for snake envenomation cases. We felt that there were numerous clinical case studies utilizing laser therapy technology that supported the beneficial effects of PBM on tissues and cells post-wounding (see Chapter 5). These effects include the local mechanisms of anti-inflammation (via an anti-edema effect, as it causes vasodilation, activation of the lymphatic drainage system, and subsequent reduction in swelling and bruising), analgesia (via decreasing nerve

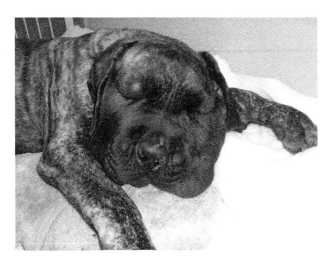

Figure 12.1 Severe swelling, edema, and ecchymosis in a mastiff puppy that suffered multiple snake-bite envenomations to the muzzle and periocular regions.

sensitivity and production of endorphins and enkephlins), accelerated tissue repair and cell growth (via increasing cellular metabolism), and improved vascular activity (via neovascularization and angiogenesis.) It seemed that these effects would prove beneficial in actively treating the local tissue damage in snake-bite envenomation cases in our veterinary center.

At the time we launched laser photobiomodulation therapy (PBMT) for snake-bite envenomation cases, there was only one clinical study in the scientific literature (Dourado *et al.*, 2003). We made an educated guess at the laser treatment protocol and have adapted it over time as we observed the clinical response to therapy. In the past decade, since we started using laser therapy as an adjuvant treatment in our snake-bite patients, the scientific literature has greatly expanded in the area of PBMT in general, and specifically in regards to Crotalinae envenomation wounds. There are now many other published studies that support our clinical findings over the past decade in utilizing PBMT for snake envenomation.

Literature Review

A review of the literature for studies on the effects of PBMT on the changes induced in tissue by snake venom reveals a number of recent publications. These publications indicate that laser therapy irradiation has a significant effect on the inflammatory response and myonecrosis of mice gastrocnemius muscles injected with Bothrops (a genus of pit viper endemic to Central and South America) snake venom. Studies have demonstrated that PBM induces an inhibition of the ability of the venom myotoxins to rapidly disrupt

the integrity of the cellular plasma membrane, thereby decreasing the amount of edema, leukocyte influx, and myonecrosis following venom inoculation (Barbosa *et al.*, 2008; Dourado *et al.*, 2003; Nadur-Andrade *et al.*, 2012, 2014). Laser irradiation does not alter the venom toxicity, but laser-only therapy does significantly reduce myonecrosis of the envenomed muscle and the neuromuscular transmission-blocking effect of the pit viper venom (Barbosa *et al.*, 2009; Doin-Silva *et al.*, 2009).

In a 2016 *in vitro* study, the effect of laser irradiation on cytotoxicity induced by crotoxin in C2C12 mouse myoblast cell line cells was examined. The mouse myoblast cells were exposed to crotoxin, and then those treated with PBMT were irradiated with either red 685 nm or infrared 830 nm light at energy densities of 2.0, 4.6, and 7.0 J/cm^2. As demonstrated in other studies, irradiation had no effect on the venom itself. In non-irradiated cells, the venom caused a decrease in cell viability and a massive release of creatine kinase and lactate dehydrogenase, indicating myonecrosis. Infrared and red laser light, at the energy densities tested, was able to cause a protective effect against the crotoxin, considerably decreasing venom-induced cytotoxicity (Silva *et al.*, 2016).

Laser therapy combined with antivenin therapy was more efficient than either therapy alone, indicating that PBMT is a potentially therapeutic approach to minimizing the severity of snake-bite envenomation and to treating the local tissue effects caused by envenomation (Barbosa *et al.*, 2008, 2009; Nadur-Andrade *et al.*, 2012, 2014).

PBMT has also been shown to increase angiogenesis by the promotion of vascular endothelial growth factor receptor 1 (VEGFR-1) expression at 3 days post-injection of venom into mouse gastrocnemius muscle. This is the first time that VEGFR-1 expression, and its modulation by PBM, has been demonstrated in endothelial and nonendothelial cells of snake-envenomed skeletal muscle (Dourado *et al.*, 2011). Laser PBMT of crotoxin-damaged mouse cranial tibialis muscles at a dose of 3 J resulted in an increased cross-sectional area of regenerating myofibers and a reduction in the previously injured muscle area compared to controls and mice receiving lower doses of 1.5 J. This suggests that laser PBMT improves skeletal muscle regeneration by accelerating the recovery of myofiber mass (Silva *et al.*, 2012).

Treatment

Our protocol for PBMT for snake-bite envenomation is currently to initiate laser therapy (810 and 980 nm, 7.2–8.0 J/cm^2) every 24 hours beginning 6–8 hours

(a)

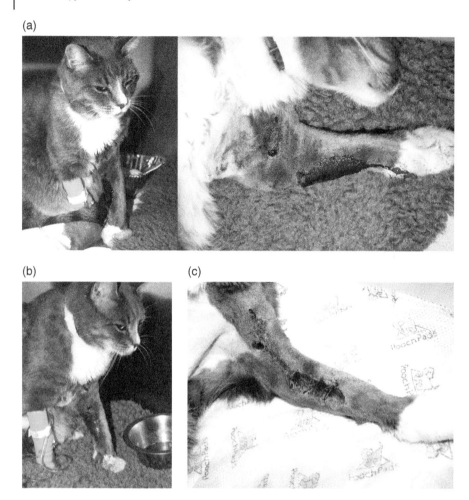

(b)   (c)

Figure 12.2 (a) Cat snake-bite envenomation of the left antebrachium before PBMT. Note severe limb and paw edema and local ecchymosis. (b) Cat snake-bite envenomation 12 hours after first PBMT. Note reduction of paw swelling, limb and paw edema, and ecchymosis. (c) Cat snake-bite 5 days post-envenomation, after receiving three PBMTs. Limb edema and bruising have resolved. The envenomation wound is healing without complications or the need for surgical intervention.

post-hospital admission. We have been reluctant to initiate laser therapy immediately in snake-envenomation patients for fear of local vasodilation created by the laser resulting in a worsening of the myotoxic effect on the tissues. The delay in commencing laser therapy allows us to better stabilize the patient with systemic crystalloids and opioids, which improves patient comfort and tolerance to any movement or positioning needed to administer the laser treatments, as well as to monitor for early onset of possible neuromuscular signs indicative of a more severe Mojave rattlesnake envenomation that could markedly worsen the overall patient prognosis. However, we are currently in the process of re-evaluating the time to commence and the frequency of laser treatments based on the current literature already cited.

We vary the PBMT dose slightly based on size and location of the wound and patient size (smaller patients, smaller wounds, or areas with less tissue density, such as

over the carpus or muzzle, receive doses at the lower end of the range). Plastic templates allow us to more accurately measure surface area for calculations without having to overmanipulate the already damaged and painful tissues.

Periocular bites can be challenging to treat in terms of adequately shielding the patient's eyes. Likewise, lingual-based bites, commonly seen in dogs, are difficult to perform PBMT on, due to the limitations of intraoral access in awake or mildly sedated patients. Many of these patients can experience significant swelling and edema of the tongue, to the point of obstructing their airway, necessitating the performance of tracheostomies until the swelling resolves.

Most snake bite-envenomation patients remain hospitalized for 2–3 days, and subsequently receive two to four laser treatments (see Figure 12.2). About 30% of patients return for continued laser treatments every 24–48 hours for two to four more sessions over the next week post-envenomation if they have wounds that are more extensive.

Anecdotally, over the past 10 years since initiating PBMT for rattlesnake envenomation, our results have shown a significant decrease in the clinical morbidity associated with the local tissue-necrosis effects of snake-bite wounds. We now very rarely have to perform major surgical reconstruction (consisting of extensive skin wound management, skin flaps, and grafts) of snake-bite wounds, and almost never perform amputations of appendages as we did routinely in the past, pre-laser therapy. The most severe cases of tissue necrosis tend to occur in those patients that delayed seeking veterinary care, or were treated at other veterinary facilities with antivenin but not PBMT.

Conclusion

Laser PBMT alone has made a significant impact not only on the overall prognosis and outcome of snake-bite patients, but also on reducing the duration and financial costs of treatment. Laser PBMT of snake bites is comfortable and well tolerated by the patient, and is easy for technical staff to administer. It is an extremely cost-effective therapy when you consider the high success rates in preventing the more extensive, complicated, and expensive surgeries required to treat the high degree of wound necrosis that is so characteristic of snake-bite envenomation. It truly is an exciting and rewarding therapy that can be offered with confidence to these patients in order to ensure the best outcomes, with the most rapid return to health.

References

Armentano, R. and Schaer, M. (2011) Overview and controversies in the medical management of pit viper envenomation in the dog. *J Vet Emerg Crit Care.* **21**(5):461–470.

Barbosa, A.M. *et al.* (2008) Effect of low-level laser therapy in the inflammatory response induced by Bothrops jararacussu snake venom. *Toxicon.* **51**(7):1236–1244.

Barbosa, A.M. *et al.* (2009) Effect of low-level laser therapy in the myonecrosis induced by Bothrops jararacussu snake venom. *Photomed Laser Surg.* **27**(4):591–597.

Doin-Silva, R. *et al.* (2009) The ability of low level laser therapy to prevent muscle tissue damage induced by snake venom. *Photochem Photobiol Sci.* **85**(1):63–69.

Dourado, D. *et al.* (2003) Effects of the Ga-As laser irradiation on myonecrosis caused by Bothrops Moojeni snake venom. *Lasers Surg Med.* **33**(5):352–357.

Dourado, D. *et al.* (2011) Low-level laser therapy promotes vascular endothelial growth factor receptor-1 expression in endothelial and nonendothelial cells of mice gastrocnemius exposed to snake venom. *Photochem Photobiol Sci.* **87**(2):418–426.

Nadur-Andrade, N. *et al.* (2012) Effects of photobiostimulation on edema and hemorrhage induced by Bothrops moojeni venom. *Lasers Med Sci.* **27**(1):65–70.

Nadur-Andrade, N. *et al.* (2014) Photobiostimulation reduces edema formation induced in mice by Lys-49 phospholipases A2 isolated from Bothrops moojeni venom. *Photochem Photobiol Sci.* **13**(11):1561–1567.

Peterson, M. (2006) Snake bite: pit vipers. *Clin Tech Small Anim Pract.* **21**(4):174–182.

Silva, L.H. *et al.* (2012) GaAs 904-nm laser irradiation improves myofiber mass recovery during regeneration of skeletal muscle previously damaged by crotoxin. *Lasers Med Sci.* **27**(5):993–1000.

Silva, L.M. *et al.* (2016) Photobiomodulation protects and promotes differentiation of C2C12 myoblast cells exposed to snake venom. *PLoS One.* **11**(4):e0152890.

Wells, R. (2012). Rattlesnake envenomation. In: *Proceedings of 84th Annual Western Veterinary Conference.* February 19–23. Las Vegas, NV.

Witsil, A. *et al.* (2015) 272 cases of rattlesnake envenomation in dogs: demographics and treatment including safety of F(ab')2 antivenom use in 236 patients. *Toxicon.* **105**:19–26.

13

Musculoskeletal Disorders and Osteoarthritis

Lisa A. Miller

Companion Animal Health by LiteCure, Newark, DE, USA

Introduction

Affecting as much as 20% of the US pet population over the age of 1 year (Johnston, 1997), osteoarthritis is a progressive, complex syndrome involving the interaction of a multitude of factors, both biochemical and biomechanical in nature, which results in the degenerative disease of the synovial joints. Regardless of the origin of the disease process, once started, the interactions of these biomechanical and biochemical factors ultimately affect all components of the joints, leading to cartilage degradation, osteophyte and enthesiophyte formation, subchondral bone sclerosis, synovial membrane inflammation, and synovial fluid alterations, as well as further changes to periarticular tissues. These changes include a thickening and increased fibrosis of the joint capsule, which results in the stiffness, pain, and decreased range of motion often observed in osteoarthritic patients. Inflammation of the synovial membrane and a secondary influx of leukocytes into the joint space further facilitate the release of prostaglandins, cytokines, free radicals, and other destructive enzymes, including metalloproteinases, all of which can change cartilage metabolism, create further inflammation, or damage cartilage matrix (McLaughlin, 2000).

Current treatment strategies in veterinary medicine are aimed primarily toward controlling pain, improving joint function, and minimizing functional incapacity in patients through pet owner education and home environmental management. Multimodal management of patients with osteoarthritis includes a therapeutic approach involving the use of a proper weight-management program (when indicated), nutraceutical supplementation, pharmacological therapy, rehabilitation therapy (including physical modalities and therapeutic exercise), and, when necessary, surgical intervention or regenerative medicine (including the use of platelet-rich plasma (PRP) or stem-cell therapy).

Increasingly, pet owners and practitioners are seeking non-pharmacological adjuncts or alternatives to standard-of-care medical therapies for the treatment of chronic painful conditions, including osteoarthritis and other musculoskeletal conditions. Photobiomodulation therapy (PBMT), delivered with a therapeutic laser, may be utilized along with any or all of these therapies, and though it may often be used as a standalone therapy, its results are better appreciated as part of a multimodal approach to pain management and rehabilitation. Utilizing PBMT for its analgesic and anti-inflammatory effects is especially important, as it may reduce or eliminate the need for medications, and the concomitant side effects that can come with their use.

Physiological Effects of PBMT

The photochemical processes initiated on a cellular level by PBMT have been described in detail in previous chapters; however, some of the analgesic and anti-inflammatory physiological effects that make this modality particularly useful in treating osteoarthritis and other musculoskeletal conditions should be reviewed. Literature supporting the use of PBMT for specific musculoskeletal conditions is detailed in the individual condition sections that follow; here, the general physiologic principles will be discussed. Unlike other physical modalities used in rehabilitation, PBMT has biomodulating effects. Several different mechanisms of action result in a reduction of inflammation and pain (Pryor and Millis, 2015), making it versatile for both short- and long-term effects.

Following PBMT application, the synthesis and secretion of inflammatory prostaglandins are inhibited (Mizutani *et al.*, 2004), and cytokines and growth factors with antioxidative, anti-inflammatory, and antiapoptotic actions are stimulated (Zhang *et al.*, 2003). PBMT has been shown to significantly reduce cyclooxygenase 2 (COX-2) production (Prianti *et al.*, 2014), as well as to reduce bradykinin levels (Jimbo *et al.*, 1998). Bradykinin is important in chronic pain states as it elicits pain by stimulating nociceptive afferents in the skin and viscera, as well as sensitizing them through the production of prostanoids or the release of other mediators (Dray and Perkins, 1993). It also reduces the production of interleukin 1 (IL1) (Lopes-Martins *et al.*, 2005) and prostaglandin E2 (PGE2) (Mizutani *et al.*, 2004).

Photobiomodulation (PBM) blocks depolarization of C-afferent fiber peripheral nerves (Wakabayashi, 1993), improves nerve cell action potential (Cambier *et al.*, 2000), promotes regeneration and recovery of injured peripheral nerves (Anders *et al.*, 2004), and promotes axonal sprouting (Rochkind *et al.*, 2009). The localized and systemic increase of beta endorphins after therapy laser irradiation has been clinically reported in multiple studies (Labajos, 1988; Montesinos, 1988), with subsequent pain reductions, and there is also PBMT-mediated analgesia via enhancement of peripheral endogenous opioids (Hagiwara *et al.*, 2007).

Increased microcirculation, and secondarily increased tissue oxygenation, are also achieved with PBMT via dilation of microvessels of all orders, effects on arteriolar vasomotions, an opening of "reserved" capillaries, and a metabolism rise in parenchymatous cells (Skobelkin *et al.*, 1990). Vasodilation is accomplished by an increase in nitric oxide (NO) in the treated area (Shiva and Gladwin, 2009), as well as an increase in serotonin release (Walker 1983), which also plays an important role in analgesia. Acceleration of neoangiogenesis occurs via release of cytokines and growth factors into the circulation, and numerous studies have examined the relationship between PBMT and vascular endothelial growth factor (VEGF) (Góralczyk *et al.*, 2015; Silva *et al.*, 2010).

There is increasing evidence that conditions characterized by an intense local or systemic inflammatory response, which can lead to maladaptive pain states if not appropriately managed, may be associated with abnormal ion transport (Schomberg *et al.*, 2012; Waxman and Zamponi, 2014). Calcium, sodium, and potassium concentrations, as well as the proton gradient over the mitochondrial membrane, are positively influenced by PBM (Chow *et al.*, 2011; Ignatov *et al.*, 2005; Karu *et al.*, 1997). After PBMT, there is an integrated and rapid modulation of ion channels. This is achieved through both direct action on photo-acceptors (such as cytochrome c oxidase, CCO) and indirect modulation via enzymes (Liebert *et al.*, 2014).

Searching for Evidence and Understanding the Literature

Literature regarding the use of PBMT in treating musculoskeletal conditions, including osteoarthritis, is prevalent, though at first glance not in the journals that might regularly come across the desk of a veterinarian in general practice. Further complicating any search for evidence are the numerous terms that have been used to describe PBM in the body of research publications. Older terms may be used, such as "cold laser" or "low-level laser therapy" (LLLT), in order to differentiate the modality from so called "hot" lasers used to thermally cut, ablate, or coagulate tissue.

Simply searching through the scientific literature for studies related to PBMT and one of the most prevalent musculoskeletal disorders, osteoarthritis, presents challenges. Certainly, there have been studies in lab animals with experimentally induced arthritis (Assis *et al.*, 2016; Carlos *et al.*, 2014; Peimani and Sardary, 2014), but it is also important to point out that larger veterinary studies in companion animals are ongoing. Human clinical studies investigating the efficacy of PBMT in naturally occurring disease models have also been published (Alfredo *et al.*, 2012; Ammar, 2014; Baltzer *et al.*, 2016; Fukuda *et al.*, 2015; Ip and Fu, 2015a).

The true effectiveness of the modality for pain relief in osteoarthritis has also been debated in the literature. It is important to take into account the possible reasons for the varying outcomes reported in some papers, which are not limited to the osteoarthritis studies alone, but also apply to much of the published research in the field of PBMT. Outcome measures used for similar conditions have varied. The laser parameters used, including wavelength, pulse frequency (Hz), energy density or fluence (J/cm^2), and power density or irradiance (mW/cm^2), have not always been reported clearly. In addition, the method of application (on-contact versus off-contact administration), anatomic areas treated (treatment of "pain points" alone versus involved periarticular soft tissues), tissue type selection (amount of melanin in treated tissue), and frequency of treatments have also varied widely and have not always been clearly reported. Though there have been meta-analyses examining the multitude of studies concluding efficacy for treating pain in osteoarthritis (Jang and Lee, 2012) and other musculoskeletal conditions (Chow *et al.*, 2009), further studies should be encouraged using consistent reported parameters to optimize outcomes and elucidate the factors necessary for effectiveness.

Of the parameters just mentioned, the differences in therapeutic outcomes with varying fluence (J/cm^2) and irradiance (W/cm^2) reported in the literature seem to be the most significant, as long as wavelengths within the therapeutic window are being used. Some studies have demonstrated clear fluence-dependent biochemical effects with PBMT (Hsieh *et al.*, 2014). Others, including the Tumilty *et al.* (2010) meta-analysis of studies on tendinopathy also supported the existence of a fluence-dependent dosing window in those trials that have had positive results. Additionally, the Chow *et al.* (2009) seminal review on PBMT for neck pain published in the *Lancet* concluded that when studies that utilized low doses or demonstrated flaws in treatment procedure were excluded, statistical heterogeneity in results disappeared.

Most importantly, when examining the literature and the dosing reported in it, one should also take into consideration whether the study described is *in vitro* or *in vivo*. As demonstrated in a 2014 study on peripheral nerve injury, doses optimized for each wavelength *in vitro* must then be translated for optimal *in vivo* parameters due to the percentage of light lost in transmission to deeper tissues from the skin surface (Anders *et al.*, 2014).

Importance of Proper Examination and Diagnostics

As for all therapeutic protocols, it should be emphasized that a proper diagnosis must be established prior to beginning treatment. All veterinary patients should undergo a thorough orthopedic and neurologic examination, as well as an investigation of their clinical history, prior to being prescribed PBMT, or, indeed, any other pharmacologic or therapeutic interventions for their osteoarthritis. The presence of comorbidities should be considered when tailoring a treatment plan for the patient, including not only the presence of other systemic or local diseases, but also any localized pain (not in the joint being treated) due to compensatory changes in biomechanics. Pain examinations should be repeated regularly on all patients, to evaluate for improvement after therapy has started and to ensure there are no "new" issues that should be treated, as well as, in the case of lack of improvement or worsening, to determine whether further diagnostics are indicated. It is also important to remember that the degree of radiographic or pathologic change discovered may not necessarily be consistent with the amount of lameness displayed by the patient or the severity of their discomfort.

Prescribed treatment areas should primarily be based on the orthopedic and pain-assessment examinations. Additionally, as part of the initial pain evaluation, and for purposes of follow-up and objective outcome measures for any treatment plan, the use of validated owner questionnaires for assessing pain in veterinary patients is strongly encouraged. At least two such pain-assessment questionnaires have been validated for dogs with chronic pain due to osteoarthritis: the Canine Brief Pain Inventory (Canine BPI) (PennVet, 2016) and the Helsinki Chronic Pain Index (HCPI) (Millis and Ciuperca, 2015). A recently published Feline Musculoskeletal Pain Index (FMPI) is also available (NC State, 2016). Not only do these evaluation tools provide the practitioner with information on the patient's behavior, demeanor, and locomotion as observed by the pet owner, but they also serve to allow the pet owners themselves to evaluate improvement or decline in their pet's quality of life with regards to their chronic pain status. Other pain-scoring systems and scales exist and may also be utilized by the practitioner for evaluation of veterinary patients. The use of one or more of these systems is in keeping with the guidelines set forth in the American Animal Hospital Association (AAHA)/American Association of Feline Practitioners (AAFP) Pain Management Guidelines for Dogs & Cats (AAHA/AAFP, 2007).

Patient Preparation and Treatment Technique

In practice, PBMT may be applied with minimal patient preparation. Patients generally experience a calming, warm sensation and relax during therapy, negating the need for sedation. The hair coat may be clipped or shaved for optimal light penetration, but it is not absolutely necessary, depending on the power capabilities of the device. PBMT units may have built-in software that can calculate a dose of energy that will help compensate for additional light losses in thick or long hair coats; alternatively, adjustment can be made manually when calculating a dose for administration (see section on Dosimetry for Musculoskeletal Conditions). The hair coat should be free of excessive debris, and any lotions, sprays, or ointments that may have been applied to the treatment area should be rinsed completely off with water prior to treatment.

A comfortable surface for the pet to lie on should be provided, such as a dog bed or pad placed on the floor or exam table. This is particularly important for patients that are old or in pain. A treatment platform may be constructed slightly elevated off the floor, to allow for comfortable seating during therapy sessions for both the laser therapist and pet owner (Figure 13.1). Laser treatment should be performed in whatever position the pet is most comfortable in that allows access to the anatomic areas being treated. Laser operators should be educated that "posture breaks" may be necessary and that repositioning from side to side should be minimized to maintain maximum patient comfort. For example, with a patient lying in lateral recumbency, the laser therapist can treat both the cranial, lateral, and caudal aspects of any joints on the "upside" limbs and the medial aspects of any joints on the "downside" limbs, without having to turn the patient over repeatedly (Figure 13.2).

As discussed in Chapter 4, the number-one safety concern with the use of any therapy laser is the protection of the eyes of the patient, the laser therapist, and anyone in the immediate treatment vicinity. For this reason, everyone should be equipped with and wear laser-safe eyewear, marked with the appropriate optical density for the wavelengths of light emitted by the laser unit being used. When treating around the head and neck, the patient should also be wearing laser-safe "doggles" (Figure 13.3), or should

Figure 13.1 Laser therapist and patient seated comfortably on a raised laser-treatment platform.

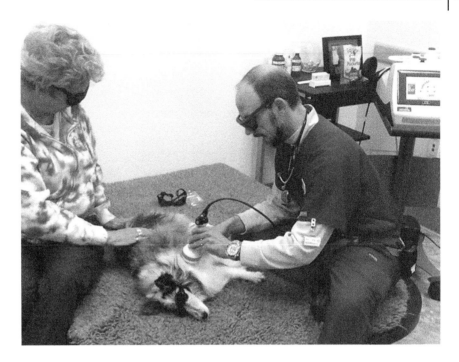

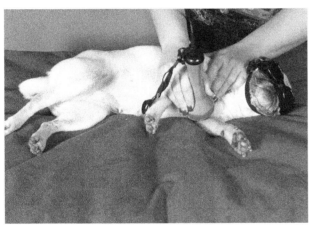

Figure 13.2 Laser therapist treating the medial aspect of the elbow on the "downside" limb.

have their eyes covered with a dark cloth (Figure 13.4) or by the hand of someone assisting in the treatment.

The patient should never be allowed to stare at the treatment area. A dark-colored Elizabethan collar may serve as a shielding device when treating caudal to the head if the patient cannot be distracted with food treats or attention, or otherwise restrained to avoid directly investigating the laser treatment area.

In general, there are two different application techniques that can be utilized, depending on the power of the laser being used (Pryor and Millis, 2015). For lower-powered devices, typically those less than 500 mW (0.5 W), a point-to-point treatment is usually used. Multiple individual points within the treatment area must be treated in order to deliver the appropriate target dose to tissues beneath the surface, and depending on the size of

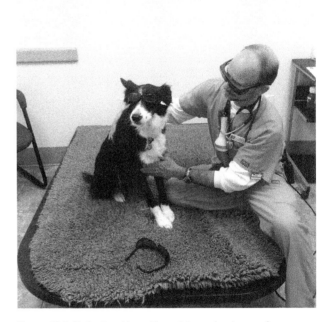

Figure 13.3 Patient and laser therapist wearing laser-safe eyewear.

the area, or when dealing with multiple treatment areas in the same patient, this may become challenging from a time perspective. Additionally, as previously discussed, irradiance (W/cm^2) plays an important role in therapeutic

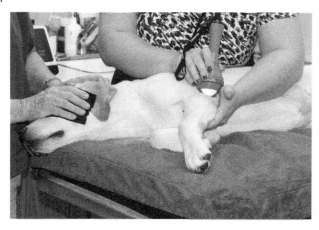

Figure 13.4 Assistant covering the patient's eyes with a dark cloth in lieu of laser-safe goggles.

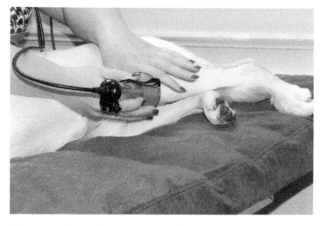

Figure 13.6 Laser therapist treating the cranial aspect of the patient's stifle joint.

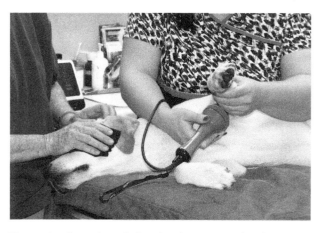

Figure 13.5 Laser therapist keeping the treatment head perpendicular to the surface of the medial aspect of the elbow.

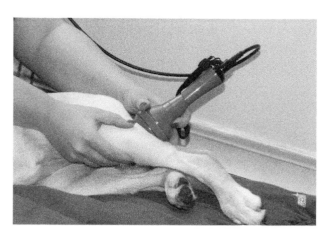

Figure 13.7 Laser therapist treating the caudal aspect of the patient's stifle joint.

outcome, especially when dealing with deep-tissue conditions, including osteoarthritis. For this reason, higher-powered devices may be able to achieve better results, in addition to being more time-efficient. For these devices (those lasers emitting more than 500 mW), a scanning technique should always be used. Even though these lasers generally have a larger spot size (depending on the optics of the treatment handpiece or head being used), thereby mitigating some of the increased power density, caution should always be used to ensure continuous movement during laser emission and good monitoring of both hair coat temperature and patient behavior during treatment. A scanning speed that maintains irradiance and fluence within the recommended safety ranges for the treatment handpiece and beam being used is recommended. For devices above 500 mW, a scanning speed of 3–7 cm/sec is usually appropriate; however, the laser operator should confirm with the manufacturer.

A "trailing finger" through the patient's fur may be used when treating with the hand on the treatment handpiece, or the laser therapist may follow the path of the handpiece with the second hand to monitor for excessive thermal buildup, and adjust treatment speed or lower treatment power as needed. If, at any time during treatment, signs of potential discomfort are noted (patient vocalizing, withdrawing the limb, or suddenly turning to look at the treatment area), this should prompt the laser therapist to check that the technique and settings being utilized are appropriate.

The laser treatment handpiece should be held perpendicular to the surface being treated (Figure 13.5) and moved in a consistent, serpentine motion, in a grid pattern evenly covering the entire area to be treated. For osteoarthritis, it is recommended to treat all of the soft-tissue structures associated with the joint biomechanically, encompassing 360° around the limb and utilizing landmarks approximately half the distance to the next joint on the limb, both proximal and distal, to demarcate a comprehensive area of treatment, which can be quite large. For example, in Figures 13.6 and 13.7, the laser

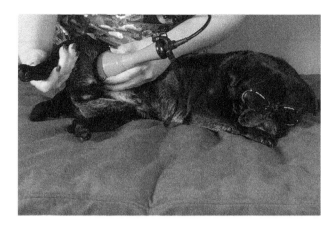

Figure 13.8 Laser therapist treating the ventral, medial aspect of the patient's coxofemoral joint.

therapist is shown treating both the cranial and caudal aspects of the stifle joint. In treating the coxofemoral joint, it is a common mistake for the laser therapist not to include the ventral, medial aspect of the hip joint in the treatment area (Figure 13.8), and to risk less than optimal therapeutic outcomes because of this omission. A smaller, more specific anatomic area of focus may of course be treated if desired, based on the anatomic knowledge of the laser therapist and utilization of appropriate dosing (see section on Dosimetry for Musculoskeletal Conditions).

Treatment is optimally applied in direct contact with the skin, using a contact handpiece or a treatment head that has been specifically designed for deep-tissue conditions. Treating in contact and applying pressure to the skin creates blanching and disperses blood from the dermis and underlying tissues (Chien and Wilhelmi, 2012). Since blood absorption is a barrier to photon penetration (via hemoglobin acting as the main absorber of light in the dermis) (Lister *et al.*, 2012), blanching improves light penetration to deeper tissues. Due to differences in the refractive index between air and skin, a large amount of light may be lost due to reflection off the skin when treating in an off-contact manner; treating on-contact minimizes these losses.

Providing passive tissue massage is another benefit of treating on-contact, though it is important to note that some patients in pain may be hypersensitive to physical contact. This is particularly true over boney prominences and in areas of thinned skin, especially of the elbow and the stifle. In these patients, as well as in any patient with a wound in the treatment area, treating in an off-contact manner may be necessary.

Lastly, particularly when administering PBMT over a joint, the limb should be placed through gentle passive range of motion during treatment to maximize light penetration to the articular surfaces and associated soft-tissue structures. Often, at the start of a course of therapy, the osteoarthritic pet may be very stiff and painful, and passive range of motion may not be possible during the first few visits. In these cases, it is best to first address the patient's pain and discomfort by treating the limb in a passive position, before attempting gentle manipulation of the limb for passive range of motion during a subsequent visit.

Use of PBMT with Metal Implants and Sutures

One of the most commonly asked questions regarding PBMT is, "Can it be applied in patient's that have metal surgical hardware, including plates, pins, and screws?" Diffuse near-infrared light will be primarily reflected by smooth metal implant surfaces, including staples, but while this means that the practitioner need not be concerned about the implants themselves heating up, there are several special considerations to be aware of:

1) Be careful when treating over implants in small patients such as small dogs or cats, or anywhere there is a superficial implant, such as a tibial plateau leveling osteotomy (TPLO) or other type of plate that is only covered by a superficial amount of tissue. These areas will effectively be receiving an increased dose, as the light reflects back off the implant into the surrounding tissue overlying or adjacent to it. The laser therapist should quickly pass over these areas when treating in a "grid-pattern" movement in order to disperse the dose evenly through the area. Adjustments may also be made to lower the treatment power (W) slightly for patient comfort.

2) Because the light does not penetrate through the metal hardware, it is equally as important to treat 360° around the limb, to ensure that the light is penetrating to all of the associated soft tissues that the therapist wishes to target. This is particularly important for osteotomy sites, such as in TPLO patients, or in fracture-repair situations.

3) When treating over staples, ensure delivery to more than "just the incision line." Treatment should include several inches of margin around the incision. Additionally, the laser therapist should quickly cross the incision line instead of "hovering" or treating back and forth directly over the line itself.

4) When treating an incision closed with sutures, the incision and the area immediately adjacent to the incision itself should be treated with the same technique just described. However, unless the optical properties of the suture itself are known, the practitioner should be aware that some darker suture materials may absorb light and heat up. Therefore, the laser operator is reminded again to continue a scanning pattern crossing the incision line and never to "hover" directly over the sutures themselves.

Dosimetry for Musculoskeletal Conditions

Laser medical procedures for musculoskeletal conditions, including osteoarthritis, usually describe recommended dosing in terms of the fluence or energy density (J/cm^2) administered to the surface of a specific anatomical area. The most practical reason for recommending doses in this manner is that it is possible to achieve the same energy density in a nearly infinite number of ways by adjusting either treatment time or power density (or irradiance, in W/cm^2).

For example, PBMT applied to the hip joint of a large-breed dog (35 kg) with a hip area of approximately 250 cm^2 (the joint itself, as well as surrounding biomechanically associated soft tissues) and a target fluence (energy density) of 10 J/cm^2 would be calculated in the following manner:

$$10J/cm^2 \times 250cm^2 = 2500J$$
$$\text{total dose over the entire hip area}$$

The question of what combination of treatment time and irradiance (or power density, in W/cm^2) is ideal for these treatments is slightly more complicated. The practitioner may conclude, for example, that this dose can be delivered in either of the following combinations:

$$100mW\left(or\ 0.1W\right) \times 25000\,sec\left(416\ minutes,\ 40\ seconds\right) = 2500J\ total$$

$$12W \times 208\,sec\left(3\ minutes,\ 28\ seconds\right) = 2500J\ total$$

Clearly, the second combination is a more efficient use of time, and allows the opportunity to treat multiple affected areas during one treatment session.

More importantly, when treating conditions, there is a minimum irradiance required that will create a clinically meaningful effect. That is, there is a certain threshold of power density at the target tissue required to ensure a therapeutic result. Below this threshold, no matter how long the treatment time, no clinical effect will be seen. Similarly, international safety standards are based upon the laser parameters of wavelength, time, and irradiance, because above a certain threshold for power density, thermal or other damage may be created. Therefore, the ideal goal for treatment is to utilize a dose that is in a window above the minimum irradiance that will produce a clinically meaningful effect and below a maximum irradiance that would produce damage (Sommer *et al.*, 2001).

Due to the percentage of light lost in transmission from the skin surface to deeper tissues, the irradiance required to produce a therapeutic effect is higher for so-called "deep-tissue" conditions, including musculoskeletal disorders, than it is for "superficial" conditions, including wounds, burns, and other dermatological conditions. This is why good clinical outcomes may be appreciated with lower irradiance when treating superficial conditions, but the results are inconsistent when treating deep-tissue conditions, even with longer treatment times.

Many studies have examined the relationship between irradiance, light penetration, and effectiveness in treating deep-tissue conditions, including peripheral nerve injury (Anders *et al.*, 2014), brain stroke (Oron *et al.*, 2006), and traumatic brain injury (Morries *et al.*, 2015), as well as conditions in ischemic skeletal (Avni *et al.*, 2005) and cardiac muscle (Oron *et al.*, 2001). As previously mentioned, not only is it important to take into account optimization of irradiance for different wavelengths, but the critical parameter is the dose delivered to target tissue. Factors including the overall depth of the target tissue being treated, the presence or absence of melanin in the skin, the presence or absence of blood vessels (and the blood contained within) in the tissues, the thickness of any bone present, and tissue hydration all play a role in the penetration of photons to the target tissue.

Calculations for clinical dosimetry for deep-tissue or musculoskeletal conditions should take as many of these factors into account as possible. Software for "preset" protocols in many commercially available PBMT units may take some into account, and the clinician should feel comfortable inquiring with the laser manufacturer to gain a more thorough understanding of the protocols in their individual PBMT devices.

When calculating clinical dosimetry for musculoskeletal conditions, a general range of energy densities (fluences) of 6–10 J/cm^2 is recommended (Gaynor, 2015) based on the size of the patient and their body condition (and consequently, the average thickness of soft tissues, including fat and muscle layers, in certain anatomic areas). Though the specifics are device- and design-dependent, the power used to achieve the desired fluence should be lower for smaller patients, areas with increased sensitivity or very little soft tissue present (e.g., over boney prominences), or relatively shallow target tissue (e.g., the Achilles tendon versus the coxofemoral joint). Table 13.1 provides a range of recommended power settings for musculoskeletal conditions in veterinary patients of various sizes. These doses should be effective and safe for most commercially available laser units, but the practitioner should *always* confirm with the laser manufacturer regarding safety specifications.

Patient comfort should be continuously monitored during treatment (see section on Patient Preparation and Treatment Technique), and adjusted as necessary. It should be noted that for conditions that are non-responsive to this standard dosing, or for those that reach a plateau in improvement, dosing with increased

Table 13.1 The recommended range of power (W) settings for treating musculoskeletal conditions in canine and feline patients. These are starting points and adjustments should be made accordingly with clinical judgment, observation of patient comfort level, consideration of anatomic area being treated, or concurrent issues.

Patients weight (kg)	Power settings (W)
<4.5	2.5–6.0
4.5–9.0	3–7
9.1–18.0	5–8
18.1–27.0	6–9
27.1–36.0	7–11
36.1–45.0	8–13
>45.0	10–15

Box 13.1 **The dose to be delivered (total joules) is easy to calculate manually, by multiplying the size of the area to be treated (cm^2) by the target energy density (J/cm^2).**

4 kg Feline Carpus

$50\,cm^2$ total area $\times 6\,J/cm^2 = 300\,J$ total
Treated at 2.5 W in continuous wave (CW)
Treatment time = 120 seconds (2 minutes)

40 kg Canine Carpus

$150\,cm^2$ total area $\times 8\,J/cm^2 = 1200\,J$ total
Treated at 8 W in continuous wave (CW)
Treatment time = 150 seconds (2 minutes, 30 seconds)

target energy densities of up to $20\,J/cm^2$ may be appropriate (by increasing treatment time, and not necessarily increasing irradiance recommended for these areas). However, prior to increasing the dose of PBMT being applied, the practitioner should ensure that a proper diagnosis is in place and that common reasons for perceived treatment failure are not present (see section on Common Reasons for Perceived Treatment Failure or Inconsistent Results).

Following these guidelines, various anatomic areas may be measured (or estimated with experience) in square centimeters (cm^2), and, given a target energy density (J/cm^2), the total energy required to treat the area can be calculated. Provided the power chosen is within the therapeutic range of irradiance discussed earlier, delivery of the dose will therefore determine the treatment time. The practitioner is encouraged to check with the laser manufacturer to confirm that parameters chosen are within this range, as this is device design-dependent. For example, compare the calculations for treating the carpus of a 4 kg feline patient and a 40 kg canine patient in Box 13.1.

It should be noted, again, that "preset" protocols in various laser units may differ from manufacturer to manufacturer. The practitioner should have a thorough understanding of the size of the areas to be treated once they are selected in the laser software. While preset guidelines are helpful for beginner laser users, they should not replace a thorough understanding of dosimetry. They should always be checked against the practitioner's calculations or estimates to ensure that an effective treatment dose is being delivered.

Treatment Session Frequency

For any acute or chronic painful condition, including osteoarthritis, an "induction phase" of initial, more frequent treatment sessions is recommended (i.e., every-other-day treatments until a significant effect is seen). For patients in acute pain that may be experiencing an overuse injury or flare-up of their arthritis pain, treating daily is optimal for faster results (Riegel, 2008). Once a significant improvement is noted in clinical signs, a "transition phase" of treatment sessions is begun. During transition, treatments are decreased to twice weekly, then once weekly, and so on as the patient improves, until the condition resolves (e.g., resolution of a soft-tissue injury) or a "maintenance phase" of treatment is established (for chronic conditions with no permanent "cure," such as osteoarthritis) usually once every 3–6 weeks, based on the patient's response. Each patient must be evaluated and treated as an individual; some take longer to respond than others. Though significant improvement may be appreciated sooner for some patients with osteoarthritis, it is usually noted between four and six treatment sessions. However, for those with severe osteoarthritis or multiple joint involvements, improvement may not be noted for seven to ten sessions. It is helpful for the practitioner to set expectations with pet owners, to avoid their becoming discouraged when they do not see immediate results.

Pet owners should also be counseled that while PBMT may help alleviate their pet's pain and decrease other clinical symptoms, it will not change anatomical biomechanical defects (such as osteochondritis dissecans lesions or dysplastic changes) or "cure" the osteoarthritic disease process permanently. PBMT is part of a long-term treatment plan for pain management. Owners should be aware that their pet will require ongoing maintenance therapy based on their clinical signs. Maintenance treatments should be scheduled before the pet experiences any deterioration in the improvements seen with their induction-phase treatments. Owners can be encouraged to schedule follow-up visits for maintenance treatments at the first sign of returning discomfort or difficulties with their pet's daily activities (e.g., decreased activity, hesitation to go up or down stairs, or difficulty laying down or getting up from the floor). Alternatively, a regular maintenance treatment session may be scheduled, at a time interval established by the practitioner and the owner. It is not uncommon, if maintenance visits are missed or delayed, to require a "mini re-induction" phase of a few, more frequent sessions in order to re-establish patient comfort, and then to wean the treatment sessions back out to a maintenance-phase interval.

It should be noted that one of the benefits of PBMT is the ability potentially to decrease the dosage or frequency of administration of chronic pain medications, including especially non-steroidal anti-inflammatories. The weaning of chronic medications is not recommended until a patient is on a regular schedule of maintenance treatments with PBMT that seems to best control their symptoms. In this way, the practitioner may appreciate changes in the patient's response and comfort level while changing only one factor at a time.

Variations in the treatment frequencies recommend here may be noted in the individual musculoskeletal condition sections that follow.

Osteoarthritis and Rheumatoid Arthritis

One of the most common uses of PBMT in veterinary medicine today is for the treatment of chronic pain associated with osteoarthritis. As previously discussed, many different animal and human trials have been performed that show the modulatory effect of PBMT on inflammatory markers (IL1β, PGE2, tumor necrosis factor alpha (TNFα)) and other aspects of the inflammatory process (reducing edema and influx of neutrophils) (Bjordal *et al.*, 2006). Others have shown the ability of PBMT to reduce significantly the total number of leukocytes and neutrophils in a treated arthritic joint cavity, as well as the concentration of IL1β and IL6 in joint fluid (Pallotta *et al.*, 2012). These results are important, since leukocyte influx to the joint is a hallmark of arthritis and IL1β and IL6 have been implicated in cartilage degradation and the stimulation of metalloproteinases, respectively. Furthermore, treatment with laser therapy has been shown to reduce the activity of metalloproteinases 2 and 9 in an experimental model involving rats with induced knee arthritis (Carlos *et al.*, 2014). More recently, studies have been published looking at the use of PBMT in treating humans with Bouchard's and Heberden's osteoarthritis (Baltzer *et al.*, 2016) and knee osteoarthritis (Fukuda *et al.*, 2015). They show that laser-treated patients experienced a significant reduction in pain and swelling, as well as a short-term increase in joint mobility and function. PBMT has also been used successfully to treat the

pain and stiffness associated with rheumatoid arthritis (Brosseau *et al.*, 2000).

Patient preparation, laser administration technique, dosing, and frequency of administration are as described earlier.

Temporomandibular Joint Disorders

The temporomandibular joint (TMJ) is a unique anatomic area that, when affected, can cause a range of clinical symptoms in veterinary patients, from difficulty opening the mouth, dysphagia, and pain to performance problems in canine and equine athletes. It is important when treating the TMJ that all structures typically associated with pain and dysfunction in this area are treated and included when calculating dose. These structures include the TMJ itself, periarticular tissues, and masticatory muscles (Figure 13.9). In human dentistry, PBMT has been used to treat disorders of the TMJ, aimed at relieving pain and improving function (Melis *et al.*, 2012); in many cases, pain-relieving effects lasted beyond the treatment period and into 1–2 years' follow-up (Ayyildi *et al.*, 2015). As with all treatments performed on or around the face, head, and neck, special care should be taken and appropriate protection for the patient's eyes should be provided (see section on Patient Preparation and Technique).

Myopathies and Myositis

PBMT for muscle injury rehabilitation and for use in myositis caused by snake-bite envenomation is covered in other chapters. When examining the literature with regard to myositis in general, however, PBMT has been used to treat experimentally induced myositis in rats (Carvalho *et al.*, 2015), resulting in a significant reduction

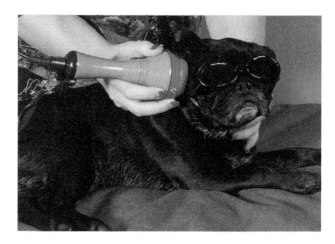

Figure 13.9 Laser therapist treating the TMJ.

in the presence of inflammatory cells and in the amount of edema present in tissue after treatment. Additional studies on experimental myopathy show significant changes in inflammatory biomarkers and oxidative stress (decreased levels of fibrinogen, L-citrulline, and superoxide dismutase (SOD)) and significant muscle recovery (Servetto *et al.*, 2010), as well as a notable reduction in the area occupied by inflammatory infiltrates (Dávila *et al.*, 2011). Though most inflammatory myopathies in dogs and cats are either idiopathic (e.g., masticatory myositis, idiopathic polymyositis) or secondarily associated with other diseases (e.g., those associated with Rickettsial or parasitic infections), both types are the result of inflammatory cells infiltrating into striated muscles (Podell, 2002). The muscle cell degeneration and necrosis seen in idiopathic inflammatory myopathies are thought to be caused by lymphocyte-mediated cytotoxic mechanisms. In particular, many of the cytokines involved in the process (including IL1β and TNFα) were mentioned in the literature review sections as those downregulated by the application of PBMT.

Current therapies for idiopathic inflammatory myopathies in veterinary medicine are aimed at reducing pain and inflammation with systemic immunosuppression and analgesics, followed by either maintenance anti-inflammatory or immune-modulatory medications when necessary. In the author's subjective experience, PBMT may be very effective, especially in managing pain in patients affected by masticatory myositis, and it has been used in several veterinary patients without any harmful sequelae noted. Dosing has been similar to that used for treating TMJ or other deep-tissue musculoskeletal disorders. Again, precautions should be taken to protect the patient's eyes during treatment around the face. Similarly, the author recommends treating all of the affected muscles of mastication (temporalis, digastricus, and masseter), any painful facial muscles, as well as the muscles in the cranial cervical area for any associated spasm or soreness. Daily treatment is recommended initially for optimal pain management, tapering as the patient improves (as for other chronic conditions). PBMT should always be used as an adjunct alongside standard-of-care treatment until further research is done to examine its effectiveness in treating these disorders in veterinary patients in a clinical setting.

Tendinopathies

Other chapters cover the treatment of acute tendon and ligament injuries with PBMT and regenerative medicine; the same mechanisms of action apply to the effectiveness of the modality for more chronic tendinopathies that occur following damage to a tendon. Histopathology of common overuse tendon conditions includes discontinuous and disorganized collagen fibers, abnormal neovascularization, and necrosis. Pain, edema, crepitus, and impaired function may be diagnosed clinically in patients with these conditions (Jozsa and Kannus, 1997; Khan *et al.*, 1999). The etiology is incompletely understood.

Treating chronic tendinopathies can be frustrating. Even though most improve with rest, a certain percentage of patients will experience reoccurrence of symptoms as soon as activities are resumed. Not unexpectedly, reports exist demonstrating a reduction in the pro-inflammatory mediators IL6, TNFα, TGFβ cytokines, and COX-2 enzyme following PBM application in a tendonitis model (Pires *et al.*, 2011). Fibroblast metabolism and proliferation are enhanced, and there is an increase in collagen fibril size and biomechanical strength (Ng *et al.*, 2004).

In a recent randomized, placebo-controlled, double-blinded clinical trial, 16 human subjects with chronic tendinopathy of the extensor carpi radialis brevis tendon (lateral epicondylitis) received eight treatments with either a sham or a real laser over a period of 18 days. The laser-treated group demonstrated improvement in handgrip strength, function, and reduction in pain continuously over a 12-month period, despite return to normal activity (Roberts *et al.*, 2013). In contrast, pain, strength, and functional impairment in the sham group remained unchanged until 12 months, when there was partial improvement in these outcomes, consistent with resolution of clinical signs of tendinopathy following 12 months of reduced use (Jozsa and Kannus, 1997). Treatment of tendinopathies in veterinary patients is optimally performed in conjunction with an excellent rehabilitation therapy program. Dosing and frequency of treatment are typical for deep-tissue musculoskeletal conditions, with consideration given to the location (depth) of the tendon being treated and of associated soft tissues when selecting power parameters. It should be noted that patients experiencing an acute exacerbation of tendonitis or tendinopathy may be very hypersensitive to pressure, temperature, or both, and that adjustments in treatment power and a choice between on-contact and off-contact treatment may need to be made according to the practitioner's clinical judgment.

Cranial Cruciate Ligament Injuries

Though literature specific to ligament injuries is described in other chapters, there are some studies that specifically examine injury of the cranial cruciate ligament (CCL) and the progression of subsequent osteoarthritis in the knee. In one rodent model, laser treatment started immediately after cruciate ligament transection was shown to prevent certain features related to articular degeneration of the knee following transection (Bublitz *et al.*, 2014). A similar rabbit model showed that at least 6 weeks of intermittent laser treatment could relieve knee pain and control synovium inflammation and cartilage damage (Wang *et al.*, 2014).

Unsurprisingly, one of the most common uses for PBMT in daily veterinary practice is in the conservative pain management of partial CCL tears. But does application of PBMT to these injuries contribute to healing or prevent further injury? Though supporting literature is more common regarding calcaneal tendon models, the principles of potential efficacy are the same. Studies have demonstrated the exertion of an anti-inflammatory effect over injured tendons, with reduction of the release of pro-inflammatory cytokines such as TNFα (Da Ré Guerra *et al.*, 2016), improvement in the remodeling of extracellular matrix (ECM) during the healing process in tendons through activation of matrix metalloproteinase 2 (MMP2), and stimulation of collagen synthesis (Guerra *et al.*, 2013). Improvement of collagen fiber organization (Oliveira *et al.*, 2009) and increased neovascularization in injured tendons exposed to PBMT (Salate *et al.*, 2005) have also been demonstrated.

For conservative management of partial CCL tears, typical dosing for deep-tissue musculoskeletal conditions should be used. It is recommended that both stifles be treated, due to compensatory weight shifting, and that treatment of the lower back be considered as well, paying particular attention to the iliopsoas muscle, to check for any pain or spasm. Treatment for the stifle should include a large area (see section on Patient Preparation and Treatment Technique), incorporating all of the important soft-tissue structures, including the insertion of the hamstring muscles and the patellar ligament. Treatment should be administered at least three times weekly until significant improvement is noted (as with all chronic conditions), with continuous reassessment, and should optimally be utilized along with an appropriate physical rehabilitation program.

Additional uses of PBMT with regards to the CCL deal with its application postoperatively for many of the surgeries used to address complete CCL tears, as well as for those pets that have not had surgery due to the owner's decision, other medical conditions, or other factors preventing surgery. It should be emphasized that PBMT is most beneficial for managing pain and decreasing inflammation associated with these conditions. Though it may also contribute to tendon healing in partial CCL tear situations, its application will not correct the structural instability in cases of complete CCL tears. It is always best utilized in combination with an appropriate physical rehabilitation program.

Treatment with PBMT should begin immediately after surgery to address the pain and inflammation created and to assist in wound healing. The incisional area and superficial soft tissues disrupted during surgery may be treated with a more superficial target energy density of $4-6\,\mathrm{J/cm^2}$ and with a lower power setting than would be used in a deep-tissue musculoskeletal dose. The deeper soft tissues of the anatomic region, which are often painful, swollen, or bruised after surgery, may be treated with a dose typical for musculoskeletal disorders (target energy density $6-10\,\mathrm{J/cm^2}$, depending on the size of the patient). The entire treatment area mentioned for partial CCL tear management (including the contralateral stifle and lower back) should be treated in postoperative cases as well. Treatment should ideally be performed daily, if possible, for the first 3 days, and then twice to three times weekly, as with other chronic conditions, tapering as the patient improves. Please note that if the patient is placed in a soft bandage after surgery, the application of PBMT should be performed during bandage changes, as PBMT cannot be performed through bandage, splint, or casting material.

Fractures and Bone Healing

PBMT may also be used to address fractures, whether freshly surgically fixated or delayed/non-union. In addition to the pain-relieving aspects that PBMT brings to these cases, there is quite a lot of evidence in the literature for its use in situations where bone healing is desired. In a recent review of 25 relevant articles regarding the use of PBMT in bone healing (13 *in vitro* and 12 animal studies), 11 *in vitro* studies showed positive results with regard to acceleration of cell proliferation and differentiation. All animal studies showed improved bone healing in laser-treated sites (Ebrahimi *et al.*, 2012). Furthermore, one paper showed that even though PBMT's effects were more prominent when treatment started during the acute phase of the injury, laser therapy still aided the bone-consolidation process and favored the physiopathologic mechanisms involved in bone tissue repair when used in the chronic phase (Mota *et al.*, 2013).

Osteopenic patients, or those with compromised bone healing, have also been looked at in the research. A study investigating bone healing of the femur in both osteopenic and normal rats with titanium implants showed an improved osseointegration process in both groups, particular in the initial phase of bone formation (de Vasconcellos *et al.*, 2014). Another study, looking at bone healing in diabetic rats with a tibial defect, showed that all laser-treated groups had a better histological pattern and a higher amount of newly formed bone than control groups in both histological and morphometric evaluation (Magri *et al.*, 2015).

Further controlled studies in veterinary patients need to be performed in order to characterize the optimal dosing and effects for bone healing, but at this time it is recommended that treatment be performed immediately after stabilization, and then proceed every other day for a total of six to eight treatments (Godbold and Arza, 2011). Fracture healing should be reassessed at this time, and treatments continued if healing is not progressing.

Please note that if the patient is placed in a soft bandage or other covering after surgery, the application of PBMT should be performed during bandage changes, as PBMT cannot be performed through bandage, splint, or casting material. Alternatively, a "window" can be created in the bandage material, through which PBMT can be performed over part of the fracture site; the window can then be re-bandaged to keep the overall bandage intact (though this is less than ideal, since the entire area may not be treated). A target energy density of $8-10\,\text{J/cm}^2$ is recommended, and the entire area to be measured or estimated for treatment should include not only the fractured area itself, but also several square centimeters of adjacent normal bone. Please note the information regarding the use of PBMT with metal implants given earlier.

Osteomyelitis

Based on *in vivo* and *in vitro* studies, which initially reported that laser energy in differing wavelengths and irradiation regimes had potential bactericidal effects on certain bacterial infections, including *Staphylococcus aureus*, one study looked at its effects on chronic osteomyelitis induced experimentally in the rat tibia. Methicillin-resistant *S. aureus* (MRSA) was used to induce osteomyelitis in the rats' tibias. After 3 weeks, rats with evidence of osteomyelitis were treated with debridement alone, treated with debridement plus laser irradiation, or not treated at all. Irradiation commenced immediately after debridement surgery with an 808 nm, 100 mW continuous-wave (CW) diode laser with an irradiance of $127.3\,\text{mW/cm}^2$ and was applied daily for five consecutive days at three different energy densities ranging from 7.64 to $22.93\,\text{J/cm}^2$. Following sacrifice, tibias were removed and analyzed histopathologically, radiographically, and microbiologically. Histopathology showed that infection levels had decreased by 37, 67, 81, and 93% in the groups treated by debridement and by debridement plus 7.64, 15.29, and $22.93\,\text{J/cm}^2$ of light therapy, respectively, compared to the negative control group (Kaya *et al.*, 2011). Further studies should be done in veterinary patients, but deep-tissue musculoskeletal dosing similar to that used for bone healing should be sufficient to achieve energy densities in this range for infections in the same

anatomic areas, should practitioners wish to attempt the use of PBMT as an adjunct to other standard-of-care osteomyelitis treatments.

Neck and Back Pain

One of the most common causes of neuropathic pain in veterinary medicine is intervertebral disk disease (IVDD). IVDD was first classified as Type I or Type II by Hansen (1951). Type I is commonly associated with chondroid disk degeneration and involves herniation of the nucleus pulposus through the annulus fibrosis, resulting in extrusion of disk material into the spinal canal and subsequently in varying degrees of compression of the spinal cord.

Typically affecting younger, small-breed, chondrodystrophic dogs, though it may also occur in larger, non-chondrodystrophic breeds, Type I disk extrusion cases usually present as an acute-onset episode, and clinical signs vary depending on the severity of the resultant spinal cord injury and neuroanatomic localization. Clinical signs include varying degrees of spinal hyperesthesia and neurological deficits from paraparesis to paraplegia, with or without deep pain perception. Thoracolumbar disk herniation is reported in 66–87% of dogs with intervertebral disk herniation (Gage, 1975; Hansen, 1951). The disks located between T12 and L3 have been shown to be at higher risk of herniation (Brisson, 2010). IVDD with extrusion can also occur in the cervical spine, and many of these patients will present with varying degrees of lowered head and neck carriage, guarding, or cervical spinal muscle spasms. Root signature may be observed with impingement of C5–C8 nerve roots.

Type II IVDD is associated with fibroid degeneration and involves a shift of the nucleus pulposus secondary to weakening and partial rupture of the annulus, causing a focal protrusion into the spinal canal. Cases usually display a slow, progressive onset of clinical signs. Type II protrusions occur more commonly in older, non-chondrodystrophic breeds; chondrodystrophic breeds *can* develop them, but it is less common (Macias *et al.*, 2002).

Disk extrusion or protrusion causes spinal cord injury. The damage is usually the most severe at the sites of occurrence, and the associated clinical signs are caused by concussion or compression. Pathologic changes progress, and the ensuing neurodegenerative process contributes to the development of inflammation, along with a complex cascade of vascular and biochemical events that contribute to secondary spinal cord injury and neuronal damage. An article on "Rehabilitation and Physical Therapy for the Neurologic Patient" by Sims *et al.* (2015) further explains, "Even in the absence of persistent compression, ischemia, or decreased perfusion, local edema and secondary oxidative damage play a key role in the extent and severity of spinal cord injury. Of these, tissue perfusion may be the most responsive to physiotherapeutic intervention; thus, physiotherapy techniques and modalities that promote circulation are often central to the rehabilitation program for patients with spinal cord injury."

If for no other reason than its positive effects on tissue perfusion, PBMT is an excellent modality to reach for in cases of IVDD, regardless of other treatments employed, conservatively or surgically. Researchers exploring the uses of PBMT in treating IVDD among other neurological conditions have not stopped there, however. One *in vitro* study investigating the inflammation induced by the interaction between macrophages and the human annulus fibrosus cells found that laser irradiation markedly suppressed IL6 and IL8 levels in a time-dependent manner (Hwang *et al.*, 2015). Another study investigating one of the major causes of pain in human degenerative lumbar spinal disease – chronic compression of the dorsal root ganglion (CCD) – examined the molecular-based irritation involving the localized release of inflammatory cytokines and the effects of laser irradiation on them. Two of the primary cytokines responsible for the hyperalgesia observed in lumbar spinal diseases are TNFα and IL1β. It has been demonstrated that herniated disk tissues release IL1β, which affects the somatosensory neural response at the dorsal root level; previous studies have also shown that TNFα in the nucleus pulposus plays an important role in radicular pain (root signature or referred pain) and that sensory neurons display increased sensitivity to TNFα in a rat CCD model. This study demonstrated not only that the expression levels of both of these cytokines are reduced by the application of laser light, but also that it promotes neural regeneration and significantly reduces CCD-mediated mechanical and thermal hyperalgesia (Chen *et al.*, 2014).

One study followed 26 human patients with chronic neck pain diagnosed as being caused by cervical disk herniation who were treated twice weekly for 4 weeks with laser irradiation over the painful area. A visual analog scale was used to determine the effects of laser on chronic pain. After the end of the treatment regimen, a significant improvement was observed (Takahashi *et al.*, 2012). These findings and others from similar studies involving the use of PBMT in treating cervical pain are consistent with Chow *et al.*'s (2009) conclusions from a meta-analysis of 16 randomized controlled trials (RCTs) including 820 patients treated with PBMT for neck pain. This review showed that laser treatment reduced pain immediately after treatment in acute neck pain and up to 22 weeks after completion of treatment in chronic neck pain.

Even diskogenic back pain patients who failed to respond to a conventional physical therapy program to avoid recourse to surgical intervention have been shown to benefit from treatment with laser. One paper reported on the long-term mean 5-year prospective follow-up of a patient group of 50 unselected patients visiting a referral pain center for diskogenic back pain. Each patient had a single-level lesion documented by magnetic resonance imaging (MRI) followed by diskography to confirm the affected disk was the source of pain. All of the patients who entered the study had failed response to a combination of non-steroidal anti-inflammatory agents, and all had at least 3 months of conventional physical therapy prior to being treated with three laser therapy treatment sessions per week for 12 consecutive weeks. At the end of treatment at 12 weeks, 49 of 50 patients had significant improvement in their Oswestry Disability Index score, which was maintained at long-term follow-up assessments 1 and 5 years later (Ip and Fu, 2015b).

Draper *et al.* (2012) examined the use of PBMT in non-ambulatory dogs with thoracolumbar IVDD following decompressive surgery compared to a control group that received hemilaminectomy alone. There was a significant difference between the two groups in the median time to ambulation (3.5 days in the PBMT-treated group versus 14 days in the control group), which was independent of age, weight, modified Frankel score, and duration of clinical signs on presentation. Even though this study demonstrated a positive effect, more information needs to be gathered in order to optimize the parameters used to treat this condition. The irradiance in this study ($25\,000\,\mathrm{mW/cm^2}$ applied "to the overlying skin of the spinal segment associated with the hemilaminectomy and the two adjacent ones (one cranial and one caudal)") is likely misreported, as this level would cause thermal damage to the tissue surface. Additionally, the calculations of irradiance and fluence "delivered to the spinal cord" are based on personal communications of unpublished data, emphasizing the need for more rigorous standards when conducting clinical laser research. Laser device parameters should be tested prior to the beginning of a clinical study to ensure that the wavelengths and power reported by a laser manufacturer are correct, and any extrapolation based on tissue modeling or other estimations should be reported.

Further studies should be done in veterinary patients, in both conservative-management models and post-surgical-application models, and in dogs that have presented with and without deep pain perception still present. However, there is certainly enough evidence in the present body of literature to support the use of PBMT as an adjunct to current standard-of-care treatment regimens for patients with IVDD. It should be noted that whether or not PBMT is available, current best practices and recommendations (whether for surgical or conservative management) should be communicated to owners after examination of the patient.

Current deep-tissue musculoskeletal dosing is appropriate for treating the cervical, thoracic, lumbar, and sacral spine. Treatment surface areas used for calculating dose should take into consideration a few spinal segments cranial to the suspected area of intervertebral disk extrusion or protrusion, and caudally the same distance. If any spasms in the paraspinal muscles are noted further caudally or if neurological deficits are present in the limbs, it is recommended to treat the remainder of the spine as well. For thoracolumbar lesions, treatment should be applied directly over the spine (Figure 13.10), as well as a few inches to either side, aiming toward the spine through the paraspinal musculature. In the neck area, a lateral and ventral approach is recommended, and the laser therapist is reminded that in order to effectively treat the caudal cervical area (Figure 13.11), manipulation of the front leg may be necessary, which is often painful for the patient due to radicular pain. This should be done with care, and a good knowledge of anatomy is critical to treating the correct areas in these patients. Patients with back and neck pain should be treated in the position that is most comfortable for them, which may involve standing, sitting, or lying down in various positions.

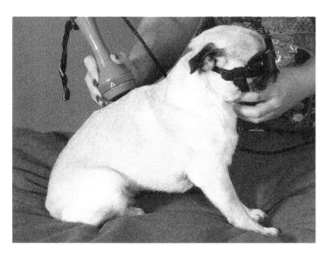

Figure 13.10 Laser therapist treating the spine.

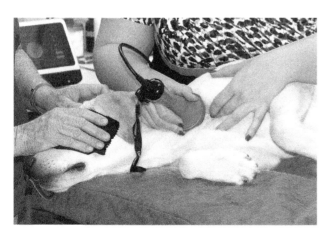

Figure 13.11 Laser therapist treating the caudal cervical area.

For patients prescribed conservative management, PBMT should begin immediately and continue daily, if possible, until significant improvement is seen. At this time, weaning to a transition phase of less frequent treatments until resolution of clinical signs, as previously described, is possible. Some patients with chronic IVDD may benefit from continued maintenance-therapy treatment, just like patients with osteoarthritis.

For patients that have undergone surgical decompression, PBMT may be started immediately after surgery for the wound area, similar to the recommendations for postoperative CCL patients. The paraspinal muscles in these patients should be treated in a similar manner to the technique described earlier, aiming toward the spine with the treatment handpiece and laser beam and using deep-tissue dosing. Since the surgical incision often has staples or sutures in place, see the recommendations given earlier regarding metal implants and suture material. Ideally, PBMT should be started daily for 3–5 days, if possible, and then continued at least three times weekly until significant improvement is seen, when the frequency of treatment can be weaned as described earlier. As always, results with PBMT are optimized when it is used in conjunction with an excellent physical rehabilitation program and other supportive care for neurologic patients.

Common Reasons for Perceived Treatment Failure or Inconsistent Results

In general, PBMT should produce consistent, reliable improvement if used in the appropriate manner (see sections describing Treatment Techniques and Dosimetry). As with any treatment modality, however, certain factors may influence the effectiveness. The most common reasons for a lack of efficacy or inconsistent results include:

1) **Treating the incorrect area:** Ensure that a recent, complete orthopedic, neurologic, and pain examination has been performed to confirm the source of problem. Often, a patient may be referred for PBMT for osteoarthritis of a specific joint, which may or may not be the primary source of discomfort. Additionally, as previously mentioned, the degree of pathologic change noted on radiographs alone may not necessarily be consistent with the amount of lameness displayed by a patient or the severity of their discomfort. To ensure that a therapeutic dose is delivered properly, ensure that the laser therapist performing the treatment knows the correct anatomical landmarks to delineate the proper treatment

area, and that these are the same as those used by the veterinarian prescribing the treatment.

2) **Not treating *all* of the problem areas:** Ensure that all sources of pain or anatomic dysfunction identified on examination are being addressed. Compensatory biomechanical changes occur commonly with chronic, painful conditions, and if they are not therapeutically addressed with PBMT and additional rehabilitation therapy, the patient may continue to experience discomfort and exhibit lameness or difficulties. For example, as previously mentioned, most animals with stifle or hip osteoarthritis usually have some degree of back pain and pain in the contralateral joint from weight shifting if both sides are not being addressed.

3) **A change in patient activity or medications:** Though more commonly seen after an initial improvement and subsequent worsening, make sure to inquire with the pet owner about any changes in medication or activity level at home. Often times after improvement with PBMT, pet owners will wean or discontinue other medications, even if this has not yet been recommended, or take their pet for a run or play session at the local dog park, which can result in increased soreness or, worse, an overuse injury.

4) **An exacerbation of the condition:** Also more commonly seen after an initial improvement and subsequent worsening, many cases of osteoarthritis may require additional pain management and further diagnostics. Some anatomical areas, particularly the elbow joint, are notoriously difficult to treat, and may require higher doses of PBMT, or the addition of other medications or therapeutics, in order to bring about improvement. It is not uncommon in some of these areas for loose or damaged pieces of articular cartilage or small pieces of osteophytes to break off with normal activity and further irritate the joint. Further diagnostics and examination should always be performed any time a patient presents with acute-on-chronic pain.

5) **The presence of an undiagnosed problem:** Ensure that there is not another pathologic process affecting the anatomic area of concern. Repeat radiographs and examinations to rule out malignancy, particularly if joint or bone pain is present and does not improve with PBMT.

6) **An inappropriate "induction phase" or the need for a "mini re-induction phase":** Ensure that an appropriate induction phase has been administered before weaning the frequency of treatments to a transition or maintenance phase (see section on Frequency of Treatment Sessions). Previously, many treatment recommendations stated that it was sufficient to treat chronic conditions with three treatments during week 1, two treatments in week 2, and one treatment in week 3. While this may be effective for some patients, many will not respond unless a more intensive and frequent induction phase is used. Patients may also fail to respond if transition- or maintenance-phase treatments are been missed due to poor owner compliance.

References

AAHA/AAFP. (2007) AAHA/AAFP pain management guidelines for dogs & cats. *J Am Anim Hosp Assoc.* **43**(5):235–248.

Alfredo, P.P. *et al.* (2012) Efficacy of low level PBMT associated with exercises in knee osteoarthritis: a randomized double-blind study. *Clinical Rehab.* **26**(6):523–533.

Ammar, T.A. (2014) Monochromatic infrared photo energy versus low level PBMT in patients with knee osteoarthritis. *J Lasers Med Sci.* **5**(4):176–182.

Anders, J.J. *et al.* (2004) Phototherapy promotes regeneration and functional recovery of injured peripheral nerve. *Neurol Res.* **26**(2):233–239.

Anders, J.J. *et al.* (2014) In vitro and in vivo optimization of infrared laser treatment for injured peripheral nerves. *Lasers Surg Med.* **46**(1):34–45.

Assis, L. *et al.* (2016) Aerobic exercise training and low-level PBMT modulate inflammatory response and degenerative process in an experimental model of knee osteoarthritis in rats. *Osteoarthritis Cartilage.* **24**(1):169–177.

Avni, D. *et al.* (2005) Protection of skeletal muscles from ischemic injury: low-level PBMT increases antioxidant activity. *Photomed Laser Surg.* **23**(3):273–277.

Ayyildiz, S. *et al.* (2015) Evaluation of low-level PBMT in TMD patients. *Case Reports in Dentistry.* **2015**:424213.

Baltzer, A.W.A. *et al.* (2016) Positive effects of low level PBMT (LLLT) on Bouchard's and Heberden's osteoarthritis. *Lasers Surg Med.* **48**(5):498–504.

Bjordal, J.M. *et al.* (2006) Photoradiation in acute pain: a systematic review of possible mechanisms of action and clinical effects in randomized placebo-controlled trials. *Photomed Laser Surg.* **24**(2):158–168.

Brisson, B. (2010) Intervertebral disc disease in dogs. *Vet Clin North Am Small Anim Pract.* **40**(5):829–858.

Brosseau, L. *et al.* (2000) Low level PBMT for osteoarthritis and rheumatoid arthritis: a metaanalysis. *J Rheumatol.* **27**(8):1961–1969.

Bublitz, C. *et al.* (2014) Low-level PBMT prevents degenerative morphological changes in an experimental model of anterior cruciate ligament transection in rats. *Lasers Med Sci.* **29**(5):1669–1678.

Cambier, D. *et al.* (2000) The influence of low intensity infrared laser irradiation on conduction characteristics of peripheral nerve: a randomised, controlled, double blind study on the sural nerve. *Lasers Med Sci.* **15**(3):195–200.

Carlos, F.P. *et al.* (2014) Protective effect of low-level PBMT (LLLT) on acute zymosan-induced arthritis. *Lasers Med Sci.* **29**(2):757–763.

Carvalho, A.F. *et al.* (2015) The low-level laser on acute myositis in rats. *Acta Cir Bras.* **30**(12):806–811.

Chen, Y.J. *et al.* (2014) Effect of low level PBMT on chronic compression of the dorsal root ganglion. *PloS One.* **9**(3):e89894.

Chien, S. and Wilhelmi, B.J. (2012) A simplified technique for producing an ischemic wound model. *J Vis Exp.* **2**(63):e3341.

Chow, R.T. *et al.* (2009) Efficacy of low level PBMT in the management of neck pain: a systematic review and meta-analysis of randomized placebo or active-treatment controlled trials. *Lancet.* **374**(9705):1897–1908.

Chow, R.T. *et al.* (2011) Inhibitory effects of laser irradiation on peripheral mammalian nerves and relevance to analgesic effects: a systematic review. *Photomed Laser Surg.* **29**(6):365–381.

Da Ré Guerra, F. *et al.* (2016) Low-level PBMT modulates pro-inflammatory cytokines after partial tenotomy. *Lasers Med Sci.* **31**(4):759–766.

Dávila, S., *et al.* (2011) Low level PBMT on experimental myopathy. *PBMT.* **20**(4):287–292.

de Vasconcellos, L.M.R. *et al.* (2014) Healing of normal and osteopenic bone with titanium implant and low-level PBMT (GaAlAs): a histomorphometric study in rats. *Lasers Med Sci.* **29**(2):575–580.

Draper, W.E. *et al.* (2012) Low-level PBMT reduces time to ambulation in dogs after hemilaminectomy: a preliminary study. *J Small Anim Pract.* **53**(8):465–469.

Dray, A. and Perkins, M. (1993) Bradykinin and inflammatory pain. *Trends Neurosci.* **16**(3):99–104.

Ebrahimi, T. *et al.* (2012) The influence of low-intensity PBMT on bone healing. *J Dent (Tehran).* **9**(4):238–248.

Fukuda, V.O. *et al.* (2015) Short term efficacy of low level PBMT in patients with knee osteoarthritis: a randomized, placebo-controlled, double-blind clinical trial. *Revista Brasileira de Ortopedia.* **46**(5):526–533.

Gage, E.D. (1975) Incidence of clinical disc disease in the dog. *J Am Anim Hosp Assoc.* **11**:135–138.

Gaynor, J. (2015) Energy modalities, therapeutic laser and pulsed electromagnetic field therapy. In: *Handbook of Veterinary Pain Management*, 3 edn., pp. 357–362. Mosby, St. Louis, MO.

Godbold, J. and Arza, R. (2011) *Reference Guide to Common Conditions for CTC, CTS.* LiteCure, Newark, DE.

Góralczyk, K. *et al.* (2015) Effect of LLLT on endothelial cells culture. *Lasers Med Sci.* **30**(1):273–278.

Guerra, F.R. *et al.* (2013) LLLT improves tendon healing through increase of MMP activity and collagen synthesis. *Lasers Med Sci.* **28**(5):1281–1288.

Hagiwara, S. *et al.* (2007) GaAlAs (830 nm) low-level laser enhances peripheral endogenous opioid analgesia in rats. *Lasers Surg Med.* **39**(10):797–802.

Hansen, H.J. (1951) A pathologic-anatomical interpretation of disc degeneration in dogs. *Acta Orthop Scand.* **20**:280–293.

Hsieh, Y.L. *et al.* (2014) Fluence-dependent effects of low-level PBMT in myofascial trigger spots on modulation of biochemicals associated with pain in a rabbit model. *Lasers Med Sci.* **30**(1):209–216.

Hwang, M.H. *et al.* (2015) Low level light therapy modulates inflammatory mediators secreted by human annulus fibrosus cells during intervertebral disc degeneration in vitro. *Photochem Photobiol.* **91**(2):403–410.

Ignatov, Y., *et al.* (2005) Effects of helium–neon laser irradiation and local anesthetics on potassium channels in pond snail neurons. *Neurosci Behav Physiol.* **35**:871–875.

Ip, D. and Fu, N.Y. (2015a) Can combined use of low-level lasers and hyaluronic acid injections prolong the longevity of degenerative knee joints? *Clin Interv Aging.* **10**:1255–1258.

Ip, D. and Fu, N.Y. (2015b) Can intractable discogenic back pain be managed by low-level PBMT without recourse to operative intervention? *J Pain Res.* **8**:253–256.

Jang, H. and Lee, H. (2012) Meta-analysis of pain relief effects by laser irradiation on joint areas. *Photomed Laser Surg.* **30**(8):405–417.

Jimbo, K. *et al.* (1998) Suppressive effects of low-power laser irradiation on bradykinin evoked action potentials in cultured murine dorsal root ganglion cells. *Neurosci Lett.* **240**(2):93–96.

Johnston, S.A. (1997) Osteoarthritis. *Vet Clin North Am Small Anim Pract.* **27**(4):699–723.

Jozsa, L.G. and Kannus, P. (1997) *Human tendons: Anatomy, Physiology, and Pathology.* Human Kinetics, Champaign, IL.

Karu T, *et al.* (1997) He–Ne laser radiation influences single-channel ionic currents through cell membranes: a patch-clamp study. *Proc. SPIE.* **3198**:57–66.

Kaya, G.Ş. *et al.* (2011) The use of 808-nm light therapy to treat experimental chronic osteomyelitis induced in rats by methicillin-resistant *Staphylococcus aureus. Photomed Laser Surg.* **29**(6):405–412.

Khan, K.M. *et al.* (1999) Histopathology of common tendinopathies. Update and implications for clinical management. *Sports Med.* **27**(6):393–408.

Labajos, M. (1988) Beta-endorphin levels modification after GaAs and HeNe laser irradiation on the rabbit. *Comparative study. Invest Clin.* **1–2**:6–8.

Liebert, A.D. *et al.* (2014) Protein conformational modulation by photons: a mechanism for laser treatment effects. *Med Hypotheses.* **82**(3):275–281.

Lister, T. *et al.* (2012) Optical properties of human skin. *J Biomed Opt.* **17**(9):90901.

Lopes-Martins, R.A. *et al.* (2005) Spontaneous effects of low-level PBMT (650 nm) in acute inflammatory mouse pleurisy induced by carrageenan. *Photomed Laser Surg.* **23**(4):377–381.

Macias, C. *et al.* (2002) Thoracolumbar disc disease in large dogs: a study of 99 cases. *J Small Anim Pract.* **43**(10):439–446.

Magri, A.M. *et al.* (2015) Photobiomodulation and bone healing in diabetic rats: evaluation of bone response using a tibial defect experimental model. *Lasers Med Sci.* **30**(7):1949–1957

McLaughlin, R. (2000) Management of chronic osteoarthritic pain. *Vet Clin North Am Small Anim Pract.* **30**(4):933–949.

Melis, M., *et al.* (2012) Low level laser therapy for the treatment of temporomandibular disorders: a systematic review of the literature. *Cranio.* **30**(4):304–312.

Millis, D.L. and Ciuperca, I.A. (2015) Evidence for canine rehabilitation and physical therapy. *Vet Clin North Am Small Anim Pract.* **45**(1):1–27.

Mizutani, K. *et al.* (2004) A clinical study on serum prostaglandin E2 with low-level PBMT. *Photomed Laser Surg.* **22**(6):537–539.

Montesinos, M. (1988) Experimental effects of low power laser in encephalin and endorphin synthesis. *J Eur Med Laser Assoc.* **1**(3):2–7.

Morries, L.D. *et al.* (2015) Treatments for traumatic brain injury with emphasis on transcranial near-infrared laser phototherapy. *Neuropsychiatr Dis Treat.* **11**:2159–2175.

Mota, F.C.D. *et al.* (2013) Low-power PBMT for repairing acute and chronic-phase bone lesions. *Res Vet Sci.* **94**(1):105–110.

NC State. (2016) Feline Musculoskeletal Pain Index (FMPI). Available from: https://cvm.ncsu.edu/research/labs/clinical-sciences/comparative-pain-research/clinical-metrology-instruments/(accessed November 30, 2016).

Ng, G.Y.F. *et al.* (2004) Comparison of single and multiple applications of GaAlAs laser on rat medial collateral ligament repair. *Lasers Surg Med.* **34**(3):285–289.

Oliveira, F.S. *et al.* (2009) Effect of low level PBMT (830 nm) with different therapy regimes on the process of tissue repair in partial lesion calcaneous tendon. *Lasers Surg Med.* **41**(4):271–276.

Oron, A. *et al.* (2006) Low-level PBMT applied transcranially to rats after induction of stroke significantly reduces long-term neurological deficits. *Stroke.* **37**(10):2620–2624.

Oron, U. *et al.* (2001) Low-energy laser irradiation reduces formation of scar tissue after myocardial infarction in rats and dogs. *Circulation.* **103**(2):296–301.

Pallotta, R.C. *et al.* (2012) Infrared (810-nm) low-level PBMT on rat experimental knee inflammation. *Lasers Med Sci.* **27**(1):71–78.

Peimani, A. and Sardary, F. (2014) Effect of low-level laser on healing of temporomandibular joint osteoarthritis in rats. *J Dent (Tehran).* **11**(3):319–327.

PennVet. (2016) Canine Brief Pain Inventory (Canine BPI). Available from: http://www.vet.upenn.edu/research/clinical-trials/vcic/pennchart/cbpi-tool (accessed November 30, 2016).

Pires, D. *et al.* (2011) Low-level PBMT (LLLT; 780 nm) acts differently on mRNA expression of anti- and pro-inflammatory mediators in an experimental model of collagenase-induced tendinitis in rat. *Lasers Med Sci.* **26**(1):85–94.

Podell, M. (2002). Inflammatory myopathies. *Vet Clin North Am Small Anim Pract.* **32**(1):147–167.

Prianti, A.C.G. *et al.* (2014) Low-level PBMT (LLLT) reduces the COX-2 mRNA expression in both subplantar and total brain tissues in the model of peripheral inflammation induced by administration of carrageenan. *Lasers Med Sci.* **29**(4):1397–1403.

Pryor, B. and Millis, D.L. (2015) Therapeutic laser in veterinary medicine. *Vet Clin North Am Small Anim Pract.* **45**(1):45–56.

Riegel, R. (2008) General therapy guidelines. In: *Laser Therapy in the Companion Animal Practice*, 1 edn., p. 7. LiteCure, Newark, DE.

Roberts, D.B. *et al.* (2013) The effectiveness of therapeutic class IV (10 W) laser treatment for epicondylitis. *Lasers in Surg Med.* **45**(5):311–317.

Rochkind, S. *et al.* (2009) Increase of neuronal sprouting and migration using 780 nm laser phototherapy as procedure for cell therapy. *Lasers Surg Med.* **41**(4):277–281.

Salate, A.C. *et al.* (2005) Effect of In-Ga-Al-P diode laser irradiation on angiogenesis in partial ruptures of Achilles tendon in rats. *Photomed Laser Surg.* **23**(5):470–475.

Schomberg, D. *et al.* (2012) Neuropathic pain: role of inflammation, immune response, and ion channel activity in central injury mechanisms. *Ann Neurosci.* **19**(3):125–132.

Servetto, N. *et al.* (2010) Evaluation of inflammatory biomarkers associated with oxidative stress and histological assessment of low-level PBMT in experimental myopathy. *Lasers Surg Med.* **42**(6):577–583.

Shiva, S. and Gladwin, M.T. (2009) Shining a light on tissue NO stores: near infrared release of NO from nitrite and nitrosylated hemes. *J Mol Cell Cardiol.* **46**(1):1–3.

Silva, T.C. *et al.* (2010) In vivo effects on the expression of vascular endothelial growth factor-A165 messenger ribonucleic acid of an infrared diode laser associated or not with a visible red diode laser. *Photomed Laser Surg.* **28**(1):63–68.

Sims, C. *et al.* (2015) Rehabilitation and physical therapy for the neurologic patient. *Vet Clin North Am Small Anim Pract.* **45**(1):123–143.

Skobelkin, O. *et al.* (1990) Blood microcirculation under laser physiotherapy and reflexotherapy in patients with lesions in vessels of low extremities. *Laser Ther.* **2**(2):69–77.

Sommer, A.P. *et al.* (2001) Biostimulatory windows in low-intensity laser activation: lasers, scanners, and NASA's light-emitting diode array system. *J Clin Laser Med Surg.* **19**(1):29–33.

Takahashi, H. *et al.* (2012) Low level PBMT for patients with cervical disk hernia. *PBMT.* **21**(3):193–197.

Tumilty, S. *et al.* (2010) Low level laser treatment of tendinopathy: a systematic review with meta-analysis. *Photomed Laser Surg.* **28**(1):3–16.

Wakabayashi, H. (1993) Effect of irradiation by semiconductor laser on responses evoked in trigeminal caudal neurons by tooth pulp stimulation. *Lasers Surg Med.* **13**(6):605–610.

Walker, J.B. (1983) Relief from chronic pain by low-power laser irradiation. *Neurosci Lett.* **43**:339–344.

Wang, P. *et al.* (2014) Effects of low-level PBMT on joint pain, synovitis, anabolic, and catabolic factors in a progressive osteoarthritis rabbit model. *Lasers Med Sci.* **29**(6):1875–1885.

Waxman, S.G. and Zamponi, G.W. (2014) Regulating excitability of peripheral afferents: emerging ion channel targets. *Nature neuroscience.* **17**(2):153–163.

Zhang, Y. *et al.* (2003) cDNA microarray analysis of gene expression profiles in human fibroblast cells irradiated with red light. *J Invest Dermatol.* **120**(5):849–857.

14

Upper and Lower Respiratory Conditions

Ray A. Arza

RSA Veterinary Technologies, Taylorsville, KY, USA

Introduction

Over the past 10 years, there has been a plethora of studies showing the beneficial effects of photobiomodulation therapy (PBMT) on upper and lower respiratory function. These studies indicate that PBMT is an effective modality in reducing pain, modulating the inflammatory response, and increasing microcirculation in both upper and lower respiratory conditions with virtually no side effects, thus alleviating symptoms and hastening recovery. Anecdotal results reported in the veterinary profession have been consistent with these findings. The addition of this modality when treating upper and lower airway disease has proven to minimize inflammatory symptoms, expedite recovery, potentiate the effects of conventional therapies, and decrease the need for pharmaceuticals with potential side effects, such as corticosteroids and non-steroidal anti-inflammatories. Practitioners are encouraged to add PBMT to their therapeutic regimens when treating conditions in the upper and lower respiratory tracts.

Upper Respiratory Conditions

The major passages and structures of the upper respiratory tract include the nose or nostrils, nasal cavity, mouth, pharynx, and larynx. Conditions affecting the mouth in relation to its function as part of the alimentary tract are discussed in Chapter 15.

General Guidelines

There are several things to consider when treating a patient in the area of the head. First is patient safety. Eye protection is recommended anytime a patient is treated, but is most important when treating in close proximity to the eyes (Figure 14.1). Exposure of direct or indirect laser light through the pupil and lens to the retina is the primary concern, so proper eye protection is vital. This may be provided by goggles (with lenses appropriate for the specific wavelengths being used) or simply by covering both eyes with dark (preferably black), dense cloth.

The second consideration is treating with a proper dose of light energy, so that an effective dose reaches the target tissue. The dose must be delivered in a way and at a rate that is comfortable to the patient and does not induce excessive heat. Some treatment areas will be relatively small (e.g., the nose or sinuses in feline patients). When treating small areas, the laser power settings should be adjusted low enough so as not to create any thermal buildup in the tissues.

It is important to note that some upper respiratory conditions may be treated as superficial conditions, through the open mouth, with direct exposure of the laser beam to the target tissue. Other conditions must be treated transcutaneously as deep-tissue conditions, with the total dose increased to account for the loss of irradiance as the photons travel through the various tissue densities to the target tissue.

Some upper respiratory structures are contained within bone, and therefore require treatment through bone. Multiple studies have verified that transcranial therapy with near-infrared laser light is possible. Transcranial near-infrared laser transmission of 800 nm laser light was demonstrated by Lapchak *et al.* (2015) in four mammalian species. As expected, they found an inverse relationship between the thickness of bone and the percentage of photonic transmission through it. In another study using intact human cadaver heads, measurement of transcranial transmission confirmed the penetration of measurable 808 nm-wavelength light through the scalp, skull, and meninges to a brain depth of 40–50 mm (Tedford *et al.*, 2015).

Since conditions that are being treated transcutaneously require much deeper penetration of light energy, treatment is optimally applied in direct contact with the skin, using a contact handpiece or a treatment head that has been specifically designed for deep-tissue conditions

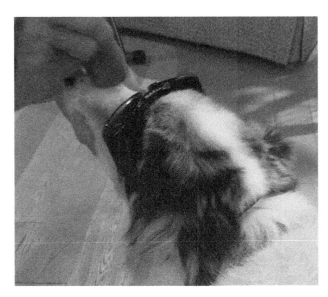

Figure 14.1 Treating the nasal cavity from a dorsal direction. Exposure of direct or indirect laser light through the pupil and lens to the retina is the primary concern, so proper eye protection is vital.

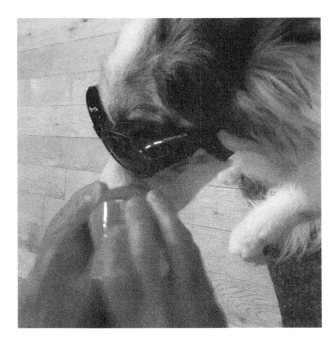

Figure 14.2 Treating the nasal cavity from a lateral direction. Treatment is optimally applied in direct contact with the skin, using a contact handpiece or a treatment head that has been specifically designed for deep tissue conditions. This will decrease reflection of light from the tissue surface, reduce potential exposure to the patient's eyes, and increase penetration of the light deep into the tissues.

(Figure 14.2). This will decrease reflection of light from the tissue surface, reduce potential exposure to the patient's eyes, and increase penetration of the light deep into the tissues (Enwemeka, 2009). Treating in contact and applying gentle pressure creates blanching and

disperses blood from the skin and underlying tissues. Since hemoglobin is the main absorber of light in the dermis (Lister *et al.*, 2012), blanching will improve light penetration to deeper tissues.

Treat with the handpiece perpendicular to the tissue. Deliver the photonic energy with movement of the handpiece so there is a uniform irradiation of the target tissues. The laser therapist should monitor the temperature of the patient's skin and hair coat with a finger placed adjacent to the handpiece on the skin, or by placing the other hand in direct proximity to the treatment area. If anything other than a gentle warming is noted, the therapist should pause and adjust the laser and treatment parameters.

Rhinitis and Sinusitis

Rhinitis is defined as any inflammation of the nasal mucous membranes. It is often associated with sinusitis, which is an inflammation of the lining of the sinuses. Both conditions are commonly presented to veterinary clinics. Of particular concern are patients with chronic rhinitis and sinusitis, since they are often challenging to treat.

In dogs, chronic nasal disease is often caused by neoplasia, followed by lympho-plasmacytic rhinitis, fungal infections, and foreign bodies. Other, less common etiologies include nasal polyps, granulomatous rhinitis, oro-nasal fistula, and naso-pharyngeal stenosis (Cohn, 2014; Lobetti, 2009; Windsor and Johnson, 2006).

In cats, like in dogs, the most common cause is neoplasia. The second most common cause, accounting for approximately 35% of feline cases, is the chronic rhino-sinusitis that follows feline herpesvirus 1 infection (Reed 2014).

Due to the prevalence of malignancies, especially with chronic rhinitis, appropriate diagnostics with radiography, rhinoscopy, cultures, and histopathology is always recommended before PBMT is added to the therapeutic regimen.

Once a diagnosis that does not include any malignancies is established, there is sound basis for including laser therapy in the clinical management of rhinitis and sinusitis. A recent pilot study showed that patients had significant improvement in symptoms from chronic rhino-sinusitis when treated with laser therapy three times a week for ten total treatments (Naghdi *et al.*, 2013). Another pilot study demonstrated that phototherapy is an effective modality for treating perennial allergic rhinitis in humans and is an option in the steroid-free management of immune-mediated mucosal diseases (Lee *et al.*, 2013). In an animal-model study, positive effects were noted after laser therapy treatment of an ovalbumin-induced model of allergic rhinitis in mice (Choi, 2013).

The role of microorganisms in rhinitis and sinusitis may be significant. Viral infections in cats are often followed by secondary bacterial infections (Reed, 2014). Sinonasal fungal infections with aspergillosis are increasingly diagnosed in both dogs (Sharman and Mansfield, 2012) and cats (Barrs and Talbot, 2014).

Studies indicate that incorporating laser therapy into therapeutics when microorganisms are present is warranted. Neutrophils from mice that received laser therapy have been shown to be more active metabolically, and to have higher fungicidal activity *in vivo* and *in vitro* (Burger *et al.*, 2015).

Laser-assisted nasal decolonization of *Staphylococcus aureus*, including methicillin-resistant *S. aureus* (MRSA), was demonstrated in human patients (Krespi and Kizhner, 2012). The study concluded that laser therapy could eradicate MRSA and potentially resensitize the bacteria to the antimicrobial effect of erythromycin.

All of these studies are consistent with clinical reports from veterinarians using laser light as an adjunct to conventional therapy for rhinitis and sinusitis in companion pets.

When developing a protocol for incorporating PBMT into the management of rhinitis and sinusitis, severity and chronicity should be considered, as should response after initiation of treatment. In acute conditions, a typical induction phase of daily or every-other-day treatment is indicated, with a gradual transition to less frequent treatment until the condition resolves. When treating chronic rhinitis or sinusitis, the author recommends three phases of treatment, as for other chronic conditions: an induction phase, a transition phase, and a maintenance phase. The induction phase will usually start with every-other-day treatment, followed, as symptoms improve, by a gradual decrease in frequency through a transition phase of treatments twice weekly, once weekly, every other week, and so on. With severe symptoms, starting with three to four daily treatments is recommended. If the condition persists, a maintenance phase may be necessary, with treatments at a frequency that maintains the clinical response achieved during the induction and transition phases. A word of caution: do not decrease treatment frequency too quickly; rather, tailor it to the patient's improvement.

The recommended target dose for treating rhinitis and sinusitis is $8–10\,J/cm^2$. The higher end of this range is recommended for larger patients with thicker bones, as the thickness of the bone affects the penetration of light. When treating small dogs or cats, especially when skin and coat color is dark, the author recommends adjusting the laser power setting to no more than 3 W to prevent excessive heat buildup. Though the area of skin overlying the nose and sinuses is small, the laser handpiece should move during treatment. When treating larger dogs, power settings may be increased to 10–12 W as long as there is constant movement of the handpiece over the entire area for the duration of treatment.

The author recommends always treating the entire area covering both nasal passages and frontal and maxillary sinuses. It is helpful to have a template to use when estimating the size of the area to be treated, in square centimeters. A $7.5 \times 12.7\,cm$ index card or a CD is almost exactly $100\,cm^2$, and because 100 is an easy multiplier, one can determine approximate dosages by visualizing the area to be treated in terms of number of index cards or CDs. The author prefers an index card to a CD, since they are readily available, flexible, and can easily be used to map out the total area to be treated. Once the area is known, the total dose in joules can easily be calculated.

Tonsillitis

Tonsillitis is common in dogs, mostly in brachycephalic or small breeds (Kaplan, 1981). Though rare in cats, it has been reported (Prescott, 1968). It seldom occurs as a primary disease; instead, it is usually secondary to other nasal, oral, or pharyngeal disorders. In brachycephalic dogs, it is thought to be associated with chronic inflammation due to elongation of the soft palate.

Clinical signs of tonsillitis are associated with pain and inflammation, and with the physical presence of the enlarged tonsils in the pharynx. Treatment is typically aimed at resolving the underlying disease. Analgesics and antibiotics are often indicated.

Laser therapy appears to be a good adjunct therapy for treating tonsillitis. Among 445 human children and teenagers (aged 2–15 years) with pollinosis (68), adenoiditis and rhino-sinusitis (198), tonsillitis (64), or otitis (115), treatment was carried out simultaneously with infrared and red laser irradiations (Gogeliia *et al.*, 2006). Positive results were achieved in 85% of patients. Another controlled study evaluated the effects of laser irradiation at the end of surgery on reduction of pain after tonsillectomy in human adults (Aghamohammadi *et al.*, 2013). In the treated group, the tonsil beds were irradiated with a 980 nm laser at a dose of $4\,J/cm^2$. The amount of pain decrease and analgesic consumption reduction were significantly higher in patients who received postoperative laser treatment than in those who did not.

Like other oropharyngeal conditions, tonsillitis may be treated as a superficial condition, with the mouth open so the light directly treats the tonsil (as in Aghamohammadi *et al.*, 2013). This is easiest if the patient is sedated or under anesthesia. Most awake patients will not tolerate prolonged opening of the mouth and displacement of the tongue, so the tonsils can be treated as deep tissues if the patient is not sedated or under anesthesia.

When treating with open mouth and direct access to the tonsils, a treatment protocol that delivers $4–6\,J/cm^2$ is recommended. A small, non-contact handpiece should be used at power setting of 2–3 W. Treatment may be somewhat easier if the handpiece collimates the laser beam and allows treatment at a greater distance from the target area.

If treating with the mouth closed, a laser setting that delivers $6–10\,J/cm^2$ is recommended. The treatment should be aimed at the pharynx from the caudal border of the mandible, with the handpiece in contact with the skin. The power setting should not exceed $3–4\,W$, as this is a relatively small area and movement of the handpiece will be limited. Initial treatments may be administered daily to decrease the severity of the pain and inflammation, then every other day until resolution.

Brachycephalic Syndrome

Animals with brachycephalic syndrome suffer from obstruction of the airways at a number of levels within the respiratory tract. The anomalies include stenotic nares, abnormally conformed turbinates, soft-palate elongation and hyperplasia, and less often hypoplastic trachea. As the condition worsens, the laryngeal saccules may evert and a secondary structural collapse of the larynx and left bronchus may occur (Dupré and Heidenreich, 2016). Secondary tonsillitis is common.

The pathological changes accompanying the syndrome result from a decrease in the lumen of the airways, which increases respiratory effort, especially on inspiration. Poiseuille's law states that as lumen radius decreases in size, the resistance to flow through the lumen increases fourfold (Sutera and Skalak, 1993). This means that even relatively small changes in the radius of the airways cause large changes in airway resistance. Thus, the significant resistance in airflow caused by the stenotic nares and elongated soft palate lead to the devastating secondary changes (Dupré *et al.*, 2012).

Most surgeons believe that early surgical intervention helps prevent development of the secondary complications (Meola, 2013). The author of the current chapter believes that this syndrome is best approached by early rhinoplasty and palatoplasty using a carbon dioxide (CO_2) surgical laser, and has performed surgical CO_2 soft-palate and stenotic nares correction in over 350 dogs. The technique has been described in multiple publications (Clark and Sinibaldi, 1994; Davidson *et al.*, 2001; Dunié-Mérigot *et al.*, 2010). However, PBMT may play an adjunctive role in brachycephalic syndrome as a means of bringing about postoperative reduction of inflammation and pain, as well as of managing the inflammatory changes that occur if early surgical intervention is not accomplished.

When laser therapy is used to treat immediately after surgical correction of brachycephalic syndrome, attention should be given to all potential areas of inflammation, including the nares, pharyngeal and laryngeal areas, and trachea. Perioperative treatment should be administered while the patient is under anesthesia so the pharyngeal area can be treated directly through the open mouth.

Depending on the degree of postoperative pain and swelling, closed-mouth treatments may be administered daily or twice daily for 3–4 days.

For the nares, a laser setting that delivers $3–4\,J/cm^2$ using a power not greater than $2\,W$ and a non-contact technique is recommended. The nasal cavity can be treated with the protocols described in the section on Rhinitis and Sinusitis. Prior to recovery from anesthesia, the visible areas of the pharynx and larynx can be treated through the open mouth with $3–4\,J/cm^2$ at $2–3\,W$, followed by closed-mouth treatment delivering $6–10\,J/cm^2$ at $4–8\,W$ using a contact technique over all of the pharyngeal and laryngeal area and the proximal trachea.

When using therapy laser as an adjunct to conventional medical therapy for the treatment of brachycephalic symptoms in lieu of surgery, the author recommends the standard three phases of laser therapy for chronic conditions. The induction phase should start with daily or every-other-day treatments until symptoms subside, with a gradual decrease in treatment frequency through a transition phase, followed by maintenance-phase treatments every 2–4 weeks at a frequency sufficient to maintain effect.

Laryngitis

Laryngitis, an inflammation of the larynx, may result from upper respiratory tract infection, foreign bodies, or irritant inhalants such as dust, smoke, or other gasses. Excessive barking or trauma from endotracheal tubes may also be a culprit. Any breed is susceptible, but as described in the section on Brachycephalic Syndrome, brachycephalic breeds are predisposed to general upper respiratory inflammation, including of the larynx. Patients with laryngeal paralysis will maintain laryngeal inflammation as well.

Treatment should address the underlying etiology, but symptomatic treatment to decrease laryngeal edema and swelling of the mucous membranes is often indicated. In addition to pharmacological agents, PBMT may be a helpful adjunctive therapy, and it is indicated for any form of laryngitis, except where malignancy is the underlying etiology. Studies in laboratory animals have demonstrated that laser therapy can successfully modulate the inflammatory response in experimental laryngitis and that it may therefore be a useful tool for the treatment of laryngitis (Marinho *et al.*, 2013a, 2013b).

A treatment protocol that delivers $6–10\,J/cm^2$ (lower doses for smaller patients and higher doses for larger patients) is recommended for the treatment of the larynx. Treatment with the handpiece in contact with the skin is indicated, and a maximum power setting of $4–8\,W$ is recommended. Depending on the degree of inflammation, laryngeal swelling, and severity of symptoms, treatments should start daily or twice daily and then decrease to every other day until resolution.

Laryngeal Collapse and Laryngeal Paralysis

Laryngeal collapse occurs when the laryngeal cartilage loses rigidity, causing the larynx to fold and collapse. This structural abnormality results in an obstruction of normal movement of air through the larynx. Laryngeal collapse can occur following trauma to the neck, but more commonly is seen in brachycephalic-syndrome patients secondary to their longstanding upper respiratory conditions.

Laryngeal paralysis differs in that it is a functional abnormality of the nerves that control the muscles and cartilage of the larynx. The paralysis results in voice changes and difficulty with eating and breathing (MacPhail, 2014).

Both conditions can result in severe respiratory distress. Surgical intervention with unilateral arytenoid lateralization is most commonly used to treat laryngeal paralysis. The same technique can be used to treat laryngeal collapse, though some severely affected patients may require a permanent tracheostomy (Monnet, 2016; Monnet and Tobias, 2012).

As described earlier, PBMT reduces pain, inflammation, and edema in the larynx regardless of the cause. Laser therapy treatment of the larynx is indicated in pre- and postoperative patients undergoing surgery for collapse or paralysis, or in patients with milder symptoms that are not deemed immediate surgical candidates (Figure 14.3).

Lower Respiratory and Thoracic Conditions

General Guidelines

Eye protection is also very important when treating conditions of the lower respiratory tract. The best options are the use of goggles (with lenses appropriate for the specific wavelengths being used) or simply covering both eyes with dark (preferably black), dense cloth.

Laser therapy treatment of lower respiratory conditions should be administered with the laser handpiece in contact with the skin, to maximize penetration of photons deep into the target areas. When treating diffuse conditions of the lower respiratory tract, the dose should be calculated based on the entire surface area of the thorax. If the trachea is involved in the condition being treated, then the neck should be considered part of the treatment area. Treatment of either the thorax or the neck should be applied from 270° (from a ventral direction, as well as both lateral sides) (Figure 14.4). Penetration into the thorax can be facilitated by following the intercostal spaces as much as possible with the handpiece. In larger patients, all of the treatment of the thoracic walls can be directed through the intercostal spaces.

When considering laser therapy for a lower respiratory or thoracic condition of unknown etiology, a complete

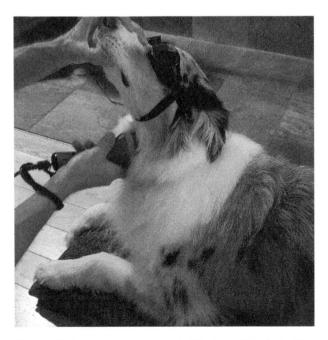

Figure 14.3 Laser therapy treatment of the larynx is indicated for laryngitis, for reduction of edema in laryngeal collapse or paralysis, and for pre- and postoperative patients undergoing surgery for laryngeal collapse or paralysis. Treatment should be administered with the laser handpiece in contact with the skin, to maximize penetration of photons deep into the target areas.

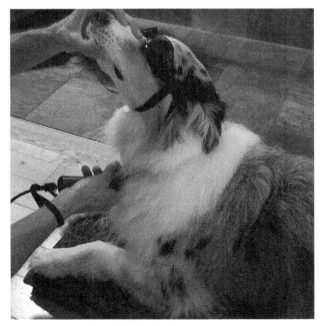

Figure 14.4 In any respiratory condition, if the trachea is involved, the neck should be considered part of the treatment area. Treatment of the cervical portion of the trachea should be administered from 270° (from a ventral direction, as well as both lateral sides) and into the cranial thoracic trachea through the thoracic inlet.

physical exam and proper diagnostic workup of the patient are strongly recommended, to rule out possible underlying malignancies.

When treating the neck, caution should be exercised to avoid prolonged, repeated treatments over the thyroid glands. Early animal studies on the effect of laser irradiation of the thyroid gland demonstrated increased mitotic activity of follicular cells and changes in the thyroid parenchyma (Parrado *et al.*, 1990, 1999). Subsequent studies indicated that lower total doses, delivered with fewer applications, result in no histological changes in the thyroid parenchyma (Azevedo *et al.*, 2005). Even more recent studies suggest that laser therapy can be used to treat thyroiditis in humans (Höfling *et al.*, 2010, 2013). These studies indicate that repetitive, high-dose treatment directly over the glands should be avoided. They also indicate that occasional inadvertent exposure of the thyroid glands when treating nearby tissue is not contraindicated.

Chronic Obstructive Pulmonary Disease

Chronic obstructive pulmonary disease (COPD), also known as chronic bronchitis, is a condition that affects the lower airways of dogs and cats. It tends to be irreversible and progressive (Rozanski, 2014). Though the etiology is not totally understood, the chronic inflammation may be caused by many factors, including inhaled irritants, allergens, and recurrent infections. As with the other respiratory conditions described in this chapter, a complete diagnostic workup is always indicated prior to starting treatment with laser therapy.

PBMT should be considered a helpful adjunctive therapy to conventional treatment protocols for COPD. A study involving 89 human patients with chronic obstructive bronchitis showed that adding laser therapy to other therapeutic modalities accelerated elimination of clinical symptoms, increased respiratory efficiency, promoted drainage function of the bronchi, and facilitated normalization of the patient's immune status (Kashanskaia and Fedorov, 2009).

Since COPD affects all of the lower airways, treatment with PBMT should be administered over the entire thorax using a treatment protocol that delivers 6–10 J/cm^2. Power settings will vary depending on the size of the patient, and may be as low as 4 W for smaller patients and as high as 15 W for the giant canine breeds. The calculated dose should be delivered with the handpiece in contact within the intercostal spaces, using a dorsal-to-ventral application technique (Figures 14.5–14.7). Since COPD is a chronic disease, the treatment should start with an induction phase of daily or every-other-day treatments, depending on the severity of symptoms, followed by a transition phase with a very gradual decrease in frequency of treatments, as dictated

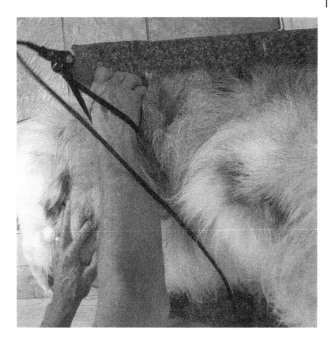

Figure 14.5 The laser handpiece should be maintained in contact with the skin when treating the lower respiratory tract with transthoracic laser application. The entire area of the thoracic walls should be treated from 270°. In this image, treatment is beginning dorsally and the treatment handpiece is moved in an arc, along the lines of the ribs, in a ventral direction.

by the improvement of symptoms. Long-term maintenance-phase treatments will be required at a frequency dictated by the patient's response. The goal of adding PBMT to conventional therapy should be to help decrease symptoms to a tolerable degree, as well as to decrease the dose and frequency of pharmacological agents that may have adverse effects on the patient.

Feline Asthma

Feline asthma is a challenging lower airway disease that can be difficult to distinguish because of the similarity of its symptoms to those of other lower airway diseases. Confirming a diagnosis of feline asthma is important because treatment and prognosis differ from those of other lower airway diseases (Reinero, 2011).

Standard pharmacological therapies for feline asthma include glucocorticoids and bronchodilators. These medications are not ideal treatments, since some cats are non-responsive and the therapies do not stop chronic airway remodeling, which leads to declining pulmonary function (Trizil and Reinero, 2014).

The application of the anti-inflammatory and immune-modulatory effects of PBMT in treating asthma is sound because of the inflammatory nature of the disease and the less-than-ideal pharmacological options. Recent studies of the effects of laser therapy on allergic asthma have shown encouraging results. One compared the effects of laser therapy on asthma in rats to that of the

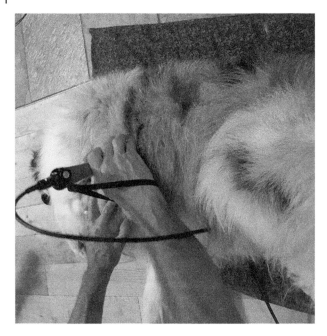

Figure 14.6 In patients of sufficient size, transthoracic treatment should be delivered through the intercostal spaces as the handpiece is moved along the lines of the ribs.

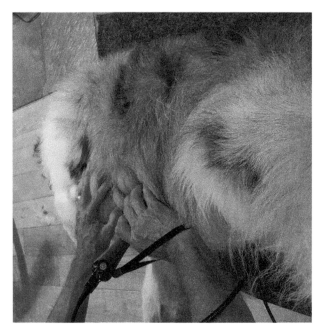

Figure 14.7 Once the handpiece has reached the ventral edge of the thoracic cavity, it should be moved back dorsally. Both sides of the thorax should be covered with a series of dorsal-to-ventral and ventral-to-dorsal movements along the lines of the ribs. The handpiece should be maintained perpendicular to the skin.

glucocorticoid budesonide and found they were similar (Wang, 2014). The findings suggest that the mechanism of laser therapy treatment of asthma is similar to that of budesonide, involving the adjustment of Th1/Th2 imbalance, which is postulated in many studies to play a major role in the pathogenesis of asthma. Another study, using mice, showed that laser therapy inhibits bronchoconstriction, Th2 inflammation, and airway remodeling in experimentally induced allergic asthma (Silva *et al.*, 2014). The results of these laboratory studies are similar to those observed in human asthma patients treated with laser therapy in clinical settings (Ailioaie and Ailioaie, 1997; Ostronosova, 2006).

The animal-model and human studies have definite cross-species application. The results are consistent with reported observations of efficacy from the veterinary community. The treatment recommendations for asthma parallel those discussed for COPD.

Tracheal Collapse

This condition, seen most often in small breeds of dogs, occurs when the C-shaped cartilage rings weaken and begin to collapse, and the trachealis muscle on the dorsal surface stretches. The collapse can extend all the way into the bronchi, resulting in severe airway compromise (Maggiore, 2014). Just as in brachycephalic syndrome, the restriction of airflow results in inflammation of the respiratory tissues. As the condition worsens, excitement or exercise will usually induce a characteristic hacking or honking cough. Treatment may include weight control, behavioral alterations (to decrease anxiety), medical treatments, and, in more severe cases, surgical intervention (Herrtage, 2009).

Though the use of laser therapy will not do anything for the anatomical abnormalities of a collapsed trachea, practitioners should consider PBMT as an adjunct to other therapies. The intent would be to help decrease the inflammatory component. The reduction of lower respiratory inflammation that results from the application of laser therapy has been demonstrated in multiple studies (Aimbire *et al.*, 2005, 2007, 2008; Miranda da Silva *et al.*, 2015; Oliveira *et al.*, 2014). Inflammation is reduced via multiple complex mechanisms, without any impairment of pulmonary function (Cury, 2015).

Because bronchi may be involved, the inflammation resulting from the anatomical abnormality will extend into deeper pulmonary tissue. It is therefore important to treat the entire lower respiratory tract with laser therapy. A contact technique should be used to deliver $6–10\,J/cm^2$ over both thoracic walls. In addition, the upper trachea should be targeted by treating the entire ventral neck area, and by aiming into the thoracic inlet. The power setting will depend on the size of the patient and of the area to be treated. When treating smaller dogs, the author recommends not exceeding 4–6 W.

Pneumonia

Bacterial pneumonia is much more commonly seen in dogs than in cats. New evidence suggests a complex relationship between respiratory viruses and the development of bacterial pneumonia in dogs (Dear, 2014). Respiratory viruses are frequently found in dogs with bacterial pneumonia and may be important in its pathogenesis (Viitanen, 2015).

With increasing evidence of the beneficial effects of PBMT on lung tissue, treatment with this modality should be considered as adjunctive therapy with any case of pneumonia. Clinical results reported by practitioners in the field have mirrored the results from many studies over the past 10 years.

One study concluded that transcutaneous laser therapy of elderly human patients with pneumonia shows an undeniable positive impact, with earlier regression of clinical symptoms and sound recovery of functional parameters (Lutaĭ, 2001). It suggested that in the absence of side effects, PBMT should be considered for rehabilitation of elderly patients with pneumonia.

In another study, laser therapy was demonstrated to be an effective method of pneumonia treatment that can be included in relevant combined schemes (Amirov, 2002). Human pneumonia patients were randomly divided into two groups: those treated with drugs and laser therapy and those treated with drugs alone. Response that was more positive was seen in the group treated with drugs and laser therapy.

A clinical study involving human patients concluded that intravenous laser therapy has a favorable effect on the clinical course of acute pneumonia, accelerates resolution, and promotes earlier and more complete restoration of the blood stream and normalization of hemostasis (Korochkin *et al.*, 1989).

When PBMT is being considered as adjunctive therapy in the treatment of pneumonia, a complete diagnostic workup is recommended to rule out malignancy. Note that a benefit of this modality is its compatibility with any other form of treatment for pneumonia, with essentially no known side effects.

A treatment protocol that delivers $6–10\,\text{J/cm}^2$ is recommended, and the author suggests treating the entire thoracic cavity. If a protocol for treating the thorax is not available in the therapy laser software, an approximate dosage can be determined by visualizing the area to be treated relative to the size of an index card or CD, as described in the section on Rhinitis and Sinusitis. A contact treatment technique is recommended, with the handpiece following the intercostal spaces. A power setting of $6–15\,\text{W}$ is recommended.

Tracheobronchitis

Tracheobronchitis is an acute or chronic inflammatory condition of the trachea and bronchial airways. The etiology is diverse, and may include viral or bacterial infection, parasites, smoke aspiration, and noxious chemical fumes. As with other airway conditions, appropriate diagnostic workup is always very important in determining the best course of therapy, though identification of a specific etiology or pathogen may not be possible in each case (Priestnall, 2014).

Tracheobronchitis is yet another condition in which laser therapy may play an adjunctive role in ameliorating the inflammatory component. The author recommends considering this modality as part of the therapeutic approach when treating tracheobronchitis in any companion pet. As with other lower respiratory conditions, laser settings that deliver $6–10\,\text{J/cm}^2$ should be used to treat all of the trachea and the entire thorax. The treatment design will be similar to that described in the section on COPD. When treating acute tracheobronchitis, daily or every-other-day treatments are indicated until the desired effects are obtained. Treatment of chronic tracheobronchitis will necessitate treating through the three phases of induction, transition, and maintenance.

Smoke Inhalation

The complex pathophysiology of smoke inhalation injury has been described in both dogs and cats (Drobatz *et al.*, 1999a, 1999b; Farrow, 1975). The formation of reactive oxygen and nitrogen species (ROS and RNS) and procoagulant and antifibrinolytic factors results in alveolar imbalance. Cast formation, bronchospasm, increased bronchial circulation, and transvascular fluid lead to massive airway obstruction (Rehberg *et al.*, 2009). Neurological signs such as stupor or non-ambulatory tetraparesis have been reported in dogs after smoke (and presumably carbon monoxide, CO) inhalation injury (Mariani, 2003). Delayed neurological sequela may be seen after the initial response to treatment.

Changes seen in the upper and lower airways following inhalation of smoke and other noxious gases may benefit from adding laser therapy to conventional treatment. A study in mice established that laser therapy reduces acute lung inflammation without provoking any deleterious effects in pulmonary function (Cury, 2015). This study concluded that transthoracic laser application reduces inflammation in acute lung injury, even when the therapy is applied after the inflammatory process is established. The reduction in inflammation occurs through inhibition of cytokine and chemokine secretion, and leads to a marked decrease in immune-cell infiltration in inflamed lungs.

Troxel (2012) reported the initial successful management of a dog with smoke inhalation. Treatment included oxygen administered via intranasal tube, intravenous (IV) lactated Ringer's solution, short-acting glucocorticoids, furosemide, theophylline, ophthalmic ointment, and infrared treatment. Though the patient recovered from the initial respiratory distress, it subsequently developed neurological signs that led to euthanasia. Necropsy and histopathology demonstrated delayed post-hypoxic leukoencephalopathy.

Anecdotal reports from small-animal practitioners indicate that in the first 24–48 hours after presentation, smoke-inhalation patients appear to breathe more comfortably following laser therapy treatments. Twice-a-day treatments are recommended, and should be dosed and applied as per the recommendations in the section on COPD.

Ischemia Reperfusion Injury-Induced Pulmonary Inflammation

Like smoke inhalation, ischemia reperfusion injuries result in complex pathophysiology (Kalogeris *et al.*, 2012). The pathophysiology may have a delayed effect on distant organs, including the lungs. Pulmonary inflammation following ischemia reperfusion injuries can be an issue in companion animals following gastrointestinal or limb ischemia. Studies in lab animals have demonstrated that PBMT can ameliorate remote-organ lung injury induced by hind-limb (Ashrafzadeh Takhtfooladi *et al.*, 2015) and gut (de Lima *et al.*, 2013a, 2013b) ischemia and reperfusion. These studies suggest that proactive treatment of the pulmonary fields is indicated following any ischemia reperfusion injury. Again, these patients should be treated twice a day with treatments dosed and applied as per the recommendations in the section on COPD.

Conclusion

PBMT is playing an ever-increasing role in thousands of veterinary practices and in the management of a variety of conditions in millions of patients. The anti-inflammatory effects of PBMT have been well established and are now being incorporated into the therapeutic approach to many inflammatory conditions in the upper and lower respiratory tracts. Based on the general and condition-specific treatment concepts presented in this chapter, veterinarians are encouraged to consider the addition of PBMT to the treatment of these conditions whenever possible.

References

Aghamohammadi, D. *et al.* (2013) Effect of low level laser application at the end of surgery to reduce pain after tonsillectomy in adults. *J Lasers Med Sci.* **4**(2):79–85.

Ailioaie, C. and Ailioaie, L. (1997) The treatment of bronchial asthma with LLLT in attack-free period in children. *Ter Arkh.* **69**(12):49–50.

Aimbire, F. *et al.* (2005) Effect of LLLT Ga-Al-As (685 nm) on LPS-induced inflammation of the airway and lung in the rat. *Lasers Med Sci.* **20**(1):11–20.

Aimbire, F. *et al.* (2007) Effect of low-level laser therapy on hemorrhagic lesions induced by immune complex in rat lungs. *Photomed Laser Surg.* **25**(2):112–117.

Aimbire, F. *et al.* (2008) Low level laser therapy (LLLT) decreases pulmonary microvascular leakage, neutrophil influx and IL-1beta levels in airway and lung from rat subjected to LPS-induced inflammation. *Inflammation.* **31**(3):189–197.

Amirov, N.B. (2002) Parameters of membrane permeability, microcirculation, external respiration, and trace element levels in the drug-laser treatment of pneumonia. *Ter Arkh.* **74**(3):40–43.

Ashrafzadeh Takhtfooladi, M. *et al.* (2015) Effect of low-level laser therapy on lung injury induced by hindlimb ischemia/reperfusion in rats. *Lasers Med Sci.* **30**(6):1757–1762.

Azevedo, L. H. *et al.* (2005) Evaluation of low intensity laser effects on the thyroid gland of male mice. *Photomed Laser Surg.* **23**(6):567–570.

Barrs, V.R. and Talbot, J.J. (2014) Feline aspergillosis. *Vet Clin North Am Small Anim Pract.* **44**(1):51–43.

Burger, E. *et al.* (2015) Low-level laser therapy to the mouse femur enhances the fungicidal response of neutrophils against *Paracoccidioides brasiliensis. PLoS Negl Trop Dis.* **9**(2):e0003541.

Choi, B. (2013) Effects of low level laser therapy on ovalbumin-induced mouse model of allergic rhinitis. *Complement Alternat Med.* **2013**:753829.

Clark, G.N. and Sinibaldi, K.R (1994) Use of a carbon dioxide laser for treatment of elongated soft palate in dogs. *J Am Vet Med Assoc.* **204**(11):1779–1781.

Cohn, L.A. (2014) Canine nasal disease. *Vet Clin North Am Small Anim Pract.* **44**(1):75–89.

Cury, V. (2015) Low level laser therapy reduces acute lung inflammation without impairing lung function. *J Biophotonics.* doi:10.1002/jbio.201500113.

Davidson, E.B. *et al.* (2001) Evaluation of carbon dioxide laser and conventional incisional techniques for resection of soft palates in brachycephalic dogs. *J Am Vet Med Assoc.* **219**(6):776–781.

Dear, J.D. (2014) Bacterial pneumonia in dogs and cats. *Vet Clin North Am Small Anim Pract.* **44**(1):143–159.

de Lima, F.M. *et al.* (2013a) Suppressive effect of low-level laser therapy on tracheal hyperresponsiveness and lung inflammation in rat subjected to intestinal ischemia and reperfusion. *Lasers Med Sci.* **28**(2):551–564.

de Lima, F.M. *et al.* (2013b) Low-level laser therapy restores the oxidative stress balance in acute lung injury induced by gut ischemia and reperfusion. *Photochem Photobiol.* **89**(1):179–188.

Drobatz, K.J. *et al.* (1999a) Smoke exposure in dogs: 27 cases (1988–1997). *J Am Vet Med Assoc.* **215**(9):1306–1311.

Drobatz, K.J. *et al.* (1999b) Smoke exposure in cats: 22 cases (1986–1997). *J Am Vet Med Assoc.* **215**(9):1312–1316.

Dunié-Mérigot, A. *et al.* (2010) Comparative use of CO_2 laser, diode laser and monopolar electrocautery for resection of the soft palate in dogs with brachycephalic airway obstructive syndrome. *Vet Rec.* **167**(18): 700–704.

Dupré, G. and Heidenreich, D. (2016) Brachycephalic syndrome. *Vet Clin North Am Small Anim Pract.* **46**(4):691–707.

Dupré, G. *et al.* (2012) Brachycephalic airway syndrome. In: *Small Animal Soft Tissue Surgery*, pp. 167–183. Wiley-Blackwell, Ames, IA.

Enwemeka, C.S. (2009) Intricacies of dose in laser phototherapy for tissue repair and pain relief. *Photomed Laser Surg.* **27**(3):387–393.

Farrow, C.S. (1975) Smoke inhalation in the dog: current concepts of pathophysiology and management. *Vet Med Small Anim Clin.* **70**(4):404–414.

Gogeliia, A. *et al.* (2006) Experience on treatment of children with otorhinolaryngological diseases by low intensity laser irradiation. *Georgian Med News.* **130**:84–86.

Herrtage, M.J. (2009) Medical management of tracheal collapse. In: *Kirk's Current Veterinary Therapy XIV*, pp. 630–635. Saunders Elsevier, St. Louis, MO.

Höfling, D.B. (2010) Low-level laser therapy in chronic autoimmune thyroiditis: a pilot study. *Lasers Surg Med.* **42**(6):589–596.

Höfling, D.B. *et al.* (2013) Low-level laser in the treatment of patients with hypothyroidism induced by chronic autoimmune thyroiditis: a randomized, placebo-controlled clinical trial. *Lasers Med Sci.* **28**(3):743–753.

Kalogeris, T. *et al.* (2012) Cell biology of ischemia/reperfusion injury *Int Rev Cell Mol Biol.* **298**:229–317.

Kaplan, B. (1981) Evaluation and management of tonsillitis & pharyngitis in dogs. *Vet Med Small Anim Clin.* **76**(11):1599–1603.

Kashanskaia, E.P. and Fedorov, A.A. (2009) Low-intensity laser radiation in the combined treatment of patients with chronic obstructive bronchitis. *Vopr Kurortol Fizioter Lech Fiz Kult.* **2**:19–22.

Korochkin, I.M. *et al.* (1989) Intravenous laser therapy in multimodal treatment of acute pneumonia. *Sov Med.* **7**:22–26.

Krespi, Y.P. and Kizhner, V. (2012) Laser-assisted nasal decolonization of *Staphylococcus aureus*, including methicillin-resistant *Staphylococcus aureus. Am J Otolaryngol.* **33**(5):572–575.

Lapchak, P.A. *et al.* (2015) Transcranial near-infrared laser transmission (NILT) profiles (800 nm): systematic comparison in four common research species. *PLoS One.* **10**(6):e0127580.

Lee, H.M. *et al.* (2013) A comparative pilot study of symptom improvement before and after phototherapy in Korean patients with perennial allergic rhinitis. *Photochem Photobiol.* **89**(3):751–757.

Lister, T. *et al.* (2012) Optical properties of human skin. *J Biomed Opt.* **17**(9):90901.

Lobetti, R.G. (2009) A retrospective study of chronic nasal disease in 75 dogs. *J S Afr Vet Assoc.* **80**(4):224–228.

Lutaĭ, A.V. (2001) Laser therapy of elderly patients with pneumonia. *Vopr Kurortol Fizioter Lech Fiz Kult.* **3**:15–18.

MacPhail, C. (2014) Laryngeal disease in dogs and cats. *Vet Clin North Am Small Anim Pract.* **44**(1):19–31.

Maggiore, A.D. (2014) Tracheal and airway collapse in dogs. *Vet Clin North Am Small Anim Pract.* **44**(1):117–127.

Mariani, C.L. (2003) Full recovery following delayed neurologic signs after smoke inhalation in a dog. *J Vet Emerg Crit Care.* **13**(4):235–239.

Marinho, R.R. *et al.* (2013a) Potentiated anti-inflammatory effect of combined 780 nm and 660 nm low level laser therapy on the experimental laryngitis. *J Photochem Photobiol B.* **121**:86–93.

Marinho, R.R. *et al.* (2013b) Potential anti-inflammatory effect of low-level laser therapy on the experimental reflux laryngitis: a preliminary study. *Lasers Med Sci.* **29**(1):239–243.

Meola, S.D. (2013) Brachycephalic airway syndrome. *Top Companion Anim Med.* **28**(3):91–96.

Miranda da Silva, C. *et al.* (2015) Low level laser therapy reduces the development of lung inflammation induced by formaldehyde exposure *PLoS One.* **10**(11):e0142816.

Monnet, E. (2016) Surgical treatment of laryngeal paralysis. *Vet Clin North Am Small Anim Pract.* **46**(4):709–719.

Monnet, E. and Tobias, K.M. (2012) Larynx. In: *Veterinary Surgery Small Animal*, pp. 1724. Elsevier, St. Louis, MO.

Naghdi, S. *et al.* (2013) A pilot study into the effect of low-level laser therapy in patients with chronic rhinosinusitis. *Physiother Theory Pract.* **29**(8): 596–603.

Oliveira, M.C. Jr. *et al.* (2014) Low level laser therapy reduces acute lung inflammation in a model of pulmonary and extrapulmonary LPS-induced ARDS. *J Photochem Photobiol B.* **134**:57–63.

Ostronosova, N.S. (2006) Outpatient use of laser therapy in bronchial asthma. *Ter Arkh.* **78**(3):41–44.

Parrado, C. *et al.* (1990) Quantitative study of the morphological changes in the thyroid gland following IR laser radiation. *Lasers Med Sci.* **5**(1):77–80.

Parrado, C. *et al.* (1999) A quantitative investigation of microvascular changes in the thyroid gland after infrared (IR) laser radiation. *Histol Histopathol.* **14**(4):1067–1071.

Prescott, C.W. (1968) A case of tonsilitis in the cat. *Aust Vet J.* **44**(7):331–332.

Priestnall, S.L. (2014) New and emerging pathogens in canine infectious respiratory disease. *Vet Pathol.* **51**(2):492–504.

Reed, N. (2014) Chronic rhinitis in the cat. *Vet Clin North Am Small Anim Pract.* **44**(1):33–50.

Rehberg, S. *et al.* (2009) Pathophysiology, management and treatment of smoke inhalation injury. *Expert Rev Respir Med.* **3**(3):283–297.

Reinero, C.R. (2011) Advances in the understanding of pathogenesis, and diagnostics and therapeutics for feline allergic asthma. *Vet J.* **190**(1):28–33.

Rozanski, E. (2014) Canine chronic bronchitis. *Vet Clin North Am Small Anim Pract.* **44**(1):107–116.

Sharman, M.J. and Mansfield, C.S. (2012) Sinonasal aspergillosis in dogs: a review. *J Small Anim Pract.* **53**(8):434–444.

Silva, V.R. *et al.* (2014) Low-level laser therapy inhibits bronchoconstriction, Th2 inflammation and airway remodeling in allergic asthma. *Respir Physiol Neurobiol.* **194**:37–48.

Sutera, S.P. and Skalak, R. (1993) The history of Poiseuille's law. *Annu Rev Fluid Mech.* **25**:1–20.

Tedford, C.E. *et al.* (2015) Quantitative analysis of transcranial and intraparenchymal light penetration in human cadaver brain tissue. *Lasers Surg Med.* **47**(4):312–322.

Trizil, J.E. and Reinero, C.R. (2014) Update on feline asthma. *Vet Clin North Am Small Anim Pract.* **44**(1):91–105.

Troxel, M. (2012) Smoke inhalation in a dog: clinician's brief (capsule). Available from: http://www.cliniciansbrief.com//column/category/column/capsules/smoke-inhalation-dog (accessed November 30, 2016).

Viitanen, S.J. (2015) Co-infections with respiratory viruses in dogs with bacterial pneumonia. *J Vet Intern Med.* **29**(2):544–551.

Windsor, R.C. and Johnson, L.R. (2006) Canine chronic inflammatory rhinitis. *Clin Tech Small Anim Pract.* **21**(2):76–81.

Wang, X.Y. (2014) Effect of low-level laser therapy on allergic asthma in rats. *Lasers Med Sci.* **29**(3):1043–1050.

15

Oral Conditions
Ray A. Arza

RSA Veterinary Technologies, Taylorsville, KY, USA

Introduction

The number of veterinary practices using therapeutic lasers has increased significantly, and photobiomodulation therapy (PBMT) has become an important treatment modality in veterinary medicine. There is now overwhelming evidence that PBMT helps control pain, modulates inflammation, and stimulates healing and tissue regeneration (Avci *et al.*, 2013; Bjordal *et al.*, 2006; Chung *et al.*, 2012). The mechanisms by which PBMT has such far-reaching effects are detailed in Chapter 5.

Veterinarians first used therapy lasers to treat musculoskeletal conditions based on the success reported in the treatment of similar conditions in human patients (Bjordal *et al.*, 2008; Chow *et al.*, 2009; Jang and Lee, 2012).

Successful treatment of wounds soon became commonly reported (Al-Watban *et al.*, 2007; Peplow *et al.*, 2010), as did the use of laser therapy for the treatment of painful conditions (Chow *et al.*, 2011; Fulop *et al.*, 2010). Veterinarians have subsequently expanded the use of this modality to treat a wide variety of medical applications, including those involving the oral cavity.

Over the past 10 years, much has been learned about the roles that proper application and dosing play in the expected results from laser therapy (Enwemeka, 2009). Increased knowledge of proper dosing and application allows practitioners to design successful treatment protocols for the oral cavity. As with other conditions that veterinarians treat with photobiomodulation therapy (PBMT), the successful treatment of oral conditions in veterinary patients mirrors what is being reported in the treatment of human oral conditions (Arany, 2016; Boras, 2013; Kathuria *et al.*, 2015; Khan and Arany, 2015; Ross, 2016). This chapter will focus on some of the common conditions that affect the oral cavity in canine and feline patients, and demonstrate how PBMT is utilized in the management of these conditions.

Oral Inflammatory Conditions

Use of laser therapy to reduce oral inflammation in both humans and animals has been widely reported (Ahmed *et al.*, 2015; Bjordal *et al.*, 2011; Chermetz *et al.*, 2014; Freire *et al.*, 2014; Ottaviani *et al.*, 2013). A pair of recent, very comprehensive review articles examined the use of PBMT in the management of the side effects of radiation and chemoradiation therapy in human head and neck cancer patients (Zecha *et al.*, 2016a, 2016b). The articles state that among the few supportive care measures available for the treatment of the side effects of radiation therapy or chemoradiotherapy in human patients, PBMT has shown the most promise. These publications emphasize the important role that laser therapy can play in the management of all oral inflammatory conditions.

In their 2016 review, Zecha *et al.* note that PBM "effectively modulates biological function is supported by a plethora of clinical and laboratory studies" (2016a). It "elicits several potentially beneficial effects, including reduction of inflammation and pain, promotion of tissue repair, reduction of fibrosis, and protection and regeneration of nerves" (2016b).

Publications reporting the successful application of PBMT in oral inflammatory conditions in humans give cross-species evidence that treatment of similar conditions is indicated in veterinary patients. Regardless of the cause of inflammation, with the exception of malignancy, therapy lasers can be used in the oral cavity with promising results and very little evidence of side effects.

Inflammation of oral tissues may be primary or secondary, and may affect many soft tissues in the mouth including the oral mucosa (stomatitis), the gingiva (gingivitis), the periodontium (periodontitis), the alveolar mucosa (alveolar mucositis), the mucosa of the tongue (glossitis), and the mucosa of the pharynx (pharyngitis) (Gorrel *et al.*, 2013a).

Laser Therapy in Veterinary Medicine: Photobiomodulation, First Edition. Edited by Ronald J. Riegel and John C. Godbold, Jr.
© 2017 John Wiley & Sons, Inc. Published 2017 by John Wiley & Sons, Inc.

Periodontal disease is the most common oral condition presented to veterinarians (Gorrel *et al.*, 2013b). It is typically an inflammatory response to the presence of bacterial plaque on adjacent tooth surfaces. Other causes of oral inflammation include infectious agents, trauma, autoimmune disease, chemical agents, metabolic disease, and burns. Traumatic stomatitis is sometimes seen when an animal has oral exposure to toxic plants or other toxic substances.

Periodontal Disease

Periodontal disease is the most common oral condition presented to veterinarians. It responds well when treated with PBMT, and should be the most common oral condition treated with PBMT. Periodontal disease is widespread in canine patients and is often associated with serious systemic diseases. It is more common in small breeds than large breeds, and increases with advancing age (Marshall *et al.*, 2014). Periodontal disease includes gingivitis (inflammation of the gums) and periodontitis (loss of soft tissue and bone around the teeth). Often ignored by clients, and often treated too late in its course, it causes companion animals significant pain and secondary health issues (AVDC, n.d.).

The diagnostic criteria and grading of gingivitis and periodontal disease have been well established in publications (Harvey *et al.*, 2008) and are specified by the American Veterinary Dental College (AVDC, 2009).

Even the earliest diagnosis, and the lowest grading (grade I gingivitis), merit attention, which should include laser therapy. Adding PBMT to the overall management plan for periodontal disease will help reduce the patient's oral pain and inflammation.

Periodontal disease may be treated as a superficial condition (when treatment can be administered with the mouth open) or as a deep condition (if the patient will not allow the mouth to be opened). Treatments are usually initiated in conjunction with dental procedures, under sedation or anesthesia. When treating with the mouth open, a laser setting that delivers 3–4 J/cm^2 is recommended, since the laser light does not have to penetrate through other tissue to get to the target tissue (Figure 15.1). The author recommends positioning the handpiece 1–2 cm from the target area. If available, a handpiece that collimates the laser beam and allows treatment at a greater distance from the tissue may be used. The laser power settings should be no more than 3 W and the handpiece should move over the entire affected area until the total dose of 3–4 J/cm^2 is delivered.

When treating with the mouth closed, laser settings that deliver 6–8 J/cm^2 are recommended (Figure 15.2). The area to be treated should include the entire dental arcades and from the ventral aspect through the intermandibular space (Figure 15.3). With the mouth closed,

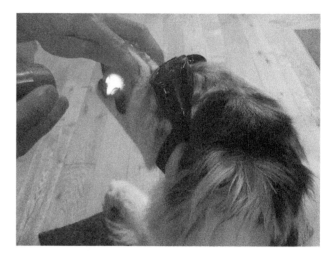

Figure 15.1 Treating periodontal disease with the mouth open.

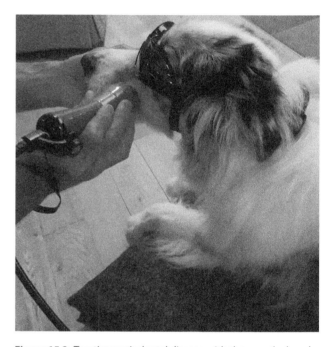

Figure 15.2 Treating periodontal disease with the mouth closed.

a higher dose is required in order to get a clinically relevant number of photons to the target tissue.

Severity, chronicity, and the patient's degree of discomfort should dictate how often the patient is treated. If the patient has low-grade periodontal disease that responds to multimodal care, therapy laser treatments may only be necessary as part of that care for a limited time.

More often, periodontal disease becomes a chronic condition, and requires long-term, open-ended treatment. When periodontal disease is chronic, three phases of treatment should be implemented: an induction phase, a transition phase, and a long-term maintenance phase. The induction phase usually starts with every-other-day

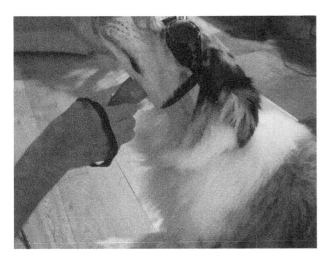

Figure 15.3 Treatment through the intermandibular space with the mouth closed. The handpiece should be placed in contact with the skin with light pressure for more effective penetration of photons.

treatments, and continues until a desirable clinical response is noted. When improvement is noted, the frequency of treatment can be reduced gradually through a transition phase of less frequent treatments, with the goal of finding a maintenance schedule that will keep the patient at the desired level of comfort.

Feline Stomatitis

Feline stomatitis, though uncommon and seen in only 3.9% of feline patients (Kornya *et al.*, 2014), can be a very serious condition that is often very difficult to manage, with severe discomfort to the patient. Affected cats present with inflammation of oral mucosal tissues that often worsens with time and becomes refractory to treatment. Typical findings are severely ulcerated, inflamed tissues, most commonly affecting the caudal aspect of the oral cavity, involving the fauces and pharyngeal areas. Severe ulceroproliferative inflammation that involves these areas bilaterally is considered pathognomonic for feline stomatitis (Crawford, 2013). The etiology of feline stomatitis is not completely understood, but a high percentage of affected cats are chronic carriers of feline calicivirus. There is also evidence that an overreaction of the immune system to antigens in dental plaque may play a role in these pathological changes (Robson and Crystal, 2011).

The most common symptom is severe pain when opening the mouth. As the condition gets worse, halitosis and dysphagia may be seen, and, with time, weight loss may be evident. Examination of the oral cavity is often difficult without sedation, due to patient discomfort and severe pain.

Diagnosis of feline stomatitis is usually made by observation of bilateral inflammation of the caudal oral cavity.

However, attempts to isolate calici and herpes viruses, as well as to evaluate other potential problems such as renal failure, are recommended. Biopsy generally reveals a predominance of lymphocytes and plasma cells.

Management of this condition requires a multimodal approach. Published data indicate that early partial or full mouth extraction is the best choice to provide long-lasting improvement (Jennings *et al.*, 2015). Medical therapy focuses on controlling inflammation, infection, and pain. This includes the use of corticosteroids, other immunosuppressants (e.g., cyclosporine or chlorambucil), antibiotics (e.g., amoxicillin-clavulanic acid, clindamycin, or azithromycin), and pain medications (e.g., buprenorphine or fentanyl). Ablating (evaporating) the abnormal tissue with a carbon dioxide (CO_2) surgical laser has been reported as an adjunctive treatment for caudal stomatitis (Lewis *et al.*, 2007).

Evidence that PBMT reduces oral pain and inflammation and the experience of veterinary practitioners support using laser therapy as an adjunct to medical and dental protocols for feline oropharyngeal inflammation. The possibility should be explored that the antiviral effects of laser therapy reported in humans may contribute to better patient outcomes in cats if viral etiologies are a factor (Navarro *et al.*, 2007).

Though practitioners report that lesions often do not improve in appearance following laser therapy, patients frequently display significantly reduced clinical signs. Treatment of this chronic and insidious condition must be tailored to the severity of the case and the patient's response to treatment.

Feline stomatitis may be treated as a superficial condition (when treatment can be administered with mouth open) or as a deep condition (if the patient will not allow the mouth to be opened). Some practitioners recommend a combination of both open- and closed-mouth protocols each time a patient is presented, and the author believes this should be considered in severely affected patients.

When treating with the mouth open, dosages in the range of 3–4J/cm^2 are recommended, since the laser light does not have to penetrate through other tissue to get to the target tissue. The author recommends using a handpiece held 1–2 cm from the target area. If available, a handpiece that collimates the laser beam and allows treatment at a greater distance from the tissue should be used. The laser power setting should be no more than 3 W and the handpiece should move over the entire affected area until the total dose of 3–4J/cm^2 is delivered.

When treating with the mouth closed, dosages in the range of 6–8J/cm^2 are recommended. The area to be treated should run from the temporomandibular joint on one side, across the front of mouth to the temporomandibular joint on the other side, as well as from the ventral aspect through the intermandibular space. The total dose should be about 2.5 times that when treating with the mouth open, to be sure a therapeutic dose reaches the target tissue. The power setting should be 3–4 W and the handpiece should move over entire area to be treated until the total dose of 6–8 J/cm^2 has been delivered.

As when treating periodontal disease, the severity, chronicity, and degree of patient discomfort should dictate how often the patient is treated. Because feline stomatitis is a chronic condition, the management plan should include induction and transition phases followed by long-term maintenance treatments. The induction phase usually starts with every-other-day treatments. It should continue until a desirable clinical response has been noted. With severely painful presentations, the author recommends treating 3–4 days in a row before moving to every-other-day treatments. When improvement is noted, the frequency of treatment can be reduced gradually through a transition phase of less frequent treatments, with the goal of finding a maintenance schedule that will keep the patient at the desired level of comfort.

It is important to note that proper, continued management of a chronic condition like feline stomatits is critical to success. A common mistake in the management of these cases is a premature reduction in the frequency of treatment, which leads to a perceived failure of PBMT.

Canine Stomatitis

Canine patients can present with severe, chronic, ulcerative, oral inflammatory lesions known as chronic ulcerative paradental stomatitis (CUPS) (or as canine chronic ulcerative stomatitis, idiopathic stomatitis, ulcerative stomatitis, or lymphocytic-plasmacytic stomatitis). As the name implies, paradental disease should be differentiated from periodontal disease (Lyon, 2005). Periodontal disease affects the tissues that attach the tooth in the socket (gingiva, alveolar bone, periodontal ligament, and cementum of the root). These structures often remain normal in the presence of paradental disease. In contrast, paradental disease affects the other soft tissues in the oral cavity, including the buccal and palatal mucosa, lips, and tongue.

Many breeds may present with CUPS, but the Maltese and cavalier King Charles spaniels appear to be overrepresented. Clinical signs usually include halitosis, inappetence or anorexia, drooling, lip-fold dermatitis, and oral pain. While diagnosis is often made by clinical observation of lesions, it is important to note that other conditions can present with similar signs and history. Other conditions which should be ruled out include immune-mediated diseases such as pemphigus and bullous pemphigoid, erythema multiforme and epitheliotropic T-cell lymphoma (Nemec *et al.*, 2012), and

Wegener's granulomatosis (Krug *et al.*, 2006). Proper diagnosis is important, since treatment of these other conditions is very different from treatment of CUPS.

The etiology of CUPS is not completely understood, but it is evident that these animals have an abnormal immune-system response, and they appear to be intolerant to the presence of bacterial plaque. Even small amounts of plaque lead to an abnormal ulcerative inflammatory response in mucous membranes in contact with the teeth (Lobprise, 2012; Niemiec, 2010).

Management of this chronic condition can be very frustrating to both the veterinarian and the patient's owner. The focus of management should be scrupulous plaque control. Teeth with concurrent periodontal disease should be extracted and home dental health care should be instituted. Medical treatment is occasionally required, with the use of appropriate antibiotics and prudential use of corticosteroids. Pain control should be considered, since these patients are often very uncomfortable.

Given the established ability of PBMT to prevent and ameliorate pain and inflammation associated with oral mucositis, laser therapy should be used in the treatment of this condition. The goal is to utilize laser therapy as part of a multimodal approach to reduce pain and inflammation, while minimizing potential adverse effects. Laser therapy should not be the sole treatment for this condition.

Laser therapy is used in the management of CUPS in a similar way to how it is used in the management of feline stomatitis, and should include induction, transition, and maintenance phases of treatment. As with feline stomatitis, the frequency of treatments should be dictated by the severity of the condition and the response to treatment.

Canine patients may be treated with the mouth open, which is the author's preference, or with the mouth closed. When treating the buccal or labial mucosal tissues, lifting of the lips without opening the jaws will often be tolerated (Figure 15.4). This technique allows direct delivery of the therapeutic light to the target tissue. When treating with the mouth open, directly on to the target tissue, administer a dose of 3–4 J/cm^2, with a power setting of no more than 4 watts. This should be accomplished with the treatment handpiece held 1–2 cm from the target tissue. The handpiece should move over the entire affected area until the total dose of 3–4 J/cm^2 has been delivered.

If a patient does not tolerate treatment with the mouth open, then the treatment can be delivered over the entire affected area through the facial tissues, at a dose of 6–10 J/cm^2 and power setting of 4–8 W. The dose should be adjusted according to the size of the patient and the thickness of the facial tissues. If possible, treat with the handpiece in contact with the facial tissues to increase photon penetration into deeper tissues.

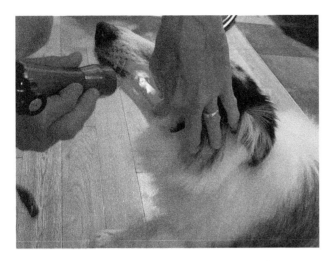

Figure 15.4 Lifting the patient's lips without opening the jaws. This technique allows direct delivery of therapeutic light to the target tissue.

Oral Wounds

PBMT has been shown to enhance wound repair and tissue regeneration by influencing the three phases of injury resolution: inflammatory, proliferative, and maturation (remodelling) (Hawkins and Abrahamse, 2006). The benefits of laser therapy application have been specifically demonstrated in oral wound healing (Arany, 2016; Khan and Arany, 2015; Wagner *et al.*, 2016). The well-established beneficial effects of PBMT on wound healing should make laser therapy a standard part of wound management in the oral cavity.

Traumatic Wounds

Though a problem in both the canine and feline patient, dogs' affinity for chewing sticks, bones, and other inanimate objects makes them more susceptible to oral injuries. Common presentations include punctures, abrasions, lacerations, burns, stings, and other traumatic wounds. Both soft and hard tissues are sometimes involved, and they need to be addressed appropriately. The rich blood supply to the oral cavity creates an environment susceptible to profuse bleeding, but one that also tends to heal much quicker than other parts of the body. In some cases, minor injuries heal quickly without medical intervention.

As with other oral conditions, treatment of oral wounds using laser therapy may be accomplished with the mouth open or closed. The author recommends treating these wounds with direct light exposure to the target tissue whenever possible. When treating with direct exposure to tissue (open mouth), administer a dose of $3–4\,J/cm^2$, with a power setting of $2–4\,W$. A lower power setting is recommended for small wounds and a higher setting for larger ones. If the patient does not allow direct treatment of the wound, then treating with the mouth closed will require higher doses of $6–10\,J/cm^2$, depending on the thickness of the tissue and the location of the wound. Power settings of $4–8\,W$ can be used.

Traumatic wounds that involve fractures of the mandible or maxilla may also benefit from PBMT. The author recommends treating immediately upon presentation to decrease inflammation and pain, then again after fracture repair, to enhance healing. The beneficial effects of PBMT on fracture healing have been well established (Kazem *et al.*, 2010; Medalha *et al.*, 2016; Son *et al.*, 2012).

There are essentially no contraindications for the use of lasers with surgical implants. The success of fixation implants will always increase if the health of surrounding soft tissues is improved by application of PBMT (Tang and Arany, 2013). Since photons are reflected by metal, the metal is not heated; however, if there is only a small amount of soft tissue superficial to the implant, one should avoid treating directly over this area to prevent heating of superficial tissues.

Dosages of $6–10\,J/cm^2$ should be used to treat fractures, with $2–8\,W$ of power depending on the size of the patient and the area to be treated. Current protocols recommend applying laser therapy at the time of fracture fixation and then two to three times a week for 3–4 weeks. After several weeks, the fracture should be assessed radiographically, and treatment should be continued for several more weeks if active healing is not noted.

Surgical Wounds

Laser therapy has become a standard of care as part of the multimodal approach to decreasing pain and inflammation in postoperative management in many practices. Studies in human medicine have shown that treating postsurgical wounds has analgesic and anti-inflammatory effects (Karlekar, 2015). Surgical wounds in the mouth, with either soft- or hard-tissue involvement, or both, can benefit from the effect of PBM (Figure 15.5). With routine soft-tissue surgery or minor extractions, the author recommends treating immediately postoperatively one time. Immediate treatment has been demonstrated to reduce postoperative inflammatory complications versus delayed treatment (Abdel-Alim *et al.*, 2015). With more extensive soft-tissue surgery, or with more involved extractions, multiple daily (or at least every-other-day) treatments should be considered. With acute inflammation and pain, daily treatments are recommended until the patient is comfortable. In some cases, treatments should be continued two to three times a week until the wound has healed.

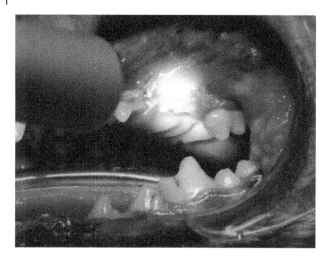

Figure 15.5 Surgical wounds in the mouth, such as with this fourth upper premolar extraction, should be treated immediately postoperatively. With more extensive soft-tissue surgery, or with more involved extractions, multiple daily or every-other-day treatments should be considered until the wound has healed. The blue-white appearance of the area being treated is a result of the camera being able to image the near-infrared wavelength. Image courtesy of Dr. John C. Godbold, Jr.

Laser settings for surgical wounds will be the same as described for inflammatory conditions. Intraoral treatment, with the mouth open at the time of surgery, is indicated. Subsequent treatments can be extraoral, with the mouth closed (Sierra *et al.*, 2016).

Other Oral Conditions

Eosinophilic Granuloma Complex

Eosinophilic granuloma complex includes three distinctly different clinical presentations that, according to William H. Miller, VMD, Professor of Dermatology at Cornell University College of Veterinary Medicine, are grouped together "because all three show the activity of eosinophils and have an apparent allergic condition as the triggering event" (Cornell University College of Veterinary Medicine, 2016). The three different forms are eosinophilic granuloma, eosinophilic ulcer (indolent ulcer), and eosinophilic plaque (Buckley and Nuttall, 2012). This chapter will only discuss the first two, since eosinophilic plaque does not occur in the oral cavity.

Treatment is dependent on the severity and the underlying cause (the source of the apparent allergic reaction), but may include corticosteroids, antibiotics (for secondary infection), antihistamines, and other immunosuppressive drugs (e.g., cyclosporine or chlorambucil).

Eosinophilic granuloma is the most commonly presented form, with a wide variation in clinical appearances that can present anywhere on the body. It is commonly seen in the oral cavity and on the hind legs. Lesions may

vary, but typically are nodular or linear raised thickened areas, red or yellowish in color, sometimes with loss of hair and ulcerations. In the oral cavity, the lesions are usually found on the tongue or palate.

Eosinophilic ulcers typically occur toward the edge of the upper lips, often close to the midline (philtrum) on one or both sides. Generally, they are well-defined ulcerated lesions with raised borders, which may become disfiguring and bleed over time. Severe lesions may cause pain and inappetence (Rees, 2011).

PBMT has been used as an adjunct to conventional medical therapy based on anecdotal reports from practitioners. The recommended dose of laser therapy for this complex of conditions has changed dramatically over the past 10 years. When a low dose (e.g., $3-4\,J/cm^2$, as is traditionally utilized for superficial conditions) is used to treat eosinophilic granulomas and ulcers, there is no appreciable clinical improvement. However, when a dosage of $30-40\,J/cm^2$ is applied, significantly better clinical results are observed. Since lesions in the mouth are usually relatively small, the power setting should not exceed 2 W. Lesions should be treated two to three times a week until resolved.

Lip-Fold Dermatitis in Dogs

Lip-fold dermatitis or lip-fold pyoderma is most commonly seen in breeds with large, saggy, floppy lips, such as St. Bernards, bloodhounds, springer spaniels, sharpeis, Neapolitan mastiffs, and bulldogs. Accumulation of saliva and food debris in the lip fold creates an environment that leads to irritation, inflammation, and, if left untreated, infection with bacteria or yeast. Treatment will depend on severity and underlying cause, but often includes medicated shampoos, topical ointments, or oral antibiotics. In severe unresponsive cases, surgical reconstruction of the lip folds may be indicated.

As with moist dermatitis found elsewhere on the body, laser therapy may play an adjunctive role in decreasing inflammation and discomfort and promoting healing. Laser settings that deliver a dosage of $3-4\,J/cm^2$ should be used, with a power setting of 2–4 W, depending on the size of area to be treated. In frequently reoccurring cases, long-term maintenance treatments every 7–10 days may help avoid acute exacerbations.

Conclusion

Laser therapy has become a standard of care in thousands of veterinary practices. PBMT is an important component of the multimodal approach to decreasing both pain and inflammation while stimulating healing in oral tissues. Many oral conditions result in similar changes in the mouth, with some variations due to the severity, chronicity, and size and thickness of the involved tissue. Regardless, all oral conditions are treated with similar laser therapy protocols. With the exception of malig-

nancies, practitioners are encouraged to utilize PBMT on any condition in the mouth that presents with inflammation, pain, or tissue damage.

References

Abdel-Alim, H.M. *et al.* (2015) A comparative study of the effectiveness of immediate versus delayed photobiomodulation therapy in reducing the severity of postoperative inflammatory complications. *Photomed Laser Surg.* **33**(9):447–451.

Ahmed, K. *et al.* (2015) Evaluation of low level laser therapy in the management of chemotherapy induced oral mucositis in pediatric and young cancer patients: a randomized clinical trial. *Eur Sci Journ.* **11**(27):209–222.

Al-Watban, F.A. *et al.* (2007) Low-level laser therapy enhances wound healing in diabetic rats: a comparison of different lasers. *Photomed Laser Surg.* **25**(2):72–77.

Arany, P.R. (2016) Craniofacial wound healing with photobiomodulation therapy: new insights and current challenges. *J Dent Res.* **95**(9):977–984.

Avci, P. *et al.* (2013) Low-level laser (light) therapy (LLLT) in skin: stimulating, healing, restoring. *Semin Cutan Med Surg.* **32**(1):41–52.

AVDC. (n.d.) Periodontal disease. Available from: http://www.avdc.org/periodontaldisease.html (accessed November 30, 2016).

AVDC. (2009) Recommendations adopted by the AVDC Board: version current as of October 2009. Available from: http://www.avdc.org/nomenclature3.html (accessed November 30, 2016).

Bjordal, J.M. *et al.* (2006) Low-level laser therapy in acute pain: a systematic review of mechanisms of action and clinical effects in randomized placebo-controlled trials. *Photomed Laser Surg.* **24**(2):158–168.

Bjordal, J.M. *et al.* (2008) A systematic review with procedural assessments and meta-analysis of low level laser therapy in lateral elbow tendonopathy (tennis elbow). *BMC Musculoskeletal Disord.* **9**:75.

Bjordal, J.M. *et al.* (2011) A systematic review with meta-analysis of the effect of low-level laser therapy (LLLT) in cancer therapy-induced oral mucositis. *Support Care Cancer.* **19**:1069–1077.

Boras, V.V. (2013) Applications of low level laser therapy. In: *A Textbook of Advanced Oral and Maxillofacial Surgery*. InTech, Rijeka.

Buckley, L. and Nuttall, T. (2012) Feline eosinophilic granuloma complex(ities): some clinical clarification. *J Feline Med Surg.* **14**(7):471–481.

Chermetz M. *et al.* (2014) Class IV laser therapy as treatment for chemotherapy-induced oral mucositis in onco-haematological paediatric patients: a prospective study. *Int J Paediatr Dent.* **6**:441–449.

Chow, R. *et al.* (2009) Efficacy of low-level laser therapy in the management of neck pain: a systematic review and meta-analysis of randomized placebo or active-treatment controlled trials. *Lancet.* **374**(9705):1897–908.

Chow, R. *et al.* (2011) Inhibitory effects of laser irradiation on peripheral mammalian nerves and relevance to analgesic effects: a systematic review. *Photomed Laser Surg* **29**:365–381.

Chung, H. *et al.* (2012) The nuts and bolts of low-level laser (light) therapy. *Ann Biomed Eng.* **40**(2):516–533.

Cornell University College of Veterinary Medicine. (n.d.) Eosinophilic granuloma complex. Available from: http://www.vet.cornell.edu/fhc/Health_Information/eosinophilic.cfm (accessed November 30, 2016).

Crawford, J. (2013) Gingivostomatitis. In: *Small Animal Dental Procedures for Veterinary Technicians and Nurses*, pp. 145–140. Wiley-Blackwell, Hoboken, NJ.

Enwemeka, C.S. (2009) Intricacies of dose in laser phototherapy for tissue repair and pain relief. *Photomed Laser Surg.* **3**:387–393.

Freire, M. *et al.* (2014) LED and laser photobiomodulation in the prevention and treatment of oral mucositis: experimental study in hamsters. *Clin Oral Investig.* **18**(3):1005–1013.

Fulop, A. *et al.* (2010) A meta-analysis of the efficacy of laser phototherapy on pain relief. *Clin J Pain.* **26**(8):729–736.

Gorrel, C. *et al.* (2013a) Common oral conditions. In: *Veterinary Dentistry for the General Practitioner*, 2 edn., pp. 81–95. Elsevier, Philadelphia, PA.

Gorrel, C. *et al.* (2013b) Periodontal disease. In: *Veterinary Dentistry for the General Practitioner*, 2 edn., pp. 97–119. Elsevier, Philadelphia, PA.

Harvey, C.E. *et al.* (2008) Scoring the full extent of periodontal disease in the dog: development of a total mouth periodontal score (TMPS) system. *J Vet Dent.* **25**(3):176–180.

Hawkins, D. and Abrahamse, H. (2006) The role of laser fluence in cell viability, proliferation, and membrane integrity of wounded human skin fibroblasts following helium-neon laser irradiation. *Lasers Surg Med.* **38**(1):74–83.

Jang, H. and Lee, H. (2012) Meta-analysis of pain relief effects by laser irradiation on joint areas. *Photomedicine and Laser Surgery.* **30**(8):405–417.

Jennings, M.W. *et al.* (2015) Effect of tooth extraction on stomatitis in cats: 95 cases (2000–2013). *J Am Vet Med Assoc.* **246**(6):654–660.

Karlekar, A. (2015) Assessment of feasibility and efficacy of class IV laser therapy for postoperative pain relief in off-pump coronary artery bypass surgery patients: a pilot study. *Ann Card Anaesth.* **18**(3):317–322.

Kathuria, V. *et al.* (2015) Low level laser therapy: a panacea for oral maladies. *Laser Ther.* **24**(3):215–223.

Kazem, S.S. *et al.* (2010) Effect of low-level laser therapy on the fracture healing process. *Lasers Med Sci.* **25**(1):73–77.

Khan, I. and Arany, P.R. (2015) Biophysical approaches for oral wound healing: emphasis on photobiomodulation. *Adv Wound Care (New Rochelle).* **4**(12):724–737.

Kornya, M.R. *et al.* (2014) Association between oral health status and retrovirus test results in cats. *J Am Vet Med Assoc.* **245**(8):916–922.

Krug, W. *et al.* (2006) Diagnosis and management of Wegener's granulomatosis in a dog. *J Vet Dent.* **23**(4):231–236.

Lewis, J.R. *et al.* (2007) Use of CO2 laser as an adjunctive treatment for caudal stomatitis in a cat. *J Vet Dent.* **24**(4):240–249.

Lobprise, H.B. (2012) Oral ulceration and chronic ulcerative paradental stomatitis. In: *Blackwell's Five-Minute Veterinary Consult Clinical Companion – Small Animal Dentistry*, 2 edn., pp. 243–247. Wiley-Blackwell, Ames, IA.

Lyon, K.F. (2005) Gingivostomatitis. *Vet Clin North Am Small Anim Pract.* **35**(4):891–911.

Marshall, M.D. *et al.* (2014) A longitudinal assessment of periodontal disease in 52 miniature schnauzers. *BMC Veterinary Research.* **10**:166.

Medalha, C.C. *et al.* (2016) Low level laser therapy accelerates bone healing in spinal cord injured rats. *J Photochem Photobiol B.* **59**:179–185.

Navarro, R. *et al.* (2007) Low-level-laser therapy as an alternative treatment for primary herpes simplex infection: a case report. *J Clin Pediatr Dent.* **31**(4):225–228.

Nemec, A. *et al.* (2012) Erythema multiforme and epitheliotropic T-cell lymphoma in the oral cavity of dogs: 1989 to 2009. *J Small Anim Pract.* **53**(8):445–452.

Niemiec, B.A. (2010) Chronic ulcerative paradental stomatitis. In: *Small Animal Dental, Oral and Maxillofacial Disease: A Color Handbook*, pp. 189–191. Manson Publishing, London.

Ottaviani, G. *et al.* (2013) Effect of class IV laser therapy on chemotherapy-induced oral mucositis: a clinical and experimental study. *Am J Pathol.* **183**(6):1747–1757.

Peplow, P.V. *et al.* (2010) Laser photobiomodulation of wound healing: a review of experimental studies in mouse and rat animal models. *Photomed Laser Surg.* **28**(3):291–325.

Rees, C.A. (2011) Eosinophilic granuloma complex. In: *The Feline Patient*, pp 154–156. Wiley-Blackwell, Hoboken, NJ.

Robson, M. and Crystal, M.A. (2011) Gingivitis-stomatitis-pharyngitis. In: *The Feline Patient*, pp 199–201. Wiley-Blackwell, Hoboken, NJ.

Ross, G. (2016) Evidence based use of photobiomodulation in periodontics – a literature search. Abstract #129 presented to the American Society for Laser Medicine and Surgery Conference. April 3, 2016. Boston, MA.

Sierra, S.O. *et al.* (2016) Choosing between intraoral or extraoral, red or infrared laser irradiation after impacted third molar extraction. *Lasers Surg Med.* **48**(5):511–518.

Son, J. *et al.* (2012) Bone healing effects of diode laser (808 nm) on a rat tibial fracture model. *In Vivo.* **26**(4):703–709.

Tang, E and Arany, P. (2013) Photobiomodulation and implants: implications for dentistry. *J Periodontal Implant Sci.* **43**(6):262–268.

Wagner, V.P. *et al.* (2016) Photobiomodulation regulates cytokine release and new blood vessel formation during oral wound healing in rats. *Lasers Med Sci.* **31**(4):665–671.

Zecha, J. *et al.* (2016a) Low-level laser therapy/photobiomodulation in the management of side effects of chemoradiation therapy in head and neck cancer. Part 1: mechanisms of action, dosimetric, and safety considerations. *Support Care Cancer.* **24**(6):2781–2792.

Zecha, J. *et al.* (2016b) Low-level laser therapy/photobiomodulation in the management of side effects of chemoradiation therapy in head and neck cancer. Part 2: proposed applications and treatment protocols. *Support Care Cancer.* **24**(6):2793–2805.

16

Abdominal Conditions

Richard L. Godine

North American Association for Light Therapy, Ruckersville Animal Hospital and Veterinary Laser Therapy Center, Ruckersville, VA, USA

Introduction

The effects of photobiomodulation (PBM) that decrease inflammation, increase microcirculation, promote tissue regeneration, modulate the immune system, and control pain makes it a useful modality for the treatment of a number of gastrointestinal and urinary tract diseases of small animals. This is particularly true when treating cats and smaller dogs. The stomach, pancreas, intestines, and urinary tract of larger dogs and humans are more difficult to reach with transcutaneous light therapy. As inflammation is a common symptom of most gastrointestinal and urinary diseases of small animals, photobiomodulation therapy (PBMT) can be a useful modality in the treatment armamentarium. The aim of most protocols is to apply a biostimulatory dose at the level of the affected organ. Also applying a biostimulatory dose to the regional lymph nodes will aid in decreasing inflammation and stimulating tissue regeneration.

Gastrointestinal Disorders

A dearth of published literature exists about the treatment of the alimentary system with PBMT. Most comes out of Russia, where both transcutaneous and intravenous light therapy have been in clinical use since the 1980s. By virtue of treating smaller patients, veterinarians can lead the medical community in discovering the applications and efficacy of using PBMT to treat diseases of the gastrointestinal system.

Oropharynx

Stomatitis and gingivostomatitis are common painful inflammatory conditions seen primarily in cats but also in dogs. Feline gingivostomatitis is an incompletely understood multifactorial disease and is thought to involve a hyper-reactive immune response against certain pathogenic periodontal bacteria (Crawford and Losey, 2013; Robson and Crystal, 2011). Best clinical results are achieved when affected teeth are extracted; it is not uncommon for whole-mouth extractions to be necessary (Jennings *et al.*, 2015). The use of the CO_2 ablative laser can be extremely helpful in eliminating residual bacteria and involved tissue following full-mouth extractions (Lewis *et al.*, 2007).

The management of other types of stomatitis can be improved by incorporating PBMT in the overall care. Laser therapy has been shown to downregulate the expression of inflammatory cytokines related to oral mucositis (tumor necrosis factor alpha, TNFα; interleukins 6 and 8, IL6 and IL8) (Basso *et al.*, 2015). It has been well established that PBMT can be used prophylactically to prevent the formation of oral mucositis in human cancer patients being treated with chemotherapy or oral radiation (Ahmed *et al.*, 2015). In cases where oral mucositis develops in human cancer patients when PBMT has not been used for prophylaxis, it can be used to treat the oral mucositis successfully (Muñoz-Corcuera *et al.*, 2013).

Stomatitis in cats and dogs that is not related to the hypersensitivity reaction to periodontal bacteria can be greatly helped by PBMT. Biostimulatory doses can be applied transcutaneously through the labia at a dose of 8–10 J per point or into an open mouth at 1–4 J per point. The submandibular and prescapular lymph nodes should be treated with biostimulatory doses, as well. Treatment frequency should be every 24–48 hours until the stomatitis has resolved. Both red and near-infrared wavelengths can be used, and both work well. A large clinical study by Russian ear, nose, and throat physicians demonstrated 85% efficacy in the treatment of pharyngeal inflammatory conditions with PBMT (Gogeliia *et al.*, 2006).

Salivary mucocele is another disease that can be helped by PBMT. Light therapy has been shown to decrease pain and swelling of the salivary glands, making it useful for treating patients prior to corrective surgery (Simões *et al.*, 2009). The affected salivary gland and associated lymph nodes should be treated with biostimulatory doses of either red or infrared light.

Stomach

Light therapy can be useful in the treatment of gastric reflux, gastric ulcers, and gastritis. Most of the published literature is from Russia and involves the use of intravenous delivery of 405 nm laser light. Intravenous laser therapy uses low doses (<5 mW) of blue, green, yellow, red, and infrared light delivered through a fiber optic catheter placed inside an intravenous catheter (Figure 16.1). Depending on the wavelength chosen, white blood cells, red blood cells, or platelets can be modulated.

Intravenous blue light (405 nm) has been successfully used in gastroesophageal reflux disease (GERD) to normalize gastric pH, increase microcirculation, and decrease inflammation of damaged esophageal tissue (Burduli and Tadtaeva, 2012a, 2012b, 2014). Benefits can also be achieved through transcutaneous application of light directed toward the gastroesophageal junction.

Researchers have shown that chronic atrophic gastritis in rats can be successfully treated with PBMT. They demonstrate a marked decrease in inflammatory cells of the gastric mucosa, as well as a return to normal gastric mucosal thickness and cellular function following laser therapy (Shao *et al.*, 2005; Yang *et al.*, 2005). This represents an opportunity for veterinarians to treat cases of chronic gastritis with light therapy when neoplasia has been ruled out as the underlying cause. Several publications have shown that the healing time of gastric ulcers can be significantly shortened through the use of endoscopic laser application, intravenous laser therapy, or transcutaneous PBMT (Alebastrov and Butov, 2005; Burduli and Gutnova, 2008). The beneficial systemic stimulation of the immune system by transcutaneous light application or intravenous laser therapy plays as much of a role in the healing of the gastric ulcer as does direct stimulation via endoscopic application of light (Alebastrov *et al.*, 2004).

Pancreatitis

Pancreatitis is a common, potentially serious disease encountered frequently in small-animal veterinary hospitals. Mild cases of edematous pancreatitis often resolve spontaneously or with medical treatment and dietary modification. Severe necrotizing pancreatitis is a life-threatening condition that can affect multiple organs. Treatment involves hospitalization, fluid and electrolyte therapy, analgesics, antiemetics, antibiotics, nutritional support, and, sometimes, surgical intervention (Steiner, 2010). It is not uncommon for these patients to be hospitalized for up to a week.

Pancreatitis is painful and involves severe inflammation and decreased microcirculation of the pancreas. PBMT is known to promote analgesia, increase microcirculation, decrease inflammation, reduce oxidative stress, and regenerate tissue (Burduli and Gutnova, 2009). It is an extremely important adjunct to the conventional treatment of pancreatitis. Not only will PBMT increase the chances of a successful outcome in pancreatitis treatment, it often also reduces the hospital stay down to 2–3 days.

The treatment involves transcutaneous application of light directed over the pancreas and surrounding organs in the right and midcranial abdomen every 12–24 hours (Figure 16.2). Initially, bioinhibitory doses (80–120 J per point) of near-infrared light are used to control pain and decrease inflammation. The dose can be decreased to the biostimulatory range (25–60 J per point) once the patient is no longer in pain. Treating the sublumbar and inguinal lymph nodes with biostimulatory doses helps speed recovery. The concurrent use of intravenous laser therapy will also improve chances of success and hasten recovery (Geïnits *et al.*, 2011). In cases of chronic pancreatitis, PBMT has been shown to increase exocrine function (Gutnova, 2011).

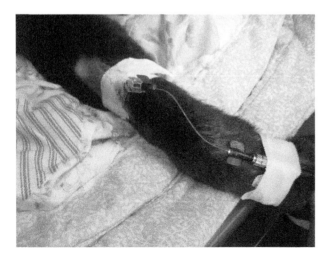

Figure 16.1 Intravenous laser therapy. The fiber optic cable is attached to a fiber optic intravenous catheter in a cephalic vein.

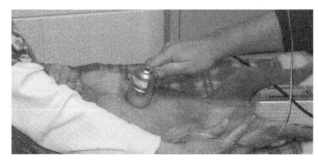

Figure 16.2 An 810 nm 500 mW × 4 multiprobe applied over the pancreas of a dog with pancreatitis.

Intestines

Inflammatory bowel disease (IBD) is a frustrating problem for the veterinarian and owner. This is because the etiology for idiopathic IBD is not completely understood and the clinical course often waxes and wanes with treatment. For those cases that do not respond to dietary modification or antibiotic therapy, immunosuppressive drugs become the hallmark for successful treatment. These drugs can have annoying side effects and can cause other diseases with long-term use.

Zigmond *et al.* (2014) showed that PBMT can induce mucosal healing in colitis of mice. It is well documented that PBMT will decrease inflammation and edema of targeted tissues. It makes sense, therefore, to use light therapy to help control inflamed bowel. This is easy to do in cats and small dogs, since the abdominal cavity is small and shallow, making the intestines accessible to light. The author has had several cases of short-term success in treating feline IBD with PBMT. It does resolve diarrhea and improve appetite, but it needs to be repeated once or twice a week in order to maintain clinical efficacy. This becomes a logistical problem for the owner, and they often want a pharmaceutical solution that will better fit their schedule and budget. However, in cases where immunosuppressive drugs are not tolerated or are contraindicated, PBMT offers a management solution. For cats, a dose of 20–25 J per point will provide biostimulatory doses to the bowel. Dogs may require two to three times that dose, depending on their size and pigmentation. The abdomen can usually be accessed with the patient in a standing position. Special attention to the mesenteric lymph nodes, as well as the sublumbar and inguinal lymph nodes, will improve efficacy, as will intravenous laser (if available).

Liver

Clinically, the author has observed that PBMT has a very positive effect on patients with both acute and chronic liver disease. Light therapy has been shown to bring down and normalize biochemical markers such as alanine transaminase (ALT), aspartate aminotransferase (AST), alkaline phosphatase (ALP), gamma glutamyl transferase (GGT), direct bilirubin, and total bilirubin (Babaev *et al.*, 2012). It also has been shown to reduce the pro-inflammatory cytokines ILβ1, IL6, and TNFα while increasing the anti-inflammatory cytokine IL4 (Burduli and Krifarid, 2011), leading to a reduction in hepatic inflammatory infiltrates (Oliveira-Junior *et al.*, 2013). A reduction in hepatic oxidative stress caused by nitric oxide (NO) free-radical metabolites was demonstrated by Burduli and Gutnova (2009) in 120 human patients with viral hepatitis, while Lim *et al.* (2009) demonstrated that PBMT induces hepatic antioxidant defense in acute and chronic diabetic rats. PBMT has also been shown to recruit mesenchaymal stem cells, induce angiogenesis, improve microcirculation, and stimulate hepatocyte regeneration in injured livers (Burduli *et al.*, 2015; Oron *et al.*, 2010).

In small-animal veterinary medicine, PBMT can be used alongside traditional medical treatment options to enhance the resolution of acute hepatic insults, as well as to improve the clinical outcomes for chronic liver conditions. In the cat and very small dog, red light can be used; however, in most patients, near-infrared light will provide optimal transcutaneous penetration to the liver. One should strive for biostimulatory doses (10–40 J per point) at the target tissue level 1–4 cm below the skin surface, depending on the size of the patient. Applying a similar dose to the inguinal and sublumbar lymph nodes prior to treating the liver is beneficial, as is the application of intravenous laser (if available). Acute cases can be treated every 24–48 hours until resolved, while chronic cases can be titrated down to being treated every other week indefinitely.

Anorectal

PBMT is useful in the treatment of anal sac disease, rectal prolapse, and perianal fistulas. Anal gland abscessation and rupture causes severe subcutaneous inflammation and infection (Culp, 2012). Administration of laser therapy can cause rapid resolution of pain and inflammation when used alongside traditional medical management. PBMT results in stimulation of tissue healing, leading to a faster resolution of this painful condition. Biostimulatory doses of red or infrared light (4–8 J per point) are applied transcutaneously over the inflamed anal gland, as well as to the inguinal and popliteal lymph nodes.

Perianal fistulas are notoriously difficult to treat and manage. They are believed to be an immune-mediated disorder and respond best to a combination of systemic immunosuppressive drugs, topical immunosuppressive drugs, and antibiotics (Craven, 2010; House, 2006; Patricelli *et al.*, 2002; Pieper and McKay, 2011; Stanley and Hauptman, 2009). High doses of immunosuppressive medications are often needed initially, and can cause unwanted side effects. The fistulous lesions will often return when immunosuppressive therapy is withdrawn.

PBMT seems to have mixed results when treating this condition. It does help control the pain and inflammation associated with the disease. In some cases, it can cause a dramatic resolution of the problem. More often, it is another useful tool in the multimodal approach to treatment. It does seem to enable the patient to improve on lower doses of immunosuppressive drugs, thereby reducing or eliminating potentially undesirable side effects. Biostimulatory doses of red or infrared light (2–4 J per point) can be applied directly over the lesion, as well as to the popliteal and inguinal lymph nodes. Lower power settings will help prevent an undesirable inhibitory effect.

Medical management of a rectal prolapse involves cleansing of the exposed mucosal lining, immediate reduction of the swelling in the rectal mucosa, and reduction of the prolapse, followed by a perianal purse string suture that will allow the passage of feces but hold the prolapse in normal anatomical position. After the prolapse has been rinsed clean, PBMT can be applied to the swollen mucosa with 4–10 J per point of red or infrared light. The sublumbar and inguinal lymph nodes should also be treated; this will assist in reducing edema from the prolapse and make it easier to reduce.

Urinary Disorders

The urinary system is quite accessible to light therapy. The kidneys, ureters, urinary bladder, and urethra usually lie 1–3 cm beneath the skin surface. Most acute and chronic conditions of the urinary system can be helped by PBMT.

Kidneys

Both acute and chronic kidney disease (CKD) will benefit from PBMT. It is especially helpful in the treatment of CKD, but can also be of significant aid in the treatment of acute renal perfusion injuries (Oron *et al.*, 2014). The roles of the vascular and tubular components of renal function are tightly intertwined, and the cause of onset of CKD often cannot be identified. Tubulointerstial nephritis is the most common histiopathological diagnosis in cats; however, glomerular damage usually exists as well. The overall process is marked by inflammation and fibrosis of the nephrons.

We know that the kidney's initial autoregulatory response to decreasing glomerular filtration rate (GFR) is to dilate afferent arterioles and constrict efferent arterioles, as well as to contract mesangial cells. The resulting nephron hypertrophy leads to GFR homeostasis. However, over time, the increased hydrostatic pressure within the glomerular corpuscle leads to glomerular capillary damage and plasma protein leakage. These cause further subsequent glomerular and tubulointerstial damage and scarring. Central regulatory mechanisms kick in as autoregulatory mechanisms fail to maintain normal GFR. The renin–angiotensin system (RAS) is activated in the juxtaglomerular complex, with a subsequent increases in antidiuretic hormone and aldosterone, as well as activation of the sympathetic nervous system.

CKD is one of the most common diseases veterinarians encounter in aging animals. Traditional management involves nutritional modifications to lower azotemia and phosphorus, improving hydration, decreasing acid secretion in the stomach, and stimulating appetite and the formation of new red blood cells.

The author has noted that adding PBMT to the traditional treatment protocols for CKD will decrease azotemia by 10–20%, and stimulate both appetite and energy levels. The PBMT protocol for treating CKD involves applying a biostimulatory dose to the kidney and regional lymph nodes (Figure 16.3).

Based upon the work of Uri Oron's lab, one can also apply 1–4 J/cm^2 to the bone marrow of the humerus or femur to stimulate the release of mesenchymal stem cells into circulation. These cells have been shown to migrate to the kidney lesions, increasing mesenchymal stem cell count 2.4-fold. Oron *et al.* (2014) found that this alone will decrease azotemia and pathological features in post-ischemic reperfusion injuries in the rat. Other beneficial mechanisms of PBMT on CKD are thought to be increasing microcirculation within the kidney, decreasing pro-inflammatory cytokines (IL1β, TNFα) (Yamota *et al.*, 2013), decreasing fibrotic factors (fibroblast-specific protein 1, FSP1; alpha smooth-muscle actin, αSMA) (Oliveira *et al.*, 2012), decreasing renal hypertension (Ucero *et al.*, 2013), and decreasing the progression of glomerular injuries (Lutoshkin *et al.*, 1993; Ucero *et al.*, 2013; Yamota *et al.*, 2013). The modulation of nephron inflammation and fibrosis by PBMT allows autoregulatory mechanisms to control GFR longer, delaying the onset of central control mechanisms, and leading to improved clinical conditions and a longer and more vibrant life. It is therefore recommended to begin PBMT as early as possible (International Renal Interest Society (IRIS) stage 1 or 2) with these patients.

The frequency of treatments starts with biweekly applications for 2 weeks, then weekly applications for

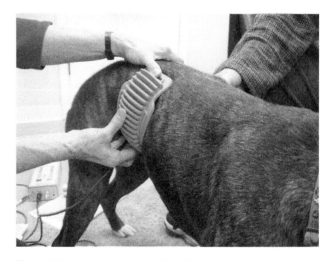

Figure 16.3 A canine patient with CKD being treated over the right kidney with a 1000 mW 840 nm superluminescent diode array.

2 weeks, then finally a continuous regimen of once every 2–3 weeks. The kidneys and sublumbar lymph nodes are treated along with the midfemur, midhumerus, or sternum for mesenchymal stem cell stimulation. Patients that experience an acute prerenal dehydration crisis can have the frequency of PBMT increased to daily while they are hospitalized for intravenous fluid therapy. It is also recommended to administer PBMT during each outpatient subcutaneous fluid (SCF) treatment visit until the crisis has passed.

Urinary Bladder

Feline lower urinary tract disease (FLUTD) is a common and frustrating problem seen daily in most small-animal hospitals. This multifactorial disease involves genetic predisposition, nutritional factors, home stressors, and a chronic pain cycle (Forrester and Roudebush, 2007; Forrester and Towell, 2015). PBMT can be quite useful in helping to downregulate the pain and inflammation associated with FLUTD. The target tissues are the bladder itself and the dorsal root ganglia, for the hypogastraic nerve (L2–4) and the pelvic and pudendal nerves (S1–3). Inflammation in the urinary bladder can be reduced with biostimulatory doses of near-infrared light. For example, 20 J of 810 nm laser light applied over the caudal abdomen will lead to 2–4 J irradiating the bladder. Wind-up of neuropathic pain is thought to play a role in the persistent and recurring nature of FLUTD. PBMT of the sympathetic, parasympathetic, and somatic dorsal root ganglia of the urinary bladder will help downregulate the acute and chronic pain associated with FLUTD.

Transitional cell carcinoma (TCC) of the canine urinary bladder is a commonly encountered cancer in small-animal practice. In the author's experience, PBMT offers an excellent palliative treatment for nonsurgical candidates. PBMT initially shrinks the tumor by 10–20% and then helps manage the hematuria, pollakiuria, and stranguria associated with the disease. Breakthroughs of hematuria commonly respond quickly to antibiotics. PBMT can be used in combination with piroxicam, but the author prefers to use PBMT only to avoid the potential gastrointestinal and renal side effects of piroxicam. Optimal results begin with treatment twice a week for 2 weeks, then once a week for 2 weeks, then every other week indefinitely. Survival times range from 8 to 30 months, with most patients living 12–18 months of good-quality life. The protocol involves applying 30–40 J of near-infrared light to the bladder tumor, from as many angles as possible, and then 10 J to the superficial inguinal lymph node. Interestingly, the author has found that PBMT does not seem to be very effective for leiomyosarcoma of the urinary bladder.

Urethra

Urethral blockage of the male cat by grit and uroliths is a common sequela to untreated FLUTD (Marshall, 2011). Distal blockages of grit can often be unobstructed by application of laser and gentle milking out of the obstruction, thus avoiding the passing of a urethral catheter. After the patient is sedated, the penis can be extruded from the prepuce and 4–10 J of red or near-infrared light can be applied over and around it. This causes a decrease in the periurethral inflammation, making it possible in some cases to unobstruct the cat. After 2–5 minutes, an attempt can be made to milk out the grit. If a good urine stream does not result after 1 minute of manipulation, a urethral catheter should be passed.

Prostate

The anti-inflammatory effects of PBMT are very effective in treating benign prostatic hyperplasia of the canine. Infrared doses of 20–40 J per point aimed at the right and left lobe of the prostate will result in biostimulatory doses to the prostate, reducing inflammation and size. One can also apply 10 J of near infrared light to the superficial inguinal lymph nodes to assist with prostate reduction. This can be quite helpful in managing dysuria until the full benefits of castration are realized. Treat daily for 2–3 days, then twice weekly for 2 months following castration. It is also possible to use a laser catheter to irradiate from the center of the prostate (Figure 16.4). This protocol is beneficial for ancillary treatment of prostatitis. Care should be taken to rule out prostatic neoplasia, though PBMT can be a useful palliative treatment

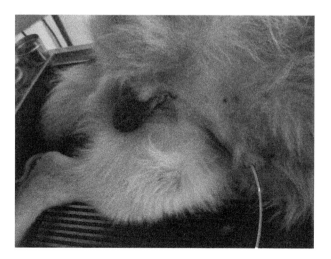

Figure 16.4 Canine prostatitis being treated post-castration with a 660 nm 100 mW laser fiber optic catheter passed proximal through a urethral catheter to the level of the center of the prostate.

for this condition when the owner elects not to pursue surgery, radiation, or chemotherapy.

Infections

PBMT for bacterial infections of the urinary bladder and kidneys can be a useful ancillary treatment to antimicrobial therapy. It aids in stimulating the immune response and reducing associated inflammation and pain. The principal is to apply biostimulatory doses of near-infrared light (2–4 J at the target tissue) to the affected organs and associated lymph nodes. Dose is important, and one should take care not to overdose and create bioinhibition, which can potentially make the infection worse. Treat every other day until resolution. Low-dose intravenous laser (5 mW) has been shown to be a potent stimulator of the immune system and can be used for pyelonepthritis (Driianskaia, 1997; Weber, 2015).

Case Studies

Canine CKD

Signalment

"Savannah," 17 years old, Jack Russell terrier, FS, 5.1 kg.

Client Complaint

The owner had recently moved to town. Savannah's previous veterinarian had diagnosed CKD 8 months previously and had been treating her for neck and shoulder pain.

History

Savannah was on 25 mg of tramadol q8h, laser therapy for neck pain, and SCF for CKD q3d. Lab parameters from the previous veterinarian 1 week prior showed a moderate azotemia.

Physical Examination

Bilateral shoulder tenderness, as well as cervical pain in the C3-4 area, a grade III/VI murmur heart, and grade III/IV periodontal disease.

Diagnosis

CKD, shoulder and neck pain, non-clinical heart murmur, periodontal disease.

Treatment Plan

Tramadol 25 mg was reduced from q8h to PRN, and famotidine 2.5 mg SID and a renal support diet were prescribed. PBMT was initiated with twice a week treatments for 2 weeks, followed by once a week for 2 weeks, and then every 2 weeks. The kidneys were treated with 660, 810, and 840 nm. The shoulder and dorsal root ganglia (C1–T1) were treated with 810 nm (Table 16.1).

Outcome

The shoulder and neck tenderness resolved after 2 months of treatments (eight treatments total) and PBMT was discontinued for those conditions. PBMT for the kidneys continued every other week until Savannah was euthanized 18 months after treatment began. After 5 months, Savannah developed dementia and a brain protocol was added to each PBMT session, which effectively reversed the signs of dementia. Her elevated renal parameters fell gradually after 5 months and remained lower until her death. Savannah developed hypertension with mild syncopal episodes toward the end of her life and the owner requested humane euthanasia.

Canine Pancreatitis

Signalment

"Mickie," 15.5 years old, longhaired Dachshund, MN, 10.7 kg.

Client Complaint

Ate two knee socks; vomiting and bloody diarrhea.

Table 16.1 PBMT protocol for treating a 17-year-old Jack Russell terrier with CKD and shoulder and neck pain.

Target tissue	Wavelength (nm)	Power (mW)	Emission and time	Power density (mW/cm²)	Energy density (J/cm²)	Total fluence (J)
Kidney	660	500	Continuous–wave (CW) 6 minutes	15	5.4	419
	840	1000	50 Hz 50% duty cycle 6 minutes			418
	810	250	CW 20 seconds	2500	50	20/kidney
Shoulder	810	250 (4× multiprobe)	CW 30 seconds	2500	60 × 12 points	180/shoulder
Dorsal root ganglion: C1–T1	810	500 (4× multiprobe)	CW 30 seconds	2500	60 × 24 points	180/side × 2 sides

History

CKD and dementia being managed with PBMT and a renal support diet; elbow luxation and surgical repair in the previous year; intervertebral disk disease 2 years ago.

Physical Examination

T = 38.2 °C (100.8 °F), overweight, dull coat, non-pliable doughy abdomen.

Differential Diagnosis

Dietary indiscretion gastroenteritis, metabolic disease, neoplasia, foreign body, pancreatitis.

Diagnostic Imaging

Abdominal radiographs showed increased radio opaqueness in the right cranial abdomen and gas in the colon. Abdominal ultrasound showed peripancreatic hyperechogenicity, mulifofocal hypoechoic pancreatic lesions, a distended gall bladder, and patches of hyperechogenicity in the liver.

Laboratory Data

A complete blood count (CBC) showed mild neutrophilia and mild lymphopenia. Amylase and lipase were very high and were accompanied by an azotemia and mild hyperkalemia.

Diagnosis

The primary problem appeared to be pancreatitis secondary to dietary indiscretion, with a secondary azotemia from prerenal exacerbation of the patient's chronic renal disease.

Treatment Plan

An intravenous catheter was placed and intravenous fluids were administered to correct the dehydration. Ampicillin (200 mg q12h) and famotidine (10 mg q24h) were administered intravenously. PBMT was administered once a day: 810 nm, 500 mW × 4 multiprobe, continuous wave (CW), 60 seconds per point × five points over the pancreas; per point: 30 J, 2.5 W/cm^2, 35 mm spot size, 150 J/cm^2; total fluence: 600 J (30 J × 4 multiprobe × 5 points) (Table 16.2).

Outcome

Mickie improved daily, had no vomiting or diarrhea in the hospital, ate the morning of day 3 and tolerated the intake, and was discharged on metronidazole, sucralfate, and a low-fat gastrointestinal diet. PBMT was repeated on days 2 and 4 following discharge, with no further symptoms of gastroenteritis. Maintenance PBMT for CKD and dementia was resumed.

Canine Transitional Cell Carcinoma of the Urinary Bladder and CKD

Signalment

"Rudy," 13 years old, bichon frise, MN, 14.5 kg.

History

Rudy presented at 11.5 years old with hematuria and was subsequently diagnosed with a bladder tumor. Histopathology after initial excision indicated the tumor was a transitional cell carcinoma with clean margins, and no further treatment was prescribed. The bladder was normal on ultrasound 2 months later, but 7 months after that the tumor reappeared. Thirteen pedunculated, friable masses were removed from the bladder. Piroxicam and misoprostol were prescribed. Symptoms returned 8 months later, and an ultrasound demonstrated diffuse infiltration of the tumor into the bladder wall. A week later, Rudy developed acute renal failure.

Treatment Plan

Medication was discontinued and Rudy was admitted for emergency intravenous fluid diuresis and PBMT. Nine PBMT treatments were administered over the kidneys and bladder every 4–6 days for 6.5 weeks. Doses averaged 5.85 J/cm^2 with 660 nm, 11.7 J/cm^2 with 840 nm, and 81 J/cm^2 with 830 nm. Rudy improved significantly after the first PBMT treatment, and after nine treatments the bladder wall was less thick and Rudy was eating well. After 6 months, PBMT was restarted at once every 5 weeks at average doses of 7 J/cm^2 with 660 nm, 18.7 J/cm^2 with 840 nm, and 64.8 J/cm^2 with 830 nm. Thirteen treatments were administered over the next 9 months, after which time Rudy rapidly deteriorated and was euthanized.

Outcome

The clinical results of using laser therapy on Rudy suggest that it may be as effective as piroxicam in palliative treatment of transitional cell carcinoma of the canine urinary bladder, without any harmful side effects

Table 16.2 PBMT protocol for treating a 15.5-year-old longhaired Dachshund with acute pancreatitis.

Target tissue	Wavelength (nm)	Power (mW)	Emission and time	Power density (mW/cm^2)	Energy density (J/cm^2)	Total fluence (J)
Pancreas	810	500 (4× multiprobe)	CW 60 seconds	2.5 × 5 points	150 × 5 points	600

(a)

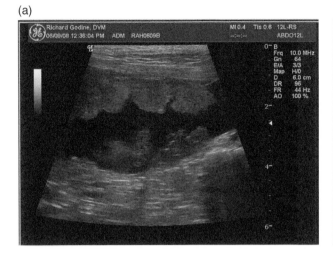

(b)

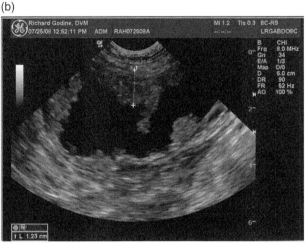

(c)

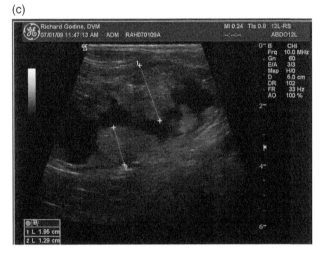

Figure 16.5 Ultrasound images showing the progression of transitional cell carcinoma of a canine urinary bladder being treated with PBMT. (a) 8 months after starting piroxicam and misoprostol therapy (ultrasound shows significant regrowth of the transitional carcinoma). (b) 8 weeks after discontinuing medication and starting PBMT. (c) 54 weeks after starting PBMT.

(Figure 16.5). In this case, piroxicam following debulking surgery resulted in 8 months (240 days) of good-quality life for Rudy, but ultimately caused acute renal failure while the mass continued to grow. Subsequent PBMT alone resulted in 15 months (465 days) of good-quality life after piroxicam was discontinued, and seemed to be beneficial in the treatment of both acute and chronic renal failure.

It is hypothesized that PBMT has a beneficial biostimulatory effect on the immune system, which results in delay of tumor growth, decreased inflammation of the tumor and surrounding tissue, decreased pain, modulation of paraneoplastic syndromes, and possibly delay of metastasis. This is due in part to a systemic immune-modulating effect, as well as the direct effect of the laser on the bladder tumor.

Conclusion

The ability of PBMT to decrease inflammation and stimulate tissue regeneration makes it a useful component in the treatment of a number of gastrointestinal and urinary tract diseases of small animals. It is particularly effective in the treatment of pancreatitis and liver diseases. One must be able to manipulate the parameters of the laser or light-emitting diode (LED) unit such that the desired power density at the level of the target tissue will be achieved. Treatment of the associated lymph nodes with biostimulatory doses will also enhance efficacy. By virtue of the accessibility of light to the internal organs of small animals, veterinarians can lead the medical community in the clinical applications of PBMT for gastrointestinal and urinary tract disorders.

References

Ahmed, K. *et al.* (2015) Evaluation of low level laser therapy in the management of chemotherapy induced oral mucositis in pediatric and young cancer patients: a randomized clinical trial. *Eur Sci Journ.* **11**(27):209–222.

Alebastrov, A.P. and Butov, MA. (2005) Potentialities of alternative non-drug therapy of gastric ulcer. *Klin Med (Mosk).* **83**(11):69–71.

Alebastrov, A.P. *et al.* (2004) Clinical and immunological aspects of low-intensity laser irradiation in patients with gastroduodenal ulcers. *Esksp Klin Gastroentero.* **4**:33–35.

Babaev, A.V. *et al.* (2012) Effect of intravenous low-intensity laser irradiation of the blood on clinical and laboratory parameters of hepatocellular insufficiency. *Bull Exp Biol Med.* **153**(5):754–757.

Basso, F.G. *et al.* (2015) Biomodulation of inflammatory cytokines related to oral mucositis by low-level laser therapy. *Photochem Photobio.* **91**(4):952–956.

Burduli, N.M. and Gutnova, S.K. (2008) Efficacy of different laser treatments in combined therapy of patients with gastroduodenal ulcer. *Ter Arkh.* **80**(2):30–33.

Burduli, NM. and Gutnova, S.K. (2009) Types of microcirculation and laser therapy and chronic pancreatitis. *Klin Med (Mosk).* **87**(8):56–61.

Burduli, N.M. and Krifaridi, A.S. (2011) The influence of low-intensity laser radiation on the vascular endothelium function in the cytokine system in patients with chronic viral hepatitis. *Vopr Kurortol Fizioter Lech Fiz Kult.* **92**(4):25–29.

Burduli, N.M. and Tadtaeva D.Y. (2012a) The influence of intravenous laser therapy on PGE2 and F2-α dynamics and the state of microcirculation in the patients presenting with gastroesophageal reflux disease. *Vopr Kurortol Fizioter Lech Fiz Kult.* **6**:17–20.

Burduli, N.M. and Tadteva D.Y. (2012b) Impact of laser therapy on PGE2 level, 24-hour pH-metry changes, and quality of life in patients with gastroesophageal reflux disease. *Ter Arkh.* **84**(12):58–61.

Burduli, N.M. and Tastaeva D.Y. (2014) The effect of low-level laser therapy on gastric mucosa microcirculation in patients with gastroesophageal reflux diseases. *Eksp Klin Gastroenterol.* **9**:35–38.

Burduli, NM *et al.* (2015) The influence of the low-frequency laser radiation on microcirculatory disorders in the patients presenting with chronic viral hepatitis. *Vopr Kurotol Fizioter Lech Fiz Kult.* **92**(4):25–29.

Craven, M. (2012) Rectoanal disease: perianal fistula. In: *Textbook of Veterinary Internal Medicine*, 7 edn., pp. 1602–1604. Saunders, St. Louis, MO.

Crawford, J. and Losey, B.J. (2013) Feline dentistry. In: *Small Animal Dental Procedures for Veterinary Technicians and Nurses*, pp. 143–160. Wiley-Blackwell, Holboken, NJ.

Culp, W.T.N. (2012) Anal sac disease. In: *Small Animal Soft Tissue Surgery*, pp. 399–405. John Wiley & Sons, Chichester.

Driianskaia, V. (1997) The clinico-immunological effects of immunotherapy in patients with acute pyelonephritis. *Lik-Sprava.* **4**:89–92.

Forrester, S.D. and Roudebush, P. (2007) Evidence-based management of feline lower urinary tract disease. *Vet Clin North Am Small Anim Pract.* **37**(3):533–558.

Forrester, S.D. and Towell, T.L. (2015) Feline idiopathic cystitis. *Vet Clin North Am Small Anim Pract.* **45**(4):783–806.

Geïnits, AV. *et al.* (2011) The use of laser beam irradiation on acute destructive pancreatitis. *Khirurgiia (Mosk).* **7**:56–61.

Gogeliia, A.L. *et al.* (2006) Experience on treatment of children with otorhinolaryngological diseases by low-intensity laser irradiation. *Georgian Med News.* **130**:84–86.

Gutnova, S.K. (2011) The evaluation of exocrinous function of pancreas in patients with chronic pancreatitis. *Klin Lab Diagn.* **12**:44–45.

House, A.K. (2006) Evaluation of the effect of two dose rates of cyclosporine on the severity of perianal fistulae lesions and associated clinical signs in dogs. *Vet Surg.* **35**(6):543–549.

Jennings, M.W. *et al.* (2015) Effect of tooth extraction on stomatitis in cats: 95 cases (2000–2013). *J Am Vet Med Assoc.* **246**(6):654–660.

Lewis, J.R. *et al.* (2007) Use of CO2 laser as an adjunctive treatment for caudal stomatitis in a cat. *J Vet Dent.* **24**(4):240–249.

Lim, J. *et al.* (2009) Effects of low-level light therapy on hepatic antioxidant defense in acute and chronic diabetic rats. *J Biochem Mol Toxicol.* **23**(1):1–8.

Lutoshkin, M. *et al.* (1993) Application of helium-neon laser for the correction of renal function in patients with chronic glomerulonephritis. *Uro Nefrol (Mosk).* **2**:17–20.

Marshall, R. (2011) Urethral obstruction. In: *The Feline Patient*, 4 edn., pp. 530–534. Wiley-Blackwell, Hoboken, NJ.

Muñoz-Corcuera, M. *et al.* (2013) Use of laser for the prevention and treatment of oral mucositis induced by radiotherapy and chemotherapy for head and neck cancer. *Med Clin (Barc).* **143**(4):170–175.

Oliveira, F.A. *et al.* (2012) Low-level laser therapy decreases renal interstitial fibrosis. *Photomed Laser Surg.* **30**(12):705–713.

Oliveira-Junior, M.C. *et al.* (2013) Low-level laser therapy ameliorates CC14-induced liver cirrhosis in rats. *Photochem Photobiol.* **89**(1):173–178.

Oron, U. et al. (2010) Enhanced liver regeneration following acute hepatectomy by low-level laser therapy. *Photomed Laser Surg.* **28**(5)675–678.

Oron U. *et al.* (2014) Autologous bone marrow stem cells stimulation reverses post-ischemic reperfusion kidney injury in rats. *Am J Nephrol.* **40**(5):425–433.

Patricelli, A.J. *et al.* (2002) Cyclosporine and ketoconazole for the treatment of perianal fistulas in dogs. *J A-M Vet Med Assoc.* **220**(7):1009–1016.

Pieper, J. and McKay, L. (2011) Perianal fistulas. *Compend Contin Educ Vet.* **33**(9):E4.

Robson, M. and Crystal, M.A. (2011) Gingivitis-stomatitis-pharyngitis. In: *The Feline Patient*, pp. 199–201. Wiley-Blackwell, Hoboken, NJ.

Shao, XH, *et al.* (2005) Effects of He-Ne laser irradiation on chronic atrophic gastritis in rats. *World J Gastroenterol.* **11**(25):3958–3961.

Simões, A. *et al.* (2009) Laser as a therapy for dry mouth symptoms in a patient with Sjögren's syndrome: a case report. *Spec Care Dentist.* **29**(3):134–137.

Stanley, B.J. and Hauptman, J.G. (2009) Long-term prospective evaluation of topically applied 0.1% tacrolimus ointment for treatment of perianal sinuses in dogs. *J Am Vet Med Assoc.* **235**(4):397–404.

Steiner, J.M. (2010) Canine pancreatic disease. In: *Textbook of Veterinary Internal Medicine: Diseases of the Dog and the Cat*, pp. 1695–1703. Elsevier, St. Louis, MO.

Ucero A.C. *et al.* (2013) Laser therapy in metabolic syndrome-related kidney injury. *Photochem Photobiol.* **89**(4):953–960.

Weber, M. *et al.* (2015) Medical low-level laser therapy-foundations and clinical applications. *Int Soc Med Laser App.* **2**:283–297.

Yamota, M. *et al.* (2013) Low-level laser therapy improves crescentic glomerulonephritis in rats. *Laser Med Sci.* **28**(4):1189–1196.

Yang, Y. *et al.* (2005) Effects of He-Ne laser on gastric mucosa in rat with chronic atrophic gastritis. *World J Gastroenterol.* **22**(5):926–929.

Zigmond, E. *et al.* (2014) Low-level light therapy induces mucosal healing in a murine model of dextran-sodium-sulfate induced colitis. *Photomed Laser Surg.* **32**(8):450–457.

17

Neurological Conditions

Richard L. Godine

North American Association for Light Therapy, Ruckersville Animal Hospital and Veterinary Laser Therapy Center, Ruckersville, VA, USA

Introduction

The central nervous system (CNS) and the nerves of the peripheral nervous system are very accessible to light therapy, usually lying less than 2 cm below the skin surface. A bioinhibitory power density of approximately $300\,mW/cm^2$ at the target tissue level will produce analgesia. Biostimulatory power densities of approximately $10\,mW/cm^2$ at the target tissue level will decrease inflammation and stimulate tissue regeneration. Thus, the use of photobiomodulation therapy (PBMT) can result in either analgesia or the repair and regeneration of damaged nervous tissue. This makes PBMT of extreme clinical importance in the treatment of a number of small-animal neurological diseases.

Pain

Pain is often the greatest concern owners have when their pets are injured or sick. Chronic pain, in particular, is a very common state for geriatric canine and feline patients. Geriatric patients often have comorbidities, which make the use of pharmaceuticals dangerous and the risk of anesthesia of great concern.

Pain produces complex chemical and neurologic changes, and untreated pain can lead to severe pathophysiologic changes that involve multiple organ systems (Silverstein, 2006). PBMT offers an effective and safe alternative to both pharmaceutical use and surgery.

Nociceptors transmit painful impulses via afferent nerves to the dorsal root ganglia (DRG), and then via ascending pathways to the thalamus. An in-depth discussion that follows the pain pathway and details the basic physiology of pain is presented in Chapter 8.

For over 4 decades, PBMT has been shown to reduce inflammation, induce analgesia, and promote healing in a range of pathologies. The use of PBMT to treat pain and the complex mechanisms involved in the body's response to PBMT have been well detailed (Cotler *et al.*, 2015).

Bioinhibitory doses of PBMT can be applied to several points along the pain pathway to block the sensation of pain. High-power density laser energy ($300\,mW/cm^2$) delivered to axons has been shown to disrupt microtubular arrays and slow fast axonal flow in Aδ fibers and C fibers (Chow *et al.*, 2012). This means that local analgesia can be achieved for 24–48 hours by applying high doses of PBMT over the area of pain perception and the associated nerve tracks. The same method can be used to block the transmission of pain by treating the associated DRG and spinal cord segment (Chow and Armati, 2007). Research is being done to see whether bioinhibitory doses applied only to the brain can downregulate chronic pain and provide analgesia for pain elsewhere in the body. It is important to note that after analgesia has been achieved for a painful condition, doses should be cut back to the biostimulatory range in order to decrease inflammation and stimulate healing.

The treatment of chronic pain should focus on decreasing inflammation and stimulating tissue health and regeneration. In addition to accomplishing those goals, PBMT has been shown to increase the release of endogenous endorphins (Labajos, 1988; Hagiwara *et al.*, 2008). Evidence has been published which shows that the increased release of beta-endorphins induced by PBMT results in a decreased need for exogenous pharmaceutical analgesics (Cramond *et al.*, 1994; Sprouse-Blum *et al.*, 2010). In addition, PBMT has been shown to modulate systemic blood levels of serotonin in humans (Magalhaes *et al.*, 2016). The effects that PBMT has on endorphins and serotonin levels explain the immediate response of contentment and relaxation seen in veterinary patients following treatment.

Laser Therapy in Veterinary Medicine: Photobiomodulation, First Edition. Edited by Ronald J. Riegel and John C. Godbold, Jr.

Intervertebral Disk Disease

Intervertebral disk disease (IVDD) is a very common condition seen by small-animal practitioners. Hansen Type 1 IVDD occurs in young to middle-age chondrodystrophic dogs and often presents as an acute-onset episode with neurological deficits. Hansen Type 2 IVDD is usually seen in older dogs of any breed, and often has a chronic, insidious progression (Hansen, 1951). Both types of IVDD can cause compression of the spinal cord and nerve roots, as well as release of superoxide radicals and pro-inflammatory cytokines.

Once the lesion has been localized and the severity has been appropriately assessed, a therapeutic plan can be instituted (LeCouteur and Grandy, 2000). Severe grade 5 lesions with paralysis and no deep pain perception are considered surgical emergencies. Less severe grade 2–4 lesions may also benefit from surgical decompression procedures, but medical treatment is often started first in these cases. Diagnosis is aided by survey radiographs; however, a definitive diagnosis requires a myelogram, a computed tomography (CT) scan, or magnetic resonance imaging (MRI). Traditional medical management of IVDD consists of 1–2 months of strict rest, analgesics, anti-inflammatories, and physical therapy (Brisson, 2010).

Traumatic and biochemical injury to axons of the spinal cord can lead to demyelination, axonal degeneration, neuronal death, cavitation, and glial scarring. PBMT has been shown to be effective in reducing pro-inflammatory cytokines and reactive oxygen species (ROS) that infiltrate the spinal cord following injury (Byrnes *et al.*, 2005). PBMT modulates inflammatory mediators secreted by human annulus fibrosus cells during intervertebral disk degeneration *in vitro* (Hwang *et al.*, 2015). Furthermore, laser light has been shown to stimulate neuronal sprouting and regrowth of severed axons (Rochkind, 2009).

A study done at the University of Florida College of Veterinary Medicine showed that dogs treated with PBMT prior to and immediately after hemilaminectomy surgery required a significantly reduced time to return to ambulation compared to those not receiving PBMT (Draper *et al.*, 2012).

Byrnes *et al.* (2005) showed that PBMT using an 810 nm laser promotes regeneration and functional recovery of rats following a T9 hemisection. Wu *et al.* (2009) demonstrated that 810 nm diode laser light applied non-invasively promoted axonal regeneration and functional recovery in the rat following experimental spinal cord injury. Moges *et al.* (2011) demonstrated a positive effect on nerve regeneration following autograft of severely injured rat median nerves using 810 nm laser light. In a randomized, double-blind, placebo-controlled study of the treatment of long-term incomplete peripheral nerve injury with 780 nm laser light, the laser-irradiated group showed statistically significant improvement in recruitment of voluntary muscle activity compared to the placebo group (Rochkind *et al.*, 2007).

Only a small percentage of the dose applied to the skin penetrates to the spinal cord 2–3 cm beneath the handpiece. In the Byrnes *et al.* (2005) study, only 6% of the 810 nm laser energy applied to the skin reached to spinal cord depth in rats. In a study by Anders *et al.* (2014), only 2.45% of the 980 nm light applied to the skin reached the depth of the peroneal nerve in anesthetized rabbits. Optimal power densities at the target tissue are thought to be relatively low at $10 \, mW/cm^2$ (Anders *et al.*, 2014). The therapeutic window is likely wider, and much research must be done before definitive optimal parameters can be recommended.

Once the IVDD lesion has been localized and the severity has been assessed, PBMT can begin being used immediately. An initial intravenous injection of a short-acting glucocorticoid should be considered alongside the first PBMT treatment. Further complementary pharmaceutical medications could include an opioid analgesic and a muscle relaxer.

The PBMT device should be directed between the dorsal spinous processes of the lesion, with additional points two intervertebral disk spaces cranially and three intervertebral disk spaces caudally (Figure 17.1). When treating cervical lesions, PBMT should be directed from the dorsolateral side toward the intervertebral foramen on both sides, as there is considerably more muscle mass between the skin surface and the spinal cord when approaching from the dorsal spinous process in the neck.

It is important to estimate the distance from the skin surface to the spinal cord. This will enable the therapist to calculate the appropriate time and other adjustable parameters in order to achieve a power density and fluence (dose) that is within the therapeutic window at the level of the target tissue. For instance, 20 J of continuous 810 nm light will provide around 0.5–1.0 J to the spinal cord of a medium-sized dog. This will be biostimulatory to the lesion. The power density at the lesion will depend on the power density of the laser and will likely be around 1–2% of the power density applied to the surface.

In acutely painful patients, the laser therapist might want to triple the time (and thus triple the dose) in order to bioinhibit pain and provide analgesia. However, once pain has been moderated, biostimulatory doses should be used as soon as possible. The patient should be treated daily until clinical progress is noted, then every 2–3 days until it is ambulating and eliminating satisfactorily, and then weekly until fully recovered.

When treating IVDD, it is also helpful to treat myofascial trigger points, regional lymph nodes, and the paraspinal muscles. Myofascial trigger points are localized by palpation and treated with bioinhibitory doses (8–15 J

(a)

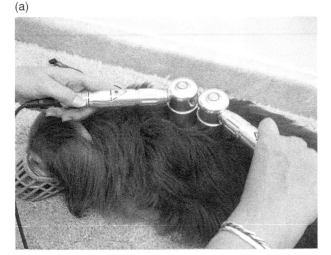

(b)

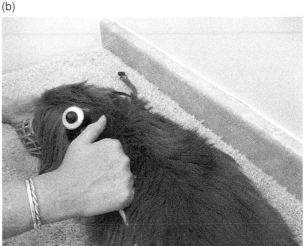

Figure 17.1 (a) Dachshund with thoracolumbar IVDD being treated over the dorsal spinous processes with dual 250 mW, 810 nm handpieces. (b) Treatment of the paraspinal muscles of the same patient with a 1390 mW, 660 and 850 nm cluster-probe handpiece.

per superficial point). The regional lymph nodes and paraspinal muscles should be treated with biostimulatory doses (6–10 J per superficial point). This will improve the patient's comfort and help control associated inflammation.

The use of PBMT in the treatment of IVDD can significantly shorten the time to functional recovery and avoid the need for surgical intervention. With careful monitoring and proper patient selection, PBMT can become a mainstay of medical management for IVDD patients.

Additional information about the treatment of IVDD is presented in Chapter 13.

Peripheral Nerve Injuries

Peripheral nerve injuries in the dog and cat are usually the result of a traumatic encounter. Brachial plexus avulsions are commonly seen in the dog, resulting in neurotmesis, axonotmesis, and neuropraxia (Inzana, 2000). Other peripheral nerve injuries can occur from fight wounds, ballistic injuries, and vehicular accidents (Mariani, 2010; Welch, 1996). Severe injuries are often permanent without proper surgical intervention, while neuropraxia will often resolve over 8 weeks (Rodkey and Sharp, 2003). The use of PBMT offers the clinician a way to increase the rate of peripheral nerve regeneration and motor neuron survival (Anders *et al.*, 2014; Rochkind *et al.*, 2007; Snyder 2002).

The optimal parameters of PBMT are the same as described for spinal cord injuries. Multiple studies indicate that 810 nm light elicits a positive response (Byrnes *et al.*, 2005; Moges *et al.*, 2011; Wu *et al.*, 2009). Using 980 nm, a power density of 10 mW/cm^2 at the level of the

injured nerve appears to be a good target dose to try to achieve (Anders *et al.*, 2014). As with spinal cord injuries, the therapeutic window is certainly slightly wider than this research-based target. Further research will help define the specific wavelengths and parameters that work best.

Ideally, the injury should be treated immediately after it occurs, as this will decrease the noxious cellular and biochemical environment, limit the extent of the damage, and increase the chances of success, while decreasing the time to healing. Treatment should be administered daily for 3 days and then every 2–3 days until resolution. Recovery of peripheral nerve injuries is a long, slow process, in which axonal growth rates may reach 1 mm/day in small nerves and 5 mm/day in large nerves (Recknor and Mallapragada, 2006). Thus, treatment with PBMT should continue for at least 8 weeks or until acceptable function has returned.

Transcranial PBMT

Transcranial PBMT is an effective way to treat a number of intracranial diseases in the dog and cat. Traumatic brain injuries, obsessive–compulsive disorders (OCDs), cognitive dysfunction, and palliation of intracranial neoplasia are all conditions that respond well to transcranial PBMT. The brain is rich in mitochondria and lies very close to the skin surface, making it an ideal recipient of the beneficial effects of light therapy. Studies have verified that effective transcranial penetration with near-infrared laser light is possible. Lapchak *et al.* (2015) demonstrated transcranial near-infrared laser transmission of 800 nm laser light in four mammalian species. The study showed an inverse relationship between the percentage of photonic transmission through the bone and the thickness of the bone. In another study, measurement of transcranial transmission into human cadaver brains confirmed the penetration of measurable 808 nm-wavelength light through the scalp, skull, and meninges to a brain depth of 40–50 mm (Tedford *et al.*, 2015).

Cognitive Dysfunction Syndrome

Cognitive dysfunction syndrome (CDS) encompasses canine cognitive dysfunction and feline cognitive dysfunction. It is becoming more common in small-animal practice as veterinarians lengthen pets' lives through better nutrition and wellness care. Confusion, disorientation, excessive panting, nocturnal pacing, agitation, circling, separation anxiety, phobias, irritability, and vocalization often characterize canine CDS. In the cat, one might see litterbox issues, wandering, increased vocalization, and nocturnal activity. The onset is gradual and the progression is insidious (Landsberg *et al.*, 2012; Ozawa *et al.*, 2016). Patients are presented to the veterinarian as the owner becomes increasingly concerned and annoyed by the behavior. Before making a diagnosis of CDS, one must rule out metabolic, infectious, arthritic, immune-mediated, and neoplastic causes for the noted behavioral changes.

A variety of supplements and pharmacological agents have been used to treat CDS (Landsberg *et al.*, 2011). These include diets fortified with antioxidants, mitochondrial cofactors, and essential fatty acids (Manteca, 2011). Enriching the environment through regular exercise and new toys is helpful in dogs but not so much in cats. Drugs such as L-deprenyl, S-Adenosyl methionine, and others are often prescribed and have inconsistent benefits. Rapid improvement of canine cognitive dysfunction with immunotherapy designed for Alzheimer's disease has been reported (Bosch *et al.*, 2013). While all these methods may be helpful, the author has observed that the use of transcranial PBMT seems to be very effective in improving the symptoms of CDS quickly.

CDS is a neurodegenerative process characterized by oxidative stress and mitochondrial dysfunction, leading to depletion of neurotransmitters and disruption of neuronal pathways. Like Alzheimer's disease in humans, it is known that beta-amyloid deposition and tauopathies occur in the canine and feline brains with CDS, leading to depletion of dopamine and altered cholinergic transmission (Gonzalez-Martinez *et al.*, 2011; Insua *et al.*, 2010). CDS no doubt can have other altered intracranial neurotransmitters and etiologies as part of its pathogenesis.

What is interesting from a PBMT standpoint is that mitochondrial dysfunction and oxidative stress are at the core of this disease process, and this happens to be where PBMT shines as a treatment modality. In two transgenic mouse models, PBMT was demonstrated to have potential as an effective, minimally invasive intervention for mitigating, and even reversing, progressive cerebral degenerations (Purushothuman *et al.*, 2014). The efficacy of PBMT in treating CDS is thought to be associated with its ability to reduce intracellular ROS, activate transcription factors, increase mitochondrial adenosine triphosphate (ATP) production, and decrease apoptosis (Gonzalez-Lima *et al.*, 2014; Liang *et al.*, 2012). In addition, PBMT decreases inflammation and increases microcirculation.

When treating CDS with PBMT, both red light in the 665 nm range and near-infrared light in the 810 nm range have been shown to be effective (Quihe *et al.*, 2012). Unless one is treating a very small animal, the 810 nm range will be more effective, because of an increased penetration potential. It has been shown that a pulsing delivery at 10 Hz has better efficacy when treating traumatic brain injuries than continuous delivery or 100 Hz. (Ando *et al.*, 2010). Pulsing will also decrease the possibility of any thermal effect within the tissues. An effective energy dose is thought to be in the range of 0.3–3.0 J/cm^2 at the level of the cortex (Naeser *et al.*, 2011).

The light source is placed on the dorsal surface of the skull, treating both the right and left hemispheres (Figures 17.2 and 17.3). If using a diode laser, treatments will include eight points per hemisphere in the dog and four in the cat. A fluence of between 10 and 20 J per point is a good starting point. It is recommended to treat the patient twice a week for 2 weeks, then once a week for 2 weeks, then every 2–3 weeks as needed for maintenance. The treatments are painless, quick, and well tolerated. The patient may seem a little tired for the first 24 hours, but resolution of clinical signs usually begins within the first one or two treatments and gets progressively better in the first month. Bimonthly maintenance treatments offer the optimal chance for continued efficacy.

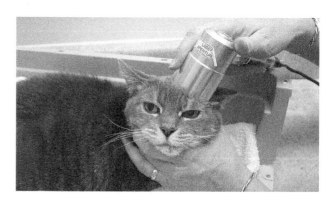

Figure 17.2 Feline patient with CDS receiving transcranial PBMT with a 500 mW, 810 nm multiprobe handpiece.

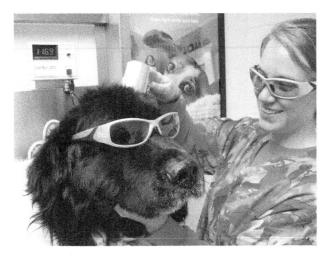

Figure 17.3 Bernese mountain dog with CDS receiving transcranial PBMT with a 500 mW, 810 nm multiprobe handpiece.

Traumatic Brain Injuries

In the case of traumatic brain injuries, it has been shown that early intervention not only assists in early resolution of clinical signs, but also can be neuroprotective against lingering symptoms (Oron *et al.*, 2012).

Animal-model studies using rats have demonstrated that transcranial near-infrared laser application may provide benefit in cases of acute traumatic brain injuries (Xuan *et al.*, 2013). The same parameters as used for treating CDS can be used to treat traumatic brain injury. The frequency of treatment should be every 12–24 hours as needed for a quick resolution of clinical signs. PBMT can decrease intracranial inflammation, decrease oxidative stress, and help stabilize damaged membranes. One must monitor for intracranial hemorrhage, since PBMT may cause a transient increase in blood flow.

Intracranial Neoplasia

In general, special considerations must be made before treating neoplasms with PBMT. As discussed in Chapter 7, PBMT can often offer significant palliative value for patients with malignancies that are beyond help of traditional treatments, or whose owners are unable or unwilling to absorb the financial cost or associated morbidity of chemotherapy, surgery, or radiation. PBMT can be an important part of hospice care of these patients. In the author's personal experience, PBMT of intracranial tumors can often provide significant temporary relief of symptoms and make the last weeks to months of these patients' lives more enjoyable and symptom-free (see Case Studies: Metastatic Neoplasia of the Brain). The same parameters as used for treating CDS can be used for palliative treatment of neoplasia of the brain.

Behavioral Disorders

PBMT can also be an alternative treatment for certain behavioral disorders and OCDs. Behavioral disorders such as aggression and urine marking are often treated with tricyclic antidepressant drugs (TCAs) or selective serotonin reuptake inhibitors (SSRIs). Likewise, compulsive behaviors, anxiety-based house soiling, and phobias are treated with TCAs and SSRIs. PBMT has been demonstrated to raise serotonin and endorphin levels (Hagiwara *et al.*, 2008; Magalhaes *et al.*, 2016). In the author's experience, transcranial PBMT, in combination with counterconditioning methods and environmental conditioning, has been successful in treating certain behavioral disorders and OCDs without the use of psychotropic drugs. The same parameters and treatment frequencies as used for treating CDS can be used to treat behavioral disorders.

Degenerative Myelopathy

Degenerative myelopathy (DM), first described in 1973, is a non-inflammatory axonal degeneration of the T3 to L3 spinal cord segments that slowly develops into pelvic limb proprioceptive ataxia, upper motor neuron paraparesis, and denervation atrophy (Averil, 1973). In advanced stages, dogs may have degenerative changes noted in the lumbar dorsal roots (Griffiths and Duncan, 1975). The disease has similarities to Lou Gehrig's disease (amyotrophic lateral sclerosis, ALS) in humans. The prognosis is poor even with empirical treatments such as the antiprotease agent aminocaproic acid, parental cobalamin, or oral tocopherol. Rigorous physiotherapy plays an important role in improving ambulation and lengthening survival times (Kathmann *et al.*, 2006).

In the author's personal experience, PBMT has not appeared to have any beneficial effects on DM. However, recent clinical experience using high doses of PBMT in conjunction with multimodal physical therapy has yielded promising results. A detailed discussion of the preliminary results of this approach to managing DM can be found in Chapter 25.

Case Studies

Canine CDS

Signalment
"Molly," 8 years old, Jack Russell terrier mix, FS.

Client Complaint
Lethargic and ataxic.

History
Molly had a history of a persistent, mild liver enzyme elevation for 2 years, with the primary rule-out being microvascular dysplasia, and intermittent diarrhea.

Current Medications
Lactulose.

Physical Examination
On physical examination, Molly showed dull mentation, a visual but blank stare, and a mild ataxia and weakness.

Differential Diagnosis
Brain disease, hepatic encephalopathy, neoplasia.

Diagnostic Imaging
Thoracic radiographs were within normal limits 4 months prior to presentation. At that time, an abdominal ultrasound showed microhepatica and hyperechoic renal medullary bands.

Laboratory Data
Laboratory work showed mild neutrophilia and monocytosis, moderate liver enzyme elevation, mild hypercalcemia, and a low T4.

Diagnosis
Canine CDS.

Treatment Plan
Molly was started on amoxicillin and a liver function support medication containing S-Adenosylmethionine and silybin. Transcranial PBMT, with an 810 nm laser at 24 J per point (eight points per hemisphere), was administered twice a week for 2 weeks, then once a week for 2 weeks, and then continued every 3 weeks. After 1 year, the protocol was changed to 20 J per point pulsed at a frequency of 10 Hz.

Outcome
Molly had a dramatic positive response to the first PBMT treatment. After the second treatment, she was clinically normal. Treatment continued sporadically over the next 3.5 years, with Molly relapsing into nocturnal pacing, circling, and blindness when the PBMT treatment interval extended beyond 1 month. She did well with PBMT treatments every 3 weeks. At times, dexamethasone injections were given at initial relapse exams. The reduced parameters begun after 1 year of treatment seemed to have no drop-off in efficacy.

Molly was euthanized after 3.5 years when she became refractory to PBMT and immunosuppressive drugs. Her brain was submitted for histopathology. Results were most consistent with a neurodegenerative disease that was not inflammatory or neoplastic.

Feline CDS

Signalment
"Maggie," 12 years old, domestic shorthair, FS, 5 kg.

Client Complaint
Nocturnal vocalization and pacing, standing by the water bowl and staring, ataxia, and weight loss.

History
Psychogenic alopecia, pancreatitis, and mild azotemia.

Physical Examination
Slightly overweight, naked belly, Grade I/VI cardiac murmur, Grade II/IV periodontal disease.

Laboratory Data
Slight increase in amylase and free T4, normal complete blood count (CBC), normal urine S.G.

Diagnosis
CDS and psychogenic alopecia. The mild elevation in free T4 was thought to be secondary to non-thyroidal illness.

Treatment Plan
PBMT to the brain was prescribed twice a week for 2 weeks, once a week for 2 week, then once every 2 weeks indefinitely. Transcranial treatment was administered at 810 nm at 16 J per point over each hemisphere of the dorsal skull.

Outcome
Maggie had a significant immediate improvement after the first treatment. She was more affectionate, only cried once during the night, and was back to her normal routine the next day. She was back to completely normal behavior after the third treatment. Treatments extended a week at a time, with long-term maintenance treatments being necessary once every 6 weeks. Maggie has been symptom-free for 4 years at the time of writing, and the owner has observed that if she does not get a PBMT treatment once every 6 weeks, the symptoms return.

Canine IVDD

Signalment
"Sassy," 8 years old, mixed breed, FS, 20.7 kg.

Client Complaint
Unable to rise in rear quarters since the day before.

History
Supraspinatus tendonitis and coxofemoral degenerative joint disease that responded well to PBMT 1 year before. Pain at T10–11 with radiographic narrowing of the disk

space that responded to rest and non-steroidal anti-inflammatories 3.5 years before.

Physical Examination

Sassy had paresis in both hind legs and was unable to ambulate. She had conscious proprioception deficits and a positive crossed extensor reflex, and her rear leg reflexes were hyper-reflexive. A complicating factor was obesity.

Diagnostic Imaging

Radiographs showed a new compressed disk space at L1–2.

Diagnosis

IVDD at L1–2.

Treatment Plan

Sassy was hospitalized and given intravenous corticosteroids. PBMT was administered twice on day 1, with treatment with 810 and 904 nm.

Outcome

Sassy was able to walk and defecate by the end of the first day, but was still weak in rear. On the second day, she was started on a tapering dose of prednisone, given another PBMT treatment, and discharged. Another PBMT treatment was administered 2 days later, at which time she was continuing to improve. A relapse developed 3 days later, after Sassy got outside and ran around. PBMT was resumed and continued every 2 days until she was finally

was able to walk almost normally after four more treatments (1 week). Twice-weekly treatments continued for 2 weeks, followed by weekly treatments for three more weeks, at which time Sassy was back to a normal gait.

Metastatic Neoplasia of the Brain

Signalment

"Duke," 14 years old, Labrador retriever, M.

Client Complaint

Depression, inappetence, wandering, circling, and panting.

History

Duke had been a healthy champion hunting dog with no previous health issues.

Physical Examination

On physical examination, Duke was anxious but showed dull mentation, was panting, would wander into corners and not be able to get out, displayed hyperesthesia around his eyes and nose, and had an occasional cough.

Differential Diagnosis

Dementia, neoplasia.

Diagnostic Imaging

Thoracic radiographs were within normal limits. An MRI of the head showed a mass in the left nasal cavity, with extension into the left cerebrum (Figure 17.4).

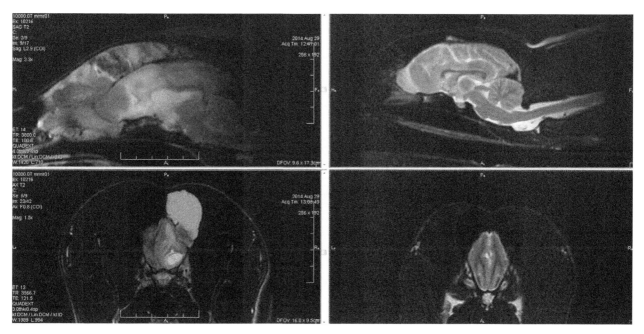

Figure 17.4 MRI of a 14-year-old Labrador retriever with changes in mentation. Note mass (nasal adenocarcinoma) in left nasal cavity with invasion into the left frontal sinus and cerebrum.

Laboratory Data

Blood chemistries and a CBC were within normal limits. A biopsy of the nasal mass and histopathology showed it be a nasal adenocarcinoma.

Diagnosis

Nasal adenocarcinoma with invasive metastasis into the left frontal sinus and cerebrum, causing ataxia, disorientation, and altered mentation.

Treatment Plan

Therapeutic options of radiation and chemotherapy were discussed with a veterinary neurologist. Due to Duke's age, potential side effects, and the extent of the metastatic involvement, the owner declined radiation and chemotherapy and elected to try PBMT to palliate for as long as possible. PBMT was administered twice a week for 2 weeks, then once a week for 2 weeks, then every other week. Therapy was administered at 810 nm to the left rostral cerebrum and left caudal nasal cavity.

Outcome

After the first treatment, Duke had a dramatic recovery to normal behavior, including long walks and fetching. When an attempt was made to reduce treatment frequency to every 2 weeks, Duke's symptoms returned. The owner elected humane euthanasia after 2 months, but was very grateful for the extra good-quality life with Duke.

Conclusion

The use of PBMT to treat neurological diseases in small animals is an exciting new modality for veterinarians. Neurological tissue is very receptive to light therapy, as well as very accessible. When used properly, PBMT is safe, inexpensive, and very effective in treating inflammatory, traumatic, and degenerative processes of the CNS and peripheral nervous system, often obviating the need for surgery or potentially harmful pharmaceuticals.

References

Anders, J.J. *et al.* (2014) In vitro and in vivo optimization of infrared laser treatment for injured peripheral nerves. *Lasers Med Surg.* **46**(1):34–45.

Ando, T. *et al.* (2010) Comparison of therapeutic effects between pulsed and continuous wave 810 nm wavelength laser irradiation for traumatic brain injury in mice. *Laser Med Surg.* **42**(6):450–466.

Averill, D.R. Jr. (1973) Degenerative myelopathy in the aging German Shepherd dog: clinical and pathological findings. *J Am Vet Med Assoc.* **162**(12):1045–1051.

Bosch, M.N. *et al.* (2013) Rapid improvement of canine cognitive dysfunction with immunotherapy designed for Alzheimer's disease. *Curr Alzheimer Res.* **10**(5):482–493.

Brisson, B. (2010) Intervertebral disc disease in dogs. *Vet Clin North Am Small Anim Pract.* **40**(5):829–858.

Byrnes, K.R. *et al.* (2005) Light promotes regeneration and functional recovery and alters the immune response after spinal cord injury. *Lasers Med Surg.* **36**:171–185.

Chow, R. and Armanti, D.M. (2007) 830 nm laser irradiation induces varicosity formation, reduces mitochondrial membrane potential, and blocks fast axonal flow in small and medium rat dorsal root ganglion neurons. *J Periph Nerv Syst.* **12**:28–39.

Chow, R. *et al.* (2012) Electrophysiological effects of a single point transcutaneous 650 and 808 nm laser irradiation of rat sciatic nerve. *Photomed Laser Surg.* **30**(9):530–535.

Cotler, H.B. *et al.* (2015) The use of low level laser therapy (LLLT) for musculoskeletal pain. *MOJ Orthop Rheumatol.* **2**(5):pii:00068.

Cramond, T. *et al.* (1994) ACTH and beta-endorphin levels in response to low level laser therapy for myofascial trigger points. *Laser Ther.* **6**(3):133–142.

Draper, W.E. *et al.* (2012) Low-level laser reduces time to ambulation in dogs after hemi- laminectomy: a preliminary study. *J Small Anima Pract.* **53**(8):465–469.

Gonzalez-Lima, F. *et al.* (2014) Mitochondrial respiration as a target for neuroprotection and cognitive enhancement. *Biochem Pharmacol.* **88**(4):584–593.

Gonzalez-Martinez, A. *et al.* (2011) Plasma β-amyloid peptides in canine aging and cognitive dysfunction as a model of Alzheimer's disease. *Exp Gerontol.* **46**(7):590–596.

Griffiths, I.R. and Duncan, I.D. (1975) Chronic degenerative radiculopathy in the dog. *J Small Anim Pract.* **16**:461–471.

Hagiwara, S. *et al.* (2008) Pre-irradiation of blood by gallium aluminum arsenide (830 nm) low-level laser enhances peripheral endogenous opioid analgesia in rats. *Anesth Anal.* **107**(3):1058–1063.

Hansen, H.J. (1951) A pathologic-anatomical interpretation of disc degeneration in dogs. *Acta Orthop Scand.* **20**:280–293.

Hwang, M.H. *et al.* (2015) Low level light therapy modulates inflammatory mediators secreted by human annulus fibrosus cells during intervertebral disc degeneration in vitro. *Photochem Photobiol.* **91**(2):403–410.

Insua, D. (2010) Dogs with canine counterpart of Alzheimer's disease lose noradrenergic neurons. *Neurobiol Aging.* **31**(4):625–635.

Inzana, K.D. (2000) Peripheral nerve disorders. In: *Textbook of Veterinary Internal Medicine*, 5 edn., pp. 662–681. Saunders, Philadelphia, PA.

Kathmann, I. *et al.* (2006) Daily controlled physiotherapy increases survival time in dogs with suspected degenerative myelopathy. *J Vet Inter Med.* **20**(4):927–932.

Labajos, M. (1988) Beta-endorphin levels modification after GaAs and HeNe laser irradiation on the rabbit. *Comparative study. Invest Clin.* **1–2**:6–8.

Landsberg, G.M. *et al.* (2011) Clinical signs and management of anxiety, sleeplessness, and cognitive dysfunction in the senior pet. *Vet Clin North Am Small Anim Pract.* **41**(3):565–590.

Landsberg, G.M. *et al.* (2012) Cognitive dysfunction syndrome: a disease of canine and feline brain aging. *Vet Clin North Am Small Anim Pract.* **42**(4):749–768.

Lapchak, P.A. *et al.* (2015) Transcranial near-infrared laser transmission (NILT) profiles (800 nm): systematic comparison in four common research species. *PLoS One.* **10**(6):e0127580.

LeCouteur, R.A. and Grandy, J.L. (2000) Diseases of the spinal cord. In: *Textbook of Veterinary Internal Medicine*, 5 edn., pp. 609–653. Saunders, Philadelphia, PA.

Liang, J. *et al.* (2012) Photobiomodulation by low-power laser irradiation attenuates Aβ-induced cell apoptosis through the Akt/GSK3β/β-catenin pathway. *Free Radic Biol Med.* **53**(7):1459–1467.

Magalhaes, M. *et al.* (2016) Light therapy modulates serotonin levels in blood flow in women with headache. A preliminary study. *Exp Biol Med (Maywood).* **241**(1):40–45.

Manteca, X. (2011) Nutrition in behavior and senior dogs. *Top Companion Anim Med.* **26**(1):33–36.

Mariani, C.L. (2010) Peripheral nerve disorders. In: *Textbook of Veterinary Internal Medicine*, 7 edn., pp. 1462–1467. Elsevier, St. Louis, MO.

Moges, H. *et al.* (2011) Effect of 810 nm light on nerve regeneration after autograft repair of severely injured rat median nerve. *Lasers Surg Med.* **43**(9):901–906.

Naeser, M.A. *et al.* (2011) Improved cognitive function after transcranial, light emitting diode treatments in chronic traumatic brain injury: two case reports. *Photmed Lasers Surg.* **29**(5):351–358.

Oron, A. *et al.* (2012) Near infrared transcranial laser therapy applied at various modes to mice following traumatic brain injury significantly reduces long-term neurological deficits. *J Neurotrauma.* **29**(2):401–407.

Ozawa, M. *et al.* (2016) The relation between canine cognitive dysfunction and age-related brain lesions. *J Vet Med Sci.* **78**(6):997–1006.

Purushothuman, S. *et al.* (2014) Photobiomodulation with near infrared light mitigates Alzheimer's disease-related pathology in cerebral cortex – evidence from two transgenic mouse models. *Alzheimers Res Ther.* **6**(1):2.

Quihe, W. *et al.* (2012) Low-level laser therapy for closed-head traumatic brain injury in mice: effect of different wavelengths. *Lasers Med Surg.* **44**(3):218–226.

Recknor, J.B. and Mallapragada, S.K. (2006) Nerve regeneration: tissue engineering strategies. In: *The Biomedical Engineering Handbook: Tissue Engineering and Artificial Organs*, pp. 48–51. Taylor & Francis: New York.

Rochkind, S. (2009) Phototherapy in peripheral nerve regeneration: from basic science to clinical study. *Neurosurg Focus.* **2**:E8.

Rochkind, S. *et al.* (2007) Laser phototherapy (780 nm), a new modality in treatment of long-term, incomplete peripheral nerve injury: a randomized double-blind placebo-controlled study. *Photmed Laser Surg.* **25**(5):436–442.

Rodkey, W. G. and Sharp, N.J.H. (2003) Surgery of the peripheral nervous system. In: *Textbook of Small Animal Surgery*, 3 edn., pp. 1218–1225. Elsevier, Philadelphia, PA.

Silverstein, D. (2006) SIRS, MODS, and sepsis in small animals. Available from: http://www.ivis.org/proceedings/scivac/2006/silverstein2_en.pdf?LA=1 (accessed November 30, 2016).

Snyder, S.K. (2002) Quantification of calcitonin gene-related peptide in RNA and neuronal cell death in facial motor nuclei following axotomy and 633 nm low-power laser treatment. *Lasers Med Surg.* **31**(3):216–222.

Sprouse-Blum, A.S. *et al.* (2010) Understanding endorphins and their importance in pain management. *Hawaii Med J.* **69**(3):70–71.

Tedford, C.E. *et al.* (2015) Quantitative analysis of transcranial and intraparenchymal light penetration in human cadaver brain tissue. *Lasers Surg Med.* **47**(4):312–322.

Welch, J.A. (1996) Peripheral nerve injury. *Semin Vet Med Surg (Small Anim).* **11**(4):273–284.

Wu, W. *et al.* (2009) 810 nm wavelength light: an effective therapy for transected or contused rat spinal cord. *Lasers Med Surg.* **41**(1):36–41.

Xuan, W. *et al.* (2013) Transcranial low level laser therapy improves neurological performance in traumatic brain injury in mice: effect of treatment repetition regimes. *PLoS One.* **8**(1):e53454.

18

Laser Therapy for the Geriatric Patient

Erin O'Leary

HEAL Mobile Veterinary Laser Therapy, Cary, NC, USA

Introduction

Geriatric pets make up a population that is steadily growing in veterinary medicine due to improved veterinary care, innovations in technology, and our ability as practitioners to catch diseases earlier in their progression. A growing population of older pets means more companion animals are suffering from age-related conditions, including organ failure, malignancies, joint disease, and cognitive deterioration. In the United States, nearly 45% of dog owners have a dog age 7 years or older, while 46% of cat owners have a cat in this oldest age bracket (PR Newswire, 2016).

It is imperative that we offer the most comprehensive treatment and maintenance options for this expanding population of patients as they age. Though we cannot prevent the process of aging, we are responsible for recognizing and minimizing its effects (both physical and cognitive) on our patients' quality of life and relationships with their families (AVMA, 2016). The purpose of this chapter is to illustrate the use and benefits of laser therapy in senior geriatric pets and offer tools to deal with this very specific and unique subset of patients. We will discuss why the introduction of laser therapy into senior protocols can be particularly rewarding and look at some special approaches that should be taken with aging patients (Rodier, 2016).

Laser therapy, now commonly called "photobiomodulation therapy" (PBMT), is one tool in a growing arsenal of methods for providing the best care for our patients. This mode of therapy, along with a focused and appropriate pain medication regimen, utilization of physical and alternative therapy options, and, most importantly, a thorough evaluation of each individual patient, allows us to provide an optimal strategy for meeting our patients' health needs. We will not go into detail in this chapter about the other therapies that are available to treat chronic pain, skin, and inflammatory conditions, but it is important to note that any of them can be used in conjunction with laser therapy.

Geriatric animals are generally defined as 7 years old and above, though this varies according to breed and species. Most such pets have been in the home for a long time and have established a strong bond with their families. Though recent studies attempt to show that cats have less secure attachment bonds (Potter and Mills, 2015) than are reported for dogs (Payne *et al.*, 2016), both species, as well as other companion animals, become well-loved family members. It therefore is crucial that you treat a senior pet with the same focus and attention that you do a new puppy whose owners are looking to you as the expert. The senior portion of life comes with a similar, if not increased, number of owner questions and concerns.

Utilizing PBMT not only provides a new option for concerned and invested pet owners, but allows them time during treatment sessions to discuss concerns, progress, and plans for their pet. The veterinarian's role in clients' decisions regarding their pets, particularly when those pets are geriatric or seriously ill, is dependent on open communication and good models of shared decision making (Christiansen *et al.*, 2016). These sessions are optimal for the veterinarian as caregiver to see their patients on a regular basis and allow time for dialogue, questions, and observations of any new conditions that might arise.

Though many of the benefits of laser therapy can be applied to the general population, some are specific and advantageous to an aging population. These include maintaining mobility and a sense of security, preserving patients' status as family members, managing and resolving long-term conditions (particularly those that can be isolating to these pets), and treating a special subset of our subset: cats.

As a mobile practitioner, I will have some additional suggestions and insights, since I do the majority of my treatments in my patients' homes. Everything detailed here can also be of use in your practice location and applied to your laser protocols.

Important PBM Effects in Geriatric Patient Management

Before we begin discussing the specific approaches to treating senior pets with laser therapy, it is worth mentioning the cellular effects of PBM that can help counteract some of the natural degeneration of physiological processes within older patients' bodies.

Application of PBMT to impaired tissue results in a number of complex and well-documented effects. The mechanisms of PBM are detailed in Chapter 5, as well as in other publications (Pryor and Millis, 2015). When considering the application of laser therapy to the specific needs of geriatric patients, a number of those mechanisms are important.

Increased Cellular Energy

PBM stimulates the production of adenosine triphosphate (ATP) in damaged and impaired cells (Hamblin and Demidova, 2006). In aging patients, this interaction can lead to healthier, more normalized cells and tissue via increased growth factor production and cellular metabolism.

Increased Blood Flow and Circulation

Vasodilation and improved circulation result in increased oxygenation of tissues, decreased effects of exposure to environmental and physical stressors, and improved response to chronic inflammation (Maegawa *et al.*, 2000).

Improved Neural Tissue Effects

As animals age, nerve cells die and are not replaced. In some cases, nerve cells malfunction or their nerve potentials or communication capabilities are altered. PBM can affect the conduction of neurotransmitters, assist in the repair of damaged nerves, and aid in the normalization of nerve potentials, leading to decreased pain sensitivity (Cambier *et al.*, 2000; Chow *et al.*, 2011; Farivar *et al.*, 2014).

Decreased Inflammation

Many geriatric patients have diseases associated with the aging process that involve chronic inflammatory changes. Dental disease, arthritis, neurological deterioration, and chronic skin inflammation are common. Prolonged inflammation can lead to a progressive destruction of the affected tissue and incite further inflammatory activity. PBM has a direct effect on the reduction of negative inflammatory processes (Cotler *et al.*, 2015; Huang *et al.*, 2015).

Improved Healing

Healing tissue fibers align themselves in a more linear and uniform direction when exposed to therapy laser light. Scarring is reduced and tissue strength improves. As aging progresses, tissues lose elasticity and become more prone to injury. PBM contributes to more normal healing and can help prevent injuries by improving tissue flexibility and elasticity (Kuffler, 2016; Medrado *et al.*, 2003; Peplow *et al.*, 2010; Tabakoglu *et al.*, 2015).

Improved Serotonin and Endorphin Release

Older pets have a decreased ability to cope with stress and can experience behavior changes, including aggression, noise phobias, and increased anxiety. PBM can help support the natural secretion of serotonin and endorphins, which can make pets feel better, happier, and less anxious (Ceylan *et al.*, 2004; Hagiwara *et al.*, 2007, 2008; Labajos, 1988; Montesinos, 1988).

Utilization of Laser Therapy in Geriatric Patients

As they have earned their place in our homes and hearts, geriatric patients come with years of ingrained desires, needs, and peculiarities that we as practitioners need to take into consideration when we initiate a laser therapy session with them. I will detail here some of those considerations, provide tools to deal with them, and assist in creating an ideal environment for treatment.

Communication

Learn Who is Under the Handpiece

First, get to know your patient. Who is this creature that will be under your handpiece? Often, you are starting a new relationship, and it helps to know a bit about your new partner. Have a thorough conversation with the pet's owner to get a good understanding of who it is. What are its idiosyncrasies, preferences, or special needs? Administering laser therapy treatments to geriatric patients is unique for most veterinarians, technicians, and nurses, since it involves relatively long contact time, one-on-one, with patients that are not sedated or under anesthesia. Taking special care to learn all you can about the patient and the owner will contribute significantly toward a successful (and peaceful) treatment. Learn from the owner and from personal observation what the patient might take as an act of aggression. Note the patient's level of sensitivity to loud noises. Confirm with the owner whether the patient's shaking is typical, or if it demonstrates a high degree of nervousness. All are valuable pieces of information that can help make everyone involved more comfortable and avoid patient aggression as the laser therapy treatment session begins.

Make the Owner a Partner in the Initial Treatment

I recommend allowing the pet owner to be present for at least the first treatment session so they can apprise you of the aforementioned information and learn exactly what takes place during a session, which will increase their (and their pet's) comfort level. In addition, this is a wonderful opportunity for you to discuss senior care, any issues they have noted, and any concerns they have. It also gives you a chance to talk with the pet owner about their bond with their pet. This will give you a very good idea of what they are looking for in terms of care and guidance, and may even open the door to future discussion of their inevitable loss as their pet continues to age.

It is rare as a veterinarian to have uninterrupted quiet time with clients in such a positive and relaxing environment. Collaborating with the client and your technician or nurse in the first treatment session can ensure all members of the pet care team are on the same page. As further treatments sessions ensue, I recommend maintaining a progress log, noting the therapist's observations – as well as the pet owner's. This will help you catch any subtle changes, positive results, or new concerns. I often find that we get one geriatric problem under control and another starts to develop. Consistent monitoring and follow-up are beneficial to all involved. Maintaining a log ensures that with each visit you are getting a true update.

The time during a laser treatment is ideal for discussions about geriatric health care topics like nutrition, weight, activity level, home environment, and supplementation. You have a captive audience and the focus is on you and the patient, your senior health care management plan, and your recommendations for the patient and owner. This is a time both for delivering care and for marketing to your current and future geriatric pet owners.

Communicate Clear Expectations

When working with geriatric patients, it is critical to discuss with the owners what their expectations are for their pet. While their pet ages, we can give them the tools they need to measure the aging process and help them take appropriate actions to improve their pet's quality of life. Laser therapy can help geriatric pets be more mobile and get them moving more comfortably. This is an incredibly beneficial element both psychologically and physically. Exercising, walking, running, and playing are among the biggest connections pets have

with their owners, and increased function and mobility will help maintain their emotional bond. In addition, laser therapy will help decrease the frequency of other unpleasant events like bed sores, accidents in the house, and skin issues, all of which can put a distance between a pet and its owners.

It is important to communicate that laser therapy is not a magic wand, however. Owner expectations should be reasonable. Laser therapists need to be clear about what this technology can and cannot achieve: age-related bone changes (the hardware) will not be reversed, but pain and inflammation (the software) can be reprogrammed. Managing expectations for owners is important when working with geriatric patients, because their conditions will often have been ongoing for long periods of time. Clients need to understand that changes may be slow and subtle. They need to not be disappointed when results take longer to appear and are not as dramatic as they might hope. The measure of success with geriatric patients is some improvement, any improvement – any increase in mobility, function, and quality of life.

Understand the Obstacles Geriatric Pets Experience at Home

As a mobile laser therapy practitioner, I have the fortune of assessing each patient's home environment and having conversations about its bedding, the obstacles to its getting around the house, its traction on hardwood floors, why area rugs may be an issue, and so on. It is important for you to have these same discussions with your geriatric pet owners so that what you accomplish with laser therapy is not reversed by falls or the home environment.

Discuss with owners where problems occur at home. Does the pet avoid parts of the house? Does it have problems making it outside for eliminations? Does it hesitate to use the litter box? Does it no longer get on the bed or sofa? Can it no longer comfortably bend over to eat and drink? Do the owners and the pet spend a lot of time in the car? Where, when, and how do they ride? How do they get in and out? These questions begin to identify what the patient's quality of life is like.

Your recommendations concerning options like booties, ramps, orthopedic bedding, lowered litterboxes, harnesses, bed stairs, and raised bowls will assist in improving your patients' quality of life, and demonstrate your partnership in ensuring their success.

Remember Your Geriatric Pet Owners are Invested

People who are interested in laser therapy for their geriatric pets will likely be your most engaged and informed clients. In addition to being the most familiar with their particular pet, they will also likely do a lot of research and have lots of propositions for alternatives to try. There are many ideas, theories, and products that promise to be the magic solution to a dog's aging problem. Don't disregard their suggestions and thoughts; be their educator, and be open to things they may come up with, while giving them good information about things that may or may not be a waste of their time and money. A large number of my clients asked their primary veterinarians about laser therapy for their pet's arthritis and were dismissed or redirected. You have the opportunity to debunk, inform, and maybe even learn something new from them.

Treating Geriatric Patients

Before Treatment Begins

As pets age, they are more likely to have impaired vision and hearing, so it is important to slow your approach, make sure they know you are coming, allow them to acclimate to the sounds the laser makes, and get used to having the handpiece in contact with their body. If pets are noise-sensitive (particularly common in cats), I recommend covering the laser with a blanket to mute the sounds of beeping. It is ideal to provide comfortable bedding or seating, a pillow for their head, or a tilted back that they can lean on. Ensure that they are in a comfortable position (according to their individual preference) during treatment.

Positioning for Laser Therapy

Laser therapy is generally easier to administer with the pet standing, giving the therapist access to all body surfaces and areas that may need to be treated. In an elderly patient, standing for a prolonged period of time may be uncomfortable or impossible. Create a pleasant, comfortable environment for geriatric patients so that they have an enjoyable experience and a complete treatment can take place. Smaller patients are frequently more comfortable in your lap, rather than on the floor or a table (Figure 18.1). Also, understand that you will likely have multiple areas to treat in an elderly animal. The patient may need to take a break and walk around rather than remain stationary for a long period of time. This applies to lying in one position for a prolonged period also. I find that older pets often have a preferred side that they tend to lie on – often their weaker side. Though getting access to this side can be tricky, it is important to do so. Do not be above using treats and bribery. As a last resort, use gentle repositioning.

Along with positioning, you have to consider the pros and cons of manipulating and putting a joint through its range of motion in pets that are severely arthritic or have pain from chronic conditions. Though it is ideal to treat joints through a passive range of motion when applying laser therapy, a geriatric patient with chronic pain may not allow manipulation of joints. After multiple treatments,

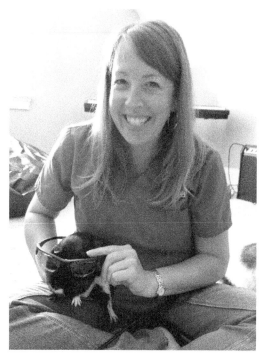

Figure 18.1 Ensure that patients are in a comfortable position during treatment. Smaller patients are frequently more comfortable in your lap, rather than on the floor or a table.

pain will reduce and flexibility will increase, and movement through range of motion may be allowed. You will want to monitor and measure these changes in range of motion and flexibility of the joint in order to have an objective measure of the progress you are making. In addition, you want to be very careful when repositioning patients during a treatment session, as they may have become protective of certain areas and they may not be used to being moved. Be gentle, be aware of the patient's responses as you move them, and protect yourself and your assistants from rogue teeth or other "weaponry."

With cats, you will sometimes have to be creative to find a good fit of position and accessibility, since their body areas are much smaller and harder to get to. With large animals, unless they are lying down or have placed themselves in a corner or against a wall, accessibility is not typically an issue. Having an experienced holder is the general solution, but again watch for "sneak" attacks if positioning upsets the patient.

Adjusting Treatment Protocols

As pets age they are less able to thermoregulate and may become more temperature-sensitive. This may require you to adjust your treatment protocols for these patients. Discuss with the pet owner whether their pet is heat-seeking or tends to choose bathroom tiles over their bed. Many pets are sensitive to heat, and you may observe increased panting or a desire to move away from the laser during treatment. Ensure that you are moving the handpiece in an appropriately consistent manner, at the correct speed, and understand that some pets will need to have the power decreased (and time increased) during their treatment. Adapt to what patients will tolerate and make appropriate changes in the therapy laser protocol to ensure that the appropriate dose is being delivered to the tissues.

Also, adjust your protocol depending on whether there has been significant muscle atrophy or a decrease in fat stores. You are more likely to have prominent bony structures in pets with these structural changes, so you need to be aware of any contact between the head of the handpiece and bone, which might be unpleasant and uncomfortable. Measure the areas that you will be treating with a cloth tape and ensure that if you are treating a 40 kg dog, the area you are treating is representative of a 40 kg dog.

Physical Barriers

As pets age and clients become more and more conscientious of their needs, you may have to deal with physical barriers that can cause difficulty during laser therapy treatment sessions. Anxiety-reducing shirts, diapers, walking harnesses, braces, booties, and a variety of bandaging and cast options can be barriers to administering laser therapy. Since our goal is to provide the most comfortable and least stressful environment for treatment, learn to navigate around these barriers.

As mentioned previously, sometimes even the position of the pet can provide an obstacle, particularly if you have a determined patient that is not going to budge from one side or a corner of a room or stall. Be prepared for these situations, work with the owner to have acceptable treats available, and have the owner prepare their pet prior to treatment when possible. Try to avoid spending valuable time having to remove a recently placed bandage or a harness that has a mystifying number of fasteners. If it is possible to perform a complete treatment with dog-appeasing pheromone collars, anxiety-reducing shirts, or anxiety wraps in place, then do so.

Incontinence

Many older pets exprience urinary or fecal incontinence, or both, and this must be taken into account during your treatment session. Often, the treatment itself will cause them to relax (gas is a very common part of my treatment sessions, particularly when I treat the back). Make sure that you are prepared for an accident or the potential need to get up and go outside during treatment. If possible, have the owner take their pet outside prior to the visit so they can relieve themselves. This is especially important for pets that are unable to walk or need help to eliminate.

Balancing Concurrent Conditions

Just by virtue of their age, older patients will have likely been diagnosed with multiple conditions that need to be balanced while treating with laser. Ensure that you have a full understanding of the medications that have been prescribed, the supplements that are being used, and the medical conditions that have been diagnosed. Knowing whether a patient is on medications or has an underlying condition like cancer or a bleeding disorder will allow you to ensure that your protocol is well calculated and appropriate. As your treatment progresses, it is also useful to begin eliminating or titrating down pain medications. Having a good method for charting progress allows you to monitor these changes, have a clear idea of what is working, and stay updated on anything else that may be affecting your progress (e.g., a change in medication could cause a backslide that appears to be orthopedic but is in fact weakness secondary to a change in blood pressure medication). It is also imperative to understand previous surgeries that have been performed and any hardware that may be present.

Cancer is still an unknown when it comes to the effects of laser therapy. The recommended approach is to avoid known cancerous regions because of a lack of knowledge about the effect PBM has on malignant tissue in companion animal species. For a full discussion of the special considerations required when considering PBMT in a patient with a malignancy, see Chapter 7. When treating an elderly patient, you will need to balance the benefits it could derive from the laser treatment with the concern of potentially worsening a present neoplastic condition. As 50% of dogs over the age of 10 are diagnosed with cancer, it is common to encounter this dilemma in senior pets. There is no right answer, other than to ensure full disclosure of the risks to the owner and to document the conversations you have about the decision to treat. I personally have not observed a perceptible increase in the rate of growth of a known cancer after PBMT. For osteosarcoma in particular, I have found laser therapy to be an invaluable tool in managing pain, but I always ensure that owners are making an informed decision to proceed with treatment.

Cats (and Other Animals for Which We Have Limited Options)

As a population, cats have benefited immensely from the arrival of laser therapy in the veterinary world. Historically, we either did not identify that cats were in pain or had to accept that if they were in pain, our options were limited. The treatment options that were available often had the negative side effect of being relatively hard to get into our patients. We are now able to increase their quality of life and avoid exacerbating some of the most common issues that we see in geriatric cats including kidney disease and gastrointestinal upset. We can

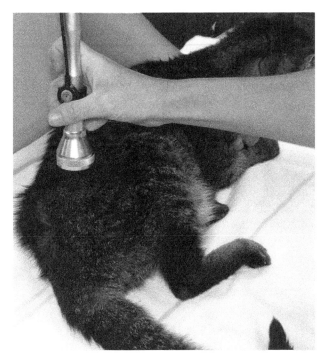

Figure 18.2 Always offer patients a comfortable surface during treatments. Cats usually require no restraint and relax within minutes of initiating treatment. Image courtesy of Dr. John C. Godbold, Jr.

address some previously unmanageable conditions, like stomatitis and nerve pain. As a bonus, we have also discovered a treatment that cats actually enjoy.

Usually, no restraint or stressful positioning is required; most cats relax within minutes of initiating treatment, and are often noted to maintain a relaxed state (Figure 18.2). When utilizing laser therapy with cats, it is important to recognize that they are particularly good at masking pain and weakness, and that some of the behaviors they demonstrate at home will respond to treatment. These behaviors include but are not limited to decreased activity, aggression, hiding, increased vocalization, pacing at night, changes in litterbox usage, decreased grooming, changes in sleep patterns, changes in eating habits, and self-mutilation. It is important to discuss any changes the owners are noting at home and to chart the cat's progress in these areas.

Senility

As pets age, they often suffer a decline in mental function. Their memory, their ability to learn, their awareness, and their senses of sight and hearing can all deteriorate. This deterioration can cause disturbances in their sleep–wake cycles, making them restless at night but sleepy during the day. It can make them forget previously learned cues (commands) or habits they once knew well. It can increase their anxiety and tendency to react aggressively (Landsberg *et al.*, 2011, 2012). It can also

change their social relationships with their owners, you, and other pets in their home. Some pets may become less interested in affection, petting, or social interaction, while others become more "attached." It is important to understand these changes as you approach any laser therapy management plan.

Treating senior patients increases the likelihood of dealing with senility or cognitive changes; be aware that you may have to adjust your protocols accordingly. You may have to slowly familiarize the pet with the laser, and you may have to do this repeatedly. You may have only short intervals of time during which the pet is accepting of laser therapy, and you may have to break up treatment times. You should be watchful of erratic and unpredictable behavior and discuss the items mentioned in this section with the owners so you can educate them on changes in sleep cycles, appetite, self-care, activity levels, relationships, and reactions to strangers or to people and pets they know. Try to determine the ideal situation that will make the patient comfortable, both physically and emotionally. (Will they feel better if their "person" is in sight or out of the room? Do they have a special blanket or toy that comforts them? Would an anxiety-reducing shirt or hormone diffuser help relax them during a treatment session?)

Many of the medications that we use for pain management in aging pets can cause some confounding side effects that are easily confused with senility. Utilizing laser therapy and minimizing or completely discontinuing the use of these medications can help create a less perplexing progress chart as you monitor the pet's "normal" state. Since cognitive function is often one of the things that veterinarians use to determine whether it may be time to recommend euthanasia, it is imperative that the signs are clear and are not based on muddled data and observations (Rodier, 2016; Schütt *et al.*, 2015).

Offering House Calls

As both pet and pet owner populations age, it may be beneficial to your practice to add house calls as an adjunct to your practice-based laser therapy. Getting large arthritic dogs and uncooperative cats into your hospital for laser therapy may be difficult for a proportion of your clientele, and offering laser therapy at home may increase the number of senior pets being served who otherwise might not be able to utilize laser therapy as an option.

Case Studies

Unilateral Coxofemoral Joint Osteoarthritis in a Feline

Signalment

"Boomer," 12 years old, domestic short hair, MN, 5.5 kg.

Client Complaint

Decreased physical activity and social interaction with family.

History

Boomer had a chondrosarcoma and amputation of his right rear leg at 6 years of age. He was being treated with chemotherapy following surgery for a gastrointestinal adenocarcinoma.

Physical Examination

Physical examination confirmed pain in the left coxofemoral joint.

Laser Therapy Treatment

Boomer's left hip was treated every other day using contact delivery and laser settings that delivered a dosage of $5 \, J/cm^2$. A total of seven treatments were administered.

Outcome

Boomer is a great example of the opportunity for laser therapy and pain management to affect the human–animal bond and increase patient well-being. The owner reported in a follow-up email, "You know, one thing I just realized yesterday about Boomer that hadn't really struck me before is that since you treated him the second time, he's continuously hanging out with the family. For months and months he's gone and laid on our bed during the day, even if I'm at home. But he now just stays in the kitchen or family room with all the dogs all the time."

Multiple-Joint Osteoarthritis in a Sheep

Signalment

"Angus," 14 years old, sheep, M.

Client Complaint

Increased difficulty in getting up and down and in moving about to graze.

History

Angus had previously been diagnosed with arthritis in the hocks and stifles. He also had chronic renal disease and was undergoing symptomatic treatment.

Physical Examination

A physical examination confirmed pain and reduced range of motion bilaterally in Angus's hocks and stifles.

Laser Therapy Treatment

A twice-weekly schedule of laser therapy treatments was initiated. The affected areas were treated with a contact delivery and laser settings that delivered a dosage of $20 \, J/cm^2$. Angus responded well to laser therapy, so treatments were continued long-term. At the time of writing, he has received 34 treatments. He also received acupuncture treatments.

Outcome

Angus showed increased mobility and the ability to get up on his own. Being able to stay mobile and graze was critical to his life on the farm. Angus was able to continue walking and to maintain muscle tone, and the potential for muscle atrophy and infections due to inactivity and pressure sores was decreased.

Though these changes can be dramatic in larger animals, this point is also very applicable to our smaller patients in terms of their ability to maintain muscle mass, mobility and flexibility. Though we feel it is normal for our older patients to sleep more and be less active, keeping exercise (though perhaps shorter and less vigorous) as a mainstay of their daily schedule is crucial to their vitality and their ability to stay healthy and active for as long as possible.

Multiple-Joint Osteoarthritis in a Canine

Signalment

"Caleb," 10 years old, border collie mix, MN, 28 kg.

Client Complaint

Caleb was an energetic dog who loved hiking, swimming, and outdoor activity. By 9 years of age, he had developed severe signs of arthritis and had slowed down substantially.

History

Caleb's regular veterinarian had diagnosed osteoarthritis of the stifles, hips, and lumbar spine.

Physical Examination

A physical examination confirmed pain and limited range of motion in both stifles and hips, and pain on deep palpation of Caleb's lumbar area.

Laser Therapy Treatment

Initial laser therapy treatments were administered every other day. After the fourth treatment, they were tapered to once a week, and then once every 2 weeks. Caleb was treated using on-contact delivery with laser settings that delivered dosages of $20 \, J/cm^2$ to his stifles, $23 \, J/cm^2$ to his hips, and $25 \, J/cm^2$ to his lumbar and sacral regions.

A total of seven treatments were administered, and then Caleb's family moved and laser therapy was continued in their new location.

Outcome

After treatments were initiated, Caleb quickly began to show an increase in activity levels, improved ability to walk up and down stairs, and renewed pleasure in playing with human and animal family members. His range of motion increased in both hips, and he demonstrated less pain on extension of his stifles.

Caleb had a very positive response to laser therapy, physically. He also demonstrated an interesting psychological response to the treatment sessions. For the first two treatments, we moved Caleb's dog bed into the den to separate him from the other pets in the house during his treatment time. During both of these sessions, he displayed visible anxiety and paced around the room between treatments of each affected body area. When I arrived for the next treatment and began discussing his progress with his owner, we observed him pulling his bed into the den! We began treating him in the den and from that point on, his anxiety level was decreased and he relaxed during his treatment sessions.

Multiple-Joint Osteoarthritis in a Canine with Chronic Renal Disease

Signalment
"Bitsy," 15 years old, cavalier King Charles spaniel, FS, 5.5 kg.

Client Complaint
Reduced activity and inability to move around comfortably.

History
Bitsy's regular veterinarian had identified severe osteoarthritis in her stifles, hips, shoulders, and spine. Bitsy had chronic renal disease, which was stable. She was unable to take any non-steroidal anti-inflammatory medications. She did not tolerate other pain management options well, in terms of the effect on both her behavior and her gastrointestinal system.

Physical Examination
A physical examination confirmed pain and reduced range of motion in Bitsy's stifles, hips, and shoulders, and pain on deep palpation of her spine.

Laser therapy Treatment
Laser therapy was initiated with every-other-day treatments. The treatments were administered using a contact delivery technique and dosages of $7 J/cm^2$ to the stifles, $8 J/cm^2$ to the shoulders and hips, and $10 J/cm^2$ to the spine. After 2 weeks of every-other-day treatments, Bitsy was tapered to once-a-week treatments. Long–term, she received a total of 84 treatments.

Outcome
Bitsy showed improved mobility, a visible decrease in pain responses on palpation and manipulation of her joints, and increased barking when I came to the house.

Laser therapy substantially decreased her level of pain, and it gave her a reprieve from the decision to euthanize that her owners had been struggling with. Due to the improvement in her ability to walk and function, Bitsy was afforded another year and a half with her family.

Multiple-Joint Osteoarthritis in an Aged Canine

Signalment
"Jelly," 17 years old, beagle, FS, 15.5 kg.

History
Jelly had a history of gradual reduction of musculoskeletal function and increased disability in getting about. Her regular veterinarian had diagnosed arthritis in the hips and shoulders, gall bladder disease, and an anal gland carcinoma.

Physical Examination
An initial physical examination verified pain and reduced range of motion in Jelly's shoulders and hips. During a treatment session several weeks later, an examination demonstrated that she was sensitive to touch in the lumbar area. That additional area was added to the areas initially being treated.

Laser Therapy Treatment
Laser therapy was initiated with two treatments the first week, two treatments the third week, then one treatment every other week. The treatments were administered using contact delivery and dosages of $10 J/cm^2$ to the shoulders and $18 J/cm^2$ to the hips.

One of the things we noted during Jelly's treatments was that she would often start panting and would shift a lot during treatment sessions. After discussion with her owners, we noted that she opted not to take long walks on warmer days and chose to lie on cold tile or wood rather than the multitude of beds she had at her disposal. At that point, we adjusted the dosage to $9 J/cm^2$ to the shoulders, $17 J/cm^2$ to the hips, and, starting with the 12th treatment, $20 J/cm^2$ to the lumbosacral area. Jelly received a total of 68 treatments long-term.

Outcome
Jelly displayed an excellent response to laser therapy. Her activity increased, she was able to jump on and off of the sofa, she was able to go for longer walks, and she generally showed an improvement of her overall attitude.

Final Considerations

Working as I have in a mobile laser therapy practice, with a majority of senior patients, it has become clear that responses to laser therapy vary greatly. In most cases, however, the response is positive and observable. Our goal with senior patients is to create an opportunity for each to experience an optimal level of physical and mental well-being, while keeping the effects of aging at bay. There are several areas in our geriatric patients' lives that we can consistently improve with the addition of laser therapy to their overall management.

Mobility

Keeping older pets mobile through appropriate exercise helps keep them healthier and decreases the loss of muscle tone. Exercise is also important for the health of the heart, digestive system, and attitude, and can be an integral part of the human–animal bond. In addition to the benefit to the patient, pet mobility also contributes to the physical activity of the owner. A study explored the associations between dog ownership, walking activity, and health outcomes in older adults and demonstrated that the relationship with one's dog may be a positive influence on physical activity for older adults (Curl *et al.*, 2016).

Cognitive Function

Supporting serotonin and endorphin release helps geriatric patients cope with stress and anxiety and lowers requirements for behavior-altering medications. Future studies will contribute to our current knowledge about direct, transcranial treatment of cognitive dysfunction (Barrett and Gonzalez-Lima, 2013; Naeser *et al.*, 2014).

Dental Disease

PBMT is ideal for addressing the inflammation and pain associated with routine dental disease, dental procedures, and difficult-to-manage conditions like stomatitis (Kathuria *et al.*, 2015).

Dermatologic Conditions

As pets age, their ability to heal becomes more and more diminished. A wound that might have taken days to heal when they were younger can now take weeks and may have many more complications associated with it. Along with the associated pain and discomfort, when pets are suffering from skin infections, they may find the amount of interaction with their humans is decreased. Wounds heal faster when laser therapy is part of their overall management (Kuffler 2016). Speeding up the healing process returns the pet to its normal surroundings, allows it to sleep with family members, and allows it to be petted regularly.

Age Is Not a Disease

Age is not a disease, but with age comes disease. Laser therapy can and should be fully utilized in managing the diseases of geriatric patients. The mindset that we have to accept a decline due to aging can be adjusted substantially by adding laser therapy to our senior conversations and management protocols. Geriatric pets offer many benefits to humans. One of the advantages of being in the veterinary profession is that we can return the favor.

References

AVMA. (2016) Senior pet care (FAQ). Available from: https://www.avma.org/public/PetCare/Pages/Caring-for-an-Older-Pet-FAQs.aspx (accessed November 30, 2016).

Barrett, D.W. and Gonzalez-Lima, F. (2013) Transcranial infrared laser stimulation produces beneficial cognitive and emotional effects in humans. *Neuroscience.* **230**:13–23.

Cambier, D. *et al.* (2000) The influence of low intensity infrared laser irradiation on conduction characteristics of peripheral nerve: a randomised, controlled, double blind study on the sural nerve. *Lasers Med Sci.* **15**(3):195–200.

Ceylan, Y. *et al.* (2004) The effects of infrared laser and medical treatments on pain and serotonin degradation products in patients with myofascial pain syndrome. A controlled trial. *Rheumatol Int.* **24**(5):260–263.

Chow, R.T. *et al.* (2011) Inhibitory effects of laser irradiation on peripheral mammalian nerves and relevance to analgesic effects: a systematic review. *Photomed Laser Surg.* **29**(6):365–381.

Christiansen, S.B. *et al.* (2016) Veterinarians' role in clients' decision-making regarding seriously ill companion animal patients. *Acta Vet Scand.* **58**(1):30.

Cotler, H.B. *et al.* (2015) The use of low level laser therapy (LLLT) for musculoskeletal pain. *MOJ Orthop Rheumatol.* **2**(5):pii:00068.

Curl, A.L. *et al.* (2016) Dog walking, the human–animal bond and older adults' physical health. *Gerontologist.* pii:gnw051.

Farivar, S. *et al.* (2014) Biological effects of low level laser therapy. *J Lasers Med Sci.* **5**(2):58–62.

Hagiwara, S. *et al.* (2007) GaAlAs (830 nm) low-level laser enhances peripheral endogenous opioid analgesia in rats. *Lasers Surg Med.* **39**(10):797–802.

Hagiwara, S. *et al.* (2008) Pre-Irradiation of blood by gallium aluminum arsenide (830 nm) low-level laser enhances peripheral endogenous opioid analgesia in rats. *Anesth Analg.* **107**(3):1058–1063.

Hamblin, M.R. and Demidova, T.N. (2006) Mechanisms of low level light therapy. *Proc of SPIE.* **6140**(612001):1–12.

Huang, Z. *et al.* (2015) The effectiveness of low-level laser therapy for nonspecific chronic low back pain: a systematic review and meta-analysis. *Arthritis Res Ther.* **17**:360.

Kathuria, V. *et al.* (2015) Low level laser therapy: a panacea for oral maladies. *Laser Ther.* **24**(3):215–223.

Kuffler, D.P. (2016) Photobiomodulation in promoting wound healing: a review. *Regen Med.* **11**(1):107–122.

Labajos, M. (1988) Beta-endorphin levels modification after GaAs and HeNe laser irradiation on the rabbit. *Comparative study. Invest Clin.* **1–2**:6–8.

Landsberg, G.M. *et al.* (2011) Clinical signs and management of anxiety, sleeplessness, and cognitive dysfunction in the senior pet. *Vet Clin North Am Small Anim Pract.* **41**(3):565–590.

Landsberg, G.M. *et al.* (2012) Cognitive dysfunction syndrome: a disease of canine and feline brain aging. *Vet Clin North Am Small Anim Pract.* **42**(4):749–768.

Maegawa, Y. *et al.* (2000) Effects of near-infrared low-level laser irradiation on microcirculation. *Lasers Surg Med.* **27**(5):427–437.

Medrado, A.R. *et al.* (2003) Influence of low level laser therapy on wound healing and its biological action upon myofibroblasts. *Lasers Surg Med.* **32**(3):239–244.

Montesinos, M. (1988) Experimental effects of low power laser in encephalin and endorphin synthesis. *J Eur Med Laser Assoc.* **1**(3):2–7.

Naeser, M.A. *et al.* (2014) Significant improvements in cognitive performance post-transcranial, red/near-infrared light-emitting diode treatments in chronic, mild traumatic brain injury: open-protocol study. *J Neurotrauma.* **31**(11):1008–1017.

Payne, E. *et al.* (2016) Exploring the existence and potential underpinnings of dog-human and horse-human attachment bonds. *Behav Processes.* **125**:114–121.

Peplow, P.V. *et al.* (2010) Laser photobiomodulation of wound healing: a review of experimental studies in mouse and rat animal models. *Photomed Laser Surg.* **28**(3):291–325.

Potter, A. and Mills, D.S. (2015) Domestic cats (*Felis silvestris catus*) do not show signs of secure attachment to their owners. *PLoS One.* **10**(9):e0135109.

PR Newswire. (2016) Packaged facts: key trends shaping the U.S. pet industry. Available from: http://www.prnewswire.com/news-releases/packaged-facts-key-trends-shaping-the-us-pet-industry-300028033.html (accessed November 30, 2016).

Pryor, B. and Millis, D.L. (2015) Therapeutic laser in veterinary medicine. *Vet Clin North Am Small Anim Pract.* **45**(1):45–56.

Rodier, L. (2016) Caring for an elderly dog: what an owner thinks of as "just old age" is often a treatable illness. Available from: http://www.whole-dog-journal.com/issues/13_1/features/Diagnosing-Older-Dogs-Illnes_16189-1.html?zkPrintable=true (accessed November 30, 2016).

Schütt, T. *et al.* (2015) Cognitive function, progression of age-related behavioral changes, biomarkers, and survival in dogs more than 8 years old. *J Vet Intern Med.* **29**(6):1569–1577.

Tabakoglu, H.O. *et al.* (2015) Assessment of circular wound healing in rats after exposure to 808-nm laser pulses during specific healing phases. *Lasers Surg Med.* **48**(4):409–415.

19

Feline-Specific Conditions

Jennifer O. Lavallee and James Olson

Cat Specialist, Castle Rock, CO, USA

Introduction

New technology and change are always feared and criticized:

> At first they said it was new, it would not work, and it would be gone in a short time; then they said it might work, but poorly, and no one would find it useful; then they said it appears to have some uses, but there are no valid studies that verify its effectiveness; then they said, it works, but with significant limitations; and finally they said it works very well, and it is in common use, but everyone has known that it would work from the start.
>
> *Anonymous*

Laser therapy in veterinary medicine has taken exactly this route, and veterinary practitioners have come to be among the technology's biggest advocates. Therapeutic and rehabilitation medicine have benefited from the reduction of pain and swelling and the increased healing responses. More long-term evidence-based studies are being driven by positive reports from individual patient outcomes.

In feline practice, our patients hide both their signs of disease and their response to treatment, which makes it harder to evaluate the efficacy of treatments. Laser therapy, or photobiomodulation therapy (PBMT) as it is increasingly being known, appears to work very well in cats as a primary or adjunct treatment modality. It is a new magic that, when combined with all the other standards of care, allows doctors to directly attack complex medical conditions. Photobiomodulation (PBM) has the benefit of potentiating response to bacterial, fungal, and viral agents, and activates a healing immune response in damaged tissue. It has become a valuable ally in the war on pain.

Smart veterinarians do not limit themselves by current "catma" (a.k.a., dogma). Giving our patients all sound medical options is why we became doctors. Most of what we do in feline practice is not backed by extensive research and evidence-based medicine, because the cat has not been thought of by the veterinary community and pharmaceutical companies as a "cash cow." In fact, an estimated 80% of the prescriptions given to felines are not Food and Drug Administration (FDA) approved in cats (at all, or for the particular condition prescribed), but as practitioners we use them off-label every day. Feline practitioners have adapted studies from other species, collected funds for specific feline research, and looked for safe and effective ways to treat feline disease.

Higher-power therapy lasers were FDA-approved for use in the United States in 2003. Since that time, they have become widely used in veterinary practice. As is presented throughout this text in the large number of references cited, there is a preponderance of publications representing laboratory bench-top studies, animal-model studies, and clinical trials in animals and humans. Cross-species applications of the knowledge from these studies continues to expand the use of PBMT in many species, including cats.

Individualized Feline Treatment Plans

For the ease of our staff and clients, we generally recommend one of four laser therapy treatment plans as an initial treatment cycle:

1) **Single-session laser treatment.**
2) **Three-session laser treatment package:** Most commonly, these treatments are spaced daily or every other day until complete.
3) **Six-session laser treatment package:** Most commonly, this is achieved with treatments three

times a week for 2 weeks, and then subsequent treatments are performed as needed.

4) **Twelve-session laser treatment package:** Most commonly, this is achieved with treatments three times a week for 4 weeks, and then subsequent treatments are performed as needed.

How to Calculate a Laser Therapy Treatment Dose

Predictable and reproducible results from PBMT are dependent on the delivery of an appropriate dose of photonic energy to the target tissue. In laser therapy, dose is expressed as a number of joules (J) delivered to a surface area of the body (cm^2) (Enwemeka, 2009). Relevant current publications from animal-model studies and clinical trials from multiple species indicate that appropriate dosing for most conditions that are superficial in tissue is in the $1-4 J/cm^2$ range (Peplow *et al.*, 2010), while dosing for most deep-tissue conditions is in the $8-20 J/cm^2$ range (Bjordal *et al.*, 2003; Roberts *et al.*, 2013).

Protocols for the treatment of specific feline conditions are available in the software of some newer-generation, veterinary-specific therapy lasers. These software-defined treatment protocols are designed to deliver an appropriate dose of laser energy. New software allows for the input of patient-specific characteristics, including body type, skin color, and coat length and color. The software uses this information to devise a protocol ensuring a correct dose is delivered with maximum photon penetration.

Treatments can also be administered using operator-defined protocols, in which the total dose is manually calculated. The steps by which to manually calculate the total dose to be delivered are as follows:

1) Determine the appropriate dose for the condition in J/cm^2 (Jenkins and Carroll, 2011).
2) Determine the size of the area to be treated in cm^2. For reference, a CD or a 3×5 in (7.6×12.7 cm) index card is roughly $100 cm^2$.
3) Multiply the dose in J/cm^2 by the area in cm^2 to calculate the total treatment dose in joules.
4) Set the laser power and treatment time to deliver the total treatment dose in joules. Using a continuous delivery (continuous wave, CW) allows for a shorter treatment time than would be provided by a pulsed delivery.

Determine the frequency of laser therapy treatments needed to achieve the treatment goals. The total number of sessions can be determined by assessing the severity and chronicity of the condition, as well as monitoring response to treatment. More severe or chronic conditions will often require a greater number of treatment sessions.

Feline-Specific Conditions

Abscess, Anal Sac

Anal sac abscesses are common. They typically develop when material within the anal sac becomes desiccated, the sac does not express well on its own, and a bacterial infection develops due to the lack of normal drainage (Zoran, 2005). Anal sacs have no functional use in the cat.

- **Diagnosis:** Appearance on physical exam is typically diagnostic. Most anal sac abscesses are discovered by the owner when a large, painful swelling is found at 4 or 8 o'clock to the anus, or when the sac ruptures, draining purulent material (Norsworthy, 2011).
- **Standard treatment:** Treatment usually consists of analgesia, anal gland expression (of residual material in both glands), topical clipping and cleaning, flushing, and systemic or topical antibiotics, or both.
- **Laser therapy:** The authors often use a short series (one to three sessions) of laser therapy applications to help treat anal gland abscesses, and have been very pleased with the outcome. The laser seems effective in reducing pain and swelling, decreasing pruritus, speeding healing, and treating the bacterial infection.
- **Prognosis:** Anal gland abscesses respond well to treatment, but recurrence is possible, so adding fiber to the diet and providing periodic anal gland expression may be indicated.
- **Dose:** $6-8 J/cm^2$.

Abscess, Cat-Bite

This common feline condition is an acute to chronic infectious process caused by a bite or puncture wound initially forming cellulitis and then forming a pocket of purulent material in the subcutaneous tissue.

- **Diagnosis:** Physical exam should identify a fluctuant to firm swelling, which is often painful. Fine-needle aspiration (FNA) of the swelling yields purulent material, and stained slides reveal bacteria and neutrophils. Many cases present with an open draining tract. Many cats with abscesses are febrile, lethargic, anorexic, and painful.
- **Standard treatment:** Closed abscesses should be lanced, drained, and flushed. Systemic antibiotics should be given (usually in the penicillin or cephalosporin groups) to combat *Pasturella* spp., *Staphylococcus* spp., and *Streptococcus* spp. Open abscesses with an existing draining tract should be clipped and cleaned. If the orifice of the draining tract is small, it may need to be opened wider to prevent closure. The owners are instructed to removed scabs and debris daily and let the wound heal from the inside out.

- **Laser therapy:** Immediate treatment of small to medium-sized puncture wounds or cellulitis swellings with only laser therapy treatment has worked well in stopping abscess formation in many patients. Most cats with an active abscess receive one to three laser treatment sessions. The authors have used therapy lasers often and quite successfully for the treatment of cat-bite abscesses.
- **Prognosis:** Cat-bite abscesses are expected to be responsive to treatment. Combining laser therapy into the treatment plan provides a more rapid response, with reduced swelling, reduced pain, and improved healing, and leaves the patient feeling better.
- **Dose:** 6–8 J/cm^2.

Allergic Dermatitis

Allergic dermatitis is an allergic skin syndrome that erupts with miliary lesions, causing pruritus, inflammation, destructive scratching, and varying degrees of discomfort. Prevalence is higher than previously suggested, and breed predispositions have been confirmed (Ravens *et al.*, 2014).

- **Diagnosis:** Physical exam will identify miliary crusts (numerous multifocal scabs), pruritus, and discomfort. Skin biopsies are rarely needed for diagnosis.
- **Standard treatment:** If an underlying allergic trigger can be identified and removed, this is the most definitive treatment. Many patients require therapy with a corticosteroid, cyclosporine, or oclacitinib.
- **Laser therapy:** Laser treatment protocols can decrease or remove dependence on medication. Laser therapy should be considered in any patient with allergic dermatitis, because it avoids drug side effects and improves long-term control. Maintenance therapy sessions can be spaced 7–60 days apart, depending on the condition and response. The authors have used laser therapy intermittently for miliary dermatitis and have been pleased with the clinical improvement. Itching is its own type of misery, so anything that helps is a positive!
- **Prognosis:** Allergic skin disease has many causes and often needs chronic treatment. Laser therapy has dramatically reduced inflammation and pruritus, and the speed of skin healing has been unexpected.
- **Dose:** 2–4 J/cm^2.

Arthritis

Arthritis is defined as chronic, progressive, degenerative joint disease, and is often seen in older patients. In cats, arthritis is most commonly found in the lumbar spine, lumbosacral junction, hips, stifles, elbows, and shoulders. One study (Slingerland *et al.*, 2011) found the large majority (90%) of cats over 12 years of age have radiographic changes of arthritis!

Feline arthritis is prone to under-diagnosis (Bennett *et al.*, 2012a). One challenge is that cats tend to hide pain and discomfort, due in part to their survival instinct. In the veterinary setting, cats may not walk around much in the exam room, especially compared with their canine counterparts, so gait dysfunction is hard to detect. Attention to owner-reported changes in mobility, particularly gait, jumping, and the use of stairs, is important (Klinck *et al.*, 2012).

> In medicine, more problems are missed by not looking than by not knowing.
>
> *Anonymous*

- **Diagnosis:** Cats may exhibit a variety of signs of arthritis, depending on the locations affected and the severity of the disease. Common signs include limping, trouble or reluctance to jump, lack of speed when getting up, short-strided gait, shuffling gait, sleeping more, playing less, and avoiding stairs. Physical exam may find muscle atrophy (from disuse), limited joint range of motion, and joint crepitus (Bennett *et al.*, 2012a). Properly positioned radiographs of suspected problem areas are needed to specifically help in the diagnosis. Note that radiographic sensitivity for arthritis is not 100%, as some arthritic change can be cartilaginous and not sufficiently ossified to be radiopaque. When in doubt, treat the patient.
- **Standard treatment:** Traditional treatment is often multimodal, as single-agent therapy can be insufficient for pain control and restoration of mobility (Bennett *et al.*, 2012b). Commonly used medications include glucosamine and chondroitin supplements, glycosaminoglycan, neuropathic pain-control medication (e.g., gabapentin), non-steroidal anti-inflammatories (with informed consent, if giving chronically), and fish oil. Acupuncture and physical therapy have also been applied. Supportive treatment can include modification of the environment: reducing joint stress by adding cat stairs to allow access to furniture, increasing traction on slippery floors with non-skid rugs, and putting food, water, and litter in relatively close proximity in the house.
- **Laser therapy:** Adding laser therapy treatments to traditional therapies reduces inflammation and reduces or eliminates pain. The authors have seen many patients show significant, rapid improvement in their mobility. Owners want to see their cat be active and play! Arthritis is one of the most frequent reasons we do long-term laser therapy treatments; the cat feels so much better.
- **Prognosis:** With a combined PBMT and traditional medical therapy plan, the treatment of arthritis is

greatly improved. Clients comment that their cat feels so much better after laser therapy treatments. Many patients may need a combination of treatments for best management of arthritis, but laser therapy has been a wonderful addition to our treatment options.

- **Dose:** 6–10 J/cm^2.

Asthma and Allergic Pulmonary Disease

Asthma and allergic pulmonary disease have eosinophilic and neutrophilic allergic inflammatory responses that cause bronchoconstriction, increased mucus production, and narrowing of the bronchi due to smooth-muscle hypertrophy. Allergic lung disease can be acute or chronic (Padrid, 2000).

- **Diagnosis:** Patients have a history of coughing, wheezing, lethargy, and dyspnea (loud, labored, tachypneic, open-mouth breathing). Physical exam may find tachypnea and crackles or wheezes on thoracic auscultation. Radiographs are usually the diagnostic test of choice and show a flat diaphragm with a classic bronchial pattern in the pulmonary parenchyma, giving the appearance of "lines and rings," representing thickened airways. Aerophagia can be found in more dyspneic cats with active clinical signs.
- **Immediate treatment:** Severely dyspneic cats need oxygen therapy and cage rest to minimize stress. Treatments such as corticosteroids and bronchodilators are commonly given.
- **Standard treatment:** The typical first-line treatment for feline asthma is a corticosteroid. The route of administration can be oral, injectable, inhaled, or transdermal. Bronchodilators are also used, both when steroids cannot be and as an additional treatment in more challenging cases. For asthmatic cats, it is important to consider the environment and look to minimize dust, perfumes, scents, second-hand smoke, and any other possible inhaled irritants.
- **Laser therapy:** Asthmatic cats have been treated with laser therapy at the thoracic inlet and both sides of the chest wall, with anecdotal response. Long-term maintenance treatments have been reported to be required as frequently as once a week after improvement from more frequent initial treatments (Thorsen, 2014). Flow cytometry assay has shown that laser therapy can help regulate T-helper 1 and T-helper 2 imbalance in asthmatic rats, having a similar effect to that of budesonide (Wang, 2014). Laser therapy inhibits bronchoconstriction, T-helper 2 inflammation, and airway remodeling in allergic asthma in mice (Silva *et al.*, 2014). Whether a similar effect occurs in cats has not been determined. The authors do not have any first-hand experience using the therapy laser for pulmonary disease.

- **Prognosis:** Feline asthma is often a chronic disease with acute flare-ups that needs ongoing treatment. The addition of laser therapy to reduce the inflammatory response in asthmatic patients could give the practitioner a powerful new tool in controlling this complex disease.
- **Dose:** 6–8 J/cm^2.

Cardiac Disease

Hypertrophic cardiomyopathy (HCM) is by far the most common cardiac disease in the cat, but others can be seen (e.g., dilated cardiomyopathy, restrictive cardiomyopathy).

- **Diagnosis:** Definitive diagnosis of cardiac disease rests on echocardiogram, often with an electrocardiogram. Clinical signs can range from asymptomatic to congestive heart failure (pulmonary edema or pleural effusion).
- **Standard treatment:** Dependent on the type and severity of cardiac disease, a multimodal medical management plan is recommended (angiotensin-converting enzyme (ACE) inhibitors, beta blockers, pimobendan, spironolactone, furosemide, clopidogrel, low-dose aspirin, and others).
- **Laser therapy:** The authors have not used laser therapy for the treatment of cardiac disease, so they cannot comment from first-hand experience. There are anecdotal reports of the use of laser therapy to reduce pain, increase muscle relaxation, and increase collateral circulation in the rear legs in cases of aortic saddle thrombus; this seems like a reasonable addition to treatment. For cardiac disease in general, the use of laser therapy over the chest wall appears to improve cardiac function when combined with standard medical therapy. On the human side, cardiac disease has been treated with laser therapy delivered intravascularly (Derkacz *et al.*, 2014).
- **Prognosis:** Cardiac disease often needs lifelong treatment and serial re-evaluation. Further investigation into laser therapy and cardiac disease is needed.
- **Dose:** 6–8 J/cm^2.

Constipation and Obstipation

Constipation is characterized by difficulty in passing stool, with straining, pain, and varying degrees of colonic distension. Studies have shown that constipation and obstipation in the cat appear to have primary pathology in the colon muscular wall.

- **Diagnosis:** Physical exam can identify firm stool in a distended colon, and radiographs can further define the extent of the problem.
- **Standard treatment:** Multiple medical treatments are often combined to achieve a successful outcome for

these patients: fluid therapy, enemas, prokinetic medications, laxatives, diets, nasogastric tube 24-hour dribble, and antibiotics (if there is concern for bacterial translocation). Some cats need to be sedated for manual de-obstipation.

- **Laser therapy:** Rapid reduction of inflammation and pain, getting the muscles of the colon to function, and promotion of a healing response can decrease the chances of chronic fibrotic scarring. These goals would seem to indicate the use of laser therapy. The authors have limited use with the therapy laser in constipated cats to date, though responses have been positive. They will continue to use laser as an adjunctive treatment in constipated cats.
- **Prognosis:** The prognosis is variable and depends on the severity, chronicity, and underlying cause of the constipation, but laser therapy treatments, diet, and medical therapy have saved many cats' lives.
- **Dose:** $6–10 J/cm^2$.

Dental Extractions, Gingivitis, and Periodontal Disease

Oral disease can include tooth resorption, tooth fractures, periodontal disease, and gingivitis.

- **Diagnosis:** Diagnosis is based on oral examination and dental radiographs, where appropriate.
- **Standard treatment:** Dental prophylaxis, procedures, antibiotics, and oral surgery are indicated.
- **Laser therapy:** The laser helps reduce pain and swelling and encourages rapid healing. The authors use laser therapy as a standard treatment following dental extractions, typically while the cat is still under anesthesia.
- **Prognosis:** The prognosis depends on the specific dental condition.
- **Dose:** $3–4 J/cm^2$ if the mouth is open; $6–8 J/cm^2$ if it is closed.

Eosinophilic Granuloma Complex

Eosinophilic granuloma complex (EGC) is a collection of ulcerated skin lesions (including indolent ulcer, eosinophilic plaques, and eosinophilic granuloma) that contain large numbers of eosinophils (Buckley and Nuttall, 2012). There may be a genetic predisposition, allergic triggers, or both.

- **Diagnosis:** The location and appearance of lesions are often suspect for EGC, but cytology or histopathology can confirm the diagnosis, if needed.
- **Standard treatment:** Treatment is aimed at reduction of inflammation and allergic triggers. It may include corticosteroids, cyclosporine, hypoallergenic diets, and flea control, with varying degrees of success. Eosinophilic granulomas on the tongue or elsewhere

in the mouth are best treated initially with CO_2 laser ablation surgery.

- **Laser therapy:** With the advent of laser therapy, EGC treatment has been improved. Traditional treatments can be combined with laser therapy to get the best healing effect. The authors have used laser therapy as part of the treatment of EGC, but not as a standalone treatment. Combining laser therapy and traditional medical therapy appears to work the best.
- **Prognosis:** Many cats with EGC need long-term treatment. Traditional treatment works very well in many patients, but the use of medications has the drawback of producing side effects and immune suppression. PBMT can lessen the amount of medication and the frequency needed.
- **Dose:** Low dose: $3–4 J/cm^2$; high dose: $20–30 J/cm^2$. Though the lesions and tissues involved seem to indicate that a low dose would be appropriate, anecdotal reports from practitioners indicate better responses have been seen clinically when treating EGC with high doses, as are recommended for some granulomatous conditions in other species, such as lick granulomas in dogs. To avoid patient discomfort when using the high dose, a low power setting of $2–4 W$ delivered over a longer time is recommend (versus a higher power over a shorter time).

Feline Acne

Feline acne, chin acne, or chin pyoderma is an acute to chronic inflammatory skin condition involving the chin and lips.

- **Diagnosis:** Location and visual appearance are usually sufficient for diagnosis. The classic milder presentation of chin acne has black debris (dirt-like in appearance) and comedones with minimal inflammation. The purulent form is painful, has pustules and furuncles, and has moderate to severe inflammation (Jazic *et al.*, 2006).
- **Standard treatment:** Clip the hair off the chin, clean thoroughly with an antimicrobial shampoo, and apply topical antibiotic ointment (often mupirocin) daily. Systemic antibiotics are used if the infection is extensive and deep.
- **Laser therapy:** Feline acne appears to have an exaggerated inflammatory response, and PBMT removes the red, sore component of the disease, often within in the first 24 hours. The authors often use a single session or a short series of laser therapy treatments for feline acne, especially if severe.
- **Prognosis:** Feline acne has a good prognosis. Some patients have complete resolution and no further need for treatment, but others require ongoing care. Laser therapy laser has been remarkably helpful in severe or recurrent cases.
- **Dose:** $3–4 J/cm^2$.

Fracture Healing

- **Diagnosis:** Physical exam and radiographs are diagnostic for most fractures, though computed tomography (CT) is helpful as well.
- **Standard treatment:** Rigid to semi-rigid stabilization of the fracture site.
- **Laser therapy:** The rate of bone healing can be increased, and in some patients has been anecdotally reported to be twice as fast as the expected healing time. Laser therapy stimulation of non-union fractures can restart the healing process and may help avoid more invasive techniques. Multiple publications have demonstrated the effect that laser therapy has on fracture healing in lab animals, improving bone healing by activating osteogenic factors and accelerating the development of newly formed bone (Jawad *et al.*, 2013; Son *et al.*, 2012; Tim *et al.*, 2014). The authors have been very pleased with the addition of laser therapy when treating patients with fractures. Laser therapy has also been demonstrated to be effective in treating experimental chronic osteomyelitis induced in rats by methicillin-resistant *Staphylococcus aureus* (MRSA) (Kaya *et al.*, 2011).
- **Prognosis:** With proper alignment, fixation, rest, and the addition of therapy laser, the prognosis for fracture healing is good.
- **Dose:** $6–10\,\mathrm{J/cm}^2$.

Hyperesthesia Syndrome

Hyperesthesia is an acute uncomfortable to painful episode characterized by frantic licking, crying, skin twitching, tail twitching, and running away (Ciribassi, 2009). Locations that show increased sensitivity are often the flanks, back, limbs, and tail base. Episode frequency varies by patient.

- **Diagnosis:** The history reported by the owner can often lead to a tentative diagnosis. Videos taken by the owner are quite helpful as well. On physical exam, there may be hypersensitivity to touch. A needle (we use a 22 gauge 1.5") can be lightly touched to the fur at a tangential angle to screen for an oversensitive response, which could be excessive skin twitching, vocalizing, or hissing or growling. Other potential causes of pain and hypersensitivity should be ruled out.
- **Standard treatment:** Corticosteroids, phenobarbital, and gabapentin have been used with variable degrees of success. Other options are calming diets or pheromone collars. Given the potential for a neurogenic etiology to this condition, injectable B-vitamins have also been tried, with modest success.
- **Laser therapy:** The authors have used laser therapy in cats with hyperesthesia with mixed results. The treatment site is usually where licking or skin twitching occurs. Some patients had complete resolution of symptoms after a single treatment, while others had minimal response after a series of treatments. Given the potential benefit, laser therapy is always offered to clients.
- **Prognosis:** Hyperesthesia is commonly a chronic condition that needs chronic therapy, but some patients appear to have been cured with laser therapy sessions.
- **Dose:** $3–4\,\mathrm{J/cm}^2$.

Inflammatory Bowel Disease

Inflammatory bowel disease (IBD) is a common immune-mediated and inflammatory disease of the small intestine.

- **Diagnosis:** IBD is a diagnosis of exclusion. Most cats have a history of chronic vomiting (including hairballs), weight loss, diarrhea, or some combination thereof. Abdominal ultrasound gives important clues to intestinal disease: diffuse or segmental thickening of the small intestine wall (>0.28 cm), with or without enlarged mesenteric lymph nodes. The diagnostic gold standard is exploratory laparotomy with multiple (three or more) biopsies of the small intestine (Norsworthy *et al.*, 2015). For cases of IBD, histopathology will identify enteritis. At this point, treatment trials need to exclude other causes (e.g., dysbiosis, food intolerance, parasitic disease, cobalamin deficiency, etc.). Surgical biopsy and histopathology will differentiate between enteritis and neoplasia. This is a very important point because enteritis can safely be treated with laser therapy and, in general, neoplasia should not be. There are clinical reports that laser therapy has been used with IBD patients to enhance quality of life by improving appetite, decreasing vomiting, decreasing nausea, decreasing pain, and improving general well-being (Karnia, 2014).
- **Standard treatment:** IBD is typically treated with corticosteroids, probiotics, a hypoallergenic diet, and B-vitamin supplementation. Some patients improve with the addition of antibiotics.
- **Laser therapy:** PBMT is a reasonable addition to treatment, as it will encourage a healing response by decreasing inflammation and allowing the intestines to return to a more normal state. The authors have used laser therapy on a handful of cases of IBD (biopsy-diagnosed cases of enteritis with exclusion of other differentials), always with other treatments given concurrently. The addition of laser therapy did not yield impressive results, so no patient continued long-term. It is hard to draw definitive conclusions, though, given the small number of cases. We did not see any adverse events, so trying laser is reasonable.

- **Prognosis:** IBD is a chronic condition where control is likely, but a cure is not expected. Most patients need long-term therapy.
- **Dose:** 6–10 J/cm^2.

Kidney Diseases

Multiple diseases can cause chronic dysfunction of the kidneys, including chronic kidney disease (CKD), congenital kidney disease, polycystic kidney disease (PKD), hydronephrosis, perinephric pseudocyst, obstructive nephrosis, pyelonephritis, infections (e.g., feline infectious peritonitis, leptospirosis), neoplasia (e.g., lymphoma), glomerulonephritis, renolithiasis, and ureterolithiasis. Multiple recent publications have attempted to clarify what is known about the diagnosis and management of feline CKD (Brown *et al.*, 2016; Sparkes *et al.*, 2016).

- **Diagnosis:** Kidney dysfunction is most often detected on blood chemistries where biomarkers are elevated (blood urea nitrogen (BUN), creatinine, symmetric dimethylarginine (SDMA)). Urinalysis is also key to renal disease, via assessment of specific gravity, microscopic sediment evaluation, urine culture and sensitivity, and urine protein–creatinine ratio. Physical exam may detect abnormalities in kidney palpation. Radiographs, ultrasound, and renal biopsy may also be helpful, depending on the underlying condition.
- **Standard treatment:** Treatment varies by the specific disease.
- **Laser therapy:** If renal neoplasia is suspected or possible, do not use laser therapy. For non-neoplastic disease, laser therapy can be considered.
- **Prognosis:** The prognosis depends on the specific underlying disease and the severity of renal dysfunction.
- **Dose:** 8–10 J/cm^2.

Liver Diseases

There are a multitude of disease processes that can create liver disease: hepatic lipidosis, cholangiohepatitis, triaditis, toxic insults, and infectious hepatopathies (toxoplasmosis, feline infectious peritonitis, liver flukes, and histoplasmosis). In the cat, primary hepatic neoplasia is seen, but metastatic disease is more common.

- **Diagnosis:** Clinical signs are non-specific: anorexia, lethargy, vomiting, and weight loss. Laboratory testing may reveal elevated liver enzymes, hyperbilirubinemia, or hypoalbuminemia. Bile acids may be normal or abnormal. Ultrasound is typically the preferred imaging modality. Definitive diagnosis of liver disease often requires biopsy or FNA with cytopathology and histopathology (Lidbury and Suchodolski, 2016).
- **Standard treatment:** Treat the specific disease or the associated clinical signs. A combination of medications can be selected as appropriate, but options include anti-inflammatories, antibiotics, antioxidants, B-vitamin supplementation, antiemetics, antacids, analgesics, fluid therapy, chemotherapeutic drugs, and nutritional support/feeding tubes.
- **Laser therapy:** If inflammatory liver disease is the primary concern then laser therapy may be added to the treatment protocol. The authors have not treated liver disease with laser therapy alone, but it is a reasonable treatment addition.
- **Prognosis:** The prognosis depends on the disease entity and response to treatment.
- **Dose:** 6–10 J/cm^2.

Musculoskeletal Acute Injury

Usually, trauma is the primary cause of acute musculoskeletal injury, but metabolic, immune-mediated, infectious, and toxic events can also cause injury.

- **Diagnosis:** Most musculoskeletal injuries are diagnosed based on history and physical exam. Imaging studies may be appropriate in some cases.
- **Standard treatment:** A specific treatment depends on the cause and extent of the problem, but often includes analgesia, anti-inflammatory medication, and rest.
- **Laser therapy:** Laser therapy can help decrease inflammation and pain, can speed the healing response, and usually makes the patient feel better sooner. The authors have been very pleased with the positive and rapid response in cats with acute injuries.
- **Prognosis:** The prognosis depends on the underlying condition.
- **Dose:** 8–10 J/cm^2.

Neuropathy, Peripheral

Feline peripheral neuropathies are an immune-mediated or secondary sequel, most often linked to poorly regulated diabetes mellitus, chemotherapy, and vitamin deficiencies (e.g., thiamine).

- **Diagnosis:** Cats with neuropathy may display dropped tarsi or carpi (most classic in diabetic peripheral neuropathy), numbness, hypersensitivity to touch, pain, ataxia, and impaired limb function. A home video taken by the owner may be helpful, as some cats do not walk normally when in the hospital – they may refuse to move or be crouched and guarded.
- **Standard treatment:** If the underlying cause is determined, then treatment is generally aimed at that cause. Specific treatments for neuropathy are not well outlined in cats. Treatment options include supplemental B$_{12}$ and B-complex vitamins (thiamine), analgesics, and anti-inflammatory medications.
- **Laser therapy:** The authors are still early in their use of laser therapy for neuropathy. This may be a

condition where it is hard to fully assess response; some symptoms of neuropathy reported in humans (itching, burning, or tingling) are difficult to assess in cats, before or after treatment. The inhibitory effects of laser therapy on peripheral mammalian nerves have been well established in multiple publications (Chow *et al.*, 2007, 2011). A human study demonstrated laser therapy was effective in reducing the symptoms of painful, diabetic peripheral neuropathy in type 2 diabetes mellitus (Cg *et al.*, 2015). Therefore, laser therapy is reasonable, especially in a cat that simply "isn't him/herself" and has a condition that may be associated with neuropathy or appropriate clinical signs. We have been pleased with clients reporting positive changes in their cats at home.

- **Prognosis:** Neuropathy can be a chronic condition, but resolution is possible. The use of laser therapy can improve function and remove discomfort. No other therapies offer the relief that laser therapy does for this condition.
- **Dose:** $6-10\,\mathrm{J/cm^2}$.

Otitis Externa

Otitis externa has multiple causes, which involve acute to chronic disease: infections (typically bacterial or fungal, or both), anatomical ear canal problems (sebaceous adenomas that narrow the ear canal), inflammation (allergies or immune-mediated), overproduction of wax, and possibly a humid environment. Due to their upright pinna, cats have fewer chronic ear problems than dog breeds with folded pinna.

- **Diagnosis:** Otitis externa is typically identified on physical exam and confirmed with cytology of otic debris. Most cats have more than one underlying issue, so defining the problems will help in developing a treatment plan (Kennis, 2013).
- **Standard treatment:** Most cats are treated with some combination of antibiotic, antifungal, and anti-inflammatory medications (as topical and additional oral medication if more severe). Analgesia is important in allowing effective at-home care. Ear cleaners and wax solvents are used when there is significant debris buildup. If foreign material is present (e.g., foxtails), this needs to be removed.
- **Laser therapy:** The use of laser therapy in feline patients with otitis externa has produced excellent results. In the short term, most patients receive standard treatment and laser therapy sessions. The authors have seen infections resolve more readily, wax production decrease, and inflammation and discomfort reduce. Hard-to-treat cases have resolved with the addition of laser treatment. Most patients receive six laser sessions during acute infections. In the authors' experience, patients afflicted by chronic recurrent otitis have been good candidates for laser therapy. When not in an acute episode, they have been treated with intermittent (every 3–4 weeks) long-term laser therapy and avoided flare-ups and the need for other medications.
- **Prognosis:** Otitis externa is often a manageable problem, but in some patients it is chronic and recurrent. Laser therapy in combination with standard therapy has been very effective in managing many patients that would otherwise be doomed to lifelong ear cleaning and ear medications.
- **Dose:** Superficial component: $3-4\,\mathrm{J/cm^2}$; deep component: $8-10\,\mathrm{J/cm^2}$. When treating otitis, two components, or anatomical areas, must be addressed. The first is the affected portion of the pinna and the visible, more distal portion of the ear canal. These tissues should be treated with a laser setting that delivers $3-4\,\mathrm{J/cm^2}$ and, usually, with a non-contact delivery. The second component is the more proximal, deeper portion of the ear canal. This deeper tissue component requires a higher target dose of $8-10\,\mathrm{J/cm^2}$ and is most commonly treated with a contact delivery.

Pancreatitis

Pancreatitis is an inflammatory disease of the pancreas that can be acute or chronic and smoldering. Compared to dogs, cats tend to have the milder, more chronic form of pancreatitis, which can be associated with concurrent triaditis. Pancreatic neoplasia and exocrine pancreatic insufficiency are uncommon in the cat.

- **Diagnosis:** Clinical signs are non-specific: anorexia, lethargy, vomiting, weight loss, and, to a lesser extent, fever and abdominal pain. Laboratory tests are available, but are imperfect (Lidbury and Suchodolski, 2016). The preferred test is feline pancreatic lipase immunoreactivity (fPLI). The gold standard for diagnosis is surgical biopsy with histopathology, but this may not be feasible.
- **Standard treatment:** There is no specific treatment for pancreatitis, but supportive care typically involves fluid therapy, pain management, nutritional support (with feeding tubes, if necessary), antiemetics, antacids, B-vitamin supplementation, and possibly antibiotics and corticosteroids.
- **Laser therapy:** Laser may be helpful in reducing inflammation and pain during the healing process. The authors have used laser therapy in conjunction with other standard treatments, so it has been hard to appreciate the specific response to laser therapy, but treatment was well tolerated.
- **Prognosis:** Prognosis can be quite variable, depending on the severity of the disease and the response to treatment.
- **Dose:** $8-10\,\mathrm{J/cm^2}$.

Rhinitis and Sinusitis

Rhinitis and sinusitis are often chronic conditions that are rooted in underlying infection (viral, bacterial, and sometimes fungal), the presence of a foreign body, tumors, polyps, and inflammation, which creates scarring of the nasal passages (Reed, 2014). In some patients, these conditions extend into the frontal sinuses.

- **Diagnosis:** Rhinitis and sinusitis are often presumptively diagnosed based on history (sneezing, oculonasal discharge, exposure to irritants, duration) and evidence of upper respiratory congestion on physical exam. Definitive diagnosis may be achieved via cytology, radiographs, biopsies, nasal flushes, rhinoscopic exam, bacterial culture and sensitivity, and polymerase chain reaction (PCR) testing.
- **Standard treatment:** Often, therapy begins with empirical treatment of the most likely cause. Upper respiratory infection is usually the first choice, and the treatments are antibiotics, antiviral medications, and supportive care. With more diagnostics, other treatment plans can be developed.
- **Laser therapy:** Laser therapy has given the practitioner the advantage of treating both infectious and inflammatory triggers in nasal disease and may be a good adjunct to standard treatments. If there is any question whether a neoplasia is present, do not use laser therapy. A recent study with human cadaver skulls demonstrated that photons of near-infrared laser therapy wavelengths do penetrate through bone (Tedford *et al.*, 2015). Protective eyewear goggles (rated for laser therapy wavelengths) must be worn by the patient for treatments around the eyes (Figure 19.1).
- **Prognosis:** Rhinitis and sinusitis are often chronic, frustrating conditions. Therefore, having laser therapy

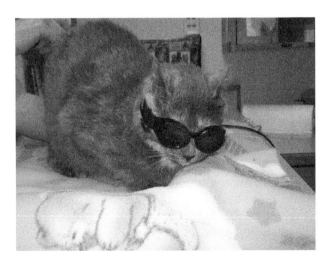

Figure 19.1 Protective eyewear goggles (rated for laser therapy wavelengths) must be worn by the patient during treatments around the eyes.

as another treatment option is helpful in challenging cases.
- **Dose:** $8-10 \, \text{J/cm}^2$.

Surgery, Treating Incisions Postoperatively

- **Standard treatment:** Appropriate analgesia is always recommended for the procedure.
- **Laser therapy:** Laser is safe for use after most surgeries; however, as detailed in Chapter 7, care should be exercised during use around eyes, thyroid glands, tumors, or testicles in breeding cats. The authors use laser therapy on all other surgical incisions. Laser can encourage more rapid healing, with a reduction in post-surgical pain.
- **Dose:** $3-4 \, \text{J/cm}^2$.

Urinary Tract Disease, Lower

There are several possible underlying diseases that can create lower urinary tract disease in the cat, including: idiopathic cystitis, urinary tract infection, urinary calculi, neoplasia (uncommon), and urethral obstruction (in males).

- **Diagnosis:** Many cats with lower urinary tract disease have a history of pollakiruia, stranguria, dysuria, vocalization, and urinating outside the litterbox. Physical exam should include palpation of the bladder and kidneys and observation of the sheath and penis. Diagnostic tests routinely include a cystocentesis for urinalysis with urine culture and ultrasound or radiographic imaging, or both. Evaluation of the urinary tract, and especially the bladder, cannot be effectively done without ultrasound!
- **Standard treatment:** Treat the specific underlying cause.
- **Laser therapy:** If inflammation, pain, or urethral obstruction is present, it is reasonable to treat with laser therapy. Many patients regain urinary function and feel better sooner. They start eating and drinking, and act like cats again. Idiopathic cystitis patients that have been unresponsive to standard forms of treatment regularly respond to laser therapy, and many patients become asymptomatic in the long term. The authors have been very impressed with the benefits of laser therapy for urethral obstruction and have repeatedly seen initial laser treatment unblock an obstructed patient before passage of a urethral catheter. Laser treatments are safe to perform with an indwelling urinary catheter. Lower urinary tract diseases in the cat seem to be very responsive to laser therapy!
- **Prognosis:** The prognosis depends on the underlying cause.
- **Dose:** $8-10 \, \text{J/cm}^2$.

Vestibular Disease, Peripheral

The vestibular system maintains the position of the head in relation to the eyes, neck, trunk, and limbs. It is the gyroscope of the body.

- **Diagnosis:** Clinical signs include head tilt, falling, rolling, nystagmus, loss of equilibrium, wide-based stance, and ataxic movements. A neurological exam can often differentiate between peripheral and central vestibular disease. Thorough examination of the ear canals and tympanum can help evaluate whether otitis media might be present as a possible cause of peripheral vestibular disease. Skull radiographs and more advanced imaging (CT or magnetic resonance imaging (MRI)) can improve diagnostic efforts.
- **Standard treatment:** Treatment depends on the cause. The use of anti-inflammatories (often corticosteroids) and antibiotics is common.
- **Laser therapy:** Laser therapy of the ear canal, middle ear, and inner ear appears to make cats feel better. Laser therapy treatment enhances immune response to bacteria and yeast, reduces swelling, decreases wax formation, and opens the ear canal for better air circulation. The authors have found laser therapy to be an excellent addition to the treatment of vestibular disease, with many cats seemingly experiencing less pain and a quicker than typical recovery.
- **Prognosis:** Outcomes are variable depending on the severity of the underlying cause and how quickly successful treatment is implemented.
- **Dose:** 4–6 J/cm^2.

Wound Healing

A 2016 literature review of the effects of laser therapy on wound healing in different animal models, *in vitro* and clinically, demonstrated that wound healing is induced by PBM despite there being some discrepancy about optimal treatment parameters (Kuffler, 2016).

- **Diagnosis:** History and visual examination of the patient are usually sufficient for diagnosis.
- **Standard treatment:** Most patients with wounds require wet or dry bandages, antibiotics, analgesics, and serial re-evaluation. Larger wounds, or those in areas of skin movement (limbs and joints), may be most challenging during the healing process. Some wounds may require surgical intervention.
- **Laser therapy:** The authors routinely use laser therapy for wound healing because of the consistent positive results. Wounds heal much faster when treated with the laser than without, which is particularly helpful when dealing with extensive tissue damage. Laser therapy should be a go-to in the treatment of trauma patients.
- **Prognosis:** Most patients with wounds have a good prognosis for long-term recovery, but restriction of activity and the need to keep wound sites clean can be challenging, depending on the extent and location of the wound.
- **Dose:** Superficial wound 3-4 J/cm^2; deep wounds 8 J/cm^2.

Case Studies

Idiopathic Cystitis

Idiopathic cystitis is a common, painful, and often recurrent disease of the lower urinary tract that can make management frustrating. The ultrasound images in Figure 19.2 show the urinary bladder of a cat with significant irregular bladder thickening on initial exam. The cat was treated with six sessions of laser therapy over 1–2 weeks, and the repeat ultrasound showed a normal thin bladder wall. Laser therapy has proven to be a nice addition to treatment of these cats.

Overgrown Nails

Nails that overgrow and puncture the digital pad can cause a persistent infection because of the structural fat in the pad. Cats' nails grow in a curve, and if they are not worn down or trimmed they can take on a ram's horn-type curl and puncture the digital paw pad (Figure 19.3). Laser therapy can minimize the chances of infection and promote quicker healing. The authors always recommend laser therapy when paw-pad injuries are identified.

Otitis Media and Peripheral Vestibular Disease

The combination of otitis media and peripheral vestibular disease is an uncommon diagnosis, but is one that requires rapid appropriate treatment if there is to be a chance of restoring normal function of the affected vestibular nerve where it courses through the middle ear. This case shows a kitten with a left-sided head tilt that was acute in onset. Physical exam found a bulging discolored tympanum on the left side. The cat was treated with oral broad-spectrum antibiotics, corticosteroids, and a series of six laser therapy sessions over 2 weeks. Figure 19.4 shows the head tilt on initial presentation and the marked improvement and resolution after laser therapy treatment sessions. The authors have found laser therapy to be a great asset in difficult cases of bacterial or yeast otitis with or without secondary vestibular disease.

Feline Acne

When the authors are presented with moderate to severe cases of feline acne, they routinely add a series of three laser therapy sessions on three consecutive days

(a) (b)

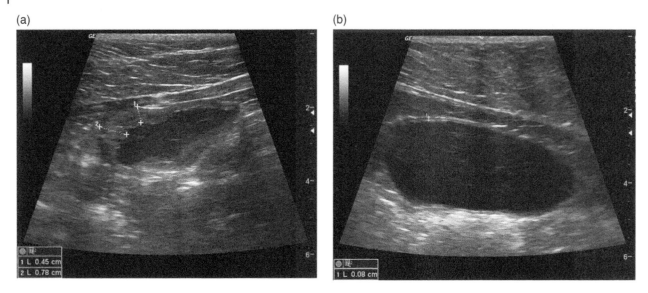

Figure 19.2 (a) Ultrasound image showing the urinary bladder of a cat with significant irregular bladder thickening on initial exam. Idiopathic cystitis was diagnosed. (b) Ultrasound image showing the urinary bladder of the same cat after six laser therapy treatments.

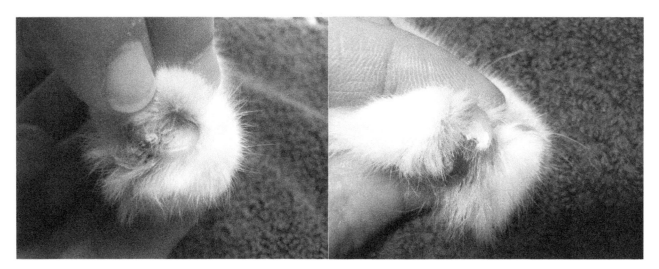

Figure 19.3 Curled nail appearance and the resulting paw-pad wound.

(a) (b)

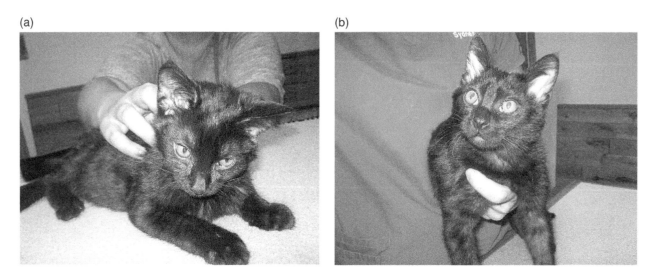

Figure 19.4 (a) Patient with head tilt from acute vestibular disease. (b) Resolution of head tilt from acute vestibular disease after six laser therapy sessions over 2 weeks.

(a)

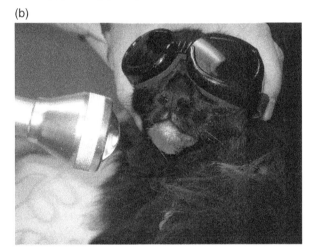

(b)

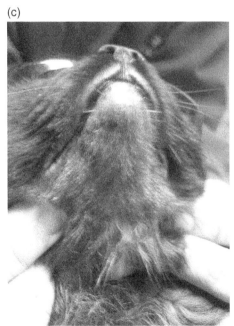

(c)

to help speed recovery. Figure 19.5 shows a case (a) upon presentation, (b) during a laser treatment session (wearing goggles), and (c) on a re-check visit 2 weeks later. This cat is a great example of the rapid positive responses seen.

Allergic Dermatitis

Allergic dermatitis can be an uncomfortable disease for the patient, and therefore one where any aid in speeding relief is important. The authors routinely use laser therapy on these cases. Figure 19.6a shows a cat with self-inflicted excoriation and dermal lesions on the belly due to allergic dermatitis. This seasonal flare-up was worse than typical; laser therapy was added as a series of three treatments over 1 week. The owner noted immediate relief of pruritus after the first treatment, and healing of skin lesions was 50% faster than expected. Figure 19.6b shows the skin without erythema and significant hair regrowth 3 weeks later.

(a)

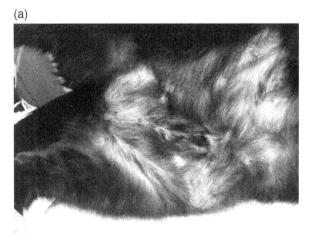

(b)

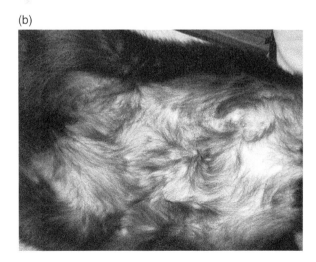

Figure 19.5 (a) Patient with feline acne lesions on presentation. (b) Laser therapy treatment of the same patient. (c) Resolution of the feline acne lesions 2 weeks after presentation, following three laser therapy sessions on three consecutive days.

Figure 19.6 (a) Self-inflicted excoriation and dermal lesions due to allergic dermatitis on presentation. (b) The same patient without erythema and with significant hair regrowth 3 weeks later, following three laser therapy treatments.

References

Bennett, D. *et al.* (2012a) Osteoarthritis in the cat: 1. How common is it and how easy to recognise? *J Feline Med Surg.* **14**(1):65–75.

Bennett, D. *et al.* (2012b) Osteoarthritis in the cat: 2. How should it be managed and treated? *J Feline Med Surg.* **14**(1):76–84.

Bjordal, J. *et al.* (2003) A systematic review of low level laser therapy with location specific doses for pain from chronic joint disorders. *Aust J Physiother.* **49**(2):107–116.

Brown, C.A. *et al.* (2016) Chronic kidney disease in aged cats: clinical features, morphology, and proposed pathogeneses. *Vet Pathol.* **53**(2):309–326.

Buckley, L. and Nuttall, T. (2012) Feline eosinophilic granuloma complex(ities): some clinical clarification. *J Feline Med Surg.* **14**(7):471–481.

Cg, S.K. (2015) Efficacy of low level laser therapy on painful diabetic peripheral neuropathy. *Laser Ther.* **4**(3):195–200.

Chow, R.T. *et al.* (2007) 830 nm laser irradiation induces varicosity formation, reduces mitochondrial membrane potential and blocks fast axonal flow in small and medium diameter rat dorsal root ganglion neurons: implications for the analgesic effects of 830 nm laser. *J Peripher Nerv Syst.* **12**(1):28–39.

Chow, R.T. *et al.* (2011) Inhibitory effects of laser irradiation on peripheral mammalian nerves and relevance to analgesic effects: a systematic review. *Photomed Laser Surg.* **29**(6):365–381.

Ciribassi, J. (2009) Understanding behavior: feline hyperesthesia syndrome. *Compend Contin Educ Vet.* **31**(3):E10.

Derkacz, A. *et al.* (2014) Effects of intravascular low-level laser therapy during coronary intervention on selected growth factors levels. *Photomed Laser Surg.* **32**(10):582–587.

Enwemeka, C.S. (2009) Intricacies of dose in laser phototherapy for tissue repair and pain relief. *Photomed Laser Surg.* **3**:387–393.

Jawad, M.M. *et al.* (2013) Effect of 940 nm low-level laser therapy on osteogenesis in vitro. *J Biomed Opt.* **18**(12):12800.

Jazic, E. *et al.* (2006) An evaluation of the clinical, cytological, infectious and histopathological features of feline acne. *Vet Dermatol.* **17**(2):134–140.

Jenkins, P.A. and Carroll, J.D. (2011) How to report low-level laser therapy (LLLT)/photomedicine dose and beam parameters in clinical and laboratory studies. *Photomed Laser Surg.* **29**(12):785–787.

Karnia, J. (2014) Feline pancreatitis and IBD. In: *Atlas of Class IV Laser Therapy – Small Animal* [CD-ROM]. Southern Digital Publishing, Jackson, TN.

Kaya, G.S. *et al.* (2011) Use of 808-nm light therapy to treat experimental chronic osteomyelitis induced in rats by methicillin-resistant *Staphylococcus aureus. Photomed Laser Surg.* **29**(6):405–412.

Kennis, R.A. (2013) Feline otitis: diagnosis and treatment. *Vet Clin North Am Small Anim Pract.* **43**(1):51–56.

Klinck, M.P. *et al.* (2012) Owner-perceived signs and veterinary diagnosis in 50 cases of feline osteoarthritis. *Can Vet J.* **53**(11):1181–1186.

Kuffler, D.P. (2016) Photobiomodulation in promoting wound healing: a review. *Regen Med.* **11**(1):107–122.

Lidbury, J.A. and Suchodolski, J.S. (2016) New advances in the diagnosis of canine and feline liver and pancreatic disease. *Vet J.* **215**:87–95.

Norsworthy, G.D. (2011) Anal sac disease. In: *The Feline Patient*, 4 edn., pp. 16–17. Wiley-Blackwell, Ames, IA.

Norsworthy, G.D. *et al.* (2015) Prevalence and underlying causes of histologic abnormalities in cats suspected to have chronic small bowel disease: 300 cases (2008–2013). *J Am Vet Med Assoc.* **247**(6):629–635.

Padrid, P. (2000) Feline asthma. Diagnosis and treatment. *Vet Clin North Am Small Anim Pract.* **30**(6):1279–1293.

Peplow, P.V. *et al.* (2010) Laser photobiomodulation of wound healing: a review of experimental studies in mouse and rat animal models. *Photomed Laser Surg.* **28**(3):291–325.

Ravens, P.A. *et al.* (2014) Feline atopic dermatitis: a retrospective study of 45 cases (2001–2012). *Vet Dermatol.* **25**(2):95–102.

Reed, N. (2014) Chronic rhinitis in the cat. *Vet Clin North Am Small Anim Pract.* **44**(1):33–50.

Roberts, D.B. *et al.* (2013) The effectiveness of therapeutic class IV (10 W) laser treatment for epicondylitis. *Lasers Surg Med.* **45**(5):311–317.

Silva, V.R. *et al.* (2014) Low-level laser therapy inhibits bronchoconstriction, Th2 inflammation and airway remodeling in allergic asthma. *Respir Physiol Neurobiol.* **194**:37–48.

Slingerland, L.I. *et al.* (2011) Cross-sectional study of the prevalence and clinical features of osteroarthritis in 100 cats. *Vet J.* **187**(3):304–309.

Son, J. *et al.* (2012) Bone healing effects of diode laser (808 nm) on a rat tibial fracture model. *In Vivo.* **26**(4):703–709.

Sparkes, A.H. *et al.* (2016) ISFM consensus guidelines on the diagnosis and management of feline chronic kidney disease. *J Feline Med Surg.* **3**:219–239.

Tedford, C.E. *et al.* (2015) Quantitative analysis of transcranial and intraparenchymal light penetration in human cadaver brain tissue. *Lasers Surg Med.* **47**(4):312–322.

Thorsen, H. (2014) Feline asthma. In: *Atlas of Class IV Laser Therapy – Small Animal* [CD-ROM]. Southern Digital Publishing, Jackson, TN.

Tim, C.R. *et al.* (2014) Low-level laser therapy enhances the expression of osteogenic factors during bone repair in rats. *Lasers Med Sci.* **1**:147–156.

Wang, X.Y. (2014) Effect of low-level laser therapy on allergic asthma in rats. *Lasers Med Sci.* **29**(3):1043–1050.

Zoran, D.L. (2005) Rectoanal disease. In: *Textbook of Veterinary Internal Medicine*, 6 edn. Elsevier Saunders, St. Louis, MO.

Part V

Clinical Applications of Laser Therapy in Canine Sports Medicine

20

Laser Therapy for the Canine Athlete

Debra Canapp

Veterinary Orthopedic and Sports Medicine Group, Orthobiologic Innovations, Annapolis Junction, MD, USA

Laser Therapy for the Canine Athlete

Laser therapy, or photobiomodulation therapy (PBMT) as it is becoming increasingly known, has been used in the treatment of sports injuries in humans for decades (Ohshiro *et al.*, 1986). Its value and importance in conditioning and exercise have also been prominent in the human literature in the last 10 years (Ishide *et al.*, 2008). With the popularity of sports in the canine world increasing exponentially, and the value and dedication of our national working dogs, canine sports medicine and rehabilitation has become a "state of the art" and a compelling area of development in veterinary medicine (Figure 20.1). The results of bench-top research in other species are now being applied to canine athletes, with significant success. Though the quantity of studies using dogs is small, the benefit of laser therapy is recognized across many species, and there is thus interest in the direct study of the canine musculoskeletal system and the use of photobiomodulation (PBM) as a therapeutic tool.

Acute, stretch-induced muscle and tendon injuries are estimated to account for over 30% of the injuries seen in a typical human sports medicine practice and have been reported to be the most common injury seen in human general practices. Until recently, however, acute muscle and tendon injuries were rarely reported in the small-animal veterinary literature. Most discussion of chronic muscle and tendon disorders in dogs continues to be limited to a handful of classical syndromes and inflammatory conditions.

Given the similarities between the human and canine musculoskeletal systems, it can be imagined that injuries common in humans would also be common in canines, especially sports-related injuries. The low reported prevalence of muscle and tendon injuries in dogs is thus likely a result of a failure to diagnose these conditions.

The trauma sustained from sporting injuries causes damage to the soft tissues, such as muscles, tendons, and ligaments. These damaged cells and tissues release enzymes and cytokines, which provoke an inflammatory response within the body. The injury cascade results in redness, swelling, warmth, and pain in the injured area. When left untreated, persistent or recurrent inflammation can predispose canine athletes to degenerative changes in their joints, resulting in premature arthritis. Rehabilitation of these conditions in the canine athlete, as in humans, involves returning to sport as quickly and efficiently as possible, while providing the most optimal outcome for the injured tissue.

Historically, laser therapy has been shown to reduce tissue inflammation (Soriano *et al.*, 2006). Additionally, it has been shown to be effective against inflammatory arthritis, and can thus help lower the risk of chronic arthritis, which is frequently seen as a result of sports injuries (Castano *et al.*, 2007). For the past decade, laser therapy has had a well-established place in human sports medicine. PBMT is used by professional sports teams and athletes to treat inflammation, aid in pain relief, and assist in minimizing athletes' downtime. This expansion of laser therapy's use in human sports has helped support the research, clinical application, and current successful use of the technology in sporting and working dogs.

Sports Injuries in the Canine Athlete and Response to Laser Therapy

Clinical research is important in determining when and how a tool can be used effectively. Researchers propose technologies that might be used in treating a broad spectrum of injuries or disease states. Veterinarians must then decide whether a particular technology might be useful in the individual case before them.

This treatment method is known as "evidence-based medicine" (Davidoff *et al.*, 1995). Using established evidence, clinicians can determine when a therapy might benefit a patient. The clinician uses his or her judgment about when and where to apply the therapy. At times,

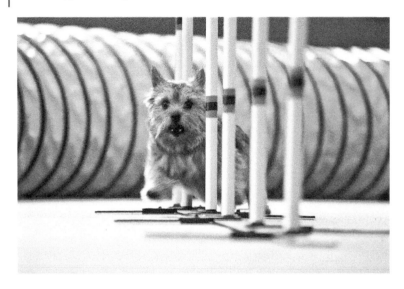

Figure 20.1 The popularity of sports in the canine world is increasing and canine sports medicine and rehabilitation has become a "state of the art" and compelling area of development in veterinary medicine.

there may be little evidence to support the use of a particular treatment in a particular species.

When considering the use of PBMT for the canine athlete, know that research specific to canine musculoskeletal injuries is limited. Many indications, protocols, and indications are taken from animal-model studies and human clinical trials and applied to our patients. Much of the research from these populations is confusing, however, since the parameters of the therapy vary from trial to trial. Even with this limitation, use of data across species has proven to be very successful clinically in the treatment of many sports-related injuries seen in the canine.

In spite of this experience, it is crucial for the veterinarian to be able to discern why a modality or treatment did or did not add benefit. It is important, for future success, that researchers describe consistently the parameters used in studies and trials. The results of treating veterinary patients should be well documented in the ongoing treatment plan.

Bjordal *et al.* (2006) made a systematic review of studies pertaining to the possible mechanism of action seen in the use of laser therapy. This meta-analysis revealed that PBM could reduce edema, post-injury bleeding, neutrophil cell influx, and cell apoptosis and improve microcirculation. Another article looked directly at tenocytes and laser therapy. It showed that the use of 660 nm at $1-2 J/cm^2$ stimulated tenocyte migration in a process that was mediated by up-regulation of dynamin 2 (Tsai *et al.*, 2012).

These basic parameters and proven theories can be applied to the successful treatment of many sports-related injuries. More clinically specific, whole-animal studies have also shown that following induction of partial tenotomies, the combination of kineseotherapy and phototherapy using 890 nm light was effective in healing sheep tendons (de Mattos *et al.*, 2015). This information

has successfully been extrapolated to dogs, with similar clinical outcomes in everyday practice.

Initial Rehabilitation Examination and Measurement

As with all initial examinations, the sports-injury examination should start with a thorough history, including how the injury occurred, what sports are played, and the patient's general attitude and energy level. This is important information by which to facilitate customization of the rehabilitation plan.

Next is a complete patient examination to determine the primary injury and any secondary or compensatory issues, and to gather as much objective information as possible in order to document the patient's progress and improvement through the rehabilitation plan (Figure 20.2). This examination also serves to determine whether there are any contraindications, special considerations, or precautions for the application of laser therapy.

Goniometric measurements of all joints, a muscle mass record of all four limbs, radiographic and diagnostic ultrasound illustrations of the injury, and a list of secondary or compensatory issues that need to be addressed throughout the rehabilitation process should all be documented. These parameters should be remeasured at least every 4 weeks in order to monitor the progress of the patient and record the effects of the modalities being used. Appropriate monitoring of data will help determine whether the patient should move into the next phase of rehabilitation, or if the rehabilitation treatment plan needs to be modified.

Overview of Sports-Injury Rehabilitation

Sports-injury rehabilitation can be broken down into four phases. For each injury, there are goals that, when

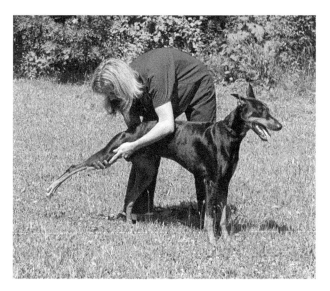

Figure 20.2 A complete physical examination is important to determine the primary injury and any secondary or compensatory issues.

and the injury is approaching a healed status. The goals of Phase III are progression of activities and exercise to prepare for return to off-lead activity and sport. The goal of increasing the strength, power, endurance, and neuromuscular control of the injured limb can be aided by more current areas of laser therapy research, which involve the support PBMT can add to muscle activity, conditioning, and strength.

Phase IV, the return to full activity, usually occurs 12 or more weeks after the injury or surgery. This phase starts when there is full, non-painful range of motion, no pain or tenderness with exercise, equal limb muscle mass and symmetry, no lameness at walk, trot, or in tight circles, and the surgical site is healed. The goals of this final phase are progressive return to full off-leash activity and training or competition, where applicable. The therapist should use a gradual-interval return to the patient's sport program to avoid re-injury. Finally, sport-specific functional exercises should be used to prepare for the stress involved with each particular activity or sport.

Laser Therapy Application in Musculoskeletal Injuries

Sports-related injuries are often accompanied by a confirmed diagnosis of a very specific afflicted area. Often, these conditions will have multiple involvements of compensatory muscles or joints contributing to the pain. It is judicious to treat the entire patient and sometimes to expose large, complete, comprehensive areas to appropriate doses of PBMT. This enables the primary injured area and the compensatory areas to be effectively treated.

Lower-power (<500 mW) laser systems (Class 2 and 3) are generally indicated for use with a point-to-point contact method of application when treating musculoskeletal conditions. Multiple points are treated in the area of injury. While performing manual massage therapy, further involved areas are identified, and these are treated in a similar point-to-point method. The dose for each treatment area is delivered in 30–60 seconds, depending on the power of the laser and the size of the treatment area. This method allows successful, precise identification and treatment of specific primary and secondary musculoskeletal issues, all in one session.

Another treatment technique is to move the laser in a scanning fashion while treating. This technique is appropriate when using therapy lasers with power >500 mW (Class 4). Administration of laser therapy by scanning over an area can be accomplished with the delivery handpiece in contact or not in contact with the tissue, depending on the patient's tolerance of being touched and

accomplished, indicate it is time to move to the next phase.

Phase I, or the acute phase, is considered the immediate motion phase, and is usually limited to 1–3 weeks after the surgery or injury. The objectives of this phase are to minimize the effects of immobilization, promote and protect the healing of the injured tissue, decrease pain and inflammation, re-establish non-painful range of motion, restore weight bearing to the injured limb, and impede muscular atrophy. Laser therapy is pivotal at this beginning stage. This is where the majority of the anti-inflammatory research data and support for PBMT currently exists.

Phase II, or the intermediate phase, usually occurs 4–6 weeks after the injury. This phase initiates when full or injury-appropriate range of motion is achieved, pain and inflammation is reduced, lameness is improved, and the surgical site, if applicable, is without complication. The goals of Phase II include enhancement of joint and patient mobility, improved muscular strength and endurance, and re-establishment of neuromuscular and proprioceptive control of the injured limb. Current data support using PBMT during this phase of healing and continuing through the next stage as reinforcement for any secondary issues arising from the increased mobility and strength training (Larkin-Kaiser *et al.*, 2015).

Phase III, or the advanced strengthening phase, is usually accomplished 7–11 weeks after the injury. This phase initiates when there is full (or as much as expected) non-painful range of motion of the affected limb, no pain or tenderness, the strength and muscle mass is 70% of the contralateral limb, any surgical implants are static, receiving massage therapy. The dose is delivered over a more comprehensive area, moving the laser beam over the entire area to be treated. Multiple areas of involvement can be treated in a therapy session.

Photon penetration into the soft tissue is much more efficient when using a contact delivery, since fewer photons are reflected from the skin surface (Enwemeka, 2009). When treating a patient with the handpiece in contact with the soft tissues, the laser therapist can massage and manipulate the tissue during treatment. Occasionally, patients will not tolerate significant tissue manipulation or massage. In these situations, the use of a non-contact delivery is recommended.

Patient comfort and positioning during the treatment session are important. Lateral recumbency will often allow the patient to relax and be comfortable, and at the same time grant access to the treatment areas. This position also allows manipulations of each limb, without the need to support or rely on the patient's balance during the treatment.

The dose and frequency of laser therapy treatments will depend on the nature of the injury and the amount of access to the patient. It is acceptable to treat every day, but this is often not realistic for owners due to limitations of time and economy. Determining the lowest frequency of laser therapy treatment that will give optimal results is ultimately the job of the therapist. This is often accomplished with a weekly or twice-weekly treatment plan for the acute phase. The time between treatments can then be gradually lengthened as the patient progresses though the rehabilitative process. Long-term maintenance therapy can usually be scheduled monthly or in conjunction with sporting events.

Treatment of Fore-Limb Sports Injuries in Canine Athletes

Sports-related injuries in the canine front limb are quite common. Each joint has its share of common injuries. The most commonly seen shoulder issues are supraspinatus tendinopathy, teres minor tendinitis, bicipital tenosynovitis, and injury to the medial shoulder compartment. These have been identified in all breeds and sports. Less commonly seen, but associated with field trial sport, is infraspinatus contracture. Fragmented coronoid process (elbow dysplasia), jump-down syndrome, and cartilage defects are often seen within the elbows. The carpus is also affected by sports-related injuries, including carpal hyperextension and flexor carpi ulnaris strains.

Shoulder Injuries
Shoulder injuries, including supraspinatus tendinopathy, infraspinatus myopathy, bicipital tenosynovitis, and medial shoulder syndrome, are common sports-related injuries, usually related to repetitive actions. At times,

they can be difficult to rehabilitate. Common secondary, compensatory issues noted alongside shoulder injuries include contralateral limb muscle trigger points and carpal laxity, scapula restrictions (especially with shoulder stabilization systems with hobble straps for medial shoulder syndrome), triceps trigger points, paraspinal tension, and diagonal hind limb sartorius and hamstring muscle stiffness. A recent systematic review of the effects of laser therapy on shoulder tendinopathies in humans revealed that such therapy can offer pain relief and "initiate a more rapid course of improvement" when used either alone or in combination with other rehabilitation modalities or techniques (Haslerud *et al.*, 2015). This meta-analysis supports similar findings from the clinical use of laser therapy in shoulder tendinopathies found in dogs, especially since they are commonly seen in our canine athletes.

Elbow Injuries
A common sports-related injury to the elbow is traumatic fragmented medial coronoid process, or "jump-down syndrome." Other elbow issues, including elbow dysplasia (fragmented coronoid process, un-united aconeal process, and osteochondrosis dessicans), can also affect many sporting breeds. Surgery is required for proper resolution of these conditions. The postoperative rehabilitation program follows similar guidelines to those for other fore-limb injuries. Common compensatory issues are similar to the ones described for shoulder injuries. In addition, excessive strain on the shoulder tendons due to external rotation of the elbow to avoid medial compartment pain is also seen as secondary irritation and inflammation. Cartilage damage is usually seen in addition to these other injuries.

In a rat model study, it was shown that laser therapy helped accelerate the initial breakdown of cartilage destroyed by the joint injury and stimulated fibroblasts to synthesize the repairing collagen III (Mangueira *et al.*, 2015). This suggests a beneficial effect of PBM on osteoarthritis involving cartilage damage, potentially reducing its long-term effects.

Unfortunately, the elbows are the most unforgiving joints in the canine patient. Therefore, an active ongoing rehabilitation program, even after full recovery, is most important in giving these patients the opportunity to return and stay active in their sport. An interesting study in human advanced knee arthritis showed that laser therapy in addition to twice-yearly hyaluronic acid intra-articular injections avoided total joint-replacement surgery due to increased and sustained comfort within the affected joint (Ip and Fu, 2015a).

Carpal Injuries
Carpal sporting injuries usually involve flexor carpi ulnaris strains or chronic carpal breakdown due to weakening of flexor tendons and ligaments as a result of

excessive, repetitive jump landings. Severe cases often lead to carpal fusion, which makes it very difficult for the patient to return to sport, due to biomechanical changes. This section will discuss only carpal strains and sprains, since they carry the best probability of return to sport, and they respond very well to laser therapy and rehabilitation.

Many carpal injuries require some form of immobilization, such as a neoprene carpal wrap with or without rigid thermoplastic, depending on the extent of injury. Immobilization causes increased secondary and compensatory changes due to the temporary change in biomechanics of the fore limb. It is important to monitor and treat these compensatory changes to avoid additional injury to the other areas of the fore limb. Laser therapy is highly indicated for use in conjunction with any condition that requires splinting or supportive wrap in the canine patient. In a 2014 study of carpal tunnel syndrome in humans, it was shown that the addition of laser therapy to subjects with a carpal orthotic, when compared to an orthotic alone, led to better nerve conduction and hand strength at the end of the study (Fusakul *et al.*, 2014).

Treatment of Hind-Limb Sports Injuries in Canine Athletes

Common hind-limb sports-related conditions include iliopsoas strains, stifle injuries such as cranial cruciate ligament (CCL) sprains and ruptures, and Achilles tendon issues, as well as hip osteoarthritis secondary to chronic, repetitive use.

Iliopsoas Strains

Iliopsoas strains are quite common, occurring when an excessive force acts on this muscle and tendon. As in humans, they are commonly associated with highly athletic activities (e.g., agility, flyball, Schutzhund) (Figure 20.3). Iliopsoas strains often occur where the muscle and tendons meet, which is the weakest part of the muscle–tendon unit. It is common to find that dogs with iliopsoas strains also have other orthopedic problems, making the strain a secondary injury. Patients that have recently undergone surgical treatment for another orthopedic condition, such as CCL rupture, often have a concurrent mild iliopsoas strain due to overuse of the hip flexor muscle, working to off-weight the injured limb.

Stifle Injuries

Rupture of the CCL is one of the most prevalent orthopedic injuries and causes of lameness in dogs, and is quite common in the canine athlete. Partial or complete CCL disruption causes stifle joint instability, leading to a cascade of inflammatory and pathologic changes, which result in synovitis, osteoarthritis, meniscal injury, and altered stifle kinematics.

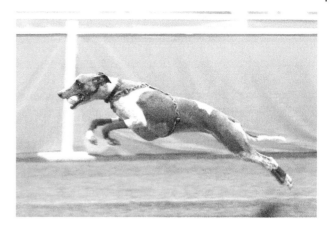

Figure 20.3 Iliopsoas strains are quite common and occur when an excessive force acts on the iliopsoas muscle and tendon. They are commonly associated with highly athletic activities like flyball.

Indications for conservative treatment of CCL injuries can be established for grade I or II sprains (partial tears). While it may be possible to rehabilitate grade I sprains back to full function with laser therapy, there is a great likelihood that a partial tear may progress to full grade III sprain (complete tear) over time. For dogs with early, mild, partial tears, strategies are focused on controlling the effects of inflammation (pain, effusion, loss of motion, and muscle atrophy). Laser therapy, using an 808 nm laser and doses of 10 and 50J/cm^2, prevented features related to articular degenerative process, such as increased release of inflammatory mediators, in the knees of rats after anterior cruciate ligament transection (Bublitz *et al.*, 2014).

If meniscal injury is diagnosed alongside CCL injury, surgical intervention is highly recommended. In addition, meniscal injury is a common cause of stifle pain and progressive degenerative joint disease even after the surgical correction of a destabilizing cruciate ligament rupture injury. To date, there is no known proven regenerative technique for the treatment of meniscal injury in the canine patient. Laser therapy is currently directed to reducing stifle inflammation, with no specific indication of healing or regenerating meniscal tissue. In canine patients that cannot have, or elect not to pursue surgical repair, laser therapy can be confidently recommended on a long-term basis, and it has been shown to significantly decrease pain in human patients with meniscal injury (Malliaropoulos *et al.*, 2013).

For the best possibility of return to sport for canine athletes with grade III sprains (complete CCL tears), corrective surgery is currently recommended, followed by 8–12 weeks of rehabilitative therapy.

Achilles Tendon Issues

Achilles tendon injury is commonly seen in sporting dogs, as both acute and chronic injury. Chronic degradation of the Achilles tendon unit is often seen in field-trial Labradors or Schutzhund-trained Dobermans. Grade I–II strains of the Achilles tendon components are often treated with laser therapy in a structured rehabilitation plan. Depending on the severity of the injury, a neoprene or rigid orthotic brace is incorporated into the treatment regime. Grade III strains or ruptures of all or part of the Achilles tendon often require surgery and an intensive postoperative rehabilitation therapy plan if the patient is to return successfully to sport.

In Wistar rats, laser therapy using 780 nm light decreased the inflammatory response in partially injured Achilles tendons at a dose of 17.5J/cm^2 once a day (de Jesus *et al.*, 2015). A recent study supports the use of PBMT in Achilles tendon healing by showing that laser therapy improves the repair process by promoting a higher percentage of collagen I fibers, the normal tendon collagen structure, and fewer collagen III fibers, which is represented by weaker, more dysfunctional fibrous tissue (de Jesus *et al.*, 2014). Another study showed that laser therapy leads to increased functional organization of collagen bundles and overall improved normal gait recovery in rats with experimentally partially tenotomized tendons (Guerra *et al.*, 2014). These same effects help accomplish the essential goals for Achilles tendon repair in canine athletes.

Sports Injury Rehabilitation

Rehabilitation for sports injuries has four phases: Phase I, or the acute phase; Phase II, or the intermediate phase; Phase III, or the advanced strengthening phase; and Phase IV, the return to full activity. With each patient and each injury, there are specific goals to be accomplished in each phase before moving to the next.

Phase I Sports Injury Rehabilitation

Phase I rehabilitation therapy for sports-related conditions usually lasts about 4 weeks. Representative findings of sports-injury conditions seen during this phase include restricted range of motion of affected joints, discomfort on range of motion, direct palpations, and static stretches of the primarily involved muscle and tendon. The patient often has a short-strided gait in the affected quadrant, including a reduced reach with the affected limb when tendinopathies are present.

In conditions such as the severe restriction seen with chronic infraspinatus contractures, gracilis contractures, or frozen shoulder, there is usually a significant amount of discomfort on direct palpation or attempts to stretch. These usually cannot be manually corrected until breakdown and healing occur. Laser therapy can assist in providing pain relief, and can improve the

clinical outcome in these instances. A recent study of frozen shoulder in human patients demonstrated that laser therapy provided significant pain relief through 8 weeks, allowing for appropriate manual therapy (Kim *et al.*, 2015).

In diseases or injuries that involve the joint, such as jump-down syndrome, osteochondritis dissecans lesions, meniscal injury, and cruciate ligament sprains and ruptures, patients will significantly off-weight the affected limb, which induces significantly more compensatory issues in the contralateral limb. Laser therapy can help keep the increased inflammation seen in the contralateral joints to a minimum and reduce unwanted synovitis or degenerative joint changes (Canapp *et al.*, 2005).

Phase I rehabilitation therapy should include the use of PBMT. Laser therapy is an important modality in shoulder injuries, and is applied to the affected primary joints, muscles, and tendons to reduce inflammation, stimulate collagen synthesis, release trigger points, and support healing (Lam *et al.*, 1986).

Significant compensatory issues often induce uncomfortable scenarios such as myofascial trigger points (MTPs). Laser therapy is an excellent tool in helping to treat and prevent the compensatory issues noted in these injuries. A study performed in oral surgery patients showed that four sessions of laser therapy treatment at a dose of 4J/cm^2 per MTP were effective for deactivating the trigger points (Uemoto *et al.*, 2013). This dosage and treatment schedule has also been shown to be successful when treating injuries and compensatory issues in canine athletes.

Laser therapy has been shown to decrease pain and disability in extensive fibrotic diseases such as frozen shoulder in both the early rehabilitative stage and later ones (Stergioulas, 2008). Laser therapy can also modulate the inflammatory mediators and reduce the degenerative changes seen in the cartilage of injured joints (Assis *et al.*, 2015; Bublitz *et al.*, 2014).

Manual therapy accompanies modality therapy in many instances, especially in the acute phase. Passive range of motion is used to assist in retaining the current range of motion. Grade I and II joint mobilizations help increase circulation, proprioception, and neuromodulation of pain by stimulating type I and type II articular receptors, with similar effects to those of laser therapy. If muscle contracture, frozen shoulder, or adhesive capsulitis is the issue, then passive range of motion is increased in this stage (including joint mobilizations up to grade III–IV) to promote significant stretching or to maintain the surgical correction and prevent contracture from returning. Laser therapy has been utilized to provide pain relief in humans with adhesive capsulitis, in addition to manual therapy and joint mobilizations aimed at restoring comfortable range of motion (Ip and Fu, 2015b). These findings are also seen in the treatment of orthopedic conditions in the dog, supporting a multimodal combination of treatments for the best overall outcome.

Phase II Sports Injury Rehabilitation

Phase II rehabilitation usually occurs between 4 and 11 weeks after the injury. This phase initiates when the patient exhibits good range of motion with minimal pain or spasm of the affected limb. The patient should have decreased lameness and an elongated stride. (When the shoulder or iliopsoas is the injured area, we often see this elongation take longer to return.)

At this stage, especially if the patient has been receiving rehabilitation from the start, fewer secondary issues should be noted, since they will have been successfully managed through manual and laser therapy. If secondary issues such as scapular restriction or contralateral limb biceps or triceps tension are still present, they should be more easily resolved. In addition, the persistent use of laser therapy should continually reduce effusion within the affected joints. Laser therapy will play a role against cartilage degradation and synovitis, as demonstrated in a study using rabbits (Wang *et al.*, 2014).

The use of laser therapy is continued throughout the rehabilitation process and is a key modality in promoting healing and maintaining the rest of the patient through the rehabilitation plan. Weekly to twice-a-week laser therapy is continued using a whole-dog, point-to-point protocol, at a dose of $5\,J/cm^2$, with either a single infrared wavelength or a combination of red and infrared wavelengths. If utilizing a higher-power therapy laser and a scanning delivery, the dose will be $5–10\,J/cm^2$, depending on the weight of the patient and the area being treated. Reputable, veterinary-specific therapy laser devices will calculate these dosages automatically when appropriate data, such as weight, skin color, hair coat color and length, body condition, clinical condition, and area to be treated, are entered.

Often, the effects seen from laser therapy give adequate comfort to allow dogs to increase their exercise protocols, such as increasing range of motion or progressing to concentric or eccentric therapeutic exercise. The effects of laser therapy on muscle tissue performance, fatigue, and repair have been well illustrated through several years of research, and documentation across species (Ferraresi *et al.*, 2012).

During Phase II, manual therapy is similar to that in Phase I, except that passive range of motion and grade III joint mobilizations (used to stretch the capsular tissue and approach end range) are performed to a greater extent.

Phase II therapeutic exercise focuses on increasing isometric exercises in static weight bearing and on introducing eccentric and concentric exercises in order to start rebuilding any loss of muscle mass. Leash walk length and intensity can be increased, usually following a guideline of 5-minute increases every 3–5 days. The owner should monitor lameness and passive range of motion, and should only increase walks if the patient is not showing any lameness at the end of a walk and does not show any restriction or discomfort on range of motion that evening or the next day. Running, jumping, playing, and plyometrics should not be allowed. Stairs can be allowed in a controlled manner, depending on how the patient manages them, barring any negative impacts such as soreness or stiffness.

Hydrotherapy often begins during this phase, 2 weeks after the absence of any muscle spasm and general resolution of lameness. These criteria will change for each patient, depending on the severity of the injury or surgery, the condition, and the patient's activity level. Underwater treadmill is preferred over swimming at this stage, since free swimming may exacerbate injuries due to its uncontrolled gait. Swimming can be introduced for fibrotic injuries such as frozen shoulder or muscle contracture, to aid in reducing circumduction or abnormal biomechanics of the limb in a non-weight-bearing manner.

It is imperative, as already discussed, that laser therapy support this increase in controlled activity and help to resolve any new inflammation it causes. In addition, laser therapy may provide additional benefit when exercise in water is initiated. Laser therapy in combination with hydrotherapy has been shown to help increase bone strength and physical properties in osteopenic rats (Muniz Renno *et al.*, 2006).

Phase III Sports Injury Rehabilitation

Phase III occurs between 7 and 14 weeks after injury, depending on the injury involved, the progress of the patient, and whether an orthotic is being utilized. This phase initiates when there is full range of motion and no spasm or discomfort on range of motion or direct palpation of the primary injury. The patient should have a normal gait at this time, and should be approaching a full weight-bearing normal stance. To begin Phase III, the muscle mass of the affected limb needs to be at least 70% that of the contralateral limb. If these criteria are met, orthotic or assistive devices can be gradually removed from the patient.

Manual and laser therapy at this time have historically focused more on maintaining what has already been accomplished. The historical approach when using laser therapy for maintenance is that the frequency of treatment is decreased to every other week. However, with current research supporting the use of laser therapy for enhancement of the musculoskeletal system during exercise, an argument can be made that this phase may incorporate more frequent treatment sessions. Positive results have been reported concerning the effect of light and laser therapy on muscle performance and repair in both

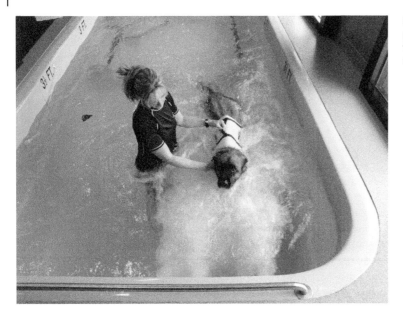

Figure 20.4 When used during the appropriate phases of rehabilitation, hydrotherapy can be a key tool and it can be continued after rehabilitation as a method of conditioning and strengthening.

acute and chronic conditions, as well as in protecting against fatigue (Ferraresi *et al.*, 2012).

Therapeutic exercise intensity increases again in Phase III. Handstands are introduced, to increase the isometric work on the front limbs. Active stretching should be used as a warm up to the more intense activity introduced during this phase. Further concentric and eccentric exercises specific to the initial muscle or tendon injury can be introduced. This adds to the controlled strength-training and muscle-building activities. Laser therapy, when associated with strength training in people, can increase muscle performance compared to strength training alone (Ferraresi *et al.*, 2011).

Achilles and carpal injury cases that use orthotics usually begin dynamization of the supportive orthotics in Phase III. This allows for key eccentric exercises to begin aiding the healing and strengthening of the carpal or Achilles tendon complex. Laser therapy, when added to eccentric Achilles exercise in healing chronic Achilles tendon injury, has been shown to accelerate clinical recovery and reduce pain and stiffness (Stergioulas *et al.*, 2008). Current dosages used in healing canine tendon injuries are $5\,J/cm^2$ at three to five points along the entire Achilles tendon or $8-10\,J/cm^2$ delivered throughout the entire tendon. Core work can progress into sit-ups, waving, begs, and begs-to-stand. Proprioception and stabilization exercises are also initiated using mattresses, obstacle courses, wobble boards, and balance balls. Passive stretching should be used after cool-down. If there is muscle tension or resistance on stretching, this is as an indicator that too much exercise or too many repetitions are being performed.

In addition to increasing speed and distance during leash walks, it is advised to add in different terrain to aid in proprioception, stamina, and balance. Gradually adding in hills and walking diagonally on hills will add in an active power component. Starting with large circles and eventually decreasing the diameter into tight circles will add in further dynamics that require strengthening prior to return to function. Plyometrics should also be introduced, primarily targeting the front end, with play bows to springing up and landing.

Hydrotherapy is a key tool during this phase, which helps strengthen and prepare for the next phase (Figure 20.4). Increasing speed and time and lowering the water height in the underwater treadmill can increase the intensity and aid in restoring normal gait animation. Medial shoulder-syndrome patients begin underwater treadmill therapy at this time. If there are no complications, then swimming can be introduced in the next 2–3 weeks (week 14 postoperative).

Phase IV Sports Injury Rehabilitation

Phase IV in sports injury rehabilitation therapy is the return-to-activity phase. In most cases, this occurs after 12–16 weeks of controlled rehabilitation. This phase initiates when the patient has full or acceptable range of motion of the injured joint, with no abnormalities noted on direct palpation or full stretching of the soft-tissue components. There should be a normal gait, with no evidence of lameness, and equal muscle mass of the limbs. Maintenance manual therapy should be used to prevent tight muscles and as a screening tool to note if any one area is reacting poorly to the new activity. Modality therapy, particularly laser therapy, can be used in a similar supportive manner, especially when a persistent spasm or restriction is evident.

Therapeutic exercise at this stage is used to address any lingering deficiencies or to continue to support any inherent insufficiencies known to the patient, such as a lack of core strength. Plyometrics are often introduced during Phase III or IV, due to their significant intensity. Laser therapy has also been shown to increase positive outcome when combined with plyometric exercise compared to either method alone. In a study involving lateral epicondylitis (tennis elbow) in humans, the combination of laser therapy and plyometric exercise was more effective than placebo or than either modality alone (Stergioulas, 2007). In canines, we see chronic tendinopathies (such as supraspinatus tendinopathy, biceps tendinopathy, and iliopsoas tendinopathy) that respond similarly when we combine laser therapy and plyometric exercise during this phase.

Exercise restrictions are gradually lifted and the therapist and owner should reintroduce free running over a 2-week period. Once this is accomplished, sport-specific re-training can be started. Evaluating performance technique and identifying any issues are key to correcting any technique that may have predisposed the patient to the injury in the first place. Hydrotherapy can be continued as a method of conditioning or of ongoing strengthening.

In very severe injuries, such as grade III–V cartilage injuries, severe chronic tendinopathies, or advanced osteoarthritis, supportive care using laser therapy can be the difference between continuing comfortably with sport and having to retire. Many canine patients, even with severe injuries, end up successfully returning to the sport they love with just laser therapy and massage administered every few weeks to once a month as a means of maintenance therapy.

Laser Therapy in Sports Training and Muscle Performance

Canine athletes are exposed to muscle damage from training and competition. This can compromise their performance for a period ranging from minutes to hours, days, weeks, or months. The intent of post-exercise or post-injury laser therapy is to reverse muscle damage. Until recent research was published, it was uncommon to attempt to prevent or attenuate exercise-induced muscle damage. However, recent studies show that laser therapy can be used as an adjunct to continued sports training and muscle performance. Multiple findings suggest that laser therapy can minimize the occurrence of injury, optimize an athlete's return to activity (possibly within a shorter period), and potentially optimize overall performance in the sport.

Laser therapy studies concerning muscle work and fatigue cover a broad spectrum of applications.

Skeletal muscle fatigue, as seen in acute conditions, decreases the capacity of the muscle to perform work by impairing its strength and affecting its overall motor coordination (Allen *et al.*, 2008). On a cellular level, muscle fatigue is a result of several metabolic changes, including consumption of adenosine triphosphate (ATP) and glycogen, local blood acidification, oxidative stress, and tissue hypoxia. Historical research findings have shown that treatment with PBM prior to work decreases inflammatory biomarkers and lactate levels in blood when compared to non-pretreated subjects following intense upper- and lower-extremity exercise (Lopes-Martins *et al.*, 2006). Laser therapy has also been shown to reduce muscle fatigue and exhaustion (Leal Junior *et al.*, 2010). These studies and similar ones have inferred that preconditioning the muscle with PBMT may increase the contractile function, decrease exercise-induced muscle fatigue, and improve post-exercise recovery.

Recent work shows that laser therapy lowers lactate levels in patients that have spasticity due to triggering muscle fatigue, therby reducing fatigue and discomfort in the muscle (dos Reis *et al.*, 2015). The data suggest that this concept may be applied to canines in a post-exercise application. In addition, research using different light sources on skeletal muscle (quadriceps) and on recovery post-exercise shows positive results, with significant increases in performance, decreases in delayed-onset muscle soreness, and improvements in biochemical markers of muscle damage (Antonialli *et al.*, 2014).

A 2012 study showed that both 660 and 830 nm light were effective in decreasing skeletal muscle fatigue and enhancing muscle performance in humans (de Almeida *et al.*, 2012). Though a formal clinical trial has not been performed on canines, positive outcomes in muscle performance appear to be attributable to laser treatment in and around performances.

In another 2012 study involving a randomized, double-blind, placebo-controlled crossover trial with 22 untrained male volunteers, laser therapy was applied to the quadriceps, hamstrings, and gastrocnemius. This treatment method is similar to established treatment protocols in post-performance tension in canines. This particular human study was performed 5 minutes before a standardized, progressive-intensity running protocol on a motor-driven treadmill until exhaustion. The use of laser therapy before this running exercise resulted in increased exercise performance, decreased exercise-induced oxidative stress, and decreased muscle damage. The measured findings suggest that PBM's effect on the redox system may be the cause of the delay in skeletal-muscle fatigue observed after the use of laser therapy (de Marchi *et al.*, 2012). This treatment protocol could easily be adapted to canine athletes for use prior to training or performance exercises.

As discussed earlier in this chapter, iliopsoas strains are a very common injury in the canine athlete, and require rehabilitative intervention with laser therapy to obtain resolution. A recent article examined the effects of laser therapy when directly applied to the iliopsoas muscle belly in a rat model, and found that a higher energy density (at $61.2 \, J/cm^2$) promoted a dose-dependent increase in oxygen consumption uptake and a performance increase (shown as distance covered) (Perini *et al.*, 2016). Another study performed in trained endurance athletes showed that laser therapy combined with endurance training led to a greater reduction in fatigue than training programs that did not incorporate laser therapy (Vieira *et al.*, 2012). Studies like these help support the use of laser therapy throughout the healing and rehabilitative process and into the supportive, retraining, and maintenance stages.

An additional approach to this application of laser therapy could be in canine sports such as herding, field trial, and sledding. In these sports, there are multiple, longer periods of exercise. Laser therapy could be applied in several sessions over the period of performance, in addition to immediately after completion. A study in people showed that laser therapy applied to the quadriceps muscle during rest intervals and immediately upon cessation of activity resulted in an increase of muscle resistance to fatigue, allowing the patient to perform longer before ultimate fatigue (de Brito Vieira *et al.*, 2014).

Research in pre-performance PBMT shows the potential ability to increase overall performance indirectly through modulation of metabolic and renal function (Ferraresi *et al.*, 2015). A controlled study in rats showed that when laser therapy was applied immediately prior to muscle injury, there was a reduction in myonecrosis and inflammatory cells after injury. This study also noted an increase in blood vessels, better organization and distribution of collagen, and new muscle fibers just 7 days after the injury (Ribeiro *et al.*, 2015). These results suggest that laser therapy before training or trials, especially in those sports with a high injury rate, carries great therapeutic value to the canine athlete.

Pain in the Canine Athlete

Eventually, pain and canine athletes will meet, in either a short- or a long-term relationship. Reduction of acute and chronic pain in the canine athlete is another area where laser therapy may be very useful and successful. Historically, there have been comprehensive studies illustrating the extensive mechanisms of action of PBM that result in pain relief. Thus, the analgesic effect of laser therapy is one of its most common applications across species.

Bjordal *et al.* (2006) found that laser therapy can modify the biochemical inflammatory response by reducing the levels of tumor necrosis factor (TNF), interleukin 1 (IL1), prostaglandin E2 (PGE2), plasminogen activator, and cyclooxygenase 2 (COX2). More recently, Jang and

Lee (2012) published a meta-analysis of pain relief effects seen with laser application on a joint. The wide spectrum of diseases covered in this review includes rheumatoid arthritis, osteoarthritis, temperomandibular disorder, low-back pain, shoulder pain, and neck pain, all of which are documented in the dog. It is important to note that in many of these meta-analysis articles, the studies reviewed use a broad spectrum of parameters of laser application. Though the frequency of use, dose, power, and wavelength of light used differs among the authors cited, these reviews confirm the efficacy of using PBMT to reduce pain caused by various conditions.

Acute pain is often found in the immediate postoperative or post-injury phase in canine patients. Looking at the effects of laser therapy immediately after injury or surgery reveals data we can extrapolate to canine athletes undergoing surgical intervention. Application of laser therapy over surgical sternotomy wounds was an effective component of postoperative analgesia when included in a multimodal approach to pain relief (Karlekar *et al.*, 2015). In a human study, laser therapy was evaluated as a tool for reducing pain post-surgically after tibial fracture repair, which could be compared to the common tibial plateau-leveling osteotomy procedure for CCL rupture in our canine athletes. Laser therapy reduced pain significantly in post-surgical fracture repair in human patients (Nesioonpour *et al.*, 2014).

In reference to chronic pain, the interaction of laser light with cells can produce several different reactions and outcomes, one of which is an increase in serotonin levels. In 1983, a study showed that repeated application of laser light produced relief of chronic pain in human subjects. In addition, the study showed a significant increase in urinary excretion of 5-hydroxyindoleacetic acid, a degradation product of serotonin (Walker, 1983). In a more recent publication, laser therapy was shown to be an effective method of relieving chronic, non-specific back pain, as measured by a visual analog scale pain-outcome score (Huang *et al.*, 2015).

Chronic stifle discomfort and other degenerative joint diseases are quite common in canine athletes. This may be caused by prior injury and continued successful engagement in sport, or by normal aging of the joint with an increased load. Laser therapy has been shown to be a useful tool in decreasing chronic knee pain in humans with osteoarthritis (Nakamura *et al.*, 2014), and in keeping elderly patients' knee pain under control, tolerable, and at a level that allows them to avoid knee-replacement surgery (Ip, 2015).

Conclusion

This chapter has looked at the relationship of laser therapy and PBM with canine athletes. There is not a lot of research involving the effects of laser therapy specifically on canine musculoskeletal injury, but there is a plethora of supportive data. Cellular responses to light in the laboratory appear to be transferable between species. With this information, it becomes obvious that PBMT is a compelling and auspicious technology that should be applied in every aspect of the canine sports-medicine world.

References

Allen, D.G. *et al.* (2008) Skeletal muscle fatigue: cellular mechanisms. *Physiol Rev.* **88**:287–332.

Antonialli, F.C. *et al.* (2014) Phototherapy in skeletal muscle performance and recovery after exercise: effect of combination of super-pulsed laser and light-emitting diodes. *Lasers Med Sci.* **29**(6):1967–1976.

Assis, L. *et al.* (2015) Aerobic exercise training and low-level laser therapy modulate inflammatory response and degenerative process in an experimental model of knee osteoarthritis in rats. *Osteoarthritis Cartilage.* **24**(1):169–177.

Bjordal, J. *et al.* (2006) Low-level laser therapy in acute pain: a systematic review of possible mechanisms of action and clinical effects in randomized placebo-controlled trials. *Photomed Laser Surg.* **24**(2):158–168.

Bublitz, C. *et al.* (2014) Low-level laser therapy prevents degenerative morphological changes in an experimental model of anterior cruciate ligament transection in rats. *Lasers Med Sci.* **29**(5):1669–1678.

Canapp, S. *et al.* (2005) The evaluation of synovial fluid and serum following intravenous injections of hyaluronan for the treatment of osteoarthritis in dogs. *Vet Comp Orthop Traumatol.* **18**(3):169–174.

Castano, A.P. *et al.* (2007) Low-level laser therapy for zymosan-induced arthritis in rats: importance of illumination time. *Lasers Surg Med.* **39**(6):543–550.

Davidoff, F. *et al.* (1995) Evidence based medicine. *BMJ.* **310**(6987):1085–1086.

de Almeida, P. *et al.* (2012) Red (660 nm) and infrared (830 nm) low-level laser therapy in skeletal muscle fatigue in humans: what is better? *Lasers Med Sci.* **27**(2):453–458.

de Brito Vieira, W.H. *et al.* (2014) Use of low-level laser therapy (808 nm) to muscle fatigue resistance: a randomized double-blind crossover trial. *Photomed Laser Surg.* **32**(12):678–685.

de Jesus. J.F. *et al.* (2014) Low-level laser therapy on tissue repair of partially injured Achilles tendon in rats. *Photomed Laser Surg.* **32**(6):345–350.

de Jesus, J.F. *et al.* (2015) Low-level laser therapy in IL-1β, COX-2, and PGE2 modulation in partially injured Achilles tendon. *Lasers Med Sci.* **30**(1):153–158.

de Marchi, T. *et al.* (2012) Low-level laser therapy (LLLT) in human progressive-intensity running: effects on exercise performance, skeletal muscle status, and oxidative stress. *Lasers Med Sci.* **27**(1):231–236.

de Mattos, L.H. *et al.* (2015) Effect of phototherapy with light-emitting diodes (890 nm) on tendon repair: an experimental model in sheep. *Lasers Med Sci.* **30**(1):193–201.

dos Reis, M.C. *et al.* (2015) Immediate effects of low-intensity laser (808 nm) on fatigue and strength of spastic muscle. *Lasers Med Sci.* **30**(3):1089–1096.

Enwemeka, C.S. (2009) Intricacies of dose in laser phototherapy for tissue repair and pain relief. *Photomed Laser Surg.* **3**:387–393.

Ferraresi, C. *et al.* (2011) Effects of low level laser therapy (808 nm) on physical strength training in humans. *Lasers Med Sci.* **26**(3):349–358.

Ferraresi, C. *et al.* (2012) Low-level laser (light) therapy (LLLT) on muscle tissue: performance, fatigue and repair benefited by the power of light. *Photonics Lasers Med.* **1**(4):267–286.

Ferraresi, C. *et al.* (2015) Muscular pre-conditioning using light-emitting diode therapy (LEDT) for high-intensity exercise: a randomized double-blind placebo-controlled trial with a single elite runner. *Physiother Theory Pract.* **31**(5):354–361.

Fusakul, Y. *et al.* (2014) Low-level laser therapy with a wrist splint to treat carpal tunnel syndrome: a double-blinded randomized controlled trial. *Lasers Med Sci.* **29**(3):1279–1287.

Guerra, F.D.R. *et al.* (2014) Pulsed LLLT improves tendon healing in rats: a biochemical, organizational, and functional evaluation. *Lasers Med Sci.* **29**(2):805–811.

Haslerud, S. *et al.* (2015) The efficacy of low-level laser therapy for shoulder tendinopathy: a systematic review and meta-analysis of randomized controlled trials. *Physiother Res Int.* **20**(2):108–125.

Huang, Z. *et al.* (2015) The effectiveness of low-level laser therapy for nonspecific chronic low back pain: a systematic review and meta-analysis. *Arthritis Res Ther.* **17**:360.

Ip D. (2015) Does addition of low-level laser therapy (LLLT) in conservative care of knee arthritis successfully postpone the need for joint replacement? *Lasers Med Sci.* **30**(9):2335–2339.

Ip D. and Fu N.Y. (2015a) Can combined use of low-level lasers and hyaluronic acid injections prolong the longevity of degenerative knee joints? *Clin Interv Aging.* **10**:1255–1258.

Ip, D. and Fu, N.Y. (2015b). Two-year follow-up of low-level laser therapy for elderly with painful adhesive capsulitis of the shoulder. *Journal of Pain Research.* **8**:247–252.

Ishide, Y. *et al.* (2008) The effect of GaAlA diode laser on pre- sports warming up and post-sports cooling down. *Laser Therapy.* **17**(4):187–192.

Jang, H. and Lee H. (2012) Meta-analysis of pain relief effects by laser irradiation on joint areas. *Photomed Laser Surg.* **30**:405–417.

Karlekar, A. *et al.* (2015) Assessment of feasibility and efficacy of Class IV laser therapy for postoperative pain relief in off-pump coronary artery bypass surgery patients: a pilot study. *Ann Card Anaesth.* **18**(3):317–322.

Kim, S.H. *et al.* (2015) Short-term effects of high-intensity laser therapy on frozen shoulder: a prospective randomized control study. *Man Ther.* **20**(6):751–757.

Lam, T.S. *et al.* (1986) Laser stimulation of collagen synthesis in human skin fibroblast cultures. *Lasers Life Sci.* **1**:61–77.

Larkin-Kaiser, K.A. *et al.* (2015) Near-infrared light therapy to attenuate strength loss after strenuous resistance exercise. *J Athl Train.* **50**(1):45–50.

Leal Junior, E.C. *et al.* (2010) Effect of low-level laser therapy (GaAs 904 nm) in skeletal muscle fatigue and biochemical markers of muscle damage in rats. *Eur J Appl Physiol.* **108**(6):1083–1088.

Lopes-Martins, R.A. *et al.* (2006) Effect of low-level laser (Ga-Al-As 655 nm) on skeletal muscle fatigue induced by electrical stimulation in rats. *J Appl Physiol.* **101**(1): 283–288.

Malliaropoulos, N. *et al.* (2013) Low-level laser therapy in meniscal pathology: a double-blinded placebo-controlled trial. *Lasers Med Sci.* **28**(4):1183–1188.

Mangueira, N.M. *et al.* (2015) Effect of low-level laser therapy in an experimental model of osteoarthritis in rats evaluated through Raman spectroscopy. *Photomed Laser Surg.* **33**(3):145–153.

Muniz Renno, A.C. *et al.* (2006) The effects of infrared-830 nm laser on exercised osteopenic rats. *Lasers Med Sci.* **21**(4):202–207.

Nakamura, T. *et al.* (2014) Low level laser therapy for chronic knee joint pain patients. *Laser Therapy.* **23**(4):273–277.

Nesioonpour, S. *et al.* (2014) The effect of low-level laser on postoperative pain after tibial fracture surgery: a double-blind controlled randomized clinical trial. *Anesth Pain Med.* **4**(3):e17350.

Ohshiro, T. *et al.* (1986) Diode laser treatment for sports pain by comparison of thermography, the second report. *J Japan Soc Laser Surg and Med.* **6**(3):383–386.

Perini, J.L. *et al.* (2016) Long-term low-level laser therapy promotes an increase in maximal oxygen uptake and exercise performance in a dose-dependent manner in Wistar rats. *Lasers Med Sci.* **31**(2):241–248.

Ribeiro, B.G. *et al.* (2015) The effect of low-level laser therapy (LLLT) applied prior to muscle injury. *Lasers Surg Med.* **47**(7):571–578.

Soriano, F. *et al.* (2006) Photobiomodulation of pain and inflammation in microcrystalline arthropathies: experimental and clinical results. *Photomed Laser Surg.* **24**(2):140–150.

Stergioulas, A. (2007) Effects of low-level laser and plyometric exercises in the treatment of lateral epicondylitis. *Photomed Laser Surg.* **25**(3):205–213.

Stergioulas, A. (2008) Low-power laser treatment in patients with frozen shoulder: preliminary results. *Photomed Laser Surg.* **26**(2):99–105.

Stergioulas, A. *et al.* (2008) Effects of low-level laser therapy and eccentric exercises in the treatment of recreational athletes with chronic achilles tendinopathy. *Am J Sports Med.* **36**(5):881–887.

Tsai, W.C. *et al.* (2012) Low-level laser irradiation stimulates tenocyte migration with up-regulation of dynamin ii expression. *PLoS ONE.* **7**(5):e38235.

Uemoto, L. *et al.* (2013) Laser therapy and needling in myofascial trigger point deactivation. *J Oral Sci.* **55**(2):175–181.

Vieira, W.H. *et al.* (2012) Effects of low-level laser therapy (808 nm) on isokinetic muscle performance of young women submitted to endurance training: a randomized controlled clinical trial. *Lasers Med Sci.* **27**(2):497–504.

Walker, J.B. (1983) Relief from chronic pain by low-power laser irradiation. *Neurosci Lett.* **43**(2–3):339–344.

Wang, P. *et al.* (2014) Effects of low-level laser therapy on joint pain, synovitis, anabolic, and catabolic factors in a progressive osteoarthritis rabbit model. *Lasers Med Sci.* **29**(6):1875–1885.

21

Discipline-Specific Canine Sports Medicine Applications

Deborah M. Gross

Wizard of Paws Physical Rehabilitation for Animals, Colchester, CT, USA

Introduction

Sports medicine has become an integral component of all canine athletic activities. The principles of sports medicine are routinely applied during conditioning, rehabilitation protocols, surgical and non-surgical treatments, and in all stages of training, and are used to maintain canine athletes at their individual peak performance levels.

Canine athletes perform in athletic endeavors that range from professional racing to recreational agility events on the weekends. Each athletic discipline is divided into amateur and professional levels, each with unique training and preparation methodology.

Irrespective of the athletic discipline, a great amount of time, effort, and attention is spent on training, trialling, and preparation. This involves a diverse range of activities, including events focused on agility, obedience, racing, flyball, water work, rally, hunting, field trialling, sledding, and conformation. It also encompasses all working endeavors, including drug and bomb detectors, protection and guard dogs, guide dogs, service dogs, and therapy dogs.

Each sporting and working dog is a unique individual in the eyes of the owner, trainer, and handler, and in its ability to excel in its distinctive task. Each discipline demands specific actions of the body relative to physiology, strength, and performance. Laser therapy, also known as photobiomodulation therapy (PBMT), provides these individuals the best probability of preventing injuries, enjoying an extended career, and experiencing a good quality of life.

The rapidly expanding number of canine athletic competitions demands canine sports medicine applications of both a proactive and a reactive nature. Proactively, PBMT is an essential component in the effort to prevent injuries (Ribeiro *et al.*, 2015), maintain the highest level of performance possible (Levine *et al.*, 2015), and provide a higher quality of life. Reactively, it is an important part of the treatment and accelerated healing of all musculoskeletal injuries (Ferraresi *et al.*, 2012). PBMT provides a higher

level of available energy, accelerated gains in strength and conditioning, and a faster recovery period after each athletic endeavor. Therefore, when PBMT is integrated into strength, conditioning, and training programs, it results in a more comfortable athlete that is easier to train and can compete at a high level.

Types of Canine Sports

Most of the canine sports involve a combination of endurance, speed, power, obedience, and explosive activities. Knowledge of balance, proprioception, and normal physiologic parameters, as well as familiarity with the sport and common sense, are needed to evaluate and support these athletes. Some of the popular sports seen in a canine sports medicine environment are listed in Box 21.1.

Additional activities many dogs perform with their owners include hiking, walking, running, guard work, and, of course, counter surfing! All of these activities are important to each individual dog, trainer, handler, and owner. Our goals as professional practitioners include injury prevention, appropriate treatment, and rehabilitation. Accomplishing these goals culminates in the dog maintaining the highest level of function and performance.

Each of the common sports can be broken down into individual components. As we split them into endurance, power, speed, and strength, we can determine what is needed for preventative activities, training, rehabilitation, and a return to activity (function). Common endurance sports and activities include hunting, field trials, sledding, and detection work. Explosive activities include flyball, protection work, agility, and dock diving. Activities requiring speed include racing, agility, protection work, flyball, and water work. Power and obedience are fundamental to all of the athletic disciplines.

Box 21.1 Popular canine sports.	
Agility	Herding
Barn hunts	Hunting
Conformation	Obedience
Disk dog	Protection work
Dock diving	Racing
Field trial	Schutzhund
Freestyle dancing	Sledding
Flyball	Tracking

Many events involve a combination of traits. For example, a dog may participate in one agility run of approximately 40 seconds that involves explosive running, turning, ascending and descending frames and obstacles, and jumping. Though the event may last only 40 seconds, the dog might participate in three to six of these runs in one day, or 15–18 runs over the course of a long weekend. Therefore, endurance also plays a significant role in participation in this explosive event.

Understanding of Individual Sports and Breeds

To provide optimal care, it is essential to have a thorough understanding of the individual sport and the unique breed-specific athletic ability to perform that sport. For example, sight hounds are very different from many working breeds in their composition of body fat and muscle. Jeusette *et al.* (2010) examined the different body compositions of greyhounds, rottweilers, standard poodles, Siberian huskies, dachshunds, and golden retrievers and found greyhounds had significantly lower levels of body fat and higher levels of muscle compared to other breeds. Golden retrievers have the distinction of having the highest percentage of body fat among all dog breeds (Raffan, 2013).

Certain sports have a much higher participation among particular breeds compared to others. For example, sighthounds commonly participate in racing events, such as straight and oval racing. Herding dogs include a predominance of border collies, German shepherds, Shetland sheepdogs, and Australian shepherds. Protection dogs normally include German shepherds, Belgian malinois, Doberman pinchers, and Russian terriers. Any dog may participate in agility, but border collies, Shetland sheepdogs, papillion, Australian shepherds, and Portuguese water dogs excel due to their natural speed and accuracy. Dogs involved in flyball are typically fast and are very ball-motivated. Water work is typically performed by breeds that can swim, including Labrador retrievers, Portuguese water dogs, Newfoundlands, and other type of retriever.

Breed clubs have specific types of activity, as well. For example, Bernese mountain dogs are common drafters and Portuguese water dogs perform water sports specific to their breeds. Newfoundlands compete in draft and water rescue. Parsons terriers and Jack Russell terriers compete in barn hunts and racing.

Since each breed has a propensity to perform different athletic activities, as the practitioner, it is important to factor breed propensity into specific considerations about treatment and preventative care in different disciplines. Our goal is to help assist with the prevention of injuries while maintaining a high level of performance. If an injury occurs, knowledge about breed propensity helps individualize the rehabilitation program to accelerate the patient's return to its previous level of competition.

General Principles of PBMT in Canine Sports Medicine

In the human field, athletic trainers and physical therapists utilize various physical, therapeutic, and electrophysical techniques and modalities as additions to the manual care of patients. They share the same goals as practitioners in the canine sports medicine field: optimum athletic performance, prevention of injuries, and accelerated recovery. Skeletal muscles utilized in high-intensity repetitive muscle activities eventually fatigue, resulting in a direct decrease in performance of the core strength and the corresponding peripheral musculature. Whether it is a person running a 5 km race or a dog running an agility course, decrease in performance is caused by fatigue.

Many factors contribute to fatigue, including nutrition, age, training, conditioning, specific exercise conditions, and the environmental temperature. Ultimately, the depletion of energy sources within the cells results in fatigue. Proper nutrition, conditioning, and exercises specifically tailored to a discipline assist the canine athlete in avoiding fatigue.

Muscle contractions are either aerobic or anaerobic in nature. Aerobic muscle contractions are oxidative and are more associated with endurance events. Anaerobic muscle contractions are lactic and alactic and are associated with short bursts of energy and strength training. Strength training or high-intensity exercise creates a metabolic change in the musculature from the anaerobic metabolic pathways. Endurance or low-intensity exercise promotes a change in the energy recruitment from the aerobic metabolism (Billat *et al.*, 2009; Sundberg and Bundle, 2015).

Successful applications and approaches in the human field can be applied in the canine world. Common techniques and protocols have included cryotherapy, moist heat, massage, hot–cold contrast baths, stretching, low-intensity exercises, neuromuscular electrical stimulation, and various combinations of the same. The results on effectiveness are varied (Barnett, 2006). The rationale behind the use of these techniques is an attempt to reduce inflammation within the tissues associated with exercise. They increase vascularization and circulation, which in turn reduce the pooling of fluids and metabolites resulting from exercise that cause muscle soreness. Though these techniques are commonly utilized, their effectiveness is limited, and there is a constant search for alternatives. PBMT has been proven effective in increasing the circulation and reducing inflammation following exercise (Antonialli *et al.*, 2014; Baroni *et al.*, 2015). These attributes make it an ideal modality for use in both the human and the canine physical therapy fields.

PBMT targets the mitochondria or "energy centers" of individual cells. Skeletal muscles are rich in mitochondria. When their photoreceptors are stimulated, there is an increase in metabolic rate. PBMT thus assists in athletic performance by facilitating muscle repair, decreasing muscle fatigue, and reducing oxidative stress, all of which reduces the incidence of injury (Avni *et al.*, 2005). It has been used to accelerate metabolic and structural changes within both the aerobic and the anaerobic metabolic cycles (Karu, 2010).

PBMT has been demonstrated to reduce inflammation on many levels (Bortone *et al.*, 2008). In addition, it increases mitochondrial function and adenosine triphosphate (ATP), ribonucleic acid (RNA), and protein synthesis (Karu, 2010). These actions assist in increasing the rate of cellular metabolism and the acceleration of the inflammatory process (Huang *et al.*, 2009; Pryor and Millis, 2015). The combination of these facts has led scientists and clinicians to study the effectiveness of laser therapy on humans and animals post exercise and activity. Scientific studies have demonstrated conclusive evidence of laser therapy reducing inflammation and accelerating muscle repair when optimal parameters of treatment are applied (Assis, 2015; Levine *et al.*, 2015; Liu *et al.*, 2009). During the recovery stage post exercise, reduction of inflammation and acceleration of healing will accelerate the training process and maintain optimal performance levels in the canine athlete (de Marchi *et al.*, 2012).

Further studies support additional benefits of PMBT. It can improve mitochondrial function, which accelerates the healing process after exercise (Avni *et al.*, 2005). It can also decrease oxidative stress and reactive oxygen species (ROS) production (Bjordal *et al.*, 2001; Silveira *et al.*, 2009). Recent studies have provided scientific evidence that PBMT is effective in preventing the development of skeletal muscle fatigue and that it enhances recovery and, therefore, helps maintain performance (Ferraresi *et al.*, 2012; Ribeiro *et al.*, 2015).

Most injuries occur secondary to muscular and physiological fatigue (Allen *et al.*, 2008). Studies have examined whether PBMT could delay the development of skeletal muscle fatigue (Avni *et al.*, 2005; Leal Junior *et al.*, 2009a, 2009b). With a delay of skeletal muscle fatigue, there should be an increase in the speed of muscle recovery, with a faster restoration (recovery) to normal, and a reduced possibility of injury (Lopes-Martins *et al.*, 2006). Leal Junior *et al.* (2009a) demonstrated a delay in skeletal muscle fatigue with laser therapy. In addition to the delay, improved biomechanical markers were noted in direct relationship with muscle recovery (Ferraresi *et al.*, 2011). While these were great initial studies, they were performed with single-diode laser therapy probes (handpieces), which irradiate only a very small area. Another study by the same group utilized a multi-diode cluster probe applied to the biceps brachii muscle (Leal Junior *et al.*, 2009b). This crossover, double-blinded, placebo-controlled trial included healthy male volleyball players between the ages of 18 and 20. PBMT was administered utilizing a wavelength of 810 nm and a dosage of 6 J per point, applied to 10 treatment areas on the biceps brachii muscle. The laser-treated group demonstrated significantly delayed development of muscle fatigue while performing active exercise and repetitions to elbow fatigue. This study was also able to demonstrate a reduction in the blood lactate concentration level at 5 minutes post exercise. Blood lactate concentration is utilized to monitor recovery and serves as a marker post exercise. Historically, modalities used in human sports medicine and physical therapy to address recovery (cryotherapy, massage, and electrical stimulation) have failed to enhance blood lactate removal (Halson *et al.*, 2008; Jarvinen *et al.*, 2005). The ability of PBMT to reduce the blood lactate concentration alone makes this a valuable modality to facilitate recovery and healing.

The studies performed by Leal Junior *et al.* (2009a, 2009b) targeted a specific muscle and demonstrated improvement within the specific movement of elbow flexion. In sports, a multitude of muscles work at the same time. In order to improve the performance level of our athletic patients, it is imperative to determine which muscles specifically to target, which will be unique to each sporting activity. This will be covered later in the chapter.

Endurance Exercises

Endurance or aerobic exercise is activity of low intensity lasting more than 30 minutes. Jogging and hiking are two examples. Since the oxidative capacity of muscle fibers is proportional to the density of the mitochondria (Coffey and Hawley, 2007), endurance exercise is a great way of promoting mitochondrial growth, which results in a decreased level of muscle fatigue. The addition of PBMT to muscle cells increases the cellular respiratory level, which results in an increase in the synthesis of ATP. This allows an increase in oxygen consumption and a reduction in the fatigue index (Silveira *et al.*, 2009). The addition of PBMT to an endurance-training program allows an increase in the ability of the muscle to function at an efficient level for long periods.

Strength Training

Strength or intensity training involves anaerobic metabolic pathways and commonly involves short exercises. Weight lifting, weight pulling, and bursts of activity are examples. PBMT increases mitochondrial activity, resulting in an increased production of ATP and a normalization of cellular respiration. Fiber recruitment occurs sequentially, first with type I fibers, then with type IIa, type IIb, and finally type IIx. Strength training involves type I fibers, and PBMT may have more of a direct effect on strengthening these fibers than endurance exercises.

PBMT applied directly to specific muscles before activity will enhance performance and decrease the rate of fatigue. Strength training demands a significant amount of ATP from the hydrolysis of phosphocreatine. The consumption of ATP is faster than the rate of phosphocreatine hydrolysis, and this produces an excessive amount of creatine. This excess of creatine is an additional cause of muscle fatigue. If ATP levels can be increased, creatine levels will ultimately be reduced; this diminishes the rate and level of muscle fatigue. PBMT will increase the production of ATP (Karu *et al.*, 1995).

Repair of Muscle Damage

Various levels of muscle damage and injuries are a common occurrence in canine sports medicine. Whether it is a significant muscle tear with bleeding, sidelining the dog for a significant period, or a minor tear in a muscle resulting in just a slight decrease in athletic performance, application of PBMT will accelerate the healing process. The regeneration of muscle tissue takes place in six phases, and typically takes 21 days (Jarvinen *et al.*, 2005). Ultimately, the faster the tissue can move through these phases, the quicker the patient can return to their previous level of activity and training. Studies have demonstrated that PBMT can increase the formation of new myofibrils that assist in filling the gap created when a muscle is injured and decrease the formation of scar tissue (Roth and Oron, 1985). Bibikova and Oron (1994) demonstrated that PBMT promotes a greater maturation of younger myofibrils. Shefer *et al.* (2009) also demonstrated an improvement in the number of young myofibrils in a group that received PBMT compared to a group that did not. These are all promising studies, demonstrating that PBMT is beneficial in decreasing the deleterious effects of strenuous exercise and training.

Secondary and Tertiary Compensations

In many sports medicine scenarios, dogs perform an array of activities. Very often, the demands on one part of their body cause compensatory effects in other parts. For example, a dog with a straight shoulder set involved in a great deal of jumping activities might place a significant amount of stress on the thoracolumbar region. A significant component of treating the canine sports athlete is treating the entire dog. Understanding where the compensatory issues are is an important part of the successful management of the recovery of the canine athlete.

Palpation, range-of-motion tests, and digital thermal imaging are useful tools for determining whether any compensatory issues exist. Palpation is extremely useful but may not always be consistent. The results can vary between practitioners or breeds. Though palpation is one of the most accurate ways of determining pain and dysfunction, it is subject to variations in knowledge, sensory ability, the dog's coat, and the depth of the problem.

Both active and passive range of motion are useful for determining pain and dysfunction. Active range of motion assists with testing the contractile units of the joint and the dog's willingness to move. Passive range of motion assists with testing the inert units, such as bones, nerves, and ligaments.

Digital thermal imaging assists in the physiological examination of a patient. Thermal imaging creates a visual image of the temperatures of the body and allows for differentiation between normal areas and areas experiencing physiological differences (Figure 21.1). With this tool, the practitioner can determine where the primary problem is, as well as the location of any secondary or tertiary issues or conditions. Digital thermal imaging also allows a visualization of the extent of an issue. It answers the questions: "Is the problem within the joint or is it both in the joint and surrounding soft tissues?" and "Is there a problem in all the soft tissues supporting a joint or just one area?" These images serve as a very accurate roadmap for the application of PBMT to all primary, secondary, and tertiary areas of concern.

In addition, digital thermal imaging can assist in identifying problems before they become major issues. For example, detecting a minor iliopsoas problem is crucial in the canine athlete. Discovering issues before they become career ending is part of the practitioner's job.

Enhancement of Performance

Regardless of the athletic activity, the goal is always to safely maintain and maximize athletes' performance levels. In human sports medicine practice, numerous studies have demonstrated the efficacy of laser therapy in improving muscle performance. Ferraresi *et al.* (2011) examined 33 male athletes performing strength training with a load for 12 weeks. The athletes were divided into a control group, a

(a)

(b)

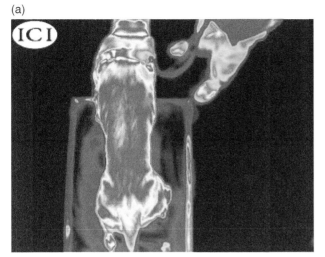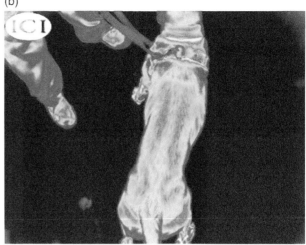

Figure 21.1 (a) Digital thermal image of a patient before PBMT. Increased thermal gradients are present throughout the thoracic and lumbar spinal musculature. Using this as a roadmap for PBMT, therapy was applied throughout all anatomical areas exhibiting an increase in thermal gradients. More energy was applied to the left side. (b) Digital thermal image taken 24 hours after PBMT of the same patient. All treated areas reveal a decrease in the thermal gradient. The patient was much more relaxed on palpation.

training group, and a training group that received laser therapy. Immediately after training, the group receiving laser therapy to the quadriceps muscle had a 55% increase in muscle performance as measured by isokinetic dynamometry. This was the only group that demonstrated an increase in muscle performance, and the study concluded that PBMT can increase muscle performance compared with strength training alone. It is easy to extrapolate this study to the world of the canine athlete when the goal is to increase the level of performance and prevent injury. Strength training combined with laser therapy is more beneficial than strength training alone.

Other studies have also demonstrated the benefits of PBMT for athletic performance. One study concluded there was a greater endurance of rotator cuff muscles in a group that received PBMT before exercise than in a group that did not (Levine *et al.*, 2015). This was a double-blind crossover study, in which the infraspinatus and teres minor musculature was treated before the initiation of exercise.

Another study showed that PBMT applied immediately prior to injury had many positive effects during the muscle regeneration processes (Ribeiro *et al.*, 2015). This study has considerable application in canine sports medicine with regards to sports where there is a constant risk of injury.

While we do not have specific measuring systems such as isokinetic dynamometry, the understanding and expansion of applications continue to grow through the tested scientific technique of trial and error coupled with collaboration with colleagues. As we continue to see the benefits and possibilities of PBMT, the opportunities for its use will continue to expand. Success is measured in the performance of canine athletes and the extension of their individual sports activities.

Application Technique

Practical applications of PBMT include performance enhancement, injury prevention, and preparation of canine athletes for their next activity. The goal is to assist with their quality of life and aid in their ability to compete safely to the best of their ability.

The first step is to understand and identify which muscles are important to an individual canine athlete's ability to perform at its maximum ability in a particular sport. The second step is to determine whether PBMT is intended for performance enhancement, injury prevention, recovery, or a combination of the three. The third step is to apply the appropriate dosage, utilizing the correct technique, at a frequency that optimizes athletic performance of the individual athlete.

Applying PBMT utilizing a contact method will help increase the blood flow, like a massage. This massage-like action potentiates the benefits of PBMT, since it actually puts the target tissue through a passive range of motion during administration. The soft tissue will be manipulated, which increases circulation. In addition, gently compressing the tissues forces the incidental absorbers hemoglobin and oxyhemoglobin away from the area. If this technique is performed properly, it is often very relaxing for the patient.

Before application of PBMT, make sure the area is clean. Clipping may not be feasible for performance dogs, so make sure the hair is clean and the laser equipment is adjusted appropriately for maximum penetration. In addition to preparing the skin, make sure the area is accessible.

Measure the treatment area to calculate the desired dose. Envisioning the area of a playing card is helpful in estimating the size of the treatment area. A single playing card is 57 cm^2; rounded up for ease of calculations, consider it 60 cm^2. Calculate the total number of playing cards needed to cover the intended area of treatment and then calculate the number of joules required to achieve the proper dosage. If a dosage of 10 J/cm^2 is desired, then administration of 600 J to an area equivalent in size to a single playing card would be correct. Always consider the patient's unique characteristics: hair color, hair length, skin color, and body mass. For example, a border collie will have pigmented and non-pigmented areas. The pigmented areas will absorb some of the photons being administered, so a higher dosage is warranted in these areas.

Treatment time is directly correlated to the power of the laser equipment. Utilizing higher power will allow you to administer the required total dose in a shorter time. A shorter treatment time will allow treatment of multiple areas in a single session in a reasonable amount of time.

To maximize penetration, hold the laser handpiece perpendicular to the muscles receiving the energy. The dog may be in lateral recumbency or in a standing position. Prior to performance, a dog will very often be excited, and standing may be the optimal position, since lying in lateral recumbency may be difficult. Handle the dog with a minimum amount of restraint. This will allow you to determine whether the treatment or positioning is painful to them.

Apply the photonic energy in a direct-contact fashion, sweeping over and massaging the targeted muscle groups. Use an overlapping pattern of movement and repeat at right angles to ensure that all areas receive the same amount of treatment. The goal of the PBMT session is to increase blood flow, increase the flow of nutrients to the muscles and surrounding tissues, increase ATP levels, prepare the body for exercise, and decrease any inflammation present. This cascade of effects from PBMT essentially results in a pre-event warm-up.

Always follow all safety precautions unique to each piece of equipment. When using a higher-power laser, keep the handpiece moving continuously. Drag a finger on the skin directly behind the handpiece to monitor the temperature of the treated area. Protective eyewear should be worn by the patient, the therapist, and anyone within the nominal hazard zone for the particular piece of equipment.

Dosages

There is always a question regarding the optimal dosage for the maximum consistent clinical response. Lopes-Martins *et al.* (2006) demonstrated a reduced fatigue in the tibialis anterior muscle in rats when a dosage of 0.5 J/cm^2 was applied, and decreased muscle damage at dosages of 1.0 and 2.5 J/cm^2. Another study examined the effects of different dosages of PBMT and found

Table 21.1 Recommended doses in canine sports medicine. Adapted from Leal Junior *et al.* (2010) and Saunders and Millis (2014).

Condition	Recommended dosage (J/cm^2)
Pain relief	
Acute injuries	2–4
Acute muscle	4–6
Acute joint	4–6
Chronic conditions	4–8
Reduction of Inflammation	
Acute	1–6
Chronic	4–8

groups of rats receiving 1 and 3 J had a higher peak force compared to groups receiving 0.1 and 0.3 J (Leal Junior *et al.*, 2010). A third study reported doses of 1–3 J/cm^2 at 660 nm and 1, 3, and 10 J/cm^2 at 905 nm provided the best results (Santos, 2014). As these studies demonstrate, there are no universal dosages. Practitioners must dose each target and each muscle to effect. One successful way to do this is to palpate the target muscle manually while administering PBMT, and continue administration until you feel the target area relax and become free of any spastic areas.

Recommended doses for clinical use in canine sports medicine vary depending upon the target area and the condition being treated. While there are no universal dosages, a range of 2–8 J/cm^2 will be very effective for most maladies (Table 21.1) (Saunders and Millis, 2014).

The physical characteristics of your patient also determine your dosage. Skin color, hair color, coat type, thick versus thin body conformation, and body mass all have to be taken into consideration when calculating the initial dose. If the target area is deep on a heavily muscled athlete, increase the dosage. If the target is on a dark-haired or dark-skinned patient with a long coat, increase the dosage. Fortunately, there are many laser units on the market with software that will do these calculations for you. The dosage can then be adjusted manually upon each re-evaluation.

Clinical Applications

Agility and Flyball

Agility and flyball are two very popular sports. Both involve short bursts of activity with jumps, quick turns, and other movements dependent on terrain. The bursts may be anywhere from 30 to 90 seconds in length, but they can be repeated several times throughout the course of a day. Therefore, recovery and preparation for the next race are significant in these activities.

Agility and flyball participants require a significant amount of power and agility, and make a significant number of turns. Thus, these athletes utilize many different muscles during their events. Due to this high demand of muscle activity, it is often necessary to determine whether one muscle group needs therapy more than others do. Because of the time constraints between events, it is often difficult to treat all muscle groups, so a priority should be established.

The adductors and abductors of the shoulders and hips provide a significant amount of power, speed, and stability. They are often injured in agility and flyball. Medial shoulder injuries are also very common. The application of laser therapy to these areas before competitions and practice has a significant effect in reducing the incidence of injuries. To provide ideal access for the application of photonic energy to the medial shoulder, the patient should be positioned in lateral recumbency.

The iliopsoas is another area that is easily warmed up with PBMT. The dog should be placed in a lateral recumbent position with the hip in slight extension. The extended position will allow better access to the entire iliopsoas muscle from origin to insertion.

The canine athlete involved with flyball or agility should receive therapy approximately 20–30 minutes prior to their activity. The length of PBMT received will depend on the number of areas requiring treatment and the size of the dog. After the appropriate amount of PBMT has been delivered, the dog should be warmed up and stretched prior to the activity. If a muscle injury is suspected after an individual heat or sprint, additional PBMT should be applied to that specific region.

One PBMT session should be sufficient warm-up for the entire day. For example, a border collie involved with agility may receive PBMT to its shoulder adductors and hip adductors prior to a competition. A 22 kg border collie's shoulder adductors are approximately $120\,\text{cm}^2$, and its hip adductors approximately $240\,\text{cm}^2$. The dosage will range from 2 to $4\,\text{J/cm}^2$, or 240–480 J to the shoulder and 480–960 J to the hip. After the dog has received PBMT, a warm-up and dynamic stretching should be performed before it participates in its activity. If, after the activity, the dog is sore in its hip flexors, additional PBMT may be applied to the iliopsoas insertion, rectus femoris, and lumbar component from the second to the seventh lumbar vertebrae.

Jumping Activities

In jumping activities, the hip extensors, hip flexors, shoulder flexors, and spinal extensors are extremely active. The spinal extensors, specifically the lumbar and cervical muscles, are also very active during protection work. In these dogs, PBMT can be applied to a combination of muscles before their activities, as part of their warm-up routine. Treatment with PBMT should include the spinal extensors, hip flexors and extensors, and shoulder flexors and extensors. If there has been a previous injury, it is important to focus on the muscles in that area as well. This results in an increase in the blood flow and flexibility of these structures, with the goal of preventing re-injury. Stretches should be applied during therapy to any areas in which there is stiffness or reduced range of motion. After PBMT, warm-up with continued movement should be continued until the activity begins.

Power Events

In power events, such as Schutzhund, agility, and flyball, the muscles that are the most active include the hip and stifle extensors and the shoulder flexors. Of course, many other muscles are also very active, but a significant amount of the power will be generated by the hip and stifle extensors as the dog propels forward. The shoulder flexors will be involved, creating the power to propel forward from extension. Very often in power events, power with reach and extension is important.

In a fast-running dog, the shoulder flexors and elbow extensors will be very active during the stride, since they increase the fore-limb extension.

PBMT should be applied to each of these muscles, from its origin to insertion.

- **Hip and stifle extensors:**
  - **Biceps femoris muscle:** Originates on the ischial tuberosity and sacrotuberous ligament, and inserts on the fascia lata, crural fascia, patellar ligament, and cranial border of the tibia.
  - **Semitendinosus muscle:** Originates on the ischial tuberosity and inserts on the distocranial border of the tibia.
  - **Semimembranosus muscle:** Arises from the ischial tuberosity and inserts into the aponeurosis of the origin of the gastrocnemius and on the medial condyle of the femur.
- **Shoulder extensors and elbow flexors:**

  - **Triceps muscle:** Originates on the caudal border of the scapula and the tricipital crest and inserts on the olecranon.
  - **Teres major muscle:** Originates on the caudal border of the scapula and inserts on the teres major tuberosity.
  - **Supraspinatus muscle:** Originates on the Supraspinous fossa and inserts on the greater tubercle of the humerus.

To maintain or enhance performance, PBMT should be applied along the entire length, origin, and insertion of the three muscles of the hip and those involved with the extension of the stifle. Application to the hind limb begins distal to the ischial tuberosity and proceeds

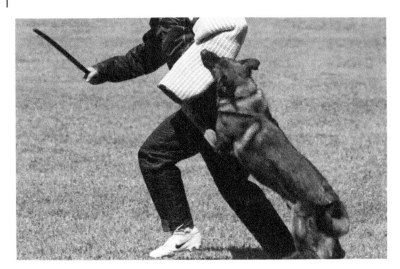

Figure 21.2 Explosion of a guard dog on to the sleeve of a decoy. The hip and spinal extensors are very active as the dog explodes up to the sleeve.

distally to the cranial stifle. Repeat the same procedure for the three muscles of the fore limb. Photonic energy should be applied from the medial and distal shoulder down to the olecranon.

Protection Work

Protection work, such as Schutzhund, French ring, or guarding, often requires powerful bursts of energy. These activities involve a number of different types of muscle contraction, including isometric, concentric, eccentric, and plyometric. Dogs that engage in protection work are often jumping over objects or jumping up to perform bite work. Bite work involves running toward a decoy or a person, with the rear legs making powerful moves to propel the dog forward. The fore-limb and spine complexes also extend and flex powerfully.

Figure 21.2 demonstrates the explosion on to the sleeve of a decoy. The hip extensors are very active as the dog explodes up to the sleeve. After the apprehension of the target, the dog requires a significant amount of control and focus to grip. The grip needs to be strong and powerful, requiring the dog to bound up in a powerful plyometric fashion and then, on release, slowly return to a guarding position. Figures 21.2 and 21.3 are from practice sessions, but in real-life situations, this is how a dog would apprehend a suspect. Police dogs, protection dogs, guard dogs, and other working dogs are familiar with this training. The combination of proper conditioning and pretreatment with PBMT has an important role in preventing injuries during this activity.

Speed Racing

Racing dogs, such as sighthounds, need increased speed and distance. The hind limb is responsible for propelling the body forward. The semitendinosus, semimembranosus, biceps femoris, and adductors also play a role in forward propulsion.

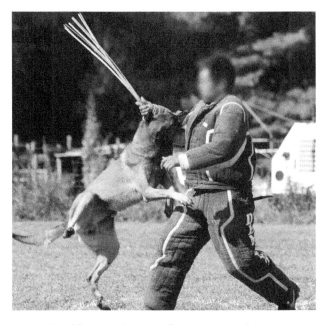

Figure 21.3 After apprehension of a target, a guard dog requires a significant amount of control and focus to maintain its grip.

The adductor group is often injured in sighthounds, since it provides stabilization within the racing motion of these breeds. The shoulder extensors work to extend the fore limb and to widen the stride. The hip, stifle, and hock extensors are responsible for forward propulsion and increasing speed. Photonic energy should be applied to all of these muscles (adductor groups, shoulder extensors, hip, stifle, and hock extensors, and hip and shoulder flexors) prior to an event. This general therapeutic protocol can be customized to an individual athlete's needs in order to maximize the clinical outcome.

Specific breeds involved in speed racing are primarily whippets, greyhounds, Rhodesian ridgebacks, and borzois. Other breeds are involved in this event, but they are in a minority. The dogs may race in a straight line or in an oval. Dogs racing in an oval require particular attention to their medial musculature on both the fore and hind limbs, as they generate more power on these muscles when they navigate turns.

Racing sighthounds are predisposed to soft-tissue injuries involving the adductor musculature in the hind limbs. Individuals who have suffered previous injuries to the adductors should be examined closely before each event and should receive additional PBMT. In order to laser the adductor group, the dog must be in a lateral recumbent position or lying on its side, with the hip abducted. It is difficult to laser this group while the dog is standing.

Optimize the beneficial effects of PBMT by applying it approximately 30–60 minutes before the event. When there is a need to apply PBMT to a variety of muscle groups, treatment time for each patient can be 10–20 minutes, depending upon the size of the dog and the areas in need of therapy. Utilize a contact method of application to impart the added benefit of a massage to the tissue. This results in a further increase in blood flow and maximizes the warm-up.

A case example is Weasel, a 4-year-old intact female whippet. Figure 21.4 shows her receiving PBMT to the hip extensor muscles, utilizing the contact method. In Figure 21.5, she is receiving treatment to the biceps femoris muscle region. This dog prefers to be standing while receiving laser therapy, but appropriate therapy could also be performed in lateral recumbency or a lying-down posture. In Figure 21.6, an on-contact application of PBMT is

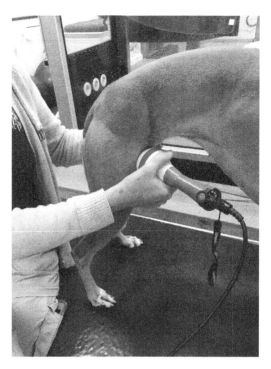

Figure 21.5 Administration of PBMT to the biceps femoris regions. To maximize photon penetration to the target tissues, the handpiece should be maintained perpendicular to the tissue and gentle pressure should be applied while moving it over the treatment area.

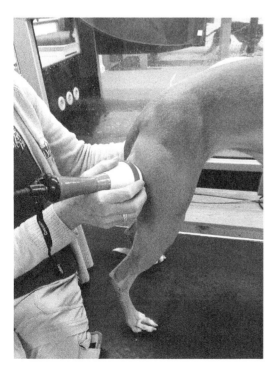

Figure 21.4 PBMT being administered to the hip extensor muscles, utilizing on-contact delivery with the handpiece in direct contact with the skin and hair coat.

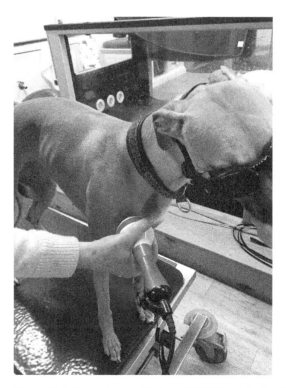

Figure 21.6 On-contact application of PBMT the right shoulder and shoulder extensors area while the patient is standing. This treatment could also be administered with the patient in lateral recumbency or a lying-down posture.

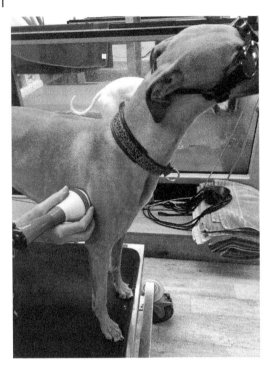

Figure 21.7 Administration of PBMT to the right triceps region. Access to the triceps region can also be gained with the patient in lateral recumbency. Gentle massage pressure should be applied along the triceps muscle and over the supraspinatus and teres major muscles.

being administered to Weasel's right shoulder and shoulder extensors while she is standing. In Figure 21.7, PBMT is being administered to her right triceps region. Access to the triceps region can also be gained when in lateral recumbency. Apply gentle pressure along the triceps muscle and over the supraspinatus and teres major muscles.

Use the playing card system when calculating the total dose to these anatomical areas. In Figure 21.4, the area to be treated is roughly four playing cards. With each playing card measuring approximately $60\,cm^2$ and a dosage of $1\text{–}4\,J/cm^2$ required to achieve a clinical response, the total dose would be 60–240 J. The triceps area in Figure 21.7 is roughly the area of two playing cards, which is approximately $120\,cm^2$. Therefore, the correct dosage would be between 120 and 480 J. A larger area would require treatment at the same dosage but an increased total number of joules; the converse applied for a smaller area.

In a racing dog, the goal of PBMT is to increase blood flow to the tissues. The vasodilation effects of PBMT

allow additional nutrients to be provided to any cells that are going to be asked for an increase in their metabolic rate during the event. The application of PBMT to the racing dog should ideally be performed before the athlete stretches and warms up. The most beneficial time is approximately 30 minutes prior to any activity. This will facilitate an increased range of motion within the limbs and greater flexibility within the muscles. Utilization of this sequence of events maximizes performance.

In some smaller dogs, it is sometimes difficult to reach certain anatomical areas when attempting to massage or stretch before exercise. The application of PBMT will provide an increased blood flow and an overall relaxation of the patient, which aids in this pre-event procedure. Particular attention should be paid to the hip region, the shoulder region, the medial muscle groups (such as the adductor and medial shoulder muscles), and the iliopsoas.

In Weasel's case, she had a previous injury to the rectus femoris and the iliopsoas muscles. She has been free of lameness for over 9 months at the time of writing, and has returned to both straight and oval racing at a very competitive level. She receives PBMT to the hip flexors, iliopsoas, and hip extensors 40 minutes prior to competition. After PBMT, she receives her warm–up, consisting of figure eights and dynamic hip extensor and flexor stretches. Movement is continued until the actual race time. The focus on the hip flexors and iliopsoas is secondary to the prior injury. An additional benefit of the application of PBMT to this area is the reduction of any pre-existing inflammation. The result of all these efforts is a safe improvement in athletic performance.

Conclusion

PBMT has been demonstrated to have numerous benefits when applied to the canine athlete. If the practitioner is able to deliver the appropriate number of joules to the target tissues, positive results will be inevitable. This modality can be utilized for the treatment and prevention of injuries, pre-event preparation, and maintenance of the canine athlete at its highest performance level. Our ultimate goal when working with animals is to allow them to live the best life they can, for the longest time possible. This includes helping them safely work and compete to the best of their ability in their athletic endeavors. PBMT is an essential tool we can use to accomplish this.

References

Allen, D.G. *et al.* (2008) Skeletal muscle fatigue: cellular mechanisms. *Physiol Rev.* **88**(1):287–332.

Antonialli, F.C. *et al.* (2014) Phototherapy in skeletal muscle performance and recovery after exercise: effect of combination of super-pulsed laser and light-emitting diodes. *Lasers Med Sci.* **29**(6):1967–1976.

Assis, L. (2015) Effect of low-level laser therapy (808 nm) on skeletal muscle after endurance exercise training in rats. *Braz J Phys Ther.* **19**(6):457–465.

Avni, D. *et al.* (2005) Protection of skeletal muscles from ischemic injury: low-level laser therapy increases antioxidant activity. *Photomed Laser Surg.* **23**(3):273–277.

Barnett, A. (2006) Using recovery modalities between training sessions in elite athletes: does it help? *Sport Med.* **36**(9):781–796.

Baroni, B.M. *et al.* (2015) Effect of low-level laser therapy on muscle adaptation to knee extensor eccentric training. *Eur J Appl Physiol.* **115**(3):639–647.

Bibikova, A. and Oron, U. (1994) Attenuation of the process of muscle degeneration in the toad gastrocnemius muscle by low energy laser irradiation. *Lasers Surg Med.* **14**(4):355–361.

Billat, V. *et al.* (2009) Differential modeling of anaerobic and aerobic metabolism in the 800-m and 1,500-m run. *J Appl Physiol.* **17**(2):478–487.

Bjordal, J.M. *et al.* (2001) Low level laser therapy for tendinopathy: evidence of a dose-response pattern. *Phys Ther Rev.* **6**(2):91–99.

Bortone, F. *et al.* (2008) Low level laser therapy modulates kinin receptor expression in the subplantar muscle of rat paw subjected to carrageenan-induced inflammation. *Int Immunopharm.* **8**(2):206–210.

Coffey, V.G. and Hawley, J.A. (2007) The molecular bases of training adaptation. *Sports Med.* **34**:663–679.

de Marchi, T. *et al.* (2012) Low-level laser therapy (LLLT) in human progressive-intensity running: effects on exercise performance, skeletal muscle status, and oxidative stress. *Lasers Med Sci.* **27**(1):231–236.

Ferraresi, C. *et al.* (2011) Effects of low level laser therapy (808 nm) on physical strength training in humans. *Lasers Med Sci.* **26**(3):349–358.

Ferraresi, C. *et al.* (2012) Low-level laser (light) therapy (LLLT) on muscle tissue: performance, fatigue and repair benefited by the power of light. *Photonics Lasers Med.* **1**(4):267–286.

Halson, S.l. *et al.* (2008) Physiological responses to cold water immersion following cycling in the heat. *Int J Sports Physiol Perform.* **3**(3):331–346.

Huang, Y.Y. *et al.* (2009) Biphasic dose response in low level light therapy. *Dose-Response.* **7**(4):358–383.

Jarvinen, T.A. *et al.* (2005) Muscle injuries: biology and treatment. *Am J Sports Med.* **33**(5):745–764.

Jeusette, *et al.* (2010) Effect of breed on body composition and comparison between various methods to estimate body composition in dogs. *Res Vet Sci.* **88**(2):227–232.

Karu, T. (2010) Mitochondrial mechanisms of photobiomodulation in context of new data about multiple roles of ATP. *Photomed Laser Surg.* **28**(2):159–160.

Karu, T.I. *et al.* (1995). Irradiation with He-Ne laser increases ATP level in cells cultivated in vitro. *J Photochem Photobiol B.* **27**(3):219–223.

Leal Junior, E.C. *et al.* (2009a) Effect of 830 nm low level laser therapy in exercise induced skeletal muscle fatigue in humans. *Lasers Med Sci.* **24**(3):425–431.

Leal Junior, E.C. *et al.* (2009b) Effect of cluster multi-diode light emitting diode therapy (LEDT) on exercise-induced skeletal muscle fatigue and skeletal muscle recovery in humans. *Lasers Surg Med.* **41**(8):572–527.

Leal Junior, E.C. *et al.* (2010) Effect of low-level laser therapy (GaAs 904 nm) in skeletal muscle fatigue and biochemical markers of muscle damage in rats. *Eur J Appl Physiol.* **108**(6):1083–1088.

Levine, D. *et al.* (2015) Effects of laser on endurance of the rotator cuff muscles. *Lasers Surg Med.* **47**(s26):44–45.

Liu, X.G. *et al.* (2009) Effects of low-level laser irradiation on rat skeletal muscle injury after eccentric exercise. *Photomed Laser Surg.* **27**(6):863–869.

Lopes-Martins, R.A. *et al.* (2006) Effect of low-level laser (Ga-Al-As 655 nm) on skeletal muscle fatigue induced by electrical stimulation in rats. *J Appl Physiol.* **101**(1):283–288.

Pryor, B. and Millis, D.L. (2015) Therapeutic laser in veterinary medicine. *Vet Clin North Am Small Anim Pract.* **45**(1):45–56.

Raffan, E. (2013) Obesity in labradors and golden retrievers. *Vet Rec.* **172**(12):320.

Ribeiro, B.G. *et al.* (2015) The effect of low-level laser therapy (LLLT) applied prior to muscle injury. *Lasers Surg Med.* **47**(7):571–578.

Roth, D. and Oron, U. (1985) Repair mechanisms involved in repair regeneration following partial excision of the rat gastrocnemius muscle. *Exp Cell Biol.* **53**(2):107–114.

Santos, L.A. (2014) Effects of pre-irradiation of low-level laser therapy with different doses and wavelengths in skeletal muscle performance, fatigue, and skeletal muscle damage induced by tetanic contractions in rats. *Lasers Med Sci.* **29**(5):1617–1626.

Saunders, D.G. and Millis, D. (2014). Laser therapy in canine rehabilitation. In: *Canine Rehabilitation and Physical Therapy*, 2 edn., pp. 359–380. Elsevier, Amsterdam.

Shefer, G. *et al.* (2009) Low-energy laser irradiation promotes the recovery of atrophied gastrocnemius skeletal muscle in rats. *Exp Physilo.* **94**(9):1005–1015.

Silveira, P.C. *et al.* (2009) Evaluation of mitochondrial respiratory chain activity in muscle healing by low level laser therapy. *J Photochem Photobiol B.* **95**(2):89–92.

Sundberg, C.W. and Bundle, M.W. (2015) Influence of duty cycle on the time course of muscle fatigue and the onset of neuromuscular compensation during exhaustive dynamic isolated limb exercise. *Am J Physiol Regul Integr Comp. Physiol.* **309**(1):R51–R61.

Part VI

Clinical Applications of Laser Therapy in Companion Animal Rehabilitation

22

Laser Therapy and Multimodal Postoperative Rehabilitation
Jeffrey J. Smith

Middletown Animal Hospital, Middletown, CA, USA

Introduction

Laser therapy is a very effective modality that is even more effective when used as a component of a multimodal management strategy. We now have many excellent pharmaceutical and non-pharmaceutical options for treating pain and facilitating healing (Box 22.1). The new standard of care calls for incorporating all of these together for maximum effectiveness and minimum side effects. This discussion will touch on several aspects of postoperative rehabilitation and will examine the role of laser therapy in that process.

When laser therapy is used as a sole modality, it is likely to require more frequent use and to deliver less optimal results, especially with advanced conditions and pathologies. When multiple modalities are used to manage pain, inflammation, and healing, with effects at different points along the healing and pain pathways, superior outcomes are the logical and scientifically proven result (Hållstam *et al.*, 2016; Jang and Lee, 2012; Van Middelkoop *et al.*, 2011; Walker, 1983).

Within a practice, the move toward offering rehabilitation services can begin with a higher–power (9–15 W) therapeutic laser as an anchor, and then add a selection of more modest rehabilitation modalities and tools, while developing protocols for their multimodal use. Eventually, the goal is to incorporate enough modalities, experience, and expertise to provide a fully fledged and fully equipped rehabilitation service (Saunders and Millis, 2014).

Why Rehabilitation?

"Veterinary physical rehabilitation" is the preferred term for the combination of non-invasive techniques in recovery from injuries, impairments, or functional limitations. "Veterinary physical therapy" would be an analogous term, but the use of "physical therapy" to describe these veterinary modalities as is proscribed by the American Physical Therapy Association (APTA) (www.apta.org). Regardless of how veterinary rehabilitation is named, the modalities included result in positive effects in patients (Millis and Ciuperca, 2015; Sims *et al.*, 2015). Rehabilitation should be recognized as good medicine and as scientifically valid.

Rehabilitation is Good Medicine

Rehabilitation services are part of the new standard of care recognized by American Animal Hospital Association (AAHA) and the American Association of Feline Practitioners (AAFP). The 2015 AAHA/AAFP Pain Management Guidelines for Dogs and Cats emphasizes the importance of multimodal management for all painful conditions (AAHA, 2015). Though patients may recover from surgeries and other interventional procedures without rehabilitation, they will recover faster and with less overall pain with rehabilitation (as similar patients do in human medicine).

Pain management is more effective and recovery is quicker after procedures when a multimodal postoperative protocol is used, because intervening in the pain and healing pathways at multiple points produces better outcomes than reliance on a single point. Laser therapy – photobiomodulation therapy (PBMT) – can be an important part of a multimodal postoperative plan for addressing pain (Enwemeka *et al.*, 2004; Fulop *et al.*, 2010; Sprouse-Blum *et al.*, 2010). Rehabilitation after invasive procedures is not just a race to return to function: it is a programmed progression toward increased activity and increased function, and it helps prevent problems like cartilage atrophy, bone loss, and loss of range of motion.

Rehabilitation is Valid

Rehabilitation is a validated modality with level III evidence to support its use. "Level III evidence" means

Laser Therapy in Veterinary Medicine: Photobiomodulation, First Edition. Edited by Ronald J. Riegel and John C. Godbold, Jr.
© 2017 John Wiley & Sons, Inc. Published 2017 by John Wiley & Sons, Inc.

Box 22.1 Therapeutic options for multimodal management of postoperative conditions.

Pharmaceutical Therapies
  Non-steroidal anti-inflammatory drugs (NSAIDs)
  Polysulfated glycosaminoglycan
  Neutraceuticals
  N-methyl-D-aspartate (NMDA) receptor antagonists
  Tricyclic antidepressants (TCAs)
  Serotoninergics
  Gabapentinoids
  Opiates
  Atypical opiates
Non-pharmaceutical Therapies
  Laser therapy
  Cold therapy
  Heat therapy
  Extracorporeal shockwave therapy
  Therapeutic ultrasound
  Electrotherapy
  Manual therapy
  Physical and proprioceptive exercises
  Aquatic exercise
  Acupuncture
Regenerative Therapies
  Platelet-rich plasma
  Stem cells

---

that publications and studies have shared evidence from well-designed controlled trials with randomization (Ebling Library, n.d.). The American Veterinary Medical Association (AVMA) recently approved board certification by the American College of Veterinary Sports Medicine and Rehabilitation (ACVSMR) (www.vsmr. org) in recognition of this area of study and care (AVMA, n.d.). Most schools of veterinary medicine now have a rehabilitation department, offer clinical rehabilitation services, and give students some exposure to rehabilitation modalities during clinical rotations.

In human medicine, rehabilitation and physical therapy is an everyday means of recovering better, faster, and with less pain after invasive procedures. That should be no different in veterinary medicine.

The Challenge and Opportunity of Rehabilitation in Veterinary Medicine

The nature of veterinary practice is changing. Regardless of location, most veterinary practices are earning less pharmacy income, administering fewer vaccinations, seeing fewer clients, seeing fewer feline patients, and doing fewer ovariohysterectomies and orchidectomies. Most authorities suggest that veterinarians need to be focused on providing expertise and technology that pet owners value and cannot find elsewhere.

Delivery of comprehensive dental services was a significant evolution in veterinary care that resulted in better patient care and improved practice income. Comprehensive dental care delivered a service that clients valued and could not find elsewhere. Rehabilitation, physical therapy, and multimodal pain management are perhaps the next great frontiers for practices.

Successful implementation of rehabilitation in a practice requires motivated veterinarians and members of staff, who are willing to comply with new protocols and procedures. Delivery of rehabilitation requires clients who comply with recommendations from the veterinary team and patients that comply with multimodal treatments as they are administered.

Veterinarian and Staff Compliance

Veterinarians and members of staff work together to deliver rehabilitation services. As in dentistry, many rehabilitation services are administered by technicians, nurses, and staff members. While maintaining a supervisory role, veterinarians can rely on support staff for hands-on treatments. From a financial standpoint, rehabilitation services can be initiated with minimal investment in equipment and space, and result in immediate economic return. Important to the success of implementation is client acceptance and increased production of expertise-based revenue. Finally, and most important to veterinarians and staff members, postoperative rehabilitation provides excellent results in terms of patient response.

Client Compliance

Pet-owning clients are preconditioned to accept veterinary prescriptions of postoperative rehabilitation, because of their own involvement in recovering from surgical procedures, either their own or those of family members. As such, clients understand the need for rehabilitative assistance in returning to function. Today, clients expect rehabilitation. They are enthusiastic about physiotherapy because they view it as drug-free (almost!) and non-invasive. What clients have experienced in their own recoveries from surgeries and injuries is readily embraced as being the standard of care for their well-loved pets. Rehabilitation sessions are appreciated and valued by clients, who love being able to participate in the "healing" of their pet.

Patient Compliance

Patients love rehabilitation because it does not involve injections, blood draws, or nail trims! In fact, much of what is done during rehabilitation feels good. Patients are able to enjoy an entirely new experience at the veterinary practice. Visits for postoperative rehabilitation mesh nicely with the emerging concept of reducing patient fear during veterinary visits.

Rehabilitation Skills

Postoperative rehabilitation will most often be a component of a comprehensive rehabilitation program. A comprehensive rehabilitation program is dependent on veterinarians and staff members having the skills necessary to prescribe, plan, and deliver rehabilitation.

Technical Rehabilitation Skills

Veterinarians and staff members involved in postoperative rehabilitation should have up-to-date training in osteology, myology, and neuroanatomy. All should be familiar with how to conduct and record orthopedic, neurological, and pain examinations. The practice should have standardized forms for recording the results of patient pain assessments. According to Robin Downing, DVM, DAAPM, DACVSMR, CVPP, CCRP, "Every single patient at every single visit needs to have a pain assessment" (Thomas, 2011). Objective pain assessment scoring systems are readily available from the University of Pennsylvania School of Veterinary Medicine (PennVet, n.d.), the Colorado State University School of Veterinary Medicine (CVMBS, n.d. a,b), and the International Veterinary Academy of Pain Management (IVAPM, n.d.).

Advanced Rehabilitation Skills

Advanced training in rehabilitation is very beneficial when conducting postoperative rehabilitation, but is not essential. A basic understanding of exercise physiology, biomechanics, and kinematics will provide additional expertise for the veterinarian directing and prescribing a patient's postoperative rehabilitation program.

Soft Rehabilitation Skills

Each rehabilitation patient is unique and will require an individualized physiotherapy regimen based on its behavior, pain level, severity of compromise, age, complicating factors, and fitness. Veterinary personnel charged with postoperative rehabilitation need to have excellent client communication skills and expertise in animal handling. Precise record keeping is mandatory. Because postoperative rehabilitation often involves assisting the movement of larger patients, an appropriate degree of physical fitness is required. Patience, kindness, perceptiveness, creativity, and self-direction are additional soft skills that are helpful.

Rehabilitation Training and Practice

Training in technical and advanced rehabilitation skills is important. It is available through several venues. In the United States, the University of Tennessee offers the Canine Rehabilitation Certificate Program (UT, n.d.), while the Universities of Florida and Colorado State offer training through the Canine Rehabilitation Institute, with a Certified Canine Rehabilitation Therapist (CCRT) program for veterinarians and physical therapists and a Certified Canine Rehabilitation Assistant (CCRA) for veterinary technicians (www.caninerehabinstitute.com).

Comprehensive textbooks on rehabilitation are available (Millis and Levine, 2013; Zink and Van Dyke, 2013). In addition, there are myriad other sources of training, including equipment manufacturers, webinars, online videos, conference lectures, specialty conferences, and the American Association of Rehabilitation Veterinarians (AARV) (www.rehabvets.org).

Postoperative Rehabilitation Modalities

Postoperative rehabilitation should be multimodal and should include appropriate, available modalities. In addition to laser therapy, postoperative rehabilitation may include cold and heat therapy, extracorporeal shockwave therapy, therapeutic ultrasound, electrotherapy, manual therapies (massage, passive range of motion, stretching, joint mobilization, acupressure), physical and proprioceptive exercises, and aquatic exercises.

Laser therapy predominates in use over ultrasound, electrotherapy, and extracorporeal shockwave therapy in most practices because of its effectiveness and ease of use, and because it doesn't require clipping of hair.

Postoperative Rehabilitation Outcomes

The gold standard for the outcome of postoperative rehabilitation is that the patient returns to function. Subjective and objective observations made by the owner can help in the evaluation of patient progress. Standardized forms for collecting owner observations are available (Valentin, 2009). Nonetheless, objective measures are an excellent and necessary method for validating progress. These methods include video images, digital thermal imaging, static weight bearing using stance analyzers, gait analysis, muscle girth measurement, and goniometry. Data and measurements should be recorded prior to initiating postoperative rehabilitation and at regular intervals during the progression to return to function.

Why Multimodal Postoperative Rehabilitation?

Multimodal therapy works better than single-modality therapy. This is because multiple issues are addressed by multiple mechanisms when additional therapies are employed. Decreased bone loss, increased range of motion in joints, and diminished adhesions are just a few examples.

Rehabilitation Tools

Much of the equipment used in postoperative rehabilitation is inexpensive. Balance boards, balance balls, peanut balls, caveletties, slings, harnesses, ice packs, hot packs, stairs, ramps, and land (dry) treadmills can all be used and all work fine. However, in order to really step into a higher-level rehabilitation program, the two most effective pieces of equipment are a therapeutic laser (9–15 W) and an underwater treadmill. The investment in these moderately expensive items will provide a very good monetary return from rehabilitation, if reliable and effective models are selected.

The Role of Laser Therapy in Postoperative Rehabilitation

Laser therapy is an ideal anchor for a rehabilitation service because of the effects of PBM on tissue: decreasing pain, decreasing inflammation, and accelerating healing (Saunders and Millis, 2014). The modality is easy to master, is effective, and is appreciated by clients. Clients view laser therapy as "high tech" and "high touch," even when their view of other rehabilitation modalities (e.g., cold therapy, massage, passive range of motion) is less enthusiastic. Clients will often accept an entire postoperative rehabilitation prescription without any objections as long as it includes laser therapy.

Postoperative Rehabilitation Protocols

The average practice will begin to incorporate rehabilitation and postoperative rehabilitation protocols into its services by starting with three common types of cases: hips (osteoarthritis, degenerative joint disease, and femoral head ostectomy surgery), knees (cranial cruciate ligament injuries and surgeries), and backs (intervertebral disk disease, IVDD). This focus on common conditions provides great experience in many rehabilitation basics and a base from which to expand into more difficult and esoteric conditions (quadriceps contracture, coronoid fractures of the elbow, iliopsoas muscle injury).

Practices should develop written protocols to use as guidelines when managing commonly seen conditions. Most practices find this approach to be less overwhelming than taking on the expectation that they must be able to do *everything* before they can do *anything*. These protocols can be modified on a case-by-case basis to individualize treatments of each particular patient. The most important concept in developing and following rehabilitation protocols is to stage therapies according to the progress of the patient. A protocol is merely an outline or guide from which to develop an individualized protocol. It should really be viewed as a menu from which to select or consider therapies.

The protocols outlined in this chapter are not definitive and can vary greatly depending on patient cooperation, progress, and owner compliance. They are presented as examples of guidelines that can help organize and direct postoperative rehabilitation. These protocols are modeled on the examples put forth in *Canine Rehabilitation and Physical Therapy*, 2 edn. (Millis and Levine, 2013). In all cases, the postoperative rehabilitation protocol actually begins with and includes the multimodal pain-management protocol initiated prior to or at the time of surgery.

Postoperative Rehabilitation Protocol: Femoral Head Ostectomy

Week 1 (Until Toe Touching)

1) Provide pain management with non-steroidal anti-inflammatory medication, opioids, and gabapentin as needed for the first 14 days minimum.
2) Apply ice for 10–20 minutes, two to four times a day for the first 48 hours after surgery, and two to three times a day thereafter (Figure 22.1).
3) Perform passive range-of-motion exercise with 10–20 slow repetitions, three times a day (60–80° to 120–135°).

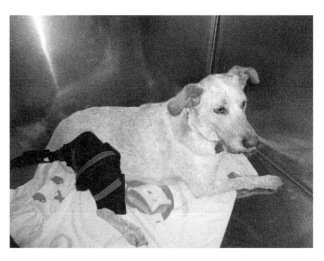

Figure 22.1 Cold compression wrap on stifle during multimodal postoperative rehabilitation.

4) Precede and follow passive range-of-motion exercises with massage of the quadriceps, biceps, and gluteal muscles for 5 minutes.
5) Begin slow leash walks of less than 10 minutes, three times a day.
6) Provide laser therapy three to five times a week.
7) Begin or continue a weight-management (careful during healing) and nutriceutical program, including omega 3 fatty acids, avocado soybean unsaponifiables, and diets formulated for joint health.

Weeks 2 and 3 (Early Weight Bearing)

1) Do a follow-up examination 2–3 weeks after surgery to evaluate the patient's range of motion, limb girth, and per cent weight bearing.
2) Continue multimodal pain management.
3) Apply ice for 10–20 minutes, two to three times a day until the swelling has resolved.
4) Continue passive range-of-motion exercises (45–160°) and massage therapy.
5) Begin proprioceptive and balance exercises: lift opposite leg, shift weight back and forth manually, implement caveletties (Figure 22.2).
6) Increase slow leash walks to 10–15 minutes, three times a day, or schedule sessions on a land treadmill or underwater treadmill for 2 minutes at 0.8 km/hr.
7) Provide laser therapy three times a week.

Weeks 4 and 5 (Consistent Weight Bearing)

1) Switch to a multimodal long-term pain-management plan, if indicated.
2) Apply an ice pack for 20 minutes, once a day.
3) Continue passive range-of-motion exercises (45–160°) and massage, and begin gentle static stretching (30-second hold).

4) Have the patient perform 10 repetitions of sit–stand exercises, three times a day.
5) Have the patient perform 10–15 repetitions of figure-of-eight walks, two to three times a day, circling to the right and left.
6) Have the patient sit against a wall for 10–15 repetitions, two to three times a day, keeping the affected side next to the wall.
7) Increase proprioceptive and balance exercises: balance boards and balls, caveletties.
8) Increase the slow leash walks to 20–30 minutes, two to three times a day, or schedule sessions on an inclined land treadmill (Figure 22.3) or an underwater treadmill (Figure 22.4) at 1.5–2.5 km/hr for 2–10 minutes, three times a week.
9) Consider initiating swimming exercises for 1–5 minutes, twice a day.
10) Provide laser therapy once a week.

Weeks 6–8 (Consistent Weight Bearing at a Trot)

1) Do a follow-up examination 6 weeks after surgery to evaluate the patient's range of motion, limb girth, and per cent weight bearing.
2) Continue the multimodal long-term pain-management plan, if indicated
3) Provide passive range-of-motion and therapeutic exercises as before (or similar).
4) Take the patient on incline walks on hills, ramps, or an inclined land treadmill for 5–10 minutes, once or twice a day.
5) Have the patient slowly go up a flight of stairs for 5–10 minutes, twice a day.
6) Have the patient swim or walk in the underwater treadmill for 10–15 minutes, every 1–3 days.

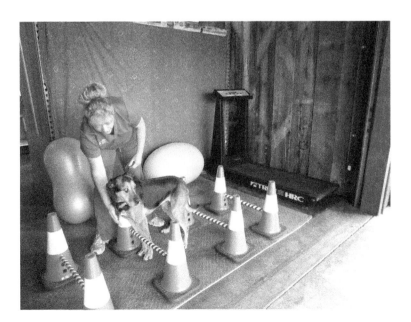

Figure 22.2 Caveletti poles of varying heights can challenge the patient's proprioceptive system, alter their walking pattern, and encourage greater range of motion in their limbs.

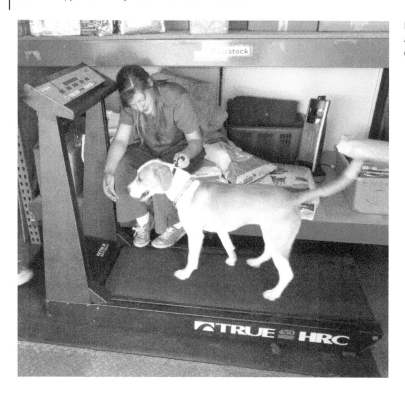

Figure 22.3 Exercise on a dry or land treadmill is an alternative to leash walks when mobility is increased during postoperative rehabilitation.

(a)

(b)

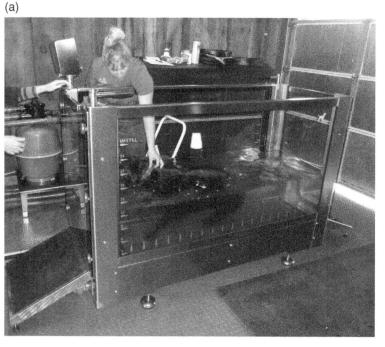

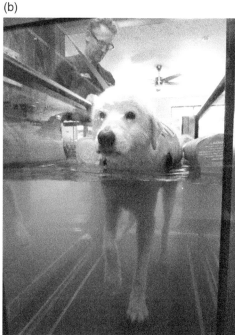

Figure 22.4 (a) An underwater treadmill, as opposed to a dry or land treadmill, allows early postoperative exercise. The buoyancy of the water reduces the strength required for early postoperative weight bearing. (b) Postoperative exercise in an underwater treadmill takes advantage of the physical properties of water so that the patient receives hydrotherapy in a controlled, comfortable environment.

7) Take the patient on leash walks for 20–30 minutes, three times a day, slow enough to ensure that the patient is weight bearing on the affected limb, but with jogging for 5–10 minutes, twice a day (or use a treadmill at 1.5–6.5 km/hr).
8) Provide laser therapy once a week.

Weeks 9–12 (Trotting at Speed with Minimal Lameness)

At this point, the patient's healing should be complete. The patient should gradually return to full activity by the end of 12 weeks. A follow-up radiograph should be obtained to confirm proper healing about 60 days after surgery.

1) Continue weight control and pain management.
2) Continue laser therapy once per month.
3) Take the patient on faster 30–40-minute walks, once or twice a day, or schedule sessions on a land treadmill or underwater treadmill at 1.5–10.0 km/hr, one to three times a week.

Postoperative Rehabilitation Protocol: Repair of Cruciate Injuries

Week 1 (Until Toe Touching)

1) Provide pain management with non-steroidal anti-inflammatory medication, opioids, and gabapentin as needed for the first 14 days minimum.
2) Apply ice for 10–20 minutes, two to four times a day for the first 48 hours after surgery, and two to three times a day thereafter.
3) Perform passive range-of-motion exercises with 10–20 slow repetitions, three times a day (60–80° to 120–135°).
4) Precede and follow the passive range-of-motion exercises with massage of the quadriceps/biceps muscles for 5 minutes.
5) Begin slow leash walks of less than 10 minutes, three times a day.
6) Provide laser therapy three to five times a week.
7) Begin or continue a weight-management (careful during healing) and nutriceutical program, including omega 3 fatty acids, avocado soybean unsaponifiables, and diets formulated for joint health.

Weeks 2 and 3 (Early Weight Bearing)

1) Do a follow-up examination 2–3 weeks after surgery to evaluate the patient's range of motion, limb girth, and per cent weight bearing.
2) Continue multimodal pain management.
3) Apply ice for 10–20 minutes, two to three times a day until the swelling has resolved.
4) Continue passive range-of-motion exercises (40–160°) and massage therapy.
5) Begin proprioceptive and balance exercises: lift opposite leg, shift weight back and forth manually, implement caveletties.
6) Increase slow leash walks to 10–15 minutes, three times a day, or schedule sessions on a land treadmill or underwater treadmill for 2 minutes at 0.8 km/hr.
7) Provide laser therapy three times a week.

Weeks 4 and 5 (Consistent Weight Bearing)

1) Switch to a multimodal long-term pain-management plan, if indicated.
2) Apply an ice pack for 20 minutes, once a day.
3) Continue passive range-of-motion exercises (40–160°) and massage, and begin gentle static stretching (30-second hold).
4) Have the patient perform 10 steps in the dancing position, three times a day.
5) Have the patient perform 10–15 repetitions of figure-of-eight walks, two to three times a day, circling to the right and left.
6) Have the patient sit against a wall for 10–15 repetitions, two to three times a day, keeping the affected knee next to the wall.
7) Increase proprioceptive and balance exercises: balance boards and balls, caveletties.
8) Increase the slow leash walks to 20–30 minutes, two to three times a day, or schedule sessions on an inclined land treadmill or an underwater treadmill (at 1.5–2.5 km/hr).
9) Consider initiating swimming exercises for 1–5 minutes, twice a day.
10) Provide laser therapy once a week.

Weeks 6–8 (Consistent Weight Bearing at a Trot)

1) Do a follow-up examination 6 weeks after surgery to evaluate the patient's range of motion, limb girth, and per cent weight bearing.
2) Continue the multimodal long-term pain-management plan, if indicated
3) Provide passive range-of-motion and therapeutic exercises as before (or similar).
4) Take the patient on incline walks on hills, ramps, or an inclined land treadmill for 5–10 minutes, once or twice a day.
5) Have the patient slowly go up a flight of stairs for 5–10 minutes, twice a day.
6) Have the patient swim or walk in the underwater treadmill for 10–15 minutes, every 1–3 days.
7) Take the patient on leash walks for 20–30 minutes, three times a day, slow enough to ensure that the patient is weight bearing on the affected limb, but with jogging for 5–10 minutes, twice a day (or use a treadmill at 1.5–6.5 km/hr).
8) Provide laser therapy once a week.

Weeks 9–12 (Trotting at Speed with Minimal Lameness)

At this point, the patient's healing should be complete. The patient should gradually return to full activity by the end of 12 weeks. A follow-up radiograph should be obtained to confirm proper healing about 60 days after surgery.

1) Continue weight control and pain management.
2) Continue laser therapy once per month.
3) Take the patient on faster 30–40-minute walks, once or twice a day, or schedule sessions on a land treadmill or underwater treadmill at 1.5–10.0 km/hr.

Postoperative Rehabilitation Protocol: IVDD

Week 1 (Until Weight Supporting – Mostly Rest!)

1) Provide pain management with non-steroid anti-inflammatory medication, opioids, and gabapentin as needed for the first 14 days minimum.

2) Apply ice for 10–20 minutes, two to four times a day.
3) Perform passive range-of-motion exercises to the rear legs with 10–20 slow repetitions, three times a day.
4) Precede and follow the passive range-of-motion exercises with massage of the muscles for 5 minutes.
5) Perform standing or floating exercises for 10 minutes, three times a day.
6) Provide laser therapy daily.
7) Provide turning and nursing care if non-ambulatory.

Weeks 2 and 3 (Early Weight Bearing – Still Lots of Rest!)

1) Do a follow-up examination to evaluate the patient's range of motion, limb girth, per cent weight bearing, and neurological status.
2) Continue multimodal pain management.
3) Apply ice for 10–20 minutes, two to three times a day.
4) Continue passive range-of-motion exercises and massage therapy to the rear legs.
5) Continue standing-in-water therapy. Consider initiating swimming exercises for 1–5 minutes, twice a day.
6) Begin easy proprioceptive and balance exercises: lift opposite leg, shift weight back and forth manually, toe tickle.
7) Begin sling-assisted walking.
8) Provide laser therapy three times a week.
9) Begin underwater treadmill therapy for up to 5 minutes, three times a week.

Weeks 4 and 5 (Initial Motor Function)

1) Switch to a multimodal long-term pain-management plan, if indicated.
2) Apply an ice pack for 20 minutes, once per day.
3) Continue passive range-of-motion exercises and massage.
4) Consider initiating swimming exercises for 1–5 minutes, twice a day.
5) Begin treadmill therapy with a sling at 0.8–1.6 km/hr.
6) Begin limb strengthening: 10 repetitions of sit–stand exercises three times a day (crawling, land treadmill, incline walking).
7) Increase proprioceptive and balance exercises: balance boards (Figure 22.5), peanut balls (Figure 22.6), toe tickle.
8) Begin slow leash walks for 5 minutes twice a day, then add zig-zags, circling, or figure-of-eights.
9) Provide laser therapy once a week.
10) Begin or continue a weight management and nutriceutical program, including omega 3 fatty acids, avocado soybean unsaponifiables, and diets formulated for weight control.
11) Increase underwater treadmill therapy to 10 minutes, three times a week.

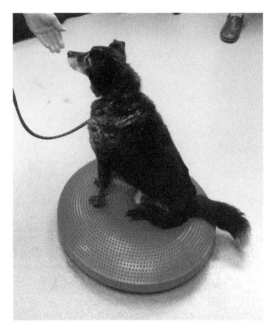

Figure 22.5 Exercise balls and balance platforms encourage weight shifting and weight bearing during postoperative rehabilitation.

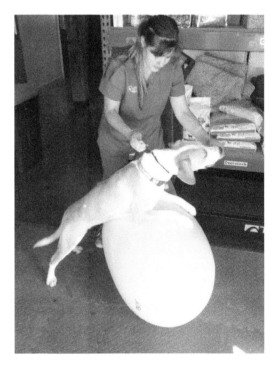

Figure 22.6 Postoperative exercise using a peanut ball helps core strengthening and encourages weight bearing on affected limbs. The peanut shape gives a larger contact base with the floor than that of a standard exercise ball, providing increased stability during use.

Weeks 6–8 (Good Motor Function but Remaining Proprioceptive Deficits)

1) Do a follow-up examination to evaluate the patient's range of motion, limb girth, per cent weight bearing, and neurological status.

2) Continue the multimodal long-term pain-management plan, if indicated.
3) Provide passive range-of-motion and therapeutic exercises as before (or similar).
4) Take the patient on incline walks on hills, ramps, or an inclined land treadmill for 5–10 minutes, once or twice a day.
5) Have the patient swim for 10–15 minutes, once a day.
6) Continue strengthening, proprioceptive, and balance exercises, with increasing challenges.
7) Increase the slow leash walks with zig-zags, circling, or figure-of-eights, and add jogging for 10 minutes, twice a day (or use a land treadmill at 0.6–2.5 km/hr). Add cavalettis.
8) Provide laser therapy once a week.
9) Increase underwater treadmill therapy difficulty for 10–15 minutes, three times a week.

Weeks 9–12 (Near-Normal Gait)

At this point, the patient's healing should be complete. The patient should gradually return to full activity by the end of 12 weeks

1) Continue weight control and pain management.
2) Continue passive range-of-motion exercises, massage, and exercises, if desired.
3) Continue laser therapy once a month.
4) Continue swimming, if possible.
5) Take the patient on faster 20-minute walks once or twice a day, or use a land or water treadmill at 0.6–3.0 km/hr.
6) Take the patient for a run (straight only, no turns) for 10 minutes, twice a day.
7) Increase underwater treadmill therapy difficulty for 10–15 minutes, three times a week.

Summary

These protocols are guidelines only and should be customized to each practice and to each patient. Additional training should definitely be pursued prior to initiating your own program. The order in which the therapies are provided generally proceeds from least difficult and most comfortable (e.g., laser therapy, passive range-of-motion exercises, massage) to more difficult and less comfortable (e.g., underwater treadmill, physical exercises). This method helps patients warm up and get ready for exercise. It is important never to hurt an animal and always to proceed with gentleness and caution. Doing so will keep patients happy and positive about their rehabilitation sessions.

Prehabilitation, Primary Therapy, and Rehabilitation

Most veterinarians accept the concept and importance of rehabilitation. The use of rehabilitation modalities, including laser therapy, for both primary therapy and prehabilitation is a valuable concept, as well. Most of this chapter deals with the primary therapeutic applications of laser therapy, but the use of laser therapy to prehabilitate tissues prior to surgical interventions should be considered as well. For example, after an acute cranial cruciate ligament rupture, there is a lot of acute inflammation in the stifle. Using laser therapy and other rehabilitation modalities (ice, compression, massage) can greatly reduce that tissue inflammation prior to surgery. "Happier" tissues will facilitate the surgery and improve the outcome and recovery from surgical trauma.

Clinical Experience

There are myriad examples of how laser therapy and rehabilitation can facilitate recovery after surgery. To illustrate, many surgeons find that with the application of laser therapy and postoperative rehabilitation, their tibial plateau-leveling osteotomy patients can progress to early weight bearing within 2 weeks, rather being merely toe touching at that time.

Treatment Plans

Postoperative rehabilitation treatment plans should incorporate all of the information provided in this chapter. It is helpful to "under-promise" and "over-deliver" when creating expectations for laser therapy.

Six, Nine, and Twelve Packs

Postoperative rehabilitation should be prescribed in packages of 6–12 treatments, just like when prescribing laser therapy as a sole modality. As with antibiotics, a full course of therapy is commonly needed to achieve the desired outcome, so providing treatments one at a time can be counterproductive. Most owners will see satisfying progress after a few sessions, so compliance is generally very high.

Expectations and Progress

Generally, patients should show noticeable incremental improvement as the postoperative rehabilitation progresses. If progress is not being made, the veterinarian should review the patient's status and the prescribed rehabilitation plan, and make appropriate changes. It is a good practice to incorporate a veterinarian consultation and recheck after every six rehabilitation sessions, to gauge progress and modify therapy as indicated.

Photos, Videos, Radiographs, and Digital Thermal Images

Records should document the postoperative rehabilitation process with visual formats like photographs, videos, radiographs, and digital thermal images.

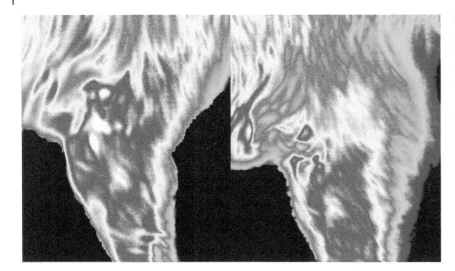

Figure 22.7 Digital thermal imaging reveals changes in temperature and circulation in injured and healing tissue. The image on the left shows an increased thermal gradient over the left stifle. The image on the right, taken 24 hours after laser therapy treatment, shows a decreased gradient.

These types of imaging are helpful to both the veterinarian and the owner, as they provide excellent before-and-after documentation of the progress being made. Photographs are particularly valuable for documenting the healing of surgical incisions and wounds. Videos are very valuable records of the return to function after orthopedic injury, and of lameness and neurologic procedures. Radiographs are appropriate for fractures and boney lesions. Digital thermal imaging is a simple and effective method of producing an image that reveals changes in temperature and circulation in injured and healing tissue (Figure 22.7). Visual formats will often help the owner see the progress being made with postoperative rehabilitation, and help enforce the validity of the treatment plan.

Postoperative Rehabilitation Fees

Both laser therapy and rehabilitation are very affordable for most clients. Both modalities are charged for based on the amount of time needed for the treatments. As an example, many practices charge in the following ranges (for either or both modalities): 20–29 minutes = $45–60; 30–39 minutes = $55–70; 40–49 minutes = $65–80. As with laser therapy alone, many patients undergoing postoperative rehabilitation will be treated three times a week initially, and transitioned to less frequent treatments as they progress.

The Biggest Obstacle

The will to take on an entirely new service and area of expertise is the biggest obstacle to embracing rehabilitation! Most practices can begin modestly or moderately, and build up to having a fully-fledged rehabilitation program as resources become available and training and experience become more advanced. Like dentistry, rehabilitation will become a service that most veterinarians offer.

References

AAHA (2015). 2015 AAHA/AAFP Pain Management Guidelines for Dogs and Cats. Available from: https://www.aaha.org/professional/resources/pain_management.aspx (accessed November 30, 2016).

AVMA. (n.d.) AVMA American Board of Veterinary Specialties. Available from: https://www.avma.org/professionaldevelopment/education/specialties/pages/default.aspx (accessed November 30, 2016).

CVMBS. (n.d. a) Canine Acute Pain Scale. Available from: http://csu-cvmbs.colostate.edu/Documents/anesthesia-pain-management-pain-score-canine.pdf (accessed November 30, 2016).

CVMBS. (n.d. b) Feline Acute Pain Scale. Available from: http://csu-cvmbs.colostate.edu/Documents/anesthesia-pain-management-pain-score-feline.pdf (accessed November 30, 2016).

Ebling Library. (n.d.) Nursing Resources: Levels of Evidence (I–VII). Available from: http://researchguides.ebling.library.wisc.edu/c.php?g=293229&p=1953406 (accessed November 30, 2016).

Enwemeka, C.S. *et al.* (2004) The efficacy of low-power lasers in tissue repair and pain control: a meta-analysis study. *Photomed Laser Surg.* **22**(4):323–329.

Fulop, A. *et al.* (2010) A meta-analysis of the efficacy of laser phototherapy on pain relief. *Clin J Pain.* **26**(8):729–736.

Hållstam, A. *et al.* (2016) Patients with chronic pain: one-year follow-up of a multimodal rehabilitation program at a pain clinic. *Scand J Pain.* **10**(10):36–42.

IVAPM. (n.d.) How We Assess a Feline's Pain Level. Available from: https://ivapm.org/for-the-public/animals-and-pain-articles/how-we-assess-your-felines-pain-level/ (accessed November 30, 2016).

Jang, H. and Lee, H. (2012) Meta-analysis of pain relief effects by laser irradiation on joint areas. *Photomed Laser Surg.* **30**(8):405–417.

Millis, D.L. and Ciuperca, I.A. (2015) Evidence for canine rehabilitation and physical therapy. *Vet Clin North Am Small Anim Pract.* **45**(1):1–27.

Millis, D.L. and Levine, D. (2013) *Canine Rehabilitation and Physical Therapy*, 2 edn. Saunders, Philadelphia, PA.

PennVet. (n.d.) Canine Brief Pain Inventory. Available from: http://www.vet.upenn.edu/docs/default-source/VCIC/canine-bpi.pdf?sfvrsn=0 (accessed November 30, 2016).

Saunders, D.G. and Millis, D. (2014). Laser therapy in canine rehabilitation. In: *Canine Rehabilitation and Physical Therapy*, 2 edn., pp. 359–380. Elsevier, Amsterdam.

Sims, C. *et al.* (2015) Rehabilitation and physical therapy for the neurologic patient. *Vet Clin North Am Small Anim Pract.* **45**(1):123–143.

Sprouse-Blum, A.S. *et al.* (2010) Understanding endorphins and their importance in pain management. *Hawaii Med J.* **69**(3):70–71.

Thomas, J. (2011) How to pinpoint pain. *Trends Magazine.* **Dec.**:17–24.

UT. (n.d.) Canine Rehabilitation Certificate Program (CCRP). UT Certification Courses and Seminars. Available from: http://ccrp.utvetce.com/ (accessed November 30, 2016).

Valentin, S. (2009) Cincinnati Orthopaedic Disability Index in canines. *Aust J Physiother.* **55**(4):288.

Van Middelkoop, M. (2011) A systematic review on the effectiveness of physical and rehabilitation interventions for chronic non-specific low back pain. *Eur. Spine J.* **20**(1):19–39.

Walker, J.B. (1983) Relief from chronic pain by low-power laser irradiation. *Neurosci Lett.* **43**:339–344.

Zink, M.C. and Van Dyke, J.B. (2013) *Canine Sports Medicine and Rehabilitation*. Wiley-Blackwell, Hoboken, NJ.

23

Laser Therapy and Injury Rehabilitation
Matthew W. Brunke

North Country Veterinary Referral Center, Queensbury, NY, USA

Introduction

Previous chapters have defined laser principles, treatment regiments, and other dynamics. Before we can apply those concepts to specific injuries, it is important to understand what injuries can be treated with laser therapy.

Injury is defined by Merriam-Webster as "an act or event that causes someone or something to no longer be fully healthy or in good condition." In veterinary medicine, we can further divide injuries between specific areas of the patient's anatomy. In this chapter, we will focus on the musculoskeletal, neurological, and dermal systems. With injury to any of these systems, the veterinary practitioner must be cognizant of the phase of the injury (acute, subacute, chronic, or acute on chronic) and the phase of wound healing (inflammatory, reparative, remodeling, or maturation) of the tissue in question before planning treatment and rehabilitation. The effects of using laser therapy in injury rehabilitation are summarized in Box 23.1.

Wound Healing

Dermal System

Dermatological injuries can be associated with some of the causes of injuries to other parts of the body. Often times, a crushing injury can affect multiple organ systems. Once the patient is properly stabilized, there is a need to address pain and inflammation from trauma to the skin, muscles, peripheral nerves, and spinal cord. Alternatively, dermal injuries can occur separately from other organ systems.

The dermal system is the organ system that benefits the most from the laser's effects of increasing the speed of healing and the host response to bacteria and viruses. Examples of dermal injuries that can be independent of the musculoskeletal or neurological system include papillomas, lick granulomas, bacterial dermatitis, decu-

bital ulcers, pressure sores, pododermatitis, nail and pad injuries, and otitis externa. Lacerations may be dermal only, or may include muscle or nerve tissue. Patients that have been burned by chemicals or fire may have extensive injury to their skin. Patients with diabetes mellitus and hyperadrenocorticism may have delayed wound-healing potential and are prone to bacterial dermatitis. Cancer patients undergoing either chemotherapy or radiation are also at risk for dermatological injuries.

The inflammatory (lag) phase of dermatologic wound healing lasts approximately 5 days. It is characterized by increased vascular permeability, chemotaxis of circulatory cells, release of cytokines and growth factors, and cell activation.

The debridement phase is dominated by white blood cell action, recruitment of mesenchymal cells, stimulation of angiogenesis, and moderate matrix production in wounds, after preventing infection and debriding the area using phagocytosis. This phase can last another 4–5 days.

The repair phase usually begins 3–5 days after injury. Macrophages stimulate DNA and fibroblast production and collagen synthesis. The amount of collagen reaches a maximum within 2–3 weeks after injury. As collagen increases, the number of fibroblasts and the rate of collagen synthesis decrease; this marks the end of the repair stage.

Depending on the nature of the wound, the fibroblastic phase of healing lasts 2–4 weeks. Careful management of wounds during this time will avoid inappropriate epithelialization and poor wound healing.

The maturation phase begins once collagen has been adequately deposited in the wounds, 17–20 days after injury, and may continue for several years. Collagen fibers remodel with alteration of their orientation and increased cross-linking, which improves wound strength (Hedlund, 2002).

Patients with compromised wound-healing abilities (e.g., obesity, diabetes mellitus, malnourishment, hepatic disease, or hyperadrenocorticism) benefit from laser therapy in the early phases of wound healing, which helps

Box 23.1 The effects of using laser therapy in injury rehabilitation.

Analgesia

Reduced pain in postoperative incisions

Decreased pain in meniscal tears

Reduced pain in arthritis

Dermatological Injuries

Wound healing	Capillary formation
Reduced tissue necrosis	Collagen formation
Increased angiogenesis	Vasodilation
Fibroblast stimulation	Lymphatic drainage

Musculoskeletal Injuries

Anti-inflammatory	Activation of osteogenic factors
Pain reduction in acute tendonitis	Improved cell proliferation and differentiation
Muscle recovery in athletes	Improved healing time
Promotion of oxygen uptake	Disruption of biofilm on implants
Promotion of exercise performance	Killing of bacteria (osteomyelitis)
Faster return to function	Reduction of acute joint inflammation
Improved collagen organization	Improved tissue organization following cruciate ligament injury
Improved biomechanical properties	Inhibition of COX-2 enzyme and prostaglandins
Improved ligament healing	Fibrous healing of cartilaginous defects
Improved bone healing	

Neurological Injuries

Immunomodulation of brain damage	Increased axon numbers
Prevention of neuron death	Improved length of axonal regrowth
Better clinical outcome with cerebral ischemia	Improved motor function in peripheral nerve injury
Faster motor evolution following spinal cord injury	Regrowth of muscle fiber in brachial plexus injuries
Maintenance of the urinary system	Increased myelinization
Preservation of neural tissue	

minimize the risks, delays, or failures of the healing process (de Loura Santana *et al.*, 2016). Additionally, those patients on corticosteroids, chemotherapeutic agents, or radiation therapy can have delayed wound healing. If the wound is over a neoplastic site, consultation with a veterinary oncologist is recommended prior to initiating laser therapy, to ensure that it will not promote proliferation of the neoplasia (Bensadoun and Nair, 2015).

Musculoskeletal System

The musculoskeletal system includes all of the bones, ligaments, tendons, cartilaginous joints, and muscles of the body. The potential for injury to these structures includes fractured bones and strained, sprained, or completely ruptured ligaments and tendons. Further, the muscle bodies themselves can be inflamed from trauma or infection. Autoimmune diseases can affect the joints or muscles and cause inflammation and pain. Articular cartilage injury can lead to osteoarthritis. Laser therapy can be beneficial at the time of injury, in preparation for surgical intervention, during postoperative pain management, and during rehabilitation.

Trauma (either acute or chronic) to both the appendicular and the axial skeleton can lead to injury of the associated muscles, tendons, ligaments, bones, and cartilage. A working knowledge of normal anatomy and physiology is essential to understanding what is abnormal for a particular patient. A full physical examination, paying attention to the orthopedic and neurologic exam, should be completed prior to initiation of laser therapy for any injury.

Injuries to muscle occur as a result of ruptures, ischemia, strains, laceration, and contusions. A strain is described as any injury to a muscle and tendon unit. Strains have a tendency to occur near the myotendinous junction. They are described as grade I–IV, with grade I strains being disruption of a few muscle fibers and grade IV being complete rupture of the muscle belly. Damage to muscle includes tearing of the fibers and disruption of vascular and connective tissue support. Severity can range from mild injury to complete rupture. Complete rupture necessitates surgical correction. Lesser injuries can take 4–6 weeks to heal, during which time the patient should have protected activity (Williams, 2004).

Injuries to tendons can occur from similar causes as their companion muscles. A similar strain grading system is used. The goal of treatment is to minimize adhesion formation and return to full function. As with muscles, complete tendon rupture requires surgical stabilization and repair prior to rehabilitation. The size, location, and stress load on a particular tendon will dictate tensile strength and speed of return to function. Full healing is normally achieved in 6–10 weeks (Williams, 2004).

Ligamentous injuries can take up to 12 months to completely remodel and to complete the maturation phase of wound healing. At that point, ligament strength will only be 50–70% of the original tensile strength (Frank *et al.*, 1991). Factors that are important for ligament healing include apposition, nutritional status, endocrine imbalance, and severity of injury. Proper blood supply and load-bearing stress are also important. Complete tears will benefit from surgery first, then rehabilitation.

Cartilage healing is directly related to the type of trauma that caused the injury. Articular cartilage is avascular in nature, and this can be a limiting factor for repair. Partial-thickness injuries are dependent on the cartilage matrix for wound healing. Full-thickness injuries to the level of the subchondral bone can benefit from the available vascular supply in the bone. Cartilage healing can take 2–6 months, but often results in arthritis due to the poor repair potential of the tissue itself (Williams, 2004).

Bone is dynamic tissue that is composed of 35% organic tissue and 65% mineral component. This complex nature dictates a prolonged healing time compared to the soft tissues. Many factors can affect bone healing. Stress at the fracture site can cause micro-motion, which can disrupt tissue healing. Surgical stabilization is thus often indicated. The application of a splint or cast can be beneficial, but does not allow for laser application unless a window is made in the material or the material is removed. Removal for laser therapy requires patient sedation to prevent the risk of motion and disruption of the healing bone.

Healing time will be dependent on the fracture location, degree of trauma, and numerous other factors. A full return to normal lamellar bone structure accommodating normal weight-bearing forces can take 4 months or longer. Disturbances in bone healing can delay healing and result in delayed unions or nonunions (Williams, 2004).

All the tissues of the musculoskeletal system will react differently to disuse and remobilization. After prolonged disuse, most tissues will atrophy and have decreased rates of new cell formation. The loss of tissue strength from atrophy can lead to further injury. Quick return to use and function through rehabilitation is almost always recommended.

Neurological System

Injuries to particular areas can result in injuries to the neurological system. The brain, spinal cord, and peripheral nerves can have different insulting injuries and different healing potentials.

The brain can be injured by trauma, infection, vascular events, inflammations, toxins, congenital defects, degenerative conditions, and neoplasia (Fenner, 2000). Laser therapy is normally not indicated for cancer, so proper diagnostic testing is essential before initiation of treatment. Additionally, the brain can be difficult to treat with laser therapy, since it is contained within the calvarium, though research is being done in this area, with potentially promising results. Data indicate that photons can penetrate human cadaver skulls to a depth of 4 cm (Tedford *et al.*, 2015).

Causes of injuries to the spinal cord include those affecting the brain and herniated intervertebral disks. Common conditions affecting the spinal cord include trauma, intervertebral disk disease (IVDD), fibrocartilagenous emboli (FCE), vascular events, cervical spondylomyelopathy (wobbler's disease), lumbosacral stenosis, discospondylitis, spondylosis deformans, syringomyelia, degenerative myelopathy, and trauma. Trauma, IVDD, and FCE can have acute onset, where the spinal cord may have better healing potential than from the more chronic conditions (e.g., lumbosacral stenosis, spondylosis deformans, and degenerative myelopathy). Proper diagnosis will aid in determining the prognosis and course of treatment (LeCouteur and Grandy, 2000).

Three basic categories of change occur after acute injury to the spinal cord: first, direct morphologic distortion of neuronal tissue, then vascular change, and finally biochemical and metabolic changes. Controversy exists regarding the relative importance of these closely related categories in the production of functional deficits.

Direct morphologic damage of the spinal cord (laceration, stretching, or compression) resulting in axonal interruption is thought to be irreversible and untreatable because central axons do not regenerate sufficiently to restore function. There may be some change in this theory with the advent of stem-cell and platelet-rich plasma therapy in both humans and animal models.

In the case of reversible spinal cord injury, a characteristic series of events occurs during the repair process. A heterogeneous population of small cells, including lymphocytes, macrophages, and plasma cells, invades the traumatized tissue 2 days after injury. This mimics the inflammatory phase, as shown in other organs. Within 7–20 days, fibroblasts appear and begin laying down scar tissue. A concurrent glial reaction consisting of astrocyte proliferation and expansion of axonal processes occurs. Depending on the extent of spinal cord injury, moderate to extensive fibrosis, nerve fiber degeneration, and multifocal malacia may be seen (Seim, 2002a).

Axons that have been severed, compressed, or stretched start to regrow, but growth will reach the edges of the scar mass and stop. Regeneration of spinal cord axons sufficient to restore function has not been achieved; however, if enough axons remain intact, return to clinically acceptable motor function may be expected.

The peripheral nervous system includes cranial nerves III–XII, the spinal nerves with their roots, peripheral nerves, and the peripheral components of the autonomic nervous system. These relay information to the central nervous system (CNS) and provide control of peripheral structures. They comprise the sole neural structure that controls skeletal muscle and are therefore essential for ambulation. A variety of diseases can affect this system, including congenital malformation, genetic diseases, metabolic conditions (diabetes mellitus, hypothyroidism), toxicities (botulism, tick paralysis), autoimmune and inflammatory diseases (acute polyradiculoneuritis, myasthenia gravis), neoplasia, trauma (brachial plexus avulsion), and vascular conditions (feline aortic thromboembolism) (Inzana, 2000).

Traumatic peripheral nerve injuries can be classified according to the degree of damage present. Class 1 is referred to as neurapraxia and includes mild or moderate focal compression. With class 2 injuries, complete recovery can occur within hours, or up to 6 weeks. Class 2 injury, axonotmesis, occurs with crushing injuries. The axons are interrupted, but the supporting connective tissue is intact and regeneration is usually effective. Axonal regeneration occurs at 1–2 mm/day, so the length of the injury will dictate the potential healing time. Classes 3–5 are varying degrees of neurotmesis. In Class 3 injuries, there is damage to the axons and endoneurium, but the perineurium is intact. Class 4 is similar, but includes disruption of the perineurium. Class 5 is complete severing of the nerve (Inzana, 2000).

A peripheral nerve sustaining neurapraxia develops transient physiological dysfunction without anatomic disruption of the axons. The nerve regains normal function within 3 months, and regeneration occurs at

3 cm/month (1 mm/day). Peripheral nerves sustaining axonotmesis or neurotmesis will undergo immediate degeneration at the site of injury. This degeneration extends toward the cell body over a distance of two to three nodes of Ranvier, and regeneration begins from that site. Nerve processes distal to the injury degenerate completely (Wallerian degeneration), and after 1 week a connective-tissue framework called the "neurilemmal sheath" remains. Within 2 days, "sprouting" of the proximal end of the severed axon occurs.

Neuron regeneration and return of function depend on several factors. If continuity of the nerve is maintained (axonotmesis), the distance from the injury site to the end organ becomes the most important variable. Little function will be achieved if the distance is more than 30 cm. The best chance for functional regeneration is a distance of less than 10 cm. If anatomic nerve continuity is not maintained (neurotmesis), recovery depends on the distance from the injury to the end organ, the wounding mechanism, the time between injury and surgical repair, the patient's age and condition, and the surgical technique. The earlier a nerve is repaired, the better the chances of healing. Clean, sharp lacerations generally heal better than avulsion, crush, open, or chronic injuries (Seim, 2002b).

Proper diagnosis of injuries, involving a consult with a veterinary neurologist and potentially an electromyelogram or advanced imaging techniques, or both, is important. Additionally, it is important to recognize that multiple types and classes of injury can occur along the same nerve.

How and Why Does Laser Therapy Work?

Studies of the successful use of laser therapy in promoting tissue repair and pain reduction are well established (Enwemeka *et al.*, 2004). Laser therapy is relatively new to our field of rehabilitation, and more studies are needed to evaluate and interpret its impact on our current treatment guidelines. Many have been done using *in vitro* models. While these are useful for establishing the fundamentals of laser treatment, they are rarely applicable in practice. As we continue to learn how to apply laser therapy in rehabilitation, it is essential that we pay proper attention to individual patient needs and responses to treatment. Precise medical records should include documentation of the areas treated, laser settings, dates, and responses. Despite a lack of species-specific clinical studies, the foundation for the use of laser therapy in veterinary rehabilitation is established (Pryor and Millis, 2015).

Laser therapy works at a cellular level to activate cytokines and other mediators along various cascades in the tissue. Chromophores and respiratory chain enzymes within the mitochondria and at the cell membrane absorb the photons. Oxygen and adenosine triphosphate (ATP) production can be enhanced. ATP may also act as a signaling molecule to enhance cell-to-cell communication (Karu *et al.*, 2010). ATP may bind with a cell receptor to allow sodium and calcium to enter, resulting in cascades of intracellular activities. This increased intracellular calcium increases mitochondrial function. ATP is also thought to be a neurotransmitter, and this may explain some of the effects of laser therapy in pain management (Baxter and McDonough, 2007).

Laser therapy stimulates collagen synthesis (Abergel *et al.*, 1984) and fibroblast development (Pourreau-Schneider *et al.*, 1990), and increases new blood vessel formation, allowing for repair of injured tissues (Corazza *et al.*, 2007). Additional studies have shown that laser therapy can lead to increased tensile strength (Vasilenko *et al.*, 2010) and faster closure of wounds (Hopkins *et al.*, 2004).

These cascades can enhance cellular growth and metabolism, and lasers therefore have the potential to accelerate tissue healing and cell growth in ligaments, tendons, skin, and muscles. Caution must be used, however, as excessively high doses of laser light may inhibit responses such as tissue healing (Huang *et al.*, 2009). Laser therapy has anti-inflammatory effects. Studies have indicated that inflammation can be reduced by using laser therapy to decrease prostaglandin E2 (PGE2) and cyclooxygenase 2 (COX-2) concentration (Honmura *et al.*, 1993; Sakarai *et al.*, 2000). This gives laser therapy the same potential treatment pathway as steroids and non-steroidal anti-inflammatory drugs (NSAIDs). For those patients that cannot take these systemic medications, and for owners looking for alternative treatment, laser therapy has been proven to be beneficial.

Reduction in inflammation and pain in both acute and chronic conditions will increase the patient's quality of life. By improving analgesia, laser therapy can be preemptive in the prevention or minimization of chronic pain or wind-up, and can help reduce dependence on medications. If medications can be avoided, there is a benefit for the patient as a whole.

Evidence for Laser Therapy in Injury Rehabilitation

Injury rehabilitation does not focus on one specific problem, but rather sees the patient as a whole. One of the main goals of rehabilitation is a return to normal or near-normal function (Millis and Ciuperca, 2015). The benefits of laser therapy for rehabilitation patients are focused in two main areas: the increase in healing times through faster, stronger tissue repair and the analgesic effect of the laser. These combine to allow the patient as a whole

to feel better and to exercise efficiently (when indicated), gain strength, and return to function with an improved quality of life.

Tendon and Ligament Conditions

Most of the research on the effects of laser therapy on tendon and ligament conditions has been done either in experimental models in laboratory animals such as rats or in people. More evidence from studies in dogs, cats, and other animals is needed. Historically, laser therapy has been recommended for tendon and ligament conditions, but its clinical efficacy remained controversial. Recent research proves that laser therapy is appropriate for these types of injury (Da Ré Guerra *et al.*, 2016; Tumilty and Baxter, 2015).

A meta-analysis evaluated the use of laser in tendinopathies in people (Tumilty *et al.*, 2010). The 25 studies reviewed had conflicting results, half being inconclusive or demonstrating no effect and the other half showing a positive effect. Positive versus negative effects appear to be related to the dose applied: those studies with positive results used doses similar to those recommended by the World Association for Laser Therapy (WALT): $1–8\,J/cm^2$ and $<100\,mW/cm^2$ for superficial tendons and $3–9\,J/cm^2$ and $600\,mW/cm^2$ for deep tendons.

One study looked at seven people with bilateral Achilles tendinitis to see whether laser therapy has an anti-inflammatory effect (Bjordal *et al.*, 2006). In those treated with laser therapy the PGE2 levels were reduced for 75–105 minutes after laser therapy, and pain pressure threshold values increased. The authors concluded that laser therapy reduces pain and inflammation in people with acute Achilles tendinitis.

Another Achilles tendon study (de Jesus *et al.*, 2015) showed that laser therapy decreased Achilles tendon inflammation. The study evaluated interleukin 1 beta (IL1β), COX-2, and PGE2 modulation in partially injured Achilles tendons of rats. The rats had a direct injury to the Achilles tendon and were placed in one of seven groups (negative control, three sham groups, and three treatment groups). The treatment groups received one, three, or seven treatments. A 780 nm laser was applied for 10 seconds once a day. The tendons were then surgically removed and assessed immunohistochemically for IL1β, COX-2 and PGE2. In the group treated three times, all three inflammatory mediators were near normal level. COX-2 and PGE2 were also near normal in the group that had seven treatments.

A randomized blinded study looked at 74 people treated with laser therapy for tendinitis, along with 68 placebo patients (Lögdberg-Andersson *et al.*, 1997). Over 3–4 weeks, all patients received three to four treatments. Pain was measured using a pain-threshold meter and a visual analog scale (VAS). Pain was measured prior to and at the end of treatment, and again 4 weeks later.

Laser therapy had a positive effect on acute tendinitis throughout the study.

Laser may also be of benefit to muscle recovery (Carvalho *et al.*, 2015). Assis *et al.* (2015) evaluated the effects of laser therapy on the biochemical markers and morphology of skeletal muscle in rats when applied after an endurance training protocol. They had a control group, a trained group, and a trained and laser group. The rats were walked on a treadmill for 1 hour per day, five days a week for 8 weeks, at 60% of maximal speed reached during a maximal-effort test. The trained and laser group showed significantly reduced lactate levels, increased tibialis anterior fiber cross-section area, and decreased fiber density. Myogenin expression was higher in both trained groups. Laser produced myogenin down-regulation as well. This suggests that laser therapy could be an effective therapeutic approach for stimulating recovery in athletes.

Another treadmill study using rats showed that laser therapy promotes an increase in maximal oxygen uptake and exercise performance in a dose-dependent manner (Perini *et al.*, 2015). Laser therapy was applied in the treated (versus placebo) rats bilaterally to the biceps femoris, gluteus, lateral and medial gastrocnemius, iliopsoas, and adductor longus muscles once a day for 10 days. All animals performed the maximal-exercise test on a metabolic treadmill, with simultaneous gas analysis. The higher-dose ($61.2\,J/cm^2$) laser group showed increased VO_2 basal, VO_2 max, and VCO_2 max levels and covered a longer distance compared to the other groups.

Conforti and Fachinetti (2013) showed that laser therapy is an effective treatment in humans with whiplash injury as compared to conventional simple segmental physical rehabilitation. They showed a reduction in VAS pain scores and a quicker recovery and return to work in the laser-treated group versus the non-laser-treated group.

Ligament healing may also benefit from laser therapy. Single-dose laser therapy has been shown to improve the healing of medial collateral ligaments in a rat model (Fung *et al.*, 2002). An earlier study demonstrated no improvement when patients were treated with suboptimal parameters (De Bie *et al.*, 1998). In a more recent animal-model study using rats, laser therapy was effective for the early improvement of the ultimate tensile strength of medial collateral ligament injuries (Bayat *et al.*, 2005). Further species-specific studies are warranted, and correct dose and treatment parameters are obviously important for successful results.

Bone and Cartilage Conditions

Bone and cartilage may also be affected by laser therapy. The focus within bone should be on healing following fracture and as an adjunct treatment for osteomyelitis.

Tim *et al.* (2014) looked at the effects of laser therapy on bone formation, immunoexpression of osteogenic factors, and biomechanical properties in a tibial bone defect model in rats. A total of 60 rats were distributed into a bone-defect control group and a laser-irradiated group. Rats were euthanized on days 15, 30, and 45 post-injury. Histological and morphometric analysis showed that the treated animals presented no inflammatory infiltrate and a better tissue organization at 15 and 30 days post-surgery. In addition, a higher amount of newly formed bone was observed at 15 days post-surgery. While this is a good reason to use laser therapy, the study also showed no statistically significant difference in COX-2 immunoexpression among the groups at 15, 30, and 45 days. Runt-related transcription factor 2 (RUNX2) was statistically higher in the treated group at 45 days. Bone morphogenetic protein (BMP-9) immunoexpression was higher in the treated group at day 30. However, there was no expressivity for this immunomarker in either group at 45 days. No statistically significant difference among the groups was observed in the maximal load at any time. This shows that laser therapy improved bone healing by accelerating the development of newly formed bone and activating osteogenic factors, but did not improve the biomechanical properties of the bone.

Another study (Barbosa *et al.*, 2014) looked at 45 rats subjected to transverse osteotomy of the right femur and divided randomly into three experimental groups. One group did not receive laser therapy; one received therapy with a 660 nm laser; and one received therapy with an 830 nm laser. Animals were sacrificed after 7, 14, and 21 days. The bone calluses were evaluated by digital x-ray and submitted to variance analysis followed by the Tukey–Kramer test. The two laser-treated groups showed significant bone development at days 7 and 14, and on day 21 a higher degree of bone repair was seen in the 830 nm group.

A 940 nm laser was used to look at osteogenesis in an *in vitro* study by Jawad *et al.* (2013). A human fetal osteoblast cell line was cultured and treated with laser and an assay was used to determine cell proliferation. Alkaline phosphatase and osteocalcin activity assays were used for cell differentiation. All treatment groups showed a significant increase in cell proliferation and differentiation compared to the control group.

A human *in vivo* study looked at wrist and hand fractures and found positive results (Chang *et al.*, 2014). It evaluated the therapeutic outcomes of administering 830 nm laser therapy to closed bone fractures of 50 patients who had not had surgery. A control group was used, and the laser-treated group was treated five times a week for 2 weeks. The pain, functional disability, grip strength, and radiographic parameters of the participants were evaluated before and after treatment, and at a 2-week follow-up. The laser group exhibited significant changes in all of the parameters compared with baseline. The results compared the two groups after treatment and at follow-up, and indicated significant differences between them. The study concluded that laser therapy relieves pain and improves the healing process in these fractures.

Laser therapy has also been studied as a treatment for infections of the musculoskeletal system. Bacteria that surround medical devices, such as orthopedic implants, can make a bacterial coating (biofilm) that prevents penetration of antibiotics. Kizhner *et al.* (2011) used laser light to disrupt this biofilm and allow conventional treatment to reach the bacteria.

Kaya *et al.* (2011) examined rats with induced, chronic methicillin-resistant *Staphylococcus aureus* (MRSA) osteomyelitis of the tibia. The rats had surgical debridement, surgical debridement and laser therapy, or no treatment. Treatment with an 808 nm laser for either 60, 120, or 180 seconds daily for five consecutive days decreased infection levels. The 180-second group had 93% less infection than the negative control, while the debridement-alone group had only 37% less. This study makes a good case for using laser as an adjunct for osteomyelitis.

A recent review of 25 articles (13 *in vitro* and 12 animal studies) evaluated the influence of laser therapy on bone healing (Ebrahimi *et al.*, 2012). All animal studies showed improved bone healing in sites irradiated with laser. It was concluded that laser therapy could accelerate bone healing in extraction sites, bone fracture defects, and distraction osteogenesis.

While the majority of the benefits of laser therapy for cartilage involve arthritis, there is evidence for the use of laser therapy in non-arthritic cases.

Dos Santos *et al.* (2014) compared the effect of two laser therapy doses on the expression of inflammatory mediators on neutrophils and macrophages in acute joint inflammation. The synovial tissue of patients with initial osteoarthritis is characterized by mononuclear cell infiltration and the production of pre-inflammatory cytokines. In this study, rats were divided into a negative-control, inflammatory injury positive-control, and two laser-treated (one at 2 J, one at 4 J) groups, after being subjected to injury. On the day of euthanasia, articular lavage was collected and centrifuged. The supernatant was analyzed for tumor necrosis factor alpha (TNFα) protein expression by enzyme-linked immunosorbent assay (ELISA) and for IL1β, IL6, and IL10 mRNA by real-time polymerase chain reaction (RT-PCR). The joint tissue was also examined histologically. Analysis of variance with Tukey's *post hoc* test was used for comparisons. All data were expressed as means ± SD ($p < 0.05$). Both laser treatment modalities

were efficient in reducing cellular inflammation and decreasing the expression of IL1β and IL6. However, the 2 J treatments led to more reduction in TNFα than the 4 J treatments. A single application of laser therapy with 2 J was more efficient in modulating inflammatory mediators and inflammatory cells. While this information proves the benefits of laser therapy, it should be pointed out that the dosing regimen reported in this study is not applicable in clinical practice. As with all such information, the practitioner must make informed decisions on how best to apply the concept to the reality.

Malliaropoulos *et al.* (2013) looked at meniscal pathology in a double-blinded, placebo-controlled study. None of the patients in the study group underwent arthroscopy or new magnetic resonance imaging (MRI). The study included only symptomatic patients, and showed that pain was significantly improved for the laser group compared to the placebo group. Pain scores were also better after laser therapy. It was concluded that laser therapy should be considered in patients with meniscal tears who do not wish to undergo surgery.

Bublitz *et al.* (2014) analyzed the effects of laser therapy in the prevention of cartilage damage after transaction of the anterior (cranial) cruciate ligament in rats' knees. They divided 30 rats into three groups (10 each): a negative control, and two groups receiving laser therapy at different doses. An 808 nm laser was used immediately after surgery and was applied for 15 sessions. To evaluate the effects of the laser treatments, qualitative and semi-quantitative histological, morphometric, and immunohistochemistry analysis were performed. Initial signs of tissue degradation were observed in the control group. The laser-treated animals presented a better tissue organization, especially at the lower ($10 J/cm^2$) settings. Laser therapy was capable of modulating some of the aspects related to the degenerative process, such as the prevention of proteoglycans loss and the increase in cartilage area. However, laser was not capable of modulating chondrocyte proliferation and the immunoexpression of markers related to the inflammatory process (IL-1 and MMP-13).

Neurological System Conditions

Brain

A study by Morries *et al.* (2015) looked at using laser therapy to treat traumatic brain injuries. In 10 patients with chronic traumatic brain injury given ten treatments over the course of 2 months, using an 810 or a 980 nm laser, symptoms of headache, sleep disturbance, cognition, mood dysregulation, anxiety, and irritability improved. Depression scales and a novel patient diary system specifically designed for this study monitored symptoms. The authors concluded that laser immunomodulates the response to brain damage.

A different study looked at the effect of laser therapy on wound healing following cerebral ischemia caused by cryogenic injury (Moreira *et al.*, 2011). This study used a 780 nm laser in rats following direct cortical cryogenic injury to look at the effects of laser treatment on inflammation and repair in the rat CNS. Wound healing in the CNS was monitored at 6 hours and 1, 7, and 14 days after laser treatment. The size of the lesions, the neuron cell viability percentages, and the distribution of lymphocytes, leukocytes, and macrophages were analyzed. Lasered lesions showed smaller tissue loss than control lesions after 6 hours. During the first 24 hours, the amount of viable neurons was significantly higher in the treated group. The lesions of the irradiated animals had fewer leukocytes and lymphocytes in the first 24 hours than those in the controls. The authors concluded that laser therapy exerts its effect in wound healing by controlling brain damage and preventing neuron death and severe astrogliosis, and could indicate the possibility of a better clinical outcome.

Spinal Cord

Another rat study looked at the effect of a 780 nm laser on locomotor functional recovery and histomorphmetric and histopathological changes of the spinal cord after moderate traumatic injury (Paula *et al.*, 2014). It divided 31 rats into seven groups: control without surgery, control surgery, laser 6 hours after surgery, laser 48 hours after surgery, medullar lesion without laser, medullar lesion with laser 6 hours after surgery, and medullar lesion with laser 48 hours after surgery. Assessment of motor function and urinary dysfunction was performed. After 21 days, the animals were euthanized for analysis of the spinal cord. The results showed faster motor evolution in rats with spinal contusion treated with laser therapy, maintenance of the effectiveness of the urinary system, and preservation of nerve tissue in the lesion area with a notorious inflammation control and increased number of nerve cells and connections.

Wu *et al.* (2009) studied two spinal cord injury models in order to show that 810 nm laser therapy was effective for transected or contused rat spinal cords. The Laser was applied transcutaneously at the lesion site immediately after injury and daily for 14 consecutive days. The daily dosage at the surface of the skin overlying the lesion was 1589 J/cm^2 (150 mW, 0.3 cm^2 spot area, 2997 seconds). Mini-ruby was used to label corticospinal tract axons, which were counted and measured from the lesion site distally. Functional recovery was assessed by footprint test for the hemisection model and open-field test for the contusion model. The average length of axonal regrowth in the rats in the treated group with hemisection and contusion injuries was significantly longer than in the comparable untreated control groups. The total axon number in the treated groups was significantly higher than in the untreated groups for both injury models. For contusion-model

rats, there was a significant functional recovery in the laser-treated groups compared to controls.

A 2015 study of human subjects with diskogenic back pain who failed to respond to a conventional physical-therapy program examined the role of laser therapy is helping patients avoid operative intervention. The study concluded that laser therapy was a viable option in the conservative treatment of diskogenic back pain, with a positive clinical result of more than 90% efficacy, not only in the short term but also in the long term, with lasting benefits (Ip and Fu, 2015).

Peripheral Nerves

A pilot study investigated the effectiveness of 780 nm laser light in the treatment of patients suffering from incomplete peripheral nerve and brachial plexus injuries for 6 months to several years (Rochkind *et al.*, 2007). It was randomized, double-blind, and placebo-controlled and used 18 patients, applying 21 consecutive daily sessions of laser or placebo transcutaneously for 3 hours to the injured peripheral nerve and for 2 hours to the corresponding segments of the spinal cord. Clinical and electrophysiological assessments were done at baseline, 21 days, and 3 and 6 months. The laser and placebo groups were in similar clinical conditions at the start of the study. Analysis of motor function during the 6-month follow-up period compared to baseline showed significant improvement in the laser-treated group compared to the placebo group. No significant difference was found in sensory function. Electrophysiological analysis showed statistically significant improvement in recruitment of voluntary muscle activity in the laser-treated group.

Another study reviewed the inhibitory effects of laser therapy on peripheral mammalian nerves and their relevance to analgesic effects (Chow *et al.*, 2011). It looked at 44 studies with variable laser settings. In 13 of 18 human studies, pulsed or continuous-wave (CW) visible and CW infrared laser application slowed conduction velocity or reduced the amplitude of compound action potentials, or both. In 26 animal experiments, infrared laser therapy suppressed electrically and noxiously evoked action potentials and pro-inflammatory mediators. Disruption of microtubule arrays and fast axonal flow may underpin neural inhibition. This could reduce acute pain through direct inhibition of peripheral nociceptors. In chronic pain, spinal cord changes induced by laser therapy may result in long-term depression of pain.

Dermatological Conditions

Calisto *et al.* (2015) randomly distributed 24 rats into two groups, control and laser-treated, to look at laser therapy's effect in the healing of traumatic wounds. An induced surgical wound was made using a scalpel, and then the treated group received five sessions of laser

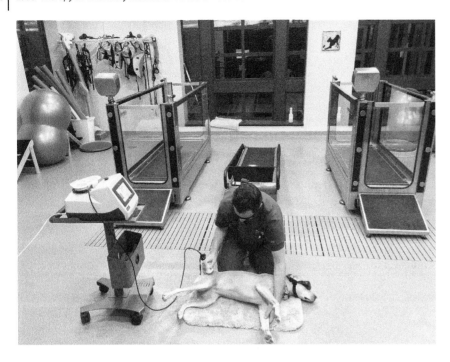

Figure 23.1 Laser therapy should be incorporated as one part of a complete rehabilitation program.

therapy on consecutive days using the following laser parameters: 660 nm, 100 mW, 10 J/cm^2. The wounds were evaluated through measurement of the area and of the depth of the wound and histological analysis. The area and depth of the wounds treated with laser therapy were significantly less than those in the control group, and the laser group presented more epithelization than the control. This shows that healing of wounds in rats was improved by the use of laser therapy.

Another study compared blue light (470 nm), red light (629 nm), and a negative control in induced ischemic abdominal flap wounds of rodents (Dungel *et al.*, 2014). Light from light-emitting diodes (LEDs) was applied for 10 minutes on five consecutive days. LED therapy of both wavelengths significantly increased angiogenesis in the sub-epidermal layer and intramuscularly, which was associated with improved tissue perfusion 7 days after ischemic insult. Accordingly, tissue necrosis was significantly reduced and shrinkage was less pronounced in the treated groups of both wavelengths. It should be noted that this study used LED and not laser therapy. LED may be efficacious when used for superficial applications: further study is needed (Opel *et al.*, 2015).

Finally, a rat study looking at induced wounds treated with 808 nm laser pulses showed good evidence for use of laser (Tabakoglu *et al.*, 2015). In this study, a control group received no treatment, while treated groups received laser treatment immediately after wounding (inflammatory group), 24 hours post-wounding (proliferative group), or 72 hours post-wounding (remodeling group). Histological analyses were performed on days 3, 7, and 14 post-wounding. On day 7, wound diameters were smaller in all treated groups versus control, with the remodeling group having the smallest wound size. At 2 weeks, dermal tissue in the inflammatory and proliferative groups closed superficially, while control and remodeling groups were open. Mean wound-healing rates for all treatment groups were found to differ significantly from the control group. Comparing the proliferative group with the other treatment groups, a significant change was found, with the proliferative group being the most efficient at wound healing. Histological and morphometric results showed that laser application had the best effect when first applied 24 hours post-wounding (late inflammatory, early proliferative stage), as demonstrated by increases in granulation tissue, fibroblasts, and collagen deposition, which lead to faster rates of wound contraction and therefore accelerated healing.

Role of Laser Therapy in Injury Rehabilitation

Based on research, case reviews, and anecdotal reports, it can be concluded that the use of laser therapy is indicated in a clinical setting (Pryor and Millis, 2015). A practical approach is also needed, which can account for many factors, including patient need, patient cooperation, cost, efficacy, and frequency and duration of treatment. Some clients may allow their pet to be treated with the laser daily; some may only be able to do so two or three times a week. It is critically important for the veterinarian to prescribe a practical and realistic treatment plan for each individual patient. Laser therapy represents only one element of comprehensive rehabilitation (Figure 23.1). While laser treatment can be safely and effectively combined with other modalities and integrated easily with other treatment approaches, it is important to prioritize the sequence of application with other modalities.

Laser Therapy as a Standalone Therapy

Examples of diagnoses that could benefit from laser treatment as a sole treatment modality include surgical incisions, wounds, lick granulomas, osteoarthritis, and tail-pull injuries.

Application of the laser therapy to every surgical incision at the end of the anesthetic period can reduce postoperative pain and swelling. This can be provided either bundled or as an option for all appropriate surgeries in a practice.

Wounds can benefit from laser therapy in the late inflammatory or early proliferative phase, and laser therapy provides continued benefit in chronic or slow-healing wounds as healing progresses.

Lick granulomas can arise from many causes and can become cycles of healing and reoccurrence. Addressing pain relief, improved circulation, and antimicrobial pathways via laser therapy can provide improvement where other treatment modalities have either failed or only address a single potential cause.

Palliative management of chronic conditions can be achieved with the laser. End-stage otitis externa in cases that are not candidates for surgical resection will benefit from a reduction of bacterial load and of inflammation and pain.

In some cases of osteoarthritis, the author has managed patients with standalone laser therapy. It is also a useful agent if other osteoarthritis management modalities need to be discontinued. An example is the severely arthritic patient on an NSAID that develops renal, hepatic, or gastrointestinal disease, meaning NSAID therapy has to be rapidly discontinued.

The therapeutic laser can be used to stimulate acupuncture points along meridians for those clinicians who practice traditional Chinese veterinary medicine (Law et al., 2015; Lorenzini et al., 2010). The author has found this helpful for anxious patients that may not sit for 20 minutes or more with acupuncture needles in place.

Neurological patients often need a comprehensive rehabilitation program (Sims et al., 2015). Such a program should be multimodal and can include laser therapy to achieve favorable results. Tail-pull injuries provide a straightforward injury for which laser treatment may be the only modality that is available, practical, and easy to achieve. Additionally, patients suffering chronic pain from tail docking will also benefit from laser therapy.

Laser Therapy in Conjunction with a Rehabilitation Program

Proper rehabilitation starts with pain management. Regardless of the injury, no patient will be able to return to function through strength training, and maintain

that outcome, if they are painful. Laser therapy is, in the author's opinion, an extremely valuable modality by which to achieve the goals of the clinician, the client, and the patient.

The release of endogenous opioids stimulated by laser therapy has applications throughout both acute and chronic conditions in injury rehabilitation (Hagiwara et al., 2008; Labajos, 1988; Montesinos, 1988). The benefit of applying laser therapy to painful muscles, tendons, ligaments, or joints before (and sometimes after) having the patient do therapeutic exercises, such as underwater treadmill workouts, cavaletti rails, or other core exercises, makes sense and has been clearly demonstrated in human patients (Levine et al., 2015).

It is important for the clinician to incorporate laser therapy as one part of a complete rehabilitation program. An example is incorporating laser therapy during the first few weeks of rehabilitation for a dog with biceps tendonitis. This aids in reducing pain and in stimulating cytokines and growth factors in order to achieve better tendon tissue healing. Laser therapy may be phased out of the rehabilitation program once the initial goals have been achieved and the patient has progressed to strength training and maintenance.

Osteoarthritis may initially require a high frequency of treatment (multiple times per week) through an induction phase. As pain and inflammation are reduced, the frequency can be reduced through a transition phase, until a maintenance-phase protocol is achieved. If an acute-on-chronic flare-up occurs, the induction phase can be easily repeated in order to keep the patient functional.

Neurological patients, such as those with brachial plexus avulsion or IVDD, may benefit from laser therapy throughout their entire rehabilitation process. It can be used early for management of pain at the insult site or in inflamed muscles. It can then be used to attempt a return of neurological function throughout recovery, and either to prevent or to manage the neuropathic pain that is a potential outcome in these cases.

Assessing Response to Laser Therapy

Based on the individual patient, diagnosis, prognosis, and plan, reassessments should be scheduled and documented appropriately by the clinician. The veterinary professionals delivering the treatment should be looking for both subjective and objective indicators of how the patient is doing.

Repeated physical examinations and photographs can be helpful in assessing patient function. Additionally, goniometry, digital thermography, and stance-analyzer measurements can be useful in providing objective data in a clinical setting.

Case Studies

Cranial Cruciate Ligament Tear in a German Shepherd

Signalment
11 years old, German shepherd, MN, 36.4 kg.

Client Complaint
Left hind limb lameness.

History
The patient had previously been diagnosed with bilateral anal sacculitis and spondylosis deformans. He had decreased mobility over the last 12 months and had become acutely lame in the left hind leg.

Current Medications
Cefpodaxime and cyclosporine were being given orally, along with topical tacrolimus for anal sacculitis. Carprofen was being given for spondylosis.

Physical Examination
The patient was bright, alert, and responsive, with appropriate hydration and a body condition score (BCS) of 4/5. He displayed stiffness and discomfort in the lumbar muscles and was 3/5 lame in the left hind leg. There was moderate left stifle effusion, partial cranial drawer movement, cranial tibial thrust, and no meniscal click. Bilateral semilunar perianal fistulas measuring 2.5 × 5.0 cm were noted. All other systems were within normal limits.

Differential Diagnosis
Cranial cruciate injury.

Diagnostic Imaging
Lateral and anteroposterior radiographs of the stifles from the referring veterinarian showed disturbance of the infrapatellar fat pad and moderate osteoarthritic changes in the left stifle, with no significant findings in the right stifle. The pelvis was within normal limits in a ventrodorsal view. The lumbar spine showed a complete ventral fusion of all lumbar vertebrae. There was no evidence of lytic or proliferative lesions or any other indication for infection or neoplasia in any of the radiographs.

Laboratory Data
Complete blood count (CBC), chemistry panel, and urinalysis showed no significant findings.

Diagnosis
Bilateral anal fistulas, obesity, spondylosis deformans with muscle pain, and a partial tear of the left cruciate ligament were diagnosed.

Treatment Plan
A weight-loss program with dietary restriction was implemented. Laser therapy was applied to the left stifle ($6-10\,J/cm^2$, contact delivery) to aid in cruciate ligament healing. The laser was applied to the right hind leg and both thoracic limbs ($6-10\,J/cm^2$, contact delivery), since increased weight bearing would occur on those limbs. The laser was also applied to the lumbar area ($8-10\,J/cm^2$, contact delivery) and to the anal fistulas ($6-8\,J/cm^2$, non-contact delivery).

Outcome
Laser therapy application was repeated twice a week for 4 weeks. During that time, the patient improved in ambulation, and lameness scores decreased. The fistulas decreased in size by 50%. The owner was then not able to bring the patient for treatment for 2 weeks, during which he became increasingly lame. Upon restarting laser therapy, the patient improved initially, but then began stumbling at home, crying out, and limping more severely. Examination revealed a complete tear of the left cranial cruciate ligament. Surgery was not an option for this patient, due to cost. The patient was fitted for a custom-made stifle brace and laser therapy was continued for another 4 weeks. During that time, the patient ambulated well and lameness scores returned to normal. The anal fistulas also resolved completely. Therapy was then discontinued due to cost and the patient was lost to follow-up.

Biceps Tendonitis in a Standard Poodle

Signalment
8 years old, standard poodle, FS, 11.8 kg.

Client Complaint
Left fore-leg lameness.

History
The owner had noted an on-and-off lameness for 4–6 weeks. It was worse after playing and running with other dogs in the household.

Current Medications
Heartworm, flea, and tick prevention medications were being given monthly.

Physical Examination
The patient was bright, alert, and responsive, with a BCS of 4/5. Moderate pain was elicited on left shoulder and biceps tendon palpation. Mild left-muscle atrophy was noted compared to the right. Mild pain was present in the right shoulder. No neck pain was noted. Neurological and other systems were within normal limits.

Differential Diagnosis

Shoulder osteoarthritis, biceps tendonitis.

Diagnostic Imaging

Lateral and anteroposterior radiographs of each shoulder were obtained. No abnormalities were found. While sedated, the patient underwent diagnostic musculoskeletal ultrasound of both shoulders, which showed inflammation and a grade I strain of both the left and the right biceps tendons.

Laboratory Data

CBC, chemistry panel, and urinalysis showed no significant findings.

Diagnosis

Bilateral biceps tendonitis.

Treatment Plan

While the patient was sedated, each tendon was injected with 10 mg of methylprednisolone acetate using ultrasound guidance. The patient was placed on restricted activity and was re-checked 7 days later. At that time, no lameness or discomfort was noted in either shoulder. An outpatient rehabilitation program was then instituted for further tissue healing and strength training. The patient was seen twice a week for 6 weeks and received laser therapy to both shoulders ($8-10 \, J/cm^2$, contact delivery, 12 treatments total) (Figure 23.2). The patient also did therapeutic exercises (cavaletti rails and core exercises on various devices) and walked on both a land and an underwater treadmill.

Outcome

The patient was sound within 2 weeks of beginning therapy. It progressed, and a full return to function occurred.

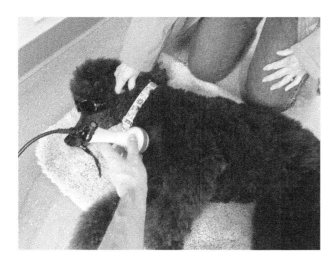

Figure 23.2 Laser therapy treatment of the shoulder for biceps tendonitis.

IVDD in a Dachshund

Signalment

7 years old, Dachshund, MN, 3.6 kg.

Client Complaint

Neurological deficits 2 weeks after T13–L1 right-sided hemilamenectomy.

History

This patient had experienced an acute disk herniation with loss of motor function and pain perception in the pelvic limbs. Within 12 hours, an MRI determined the diagnosis and surgery was performed to remove the herniated disk. The patient regained pain perception after surgery, but not motor function.

Current Medications

Gabapentin 100 mg BID.

Physical Examination

The thoracic limbs were within normal limits. Grade I motor function was present in the pelvic limbs. Pain and withdrawal reflexes were present in both hind legs. Upper motor neuron bladder function was noted, with the bladder requiring manual expression three times a day.

Treatment Plan

The patient received electroacupuncture treatments weekly for 6 weeks. He also had therapeutic laser, underwater treadmill, and other physical-therapy modalities three times a week for 4 weeks, then twice a week for 6 weeks. Laser therapy was used on the thoracic spine, lumbar spine, and pelvic limbs. Laser settings delivered $8-10 \, J/cm^2$ to the thoracic spine, lumbar spine, and pelvic limbs. Treatments were delivered with a handpiece in contact with the skin. When treating the pelvic limbs, the joints were taken through a passive range of motion to facilitate photon penetration into the joint spaces.

Outcome

Over the course of 4 weeks, the patient regained all motor function but was ataxic and had conscious proprioceptive deficits in both hind legs. In the following 6 weeks, the patient made a full recovery.

Presumed IVDD in a Jack Russell Terrier

Signalment

12 years old, canine Jack Russell terrier, MN, 8.2 kg.

Client Complaint

Acute non-ambulatory paraplegia.

History

The patient was boarding, had been normal one evening, and in the morning could not use his hind legs. There was no evidence of trauma.

Current Medications

Famotidine 2.5 mg BID, prednisone 5 mg BID, gabapentin 100 mg BID.

Physical Examination

The thoracic limbs were within normal limits. Pain, withdrawal, and patellar reflexes were present in the hind legs. The patient had no motor function in either hind leg. His cutaneous trunci reflex stopped at approximately the second lumbar vertebrae. His bladder was large and turgid, but expressible.

Diagnostic Imaging

Survey radiographs did not show any fracture, lytic area, or other concerns.

Laboratory Data

CBC, chemistry panel, and urinalysis showed no significant findings.

Differential Diagnosis

IVDD was most likely. Fibrocartilagenous emboli and neoplasia were felt to be less likely.

Treatment Plan

This patient was treated as IVDD. Laser therapy was applied twice a week for 6 weeks as part of a full rehabilitation program. The patient also received transcutaneous electrical nerve stimulation, underwater treadmill therapy, massage, and range-of-motion and weight-bearing exercises. Laser settings delivered 8–10 J/cm^2 to the thoracic spine, lumbar spine, and pelvic limbs.

Outcome

Over the course of 4 weeks, the patient regained motor function in the pelvic limbs but was ataxic. This improved over the next 8 weeks.

Conclusion

Injury rehabilitation in veterinary medicine is an expanding field that requires both a practical approach and a commitment to staying on the cutting edge of available treatment options. Laser therapy is a vital tool in the veterinary professional's armament. Its variability, ease of administration, and proven benefits allow many types of patient to recover faster and more effectively. Further research is needed to find other types of injury that may benefit from laser therapy, as well as to further verify treatment settings and time frames.

References

Abergel, R.P. *et al.* (1984) Control of connective tissue metabolism by lasers: recent developments and future prospects. *J Am Acad Dermatol.* **11**(6):1142–1150.

Assis, L. *et al.* (2015) Effect of low level laser therapy (808 nm) on skeletal muscle after endurance exercise training in rats. *Braz J Phys Ther.* **19**(6):457–465.

Barbosa, D. *et al.* (2014) Laser therapy in bone repair in rats: analysis of bone optical density. *Acta Ortop Bras.* **22**(2):71–74.

Baxter, G.D. and McDonough, S.M. (2007) Principles of electrotherapy in veterinary physiotherapy. In: *Animal Physiotherapy: Assessment, Treatment and Rehabilitation of Animals*, pp. 182–184. Blackwell, Oxford.

Bayat, M. *et al.* (2005) Low-level laser therapy improves early healing of medial collateral ligament injuries in rats. *Photomed Laser Surg.* **23**(6):556–560.

Bensadoun, R.J. and Nair, R.G. (2015) Low-level laser therapy in the management of mucositis and dermatitis induced by cancer therapy. *Photomed Laser Surg.* **33**(10):487–491.

Bjordal, J.M. *et al.* (2006) A randomized, placebo controlled trial of low level laser therapy for activated Achilles tendinitis with microdialysis measurements of peritendinous prostaglandin E2 concentrations. *Br J Sports Med.* **40**(1):76–80.

Bublitz, C. *et al.* (2014) Low level laser therapy prevents degenerative morphological changes in an experimental model of anterior cruciate ligament transection in rats. *Lasers Med Sci.* **29**(5):1669–1678.

Calisto, F.C. *et al.* (2015) Use of low-power laser to assist the healing of traumatic wounds. *Acta Cir Bras.* **30**(3):204–208.

Carvalho, A.F. *et al.* (2015) The low-level laser on acute myositis in rats. *Acta Cir Bras.* **30**(12):806–811.

Chang, W. *et al.* (2014) Therapeutic outcomes of low-level laser therapy for closed bone fracture in the human wrist and hand. *Photomed Laser Surg.* **32**(4):212–218.

Chow, R. *et al.* (2011) Inhibitory effects of laser irradiation on peripheral mammalian nerves and relevance to analgesic effects: a systematic review. *Photomed Laser Surg.* **29**(6):365–381.

Conforti, M. and Fachinetti, G.P. (2013) High power laser therapy treatment compared to simple segmental physical rehabilitation in whiplash injuries (1 and 2 grade of the Quebec Task Force classification) involving muscles and ligaments. *Muscles Ligaments Tendons J.* **3**(2):106–111.

Corazza, A.V. *et al.* (2007) Photobiomodulation of the angiogenesis of skin wounds in rats using different light sources. *Photomed Laser Surg.* **25**(2):102–106.

Da Ré Guerra, F. *et al.* (2016) Low-level PBMT modulates pro-inflammatory cytokines after partial tenotomy. *Lasers Med Sci.* **31**(4):759–766.

De Bie, R.A. *et al.* (1998) Low-level laser therapy in ankle sprains: a randomized clinical trial. *Arch Phys Med Rehabil.* **79**(11):1415–1420.

de Jesus, J.F. *et al.* (2015) Low-level laser therapy in IL-1B, COX-2 and PGE2 modulation in partially injured Achilles tendon. *Lasers Med Sci.* **30**(1):153–158.

de Loura Santana C. *et al.* (2016) Effect of laser therapy on immune cells infiltrate after excisional wounds in diabetic rats. *Lasers Surg. Med.* **48**(1):45–51.

dos Santos, S.A. *et al.* (2014) Comparative analysis of two low-level laser doses on the expression of inflammatory mediators and on neutrophils and macrophages in acute joint inflammation. *Lasers Med Sci.* **29**(3):1051–1058.

Dungel, P. *et al.* (2014) Low level light therapy by LED of different wavelength induces angiogenesis and improves ischemic wound healing. *Lasers Surg Med.* **46**(10):773–780.

Ebrahimi, T. *et al.* (2012) The Influence of low-intensity laser therapy on bone healing. *J Dent (Tehran).* **9**(4):238–248.

Enwemeka, C.S. *et al.* (2004) The efficacy of low-power lasers in tissue repair and pain control: a meta-analysis study. *Photomed Laser Surg.* **22**(4):323–329.

Fenner, W.R. (2000) Diseases of the brain. In: *Textbook of Veterinary Internal Medicine*, 5 edn., pp. 552–556. Saunders, Philadelphia, PA.

Frank, C. *et al.* (1991) Normal ligament: structure, function and composition. In: *Injury and Repair of the Musculoskeletal Soft Tissues.* American Academy of Orthopedic Surgeons Symposium: Park Ridge, IL.

Fung, D.T. *et al.* (2002) Therapeutic low energy laser improves the mechanical strength of repairing medial collateral ligament. *Lasers Surg Med.* **31**(2):91–96.

Hagiwara, S. *et al.* (2008) Pre-irradiation of blood by gallium aluminum arsenide (830 nm) low-level laser enhances peripheral endogenous opioid analgesia in rats. *Anesth Analg.* **107**(3):1058–1063.

Hedlund, C.S. (2002) Surgery of the integumentary system. In: *Small Animal Surgery*, 2 edn., pp. 134–137. Mosby, St. Louis, MO.

Honmura, A. *et al.* (1993) Analgesic effect of GaA1As diode laser irradiation on hyperalgesia in carrageenin-induced inflammation. *Lasers Surg Med.* **13**(4):463–469.

Hopkins, J.T. *et al.* (2004) Low-level laser therapy facilitates superficial wound healing in humans: a triple-blind, sham-controlled study. *J Athl Train.* **39**(3):223–229.

Huang, Y.Y. *et al.* (2009) Biphasic dose response in low level light therapy. *Dose-Response.* **7**(4):358–383.

Inzana, K.D. (2000) Peripheral nerve disorders. In: *Textbook of Veterinary Internal Medicine*, 5 edn., pp. 662–681. Saunders, Philadelphia, PA.

Ip, D. and Fu, N.Y. (2015) Can intractable discogenic back pain be managed by low-level PBMT without recourse to operative intervention? *J Pain Res.* **8**:253–256.

Jawad, M.M. *et al.* (2013) Effect of 940 nm low-level laser therapy on osteogenesis in vitro. *J Biomed Opt.* **18**(12):128001.

Karu, T. (2010) Mitochondrial mechanisms of photobiomodulation in context of new data about multiple roles of ATP. *Photomed Laser Surg.* **28**(2):159–160.

Kaya, G.S. *et al.* (2011) Use of 808-nm light therapy to treat experimental chronic osteomyelitis induced in rats by methicillin-resistant *Staphylococcus aureus*. *Photomed Laser Surg.* **29**(6):405–412.

Kizhner, V. *et al.* (2011) Laser-generated shockwave for clearing medical device biofilms. *Photomed Laser Surg.* **29**(4):277–282.

Labajos, M. (1988) Beta-endorphin levels modification after GaAs and HeNe laser irradiation on the rabbit. *Comparative study. Invest Clin.* **1–2**:6–8.

Law, D. *et al.* (2015) Laser acupuncture for treating musculoskeletal pain: a systematic review with meta-analysis. *J Acupunct Meridian Stud.* **8**(1):2–16.

LeCouteur, R.A. and Grandy, J.L. (2000) Diseases of the spinal cord. In: *Textbook of Veterinary Internal Medicine*, 5 edn., pp. 609–653. Saunders, Philadelphia, PA.

Levine, D. *et al.* (2015) Effects of laser on endurance of the rotator cuff muscles. *Lasers Surg Med.* **47**(S26):44–45.

Lögdberg-Andersson, M. *et al.* (1997) Low level laser therapy (LLLT) of tendinitis and myofascial pains – a randomized, double-blind, controlled study. *Laser Ther.* **9**:79–86.

Lorenzini, L. *et al.* (2010) Laser acupuncture for acute inflammatory, visceral and neuropathic pain relief: An experimental study in the laboratory rat. *Res Vet Sci.* **88**(1):159–165.

Malliaropoulos, N. *et al.* (2013) Low-level laser therapy in meniscal pathology: a double-blinded placebo controlled study. *Lasers Med Sci.* **28**(4):1183–1188.

Millis, D.L. and Ciuperca, I.A. (2015) Evidence for canine rehabilitation and physical therapy. *Vet Clin North Am Small Anim Pract.* **45**(1):1–27.

Montesinos, M. (1988) Experimental effects of low power laser in encephalin and endorphin synthesis. *J Eur Med Laser Assoc.* **1**(3):2–7.

Moreira, M.S. *et al.* (2011) Effect of laser phototherapy on wound healing following cerebral ischemia by cryogenic injury. *J Photochem Photobiol B.* **105**(3):207–215.

Morries, L.D. *et al.* (2015) Treatments for traumatic brain injury with emphasis on transcranial near-infrared laser phototherapy. *Neuropsychiatr Dis Treat.* **11**:2159–2175.

Opel, D.R. *et al.* (2015) Light-emitting diodes. a brief review of clinical experience. *J Clin Aesthet Dermatol.* **8**(6):36–44.

Paula, A.A. *et al.* (2014) Low-intensity laser therapy effect on the recovery of traumatic spinal cord injury. *Lasers Med Sci.* **29**(6):1849–1859.

Perini, J.L. *et al.* (2015) Long-term low-level laser therapy promotes an increase in maximal oxygen uptake and exercise performance in a dose-dependent manner in Wistar rats. *Lasers Med Sci.* **31**(2):241–248.

Pourreau-Schneider, N. *et al.* (1990) Helium-neon laser treatment transforms fibroblasts into myofibroblasts. *Am J Pathol.* **137**(1):171–178.

Pryor, B. and Millis, D.L. (2015) Therapeutic laser in veterinary medicine. *Vet Clin North Am Small Anim Pract.* **45**(1):45–56.

Rochkind, S. *et al.* (2007) Laser phototherapy (780 nm), a new modality in treatment of long-term incomplete peripheral nerve injury: a randomized double-blind placebo-controlled study. *Photomed Laser Surg.* **25**(5):436–442.

Sakarai, Y. *et al.* (2000) Inhibitory effect of low-level laser irradiation on LPS-stimulated prostaglandin E2 productions and cyclooxygenase-2 in human gingival fibroblasts. *Eur J Oral Sci.* **108**(1):29–34.

Seim, H.B. (2002a) Surgery of cervical spine. In: *Small Animal Surgery*, 2 edn., p. 1227. Mosby, St. Louis, MO.

Seim, H.B. (2002b) Surgery of the lumbosacral spine. In: *Small Animal Surgery*, 2 edn., pp. 1304 and 1349. Mosby, St. Louis, MO.

Sims, C. *et al.* (2015) Rehabilitation and physical therapy for the neurologic patient. *Vet Clin North Am Small Anim Pract.* **45**(1):123–143.

Tabakoglu, H.O. *et al.* (2015) Assessment of circular wound healing in rats after exposure to 808-nm laser pulses during specific healing phases. *Lasers Surg Med.* **48**(4):409–415

Tedford, C.E. *et al.* (2015) Quantitative analysis of transcranial and intraparenchymal light penetration in human cadaver brain tissue. *Lasers Surg Med.* **47**(4):312–322.

Tim, C.R. *et al.* (2014) Low-level laser therapy enhances the expression of osteogenic factors during bone repair in rats. *Lasers Med Sci.* **29**(1):147–156.

Tumilty, S. and Baxter, D. (2015) Effectiveness of class IV lasers for Achilles tendinopathy. *Lasers Surg Med.* **47**(S26):38.

Tumilty, S. *et al.* (2010) Low level laser treatment of tendinopathy: a systematic review with meta-analysis. *Photomed Laser Surg.* **28**(1):3–16.

Vasilenko, T. *et al.* (2010) The effect of equal daily dose achieved by different power densities of low-level laser therapy at 635 and 670 nm on wound tensile strength in rats: a short report. *Photomed Laser Surg.* **28**(2):281–283.

Williams, J. (2004) Wound healing: tendons, ligaments, bone, muscles and cartilage. In: *Canine Rehabilitation and Physical Therapy*, pp. 100–110. Saunders, St. Louis, MO.

Wu, X. *et al.* (2009) 810 nm wavelength light: an effective therapy for transected or contused rat spinal cord. *Lasers Surg Med.* **31**(1):36–41.

24

Laser Therapy and Multimodal Performance Maintenance

Deborah M. Gross

Wizard of Paws Physical Rehabilitation for Animals, Colchester, CT, USA

Introduction

As photobiomodulation therapy (PBMT) continues to expand in veterinary rehabilitation and progressive veterinary medicine, the scope of additional applications and utilizations broadens. Other chapters discuss the mechanisms and benefits of using PBMT in practice, demonstrating that laser therapy is a key component in a large array of treatments for animals. This chapter will focus on the incorporation of PBMT in the multimodal performance maintenance of canine athletes and working dogs.

The multimodal approach to therapeutics is considered the standard of care in veterinary medicine; it includes a comprehensive approach. Dr. Steven Fox, the direction of pain management at Novartis Animal Health, stated, "The multimodal management of canine osteoarthritis is rapidly becoming the standard of care. This approach integrates nonmedical modalities – weight control, EPA [eicosapentaenoic acid] rich diets and physical rehabilitation – with medical modalities, such as non-steroidal anti-inflammatories, chrondroprotectants, and adjunct drugs" (Fox, 2014). PBMT is one of the integral nonmedical modalities, playing a significant role in the management of osteoarthritis, as well as many other common conditions seen in companion-animal practice.

The Role of PBMT in the Multimodal Approach

The multimodal approach is key to the successful management of pain and inflammation and the improvement of strength and function. Improvement of strength and function cannot be obtained without the reduction of pain and inflammation. This is a simple concept and needs to be addressed on a continued basis for the successful treatment and maintenance of many common conditions. PBMT has been demonstrated to be a very successful approach to the treatment of pain, inflammation, and dysfunction. Thus, in the successful rehabilitation of animals, PBMT plays a significant role in the multimodal approach.

Many laser technologies are incorporated into medical applications in order to contribute to the multimodal management of conditions. Though different from PBMT in that it requires a non-endogenous chromophore to be present in the tissue, photodynamic therapy is an example. Maier *et al.*, (2000) demonstrated the effects of photodynamic therapy in a multimodal approach to the management of carcinoma of the gastroesophageal junction.

Ultimately, the goal for each patient is to restore the highest level of function possible. Improved function will be obtained through the appropriate range-of-motion and stretching gains and through strengthening, balance, proprioceptive, and endurance exercises. However, an increase or maintenance of strength and function cannot be obtained without achieving one of the first goals in rehabilitation: the reduction of pain and inflammation. Without a reduction of noxious levels of pain and inflammation, a successful progression will not be achieved. The healing properties of PBMT outlined in other chapters will facilitate the successful multimodal approach.

Once pain and inflammation are reduced through PBMT, appropriate range-of-motion, stretching, and strengthening exercises may be performed. Ideally, a rehabilitative session should include an initial application of laser therapy to the primary, secondary, and any tertiary areas of pain and inflammation. Range-of-motion exercises may be performed concurrently with the laser treatment or directly after the laser treatment for optimal benefit.

An excellent example is the treatment of a dog with canine hip dysplasia presenting with pain, limited hip extension and abduction, and decreased strength and proprioception. The first goal is to determine whether

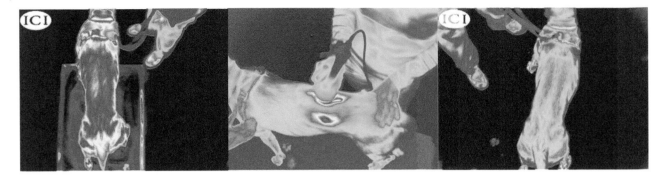

Figure 24.1 Left: Digital thermal image of a patient with increased thermal gradients throughout the thoracic and lumbar spinal musculature. Center: Using this as a road map for PBMT, therapy was applied throughout all anatomical areas exhibiting an increase in thermal gradients. More energy was applied to left side. Right: 24 hours after PBMT, the patient had less pain and was more relaxed on palpation, and all treated areas revealed a decrease in the thermal gradient.

there is compensatory pain elsewhere in the body. Digital thermal imaging (Figure 24.1), palpation, and function analysis can all be utilized to determine whether there are areas of secondary and tertiary compensation. In many cases of canine hip dysplasia, the dog has secondary pain in the lumbar and lumbosacral spine secondary to the loss of range of motion in hip extension and the body's need to increase the motion. A full multimodal approach will include laser treatment to the bilateral hips, lumbar, and lumbosacral spines.

If the treatment is applied with the dog in a lateral recumbent position, passive pain-free hip extension may be performed while the dog receives the laser treatment. Application with the treatment handpiece in contact with the skin is favored when treating the canine hip. The circumference of the hip should be treated. A dose of $8-10\,\mathrm{J/cm^2}$ is recommended. Application beginning at the greater trochanter and moving cranially, medially, and then caudally ensures photonic saturation within all of the involved structures. While the medial component of the hip is treated, a stretch into hip abduction may be performed. Contact application to the adductors, including the pectineus muscle, will facilitate stretching of the hip into hip abduction. While the laser is applied to the cranial component of the hip, or to the hip flexors and the quadriceps, the hip may easily be stretched into extension. To stretch into hip flexion, perform a simultaneous application of laser therapy to the caudal surface of the hip or the gluteal muscles and proximal hamstrings.

If stretching and range of motion are not applied simultaneously with laser therapy, they should be added after the laser treatment. Passive range of motion will stretch the inert structures, but it should only be approached after evaluation of pain and determination of a comfortable range of motion. As already mentioned, hip extension and abduction are commonly limited.

Once passive range of motion has been performed, active range of motion should be encouraged. Active range of motion stretches the contractile units and

demonstrates the dog's willingness to move. Active motion may be encouraged by asking the dog to place its front limbs on a step in order to move the hip into extension. Walking over cavaletti rails will actively increase both hip flexion and extension. Lateral stepping will increase both hip abduction and hip adduction.

Another example is elbow dysplasia. One of the key factors in the improvement of canine elbow dysplasia is a decrease in pain and inflammation (Michelson, 2013), which can be easily accomplished with PBMT. PBMT will also serve to exert a positive effect on bone regeneration (Nagasawa *et al.*, 1991). An increase in microcirculation and vascularization is also a known benefit of laser therapy, and is very helpful in the multimodal treatment of the dysplastic elbow (Barushka *et al.*, 1995).

Like the hip, the elbow is treated with the treatment handpiece in contact with the skin, delivering a dose of $8-10\,\mathrm{J/cm^2}$. The elbow should be treated circumferentially for best effect. In addition, the shoulder and carpus should be treated, due to their potential compensatory movements and altered biomechanics. Digital thermal imaging can help confirm any other associated areas of pain and discomfort.

In addition to treating the pain and inflammation of elbow dysplasia, it is also advisable to treat range-of-motion losses (Innes, 2009). Functional losses of motion in the end ranges of extension and flexion are debilitating. PBMT has shown numerous benefits in improving range-of-motion loss (Baltzer *et al.*, 2016). If possible, passive range-of-motion movement and prolonged stretching should be applied while the laser treatment is administered. If this is not possible, range of motion and prolonged stretching may be applied directly after treatment.

In the treatment approach, after an assessment with objective tools such as palpation, pain scales, a gait evaluation, and digital thermal imaging, PBMT will be the next step. As previously mentioned, PBMT is directed at the dysplastic elbows, as well as any of the other

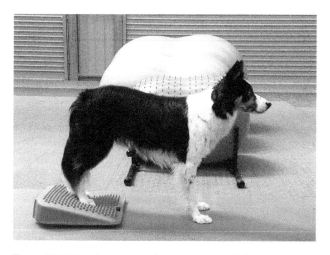

Figure 24.2 Standing on a wedge to improve stability.

compromised joints. In addition to the shoulder and carpal region being affected secondary to altered gait biomechanics, the cervical region may also demonstrate adaptations and warrant PBMT.

If the PBMT treatment is not performed concurrently with the range of motion and prolonged stretching in elbow flexion and extension, it should be performed immediately afterward. Joint mobilization may be applied at this stage as well, if the practitioner is skilled in mobilization. Balance and proprioceptive exercises can then be applied. Increasing stability in the dysplastic elbow is key, regardless of whether or not there has been a surgical intervention. Balance, weight bearing, and low-level therapeutic exercises are beneficial in improving stability. Examples include standing on an uneven surface with weight shifting (Figure 24.2), and active movements. In addition, walking in an underwater treadmill is beneficial in reducing the stress on the elbow while increasing the strength of the surrounding musculature. If lameness persists after treatment, cryotherapy or a second laser therapy treatment, or both, may be applied to the elbow region. This will enhance the anti-inflammatory effects.

The Role of PBMT in Osteoarthritis

Osteoarthritis is one of the more common conditions seen in the small-animal rehabilitation clinic. As the length of pets' lives increase, the incidence of osteoarthritis continues to increase in the pet population. PBMT is an important component of the multimodal approach to the management of osteoarthritis. On a basic level, the goals of managing osteoarthritis include reducing pain and inflammation, improving range of motion and strength, and bringing about return of function. More specifically, the stimulation of healing, improvement of mitochondrial respiration, improvement in adenosine

triphosphate (ATP) production, and reduction of inflammatory cells are among the actions needed for the appropriate treatment of osteoarthritis (Cheng and Visco, 2012).

A multitude of studies have demonstrated the effectiveness of laser therapy in treating inflammation and bringing about a reduction in inflammatory cells such as neutrophils, macrophages, lymphocytes, and mast cells (Chung *et al.*, 2012). Alves *et al.* (2013) examined a model of osteoarthritis in the rat stifle and concluded that a single application of 4 J to both the medial and the lateral aspects of the stifle caused a reduction in inflammatory cells.

PBMT decreases the pain and inflammation in the affected joints, as well as the surrounding ones. It demonstrates a positive influence on the fibroblasts in osteoarthritis, osteoblast proliferation, collagen synthesis, and bone regeneration (Nagasawa *et al.*, 1991). Mokmeli *et al.* (2006) demonstrated the effectiveness of laser therapy on osteoarthritis of the knee, while Hegedus *et al.* (2009) demonstrated in a double-blinded, randomized, placebo-controlled trial that laser therapy reduces pain in knee osteoarthritis and improves microcirculation. The latter study assessed pain, thermographic measurements, and range of motion. In the group treated with laser therapy, a significant improvement was observed in pain, sensitivity, flexion range of motion, and thermographic measurements, demonstrating an increase in circulation compared to the original values.

Laser therapy will assist in the repair of cartilage and the promotion of angiogenesis. Da Rosa *et al.* (2012) examined the effects of different wavelengths of laser therapy on osteoarthritis and found 808 nm to be superior compared to 660 nm. In addition, they demonstrated a limitation in the development of fibrosis in osteoarthritic rodents.

When treating the osteoarthritic patient, it is imperative to examine and identify secondary and tertiary areas of pain and compensations. For example, in the case of osteoarthritis of the stifle, a dog often may not extend its hip fully during the walk and trot gait cycle. This can cause secondary pain and discomfort in the hip and lumbar region. A comprehensive evaluation, including digital thermal imaging, will determine whether there are secondary and tertiary compensations.

When treating osteoarthritis, it is the author's opinion that using a continuous-wave (CW) laser delivery (as opposed to a pulsed delivery) is most effective. A dose of at least 10 J/cm^2 is a good starting point. Many dogs with osteoarthritis benefit from the application of laser therapy with the treatment handpiece in contact with the skin, which gives a massaging effect that provides the benefit of increased blood flow and tactile sensation. If dogs in too much pain for the contact approach, then a non-contact method may be utilized.

The goal of using PBMT is to decrease the pain and inflammation associated with the osteoarthritis in order to increase strength, range of motion, and, ultimately, the highest level of function possible for the patient. Laser treatments to the primary, secondary, and any tertiary areas are best performed during the initial phase of treatment, in order to assist with the reduction in pain and inflammation. The identification of the primary problem areas should be ascertained via the appropriate medical history, inclusive of radiographs, history, and additional diagnostic tests. Clinical history should include functional limitations, range-of-motion limitations, strength deficits, palpation, and digital thermal imaging. Radiographs may indicate limitations in one area, while clinically the dog presents with functional limitations in another. It is imperative to treat both clinical and functional limitations, and fortunately, this may be easily accomplished with PBMT. An example is osteoarthritic stifle secondary to cruciate disease. Functional limitations may be present in the ipsilateral hip, hock, and lumbar region, in addition to the contralateral hip, stifle, hock, and perhaps fore limb. To assist the dog in returning to the highest level of function, it will be imperative to treat all affected areas.

Once the painful areas are identified, the initial treatments may be started. In a circumferential or sweeping method, laser treatments should be applied to the areas identified. Dosages of $10–12\,J/cm^2$ may be utilized. If treating acute pain or a smaller patient, a lower dose may be used. If treating larger patients or more chronic pain, use higher doses. The area treated should encompass the area surrounding the joint in addition to the joint itself. For example, the stifle of a Labrador retriever might require treatment of an area of $300–400\,cm^2$. The distal hamstrings, proximal quadriceps, abductors, and adductors may add an additional $200–300\,cm^2$.

If possible, range of motion or stretching should be attempted as the laser treatment is being applied. The dog will benefit from the positive effects of laser and begin to relax, which will assist with the range of motion and stretching. Pain and limitations should be respected. The goal is to facilitate a pain-free increase in range of motion.

Treatments for osteoarthritis should initially be applied two to three times per week. Functional objective outcomes, in addition to pain scales, should be utilized to determine the amount of progress. Examples include assessment of static weight bearing, dynamic gait analysis, range of motion, functional sit–stand scores, client perceptions, and home functional goals. Ideally, the dog should demonstrate an improvement within two or three visits. One of the more common errors in treating dogs with osteoarthritis is not treating with a high enough dosage. Beginning with a low dosage

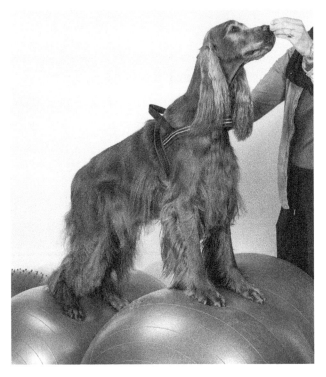

Figure 24.3 Uneven peanut balls can facilitate the gain of balance and strength.

may be indicated, but the practitioner should make sure the it is appropriate for the goals and expectations.

In addition to laser treatments, range of motion, and stretching, functional and strengthening exercises need to be performed in order to assist with the functional goals (Figure 24.3). Appropriate short- and long-term goals established during the initial evaluation will assist in determining the appropriate treatments. Strengthening exercises will come in the form of balance, proprioception, specific therapeutic exercises, ambulation, aquatic therapy, and functional exercises (Figure 24.4).

PBMT and the Approach to Treatment

The common goal of animal rehabilitation is the maximum possible improvement in the quality of life of the animal. Whether the dog has had a recent orthopedic surgery or is a senior with multiple areas of osteoarthritis, the practitioner's goals should include pain relief, reduction of inflammation, restoration of strength and range of motion, and return of function. Function will be determined by the individual animal's ability and by the owner's goals. Companion animals rely on their owners for much of their movement, and thus the owner's expectations and goals need to be factored in to the treatment approach. The psychological effects for both the owner and the animal of PBMT within a multimodal treatment can be great. Owners are cognizant of their animal's

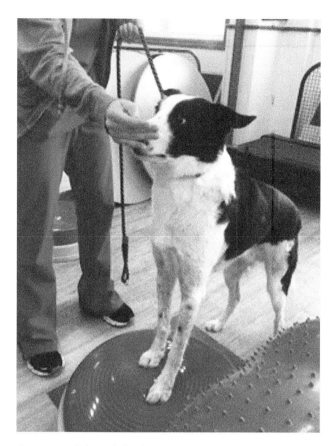

Figure 24.4 Balance balls play an important role in achieving strengthening goals.

limitations in a functional environment. For example, an owner will recognize if their dog does not rise to greet them at the door when they come in – and will also recognize when it does happily greet them the day after a treatment.

The first step in treating with PBMT is to provide a specific diagnosis and a list of problems. Every treatment intervention should have a target inclusive of pharmaceutical and non-pharmaceutical interventions. Once the area to be treated is confirmed, the problem list should be developed. This may be inclusive of pain rated on an individual score, limitation of range of motion with specific goniometric measurements, gait deviations measured on a gait scale or a dynamic gait analysis, strength deficits, and functional deficits. Once the problems are established, a treatment plan may be designed, with both short- and long-term goals. The short-term goals should be met within 2–4 weeks, and the long-term goals within a few months. Examples of short-term goals include reduction of pain from 4/10 to 2/10 on a pain scale, an increase of range of motion of 10°, and an increase of independent ambulation to 1000 feet without lameness. Long-term goals might include returning to 1-mile walks with the owner, getting in and out of the car independently, and walking up and down a flight of stairs

on a regular basis. Individual goals will vary depending upon the age of the dog, the condition, and the goals of the owner.

Once the problems and goals are established, the appropriate treatments can be chosen. PBMT is a diverse modality and may be used to treat a wide array of conditions. As described throughout this book, it has many applications. In the multimodal approach, it should be used to complement and assist in the achievement of the goals.

Maintenance in Postoperative Cases

Postoperative cases are one of the most common applications of laser therapy. The goal will be to treat the wound and incision as quickly as possible in order to facilitate the healing process. Surgical wounds, whether deep or superficial, have a common inflammatory process. The granulation process then goes through multiple stages, inclusive of fibroblast proliferation and collagen and elastin synthesis. The entire wound area is flooded with macrophages and leukocytes to speed the process of connective-tissue regeneration.

Primary healing is a process lasting approximately 8–12 days. This is typically when sutures are removed. However, the complete healing continues for at least 3 weeks. PBMT is one of the methods utilized to facilitate the healing process. The effect on wound healing is one of the most researched areas of PBMT. Hopkins *et al.* (2004) examined the effects of healing on human sports medicine wounds and demonstrated an improvement and reduction in healing time. Abergel *et al.* (1984) demonstrated an increase in fibroblast proliferation, and Herascu *et al.* (2005) demonstrated an improvement in the stimulation of the healing of postoperative aseptic wounds and early scars.

Immediate postoperative application of laser therapy to the incision will facilitate the healing process. A grid pattern of application may be utilized to assist in the treatment of the wound. Treatment with the handpiece not in contact with the tissue is recommended. The dose for an open wound is $0.5–1.0 J/cm^2$, and $2–4 J/cm^2$ for the surrounding skin. Depending on the size of the wound, the surrounding skin should be treated 1–2 cm from the wound. For example, if the incision is 4 cm long, the length of the entire treated area might be 6–8 cm, and the width 2–4 cm.

Post-surgical wounds are inclusive of orthopedic, neurological, spay, neuter, dewclaw removals, and other surgical interventions that do not involve the removal of malignancies or potential malignant areas. Immediate laser treatment of the incision while the animal is still on the operating table or in recovery is advantageous. Immediate PBMT is recommended, in order to begin the reduction of pain and inflammation and the stimulation of the healing process as early as possible (Abdel-Alim *et al.*, 2015). Since primary healing lasts approximately 8–12 days, laser therapy should be applied daily to the incision and surrounding structures for at least 7–10 days. Realistically, many owners may not be able to bring their animal in for laser therapy on a daily basis, but the more frequent, the more beneficial. If the animal is staying as an inpatient, this gives the opportunity for daily treatment.

In addition to the incision in postoperative cases, PBMT will also be significantly beneficial if used to treat the surrounding area. For example, if a dog has undergone a tibial plateau-leveling osteotomy, the entire stifle should be circumferentially treated in order to diminish the postoperative pain and inflammation and initiate the healing process, as outlined in other chapters. Due to pain, a non-contact delivery may be required initially. Passive range of motion should be attempted either during or immediately after treatment. Once the animal's pain level is lower, a contact delivery should be used to give a massage effect, which increases circulation and blood flow to the area.

Following orthopedic surgeries, it is highly recommended that laser therapy be performed as part of the initial sequence of postoperative care in order to facilitate a more progressive multimodal treatment. The reduction of pain and inflammation will allow an increase in range of motion, and an additional increase in strength through functional activities. A full multimodal approach can include evaluation of range of motion and functional testing, laser therapy of the involved joint (as well as secondary and tertiary areas), passive range of motion, active range of motion, balance and proprioceptive exercises, core exercises, and endurance exercises.

Multimodal treatments will enhance the progression of functional motion. A progression is important in rehabilitation. PBMT will play a key role in the healing process and allow for increased passive range of motion. Active range of motion and function should be the last step.

Osteoarthritis Treatment and Maintenance

Osteoarthritis is characterized by a potential initial episode of acute pain and inflammation. There are different causes of osteoarthritis, and a variety of types. Osteoarthritis is a progressive disease of the synovial joint typified by synovitis, osteophyte formation, a progressive loss of cartilage, and remodeling of subchondral bone. In addition, instability, loss of range of motion, and pain all exist (Hunter, 2011). Regardless of the cause or type, one of the hallmarks is the presence of pain and

inflammation. Continued pain and inflammation cause muscle weakness, muscle spasm, a decrease in function, a decrease in ambulation, possible aggression, and possible patient depression. Additional complicating factors include weight gain, owner depression, and decreased quality of life.

A multimodal approach is established as the standard of care for cases of osteoarthritis. Three of the fundamental goals of the management of osteoarthritis are:

1) Reduction of pain and inflammation.
2) Restoration of range of motion and flexibility.
3) Restoration of strength and function.

There are many methods by which to achieve these goals. PBMT has been demonstrated to have an impact on each of them and to be an effective non-medical treatment for osteoarthritis and its ramifications.

A study on human knees demonstrated that laser therapy with an 830 nm diode laser was an effective method of reducing the pain related to osteoarthritis (Nakumara *et al.*, 2014). A visual analog scale (VIS) and range-of-motion tests were performed to determine the outcome. Four points were treated in the human knee at 20J/cm^2, twice a week for 4 weeks. Gao and Xing (2009) and Pallotta *et al.* (2012) demonstrated positive effects of the use of laser therapy on osteoarthritic joints in modulating inflammation and reducing pro-inflammatory mediators.

A randomized study demonstrated that human patients with low back pain responded better to laser therapy combined with exercise than to exercise alone (Djavid *et al.*, 2007). Gur *et al.* (2003) also concluded that the efficacy of the combination of laser therapy and exercise was greater than that of exercise alone in treatment of low back pain in humans. Jang and Lee (2012) conducted a meta-analysis of 22 trials of the pain relief effects of laser irradiation of joint areas. They concluded that investigations relating to laser therapy indicated that it could be an effective pain-relief treatment when appropriate dosages are selected.

The treatment of osteoarthritic joints with PBMT should include the entire joint. A contact method of treatment is preferred to increase the circulation and range of motion. However, if the joint is too painful, a non-contact method may be utilized. The preference is to laser the joint circumferentially, beginning and ending in the same area. The joint line, in addition to the area above and below the joint, should be treated in order to assist with the mechanical compensations, muscle spasms, inflammation, and additional areas of discomfort.

A key component of the successful treatment of osteoarthritis is the treatment of any compensatory areas that have soreness or pain. A thorough evaluation, including investigation of range of motion, palpation, and digital thermal imaging, will help determine where additional areas of pain and compensatory soreness are located. For

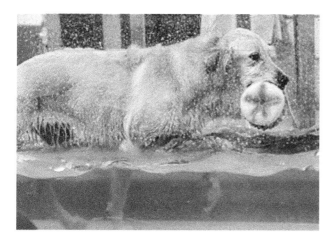

Figure 24.5 Walking in an underwater treadmill is beneficial in reducing the stress on joints while increasing the strength of the surrounding musculature.

example, a dog with osteoarthritis of the elbow will most likely experience compensatory pain and inflammation in the elbow, ipsilateral shoulder, and carpal region, and possibly in the contralateral shoulder and lower cervical and upper thoracic spine. Range-of-motion losses may also be seen in these areas, in addition to muscular losses in the scapular and humeral regions. To effectively treat the dog, PBMT should be applied to both of the shoulders, both elbows, and the upper thoracic and lower cervical regions.

The initial treatments of an osteoarthritic dog might consist of a longer treatment of PBMT and range of motion, and less therapeutic exercise consisting of balance, proprioception, and strengthening. As the pain and inflammation level decrease, the amount of PBMT can be decreased.

Additional treatments should include range of motion and stretching of the shoulders, elbows, and cervical and thoracic regions. After stretching and range of motion are performed, rhythmic stabilization and weight shifting should be imitated to begin the strengthening process in a weight-bearing position. Objective and functional testing should reveal an improvement in the compensatory areas. The practitioner may then reduce the amount of PBMT to the affected elbow and shoulder, and increase range-of-motion and strengthening exercises. An increase in therapeutic exercises may be added to include an increase in walking, cavaletti work, underwater treadmill (Figure 24.5), and core and balance activities.

Performance Issues and PBMT

Performance events continue to become popular worldwide and include many sports and many levels.

The American College of Veterinary Sports Medicine and Rehabilitation (ACVSMR) recognizes a variety of injuries in recreational and professional canine athletes and working dogs. Prevention through injury recognition, appropriate strengthening and stretching, training, and safety is utilized in human sports medicine, and the same approach may be applied in veterinary medicine for sporting and working dogs.

The first step in prevention is to appropriately condition and train the animal for the event or task. Appropriate strength training and warm-up and cool-down are important for successful performance. PBMT may be utilized for strength enhancement and the facilitation of stretching. Laser therapy can improve mitochondrial function, accelerating the healing process after exercise (Avni *et al.*, 2005). Studies suggest that laser therapy can also decrease oxidative stress and reactive oxygen species (ROS) production (Bjordal *et al.*, 2001). It has also been suggested that PBMT is effective in preventing the development of skeletal muscle fatigue, in enhanced recovery, and in providing overall enhanced performance (Ferraresi *et al.*, 2012; Leal Junior *et al.*, 2009a, 2009b, 2010; Ribeiro *et al.*, 2015). Given these studies, PBMT is a highly recommended component of the successful management of a performance dog.

Early recognition and appropriate treatment of soft-tissue injuries and other related performance issues are paramount. PBMT will assist with the rapid reduction of the pain and inflammation associated with performance injuries. In addition, there are benefits to improving muscular contractions with the addition of PBMT. Its application before exercise has been demonstrated to improve strength performance (de Marchi *et al.*, 2012; Santos, 2014).

Degenerative Myelopathy

Degenerative myelopathy is a condition that many rehabilitation and small-animal practitioners will see in the course of their career. Degenerative myelopathy was first described in 1973 as a specific disease of the spinal cord affecting dogs (Averil, 1973). The hallmarks are hind-limb weakness, exaggerated proprioceptive deficits, exaggerated spinal reflexes, and a decreased ability to walk. Degenerative myelopathy, with its movement deficits, is a difficult disease process for the owner to observe and to manage physically.

Kathmann *et al.* (2006) demonstrated that daily physiotherapy increases survival time in dogs with suspected degenerative myelopathy from approximately 130 to 255 days. In addition to the increase in mean survival time, dogs also remained mobile and ambulatory longer than those not receiving physiotherapy. Physiotherapy consisted of active exercises, passive exercises, massage, hydrotherapy, and paw protection. This study emphasizes how promising physical therapy is to the improvement of quality of life for dogs with degenerative myelopathy.

Laser therapy has been reported to improve many aspects of neurological healing in the literature. While degenerative myelopathy is a chronic condition, improvements in function, quality of life, and movement are possible. An examination of the literature on the improvement of peripheral nerve injuries and central nervous system (CNS) lesions shows that PBMT should be a part of the multimodal approach to managing dogs with degenerative myelopathy.

Laser therapy increases angiogenesis, blood circulation through vasodilation, release of cytokines, and fibroblast activity. A study on the effects of early and delayed laser application on nerve regeneration demonstrated an increase in neural activity (Akgul *et al.*, 2014). Another study examined the effect of laser therapy on injured peripheral nerves and demonstrated an increase in neurological activity and angiogenesis (Anders *et al.*, 2013).

Rochkind *et al.* (1990) examined the spinal cord response after laser treatments to crush injuries of the sciatic nerve in rats. Laser treatment was found to allay degenerative changes in the corresponding neurons of the spinal cord and to induce proliferation of neuroglia. The study's summary proposes higher metabolism in the neurons and an improved myelin production with PBMT. A follow-up study by Rochkind and Quaknine (1992) examined further potential of laser therapy treatment of the central nervous system as well as peripheral nerves. Laser irradiation was demonstrated to maintain the electrophysiological activity of severely injured peripheral nerves in rats and to prevent scar formation and degenerative changes in the corresponding motor neurons. This corresponded to an induction of axonal sprouting in the injured area and restoration of locomotor function. The study also concluded that laser irradiation might improve neuronal metabolism, prevent neuronal degeneration, and promote improved spinal cord function.

Awano *et al.* (2009) described a superoxidase dismutase-1 (SOD1) gene mutation in dogs with degenerative myelopathy (which resembles amyotrophic lateral sclerosis, ALS). Originally described in German shepherds, the disease is now known to occur in many other dog breeds. A recent study of dogs in a referral population of German shepherds from the United Kingdom suggests that genotyping for the SOD1 mutation is clinically applicable (Holder *et al.*, 2014). The study demonstrates that the mutation has a high degree of penetrance in the population considered.

SOD is responsible for repairing oxidative changes in cells. Cells that are particularly vulnerable to oxidative damage include those high in lipids, such as myelin. Myelin-rich white matter in the nervous system would be expected to be one of the most sensitive tissues in the body to oxidative damage, the exact pathology seen in dogs with degenerative myelopathy. The spinal cords of dogs with degenerative myelopathy have been demonstrated to contain mutant SOD1, which increases with disease severity (Crisp *et al.*, 2013).

As demonstrated in other chapters, laser therapy has been successful in increasing the blood supply, axonal growth, and potential nerve regeneration, and in decreasing pain and inflammation. The photonic energy of laser light stimulates the photoreceptors in mitochondria to decrease the reaction time for cytochrome c to become cytochrome c oxidase (CCO). This facilitates an increase in the cellular respiration rate and increases the blood flow to the region. With these effects, it may be deduced that the application of laser therapy directly to the thoracic and lumbar spine of dogs with degenerative myelopathy will increase blood flow and circulation to this region, improving oxygenation of the tissue.

The significant effect of PBM on spinal tissue has been clearly demonstrated. A study examined two groups of dogs that had undergone surgery for a herniated disk, with modified Frankel scores of 0–3 (Draper *et al.*, 2002). One of the groups received laser therapy for five consecutive days, or until the dogs had a Frankel score of 4. The other group did not receive laser therapy. The results indicated that the dogs that received laser therapy achieved ambulation in a significantly shorter time than those that did not.

The anatomical location of degenerative myelopathy is between the third thoracic and the third lumbar segments, and between the third lumbar and the third sacral segments. Increased circulation and stimulation of the appropriate neural pathways in these areas is beneficial for degenerative myelopathy patients' overall circulation, function, and ambulatory status. Dogs with advanced degenerative myelopathy have degenerative changes noted in the lumbar dorsal roots (Griffiths and Duncan, 1975). Some of the known effects of PBM are a decrease in inflammation and a reduction in degenerative changes. Thus, an interesting hypothesis involves using laser therapy to decrease the rate of progression of degenerative myelopathy and delay the neurological impact on quality of life.

Based on reports that affected dogs that receive physiotherapy remain ambulatory longer those that do not (Kathmann *et al.*, 2006), the author is currently involved in a review of the impact of PBMT and physiotherapy on patients with degenerative myelopathy. At the beginning of this study, all of the patients had symptoms of degenerative myelopathy and tested positive for the SOD1 mutation. Each dog was individually evaluated neurologically for loss of function, and each was assigned a modified Frankel score. A specific program of physical therapy was established for each. Therapy included balance and proprioceptive exercises, range of motion and stretching, proprioceptive neuromuscular facilitation, therapeutic exercise, core strengthening, controlled walking, activities in an underwater treadmill, owner education, and a home exercise program. In addition to the specified physical therapy program, all of the dogs received laser therapy to the anatomical location of degenerative myelopathy, from the second thoracic segment through the sacral segments.

The laser therapy dose was increased from the normally recommended dose of 8–12 J/cm^2 to a higher dose of 25–45 J/cm^2. All of the treatments were administered with the laser handpiece in contact with the skin. Treatments were administered one to two times a week, along with the specific exercise program and a home exercise program. At each laser and physiotherapy session, laser therapy was administered before other modalities.

Progress was based on clinical objective data, including the modified Frankel score, function, sit–stand, stand–down, standing, owner's perception, skin integrity, and ambulation. Preliminary results indicate that the dogs receiving PBMT along with physiotherapy remain ambulatory for a longer time compared to those in the study performed by Kathmann *et al.* (2006). Most continue a high quality of life and functional ambulation to at least 18 months past the initial treatment. These preliminary results are very promising for the future use of PBMT for dogs with degenerative myelopathy.

Maintenance When the Pain is Gone

Practitioners want to help patients maintain the highest possible quality of life. For sporting and working dogs, this means maintaining strength, coordination, acceptable range of motion, and privation of pain. Laser therapy and PBMT can help accomplish this. PBMT is an integral component of the multimodal approach to many common conditions seen in small-animal companion practice and should be a component of performance maintenance. The many benefits of PBMT include pain relief, diminished inflammation, provision of an alternative treatment to pharmaceutical interventions and surgery, facilitated healing, and an overall improvement in the quality of life.

Once a patient has met the short- and long-term goals of multimodal therapy, it is part of the practitioner's responsibility to maintain this status. A scheduled monthly maintenance appointment allows the practitioner to reassess the patient to determine whether long-term goals are being maintained. The reassessment should include digital thermal imaging and other objective tests, which should be compared to the previous visit. During this visit, a review of home instructions may be processed, and a maintenance PBMT treatment should be provided.

References

Abdel-Alim, H.M. *et al.* (2015) A comparative study of the effectiveness of immediate versus delayed photobiomodulation therapy in reducing the severity of postoperative inflammatory complications. *Photomed Laser Surg.* **33**(9):447–451.

Abergel, R.P. *et al.* (1984) Control of connective tissue metabolism by lasers: recent developments and future prospects. *J Am Acad Dermatol.* **11**(6):1142–1150.

Akgul, T. *et al.* (2014) Effects of early and delayed laser application on nerve regeneration. *Lasers Med Sci.* **29**(1):351–357.

Alves, A.C. *et al.* (2013) Effect of low level laser therapy on the expression of inflammatory mediators and on neutrophils and macrophages in acute joint inflammation. *Arthritis Res Ther.* **15**(5):R116.

Anders, J.J. *et al.* (2013) In vitro and in vivo optimization of infrared laser treatment for injured peripheral nerves. *Lasers Surg Med.* **46**(1):34–45.

Averill, D.R. Jr. (1973) Degenerative myelopathy in the aging German shepherd dog: clinical and pathological findings. *J Am Vet Med Assoc.* **162**(12):1045–1051.

Avni, D. *et al.* (2005) Protection of skeletal muscles from ischemic injury: low-level laser therapy increases antioxidant activity. *Photomed Laser Surg.* **23**(3):273–277.

Awano, T. *et al.* (2009) Genome-wide association analysis reveals a SOD1 mutation in canine degenerative myelopathy that resembles amyotrophic lateral sclerosis. *Proc Natl Acad Sci USA.* **106**(8):2794–2799.

Baltzer, A.W. *et al.* (2016) Positive effects of low level laser therapy (LLLT) on Bouchard's and Heberden's osteoarthritis. *Lasers Surg Med.* **48**(5):498–504.

Barushka, O. *et al.* (1995) Effect of low-energy laser (He-Ne) irradiation on the process of bone repair in the rate tibia. *Bone.* **16**(1):47–55.

Bjordal, J.M. *et al.* (2001) Low level laser therapy for tendinopathy: evidence of a dose-response pattern. *Phys Ther Rev.* **6**:91–99.

Cheng, D.S. and Visco, C.J. (2012) Pharmaceutical therapy for osteoarthritis. *PM R.* **4**(5 Suppl.):S82–S88.

Chung, H. *et al.* (2012) The nuts and bolts of low level laser (light) therapy. *Ann Biomed Eng.* **40**(2):516–533.

Crisp, M.J. *et al.* (2013) Canine degenerative myelopathy: biochemical characterization of superoxide dismutase 1 in the first naturally occurring non-human amyotrophic lateral sclerosis model. *Exp Neurol.* **248**:1–9.

da Rosa, A.S. *et al.* (2012) Effects of low-level laser therapy at wavelengths of 660 and 808 nm in experimental model of osteoarthritis. *Photochem Photobiol.* **88**(1):161–166.

de Marchi, T. *et al.* (2012) Low-level laser therapy (LLLT) in human progressive-intensity running: effects on exercise performance, skeletal muscle status, and oxidative stress. *Lasers Med Sci.* **27**(1):231–236.

Djavid, G.E. *et al.* (2007) In chronic low back pain, low level laser therapy combined with exercise is more beneficial than exercise alone in the long term: a randomized trial. *Aust J Physiother.* **53**(3):155–160.

Draper, W.E. *et al.* (2012) Low-level laser therapy reduces time to ambulation in dogs after hemilamectomy: a preliminary study. *J Small Anim Pract.* **53**(8):465–469.

Ferraresi, C. *et al.* (2012) Low-level laser (light) therapy (LLLT) on muscle tissue: performance, fatigue and repair benefited by the power of light. *Photonics Lasers Med.* **1**(4):267–286.

Fox, S.M. (2014) Multimodal management of canine osteoarthritis. In: *Pain Management in Small Animal Medicine*, pp. 223–242. CRC Press, Boca Raton, FL.

Gao, X. and Xing, D. (2009) Molecular mechanisms of cell proliferation induced by low power laser irradiation. *J Biomed Sci.* **16**:4.

Griffiths, I.R. and Duncan, I.D. (1975) Chronic degenerative radiculopathy in the dog. *J Small Anim Pract.* **16**:461–471.

Gur, A. *et al.* (2003) Efficacy of low power laser therapy and exercise on pain and functions in chronic low back pain. *Lasers Surg. Med.* **32**(3):233–238.

Hegedus, B. *et al.* (2009) The effect of low-level laser in knee osteoarthritis: a double blind, randomized, placebo-controlled trial. *Photomed Laser Surg.* **27**(4):577–584.

Herascu, N. *et al.* (2005) Low-level laser therapy (LLLT) efficacy in post-operative wounds. *Photomed Laser Surg.* **23**(1):70–73.

Holder, A.L. *et al.* (2014) A retrospective study of the prevalence of the canine degenerative myelopathy associated superoxide dismutase 1 mutation (SOD1:c.118G > A) in a referral population of German shepherd dogs from the UK. *Canine Genet Epidemiol.* **1**:10.

Hopkins, J.T. *et al.* (2004) Low-level laser therapy facilitates superficial wound healing in humans: a triple-blind, sham controlled study. *J Ath Training.* **39**(3):223–229.

Hunter, D.J. (2011) Osteoarthritis. *Best Pract Res Clin Rheumatol.* **25**(6):801–814.

Innes, J. (2009) Getting the elbow: diagnosis and management of elbow disease in dogs. *J Small Anim Pract.* **50**(6):18–20.

Jang, H. and Lee, H. (2012) Meta-analysis of pain relief effects by laser irradiation on joint areas. *Photomed Laser Surg.* **30**(8):405–417.

Kathmann, I. *et al.* (2006) Daily controlled physiotherapy increases survival time in dogs with suspected degenerative myelopathy. *J Vet Intern Med.* **20**(4):927–932.

Leal Junior, E.C. *et al.* (2009a) Effect of 830 nm low level laser therapy in exercise induced skeletal muscle fatigue in humans. *Lasers Med Sci.* **24**(3):425–431.

Leal Junior, E.C. *et al.* (2009b) Effect of cluster multi-diode light emitting diode therapy (LEDT) on exercise-induced skeletal muscle fatigue and skeletal muscle recovery in humans. *Lasers Surg. Med.* **41**(8):572–527.

Leal Junior, E.C. *et al.* (2010) Effect of low-level laser therapy (GaAs 904 nm) in skeletal muscle fatigue and biochemical markers of muscle damage in rats. *Eur J Appl Physiol.* **108**(6):1083–1088.

Maier, A. *et al.* (2000) Effect of photodynamic therapy in a multimodal approach for advanced carcinoma of the gastro-esophageal junction. *Lasers Surg Med.* **26**(5):461–466.

Michelson, J. (2013) Canine elbow dysplasia: aeitopathogenesis and current treatment recommendations. *Vet J.* **196**(1):12–19.

Mokmeli, S. *et al.* (2006) Low level laser therapy (LLLT) for knee osteoarthritis: (a clinical study on 386 patients). *Proceedings of the 6th International Congress of the World Association of Laser Therapy.* October 25–28, 2006. Limassol.

Nagasawa, A. *et al.* (1991) Bone regeneration effect on low level lasers including argon laser. *Laser Ther.* **3**:59–62.

Nakumara, T. *et al.* (2014) Low level laser therapy for chronic knee joint pain patients. *Laser Ther.* **23**(4):273–277.

Pallotta, R.C. *et al.* (2012) Infrared (810-nm) low-level laser therapy on rat experimental knee inflammation. *Lasers Med Sci.* **27**(1):71–78.

Ribeiro, B.G. *et al.* (2015) The effect of low-level laser therapy (LLLT) applied prior to muscle injury. *Lasers Surg Med.* doi:10.1002/lsm.22381.

Rochkind, S. and Quaknine, G.E. (1992) New trend in neuroscience: low-power laser effect on peripheral and central nervous system (basic science, preclinical and clinical studies). *Neurol Res.* **14**(1):2–11.

Rochkind, S. *et al.* (1990) Spinal cord response to laser treatment of the injured peripheral nerve. *Spine.* **5**(1):6–10.

Santos, L.A. (2014) Effects of pre-irradiation of low-level laser therapy with different doses and wavelengths in skeletal muscle performance, fatigue, and skeletal muscle damage induced by tetanic contractions in rats. *Lasers Med Sci.* **29**(5):1617–1626.

25

Laser Therapy and Geriatric Rehabilitation

Dianne Adjan Logan

Wilmington Animal Fitness & Rehabilitation Center at Needham Animal Hospital, Wilmington, NC, USA

Introduction

Rehabilitation in the geriatric patient is challenging because often there are multiple diagnoses and medical issues to be addressed. The increased likelihood of multiple conditions being present in a geriatric patient warrants a thorough medical evaluation before a rehabilitation program is designed (Taylor *et al.*, 2004).

Many older patients come to the rehabilitation center with a suspected diagnosis of osteoarthritis but no diagnostics such as radiographs to confirm this. In some cases, owners decline radiographs because of the expense. A mindset still exists that, when dogs and cats grow old, "old age" is a medical condition rather than a stage of life during which some common medical conditions may occur. It is our job in the rehabilitation center to determine whether the diagnosis that accompanies a particular patient is the entirety of the patient's issues. There may be additional problems that the referring veterinarian needs to evaluate before a rehabilitation plan can be developed.

Even when a complete medical evaluation has determined a definitive diagnosis, changes can occur over time during treatment, so it is important to reassess the patient regularly to ensure treatment protocols remain appropriate and effective. In the vast majority of geriatric patients being treated at our rehabilitation center, a multimodal approach to their rehabilitation, which includes laser therapy, has shown to give the most promising long-term results (Millis and Ciuperca, 2015; Pryor and Millis, 2015; Saunders and Millis, 2014).

Geriatric Rehabilitation

The most common problem of the musculoskeletal system in aged dogs is osteoarthritis. Dogs may have difficulty rising, and obesity compounds the effects of arthritis (Taylor *et al.*, 2004). Our focus is first on treating pain and then, when the pain is controlled,

introducing low-impact exercise to strengthen and build muscle mass in order to help support joints.

We are reluctant to exercise patients if they are in pain. Unless contraindicated by compromised organs, or the patient is prone to gastrointestinal upset, we normally recommend the owner give non-steroidal anti-inflammatory drugs (NSAIDs) or other pain medications prescribed by their veterinarian. We are always amazed by the number of owners who do not give these medications because they are concerned they may do more harm than good. These owners seem much more likely to want to treat their pet's pain with laser therapy. In some cases, we find that owners simply prefer an alternative to pain medications. Many times, owners give medications as prescribed and the result is just not good enough to make the patient comfortable. We have found laser therapy to negate the need for NSAIDs and pain medications in some patients, and to reduce the amount of medications needed in others.

Several modalities, rather than one, are required in geriatric rehabilitation to produce a notable result and an improvement in the patient's comfort and mobility. Each rehabilitation plan is tailored to the patient, their individual needs, their abilities, and the anticipated owner compliance. Owners must participate in the overall plan for rehabilitation to have success. Changing the patient's home environment to include padded bedding, warmth, and carpet runners is relatively simple and can make a big difference in the patient's comfort.

Weight loss is one of the most important factors in successful osteoarthritis management, and we offer nutritional counseling toward that end. In a 2000 study, weight loss improved clinical signs of lameness among overweight dogs with clinical and radiographic signs of hip osteoarthritis (Impellizeri *et al.*, 2000). Mlacnik *et al.* (2006) demonstrated that caloric restriction combined with intensive physical therapy improved mobility and facilitated weight loss in overweight dogs with osteoarthritis. It is essential that owners participate in the weight-loss objectives. Marshal *et al.* (2010) confirmed

Laser Therapy in Veterinary Medicine: Photobiomodulation, First Edition. Edited by Ronald J. Riegel and John C. Godbold, Jr.

that weight loss should be presented as an important treatment modality to owners of obese dogs with osteoarthritis. In their study, noticeable improvement was seen after modest weight loss of as low as 6.10–8.85% of body weight.

Common modalities used for managing osteoarthritis are low-impact exercise in the underwater treadmill, warming the joints, passive range of motion, controlled short leash walks, massage, therapeutic ultrasound, transcutaneous electrical nerve stimulation, Cavaletti rails, swimming, and laser therapy. We are always careful to advise owners that managing osteoarthritis is an ongoing process and that the management plan will change as the patient's needs change. For example, in a case where laser therapy is recommended, after the initial induction phase, we begin a pain-management maintenance schedule with the patient returning weekly, biweekly, or monthly, depending on need. Our goal is to treat the patient no more than is needed for its comfort. Most of our geriatric patients return monthly for laser therapy.

The Geriatric Rehabilitation Visit

Older patients coming in for their initial evaluation appointment are led to an area where the tile flooring is covered with rubber fatigue mats. This enables us to evaluate them as they rise, or attempt to rise, from a recumbent position without the problem of negotiating slick floors. The rehabilitation room flooring is rubber-padded, and a comfortable orthopedic bed is available. During our examination, we take care to check paws to assess worn nails, particularly in the hind feet. Nail wear can be an excellent indicator of limb dragging and of the severity of impairment in daily life. Overgrown nails are trimmed to prevent them from impeding ambulation. We always trim the fur from paw pads to create more traction and less sliding on floors.

Giving owners a home exercise program is part of our initial evaluation appointment. Assessing owner expectations of rehabilitation, and getting them involved in the program, is crucial to success. After our initial evaluation, we meet with the client, share our findings, and learn their expectations and their willingness to engage in the rehabilitation plan. At this point, it is important to advise the client if we feel their expectations for the patient are reasonable. There are occasional instances when degenerative joint disease or other medical conditions are so advanced that our focus is merely on palliative care, or keeping the patient comfortable, for the remainder of its life. Most owners are relieved that at least something can be done to help them help their geriatric pet.

Case Studies

The following case studies are examples where laser therapy has played an active role in our rehabilitation plan for geriatric patients.

Rottweiler with Multiple-Joint Osteoarthritis

Signalment
"Toby," 12 years old, Rottweiler, NM, 40.9 kg.

Client Complaint
Toby was presented to the rehabilitation center with a diagnosis of multiple-joint osteoarthritis, spondylosis, and bilateral hind-limb conscious proprioception deficits, having been examined by his regular veterinarian a few days earlier.

Current Medications
The veterinarian had prescribed gabapentin for pain. This patient had a history of gastric upset due to prior use of NSAIDs.

Physical Examination
Our initial examination showed Toby to be grade 2/4 lame at a stance and a walk, with widely placed fore and hind limbs and a stiff gait, more in the right hind limb than in the left. Conscious proprioception appeared absent bilaterally in the hind limbs, but it was unclear if this was due to muscle atrophy and general weakness or a neurologic condition. He was unable to stand from a recumbent position on slick flooring, and needed minimal assistance to do so on a non-skid surface. He exhibited discomfort upon palpation of the spine at T13–L1, which was consistent with radiographs confirming spondylosis from T13 to L5. Toby was grade 2/5 painful and exhibited decreased range of motion upon flexion and extension of the elbows bilaterally. Crepitus was noted in the left elbow. He was grade 3/5 painful upon manipulation of the left tarsus, which was thickened medially and stiff with limited flexion. He was grade 4/5 painful upon external rotation of the hips bilaterally. Medial buttress was noted in the right stifle, with a mild, "spongy" anterior drawer sign present. Hind-limb circumference measurements showed a 6 cm deficit in the right hind limb weight-bearing muscles in comparison to the left. Withdrawal reflexes and deep pain were normal in all limbs.

Laboratory Data
Testing for degenerative myelopathy, a condition that is not uncommon in this breed, had not been performed prior to Toby's referral to the rehabilitation center.

Treatment Plan
The owner's expectations of rehabilitation were for the patient to have an improved quality of life and,

specifically, to retain the ability to navigate the stairs at home. Our goals for Toby were to control pain and inflammation, strengthen and build his right hind-limb muscle mass, and increase his mobility.

We recommended to the referring veterinarian that Toby be prescribed oral and injectable chondroprotective agents (Gallagher *et al.*, 2015; Ip and Fu, 2015; Verbruggen, 2006), and we began laser therapy treatments to help relieve his pain. A double-blind, randomized, placebo-controlled trial (Hegedűs *et al.*, 2009) and a descriptive, prospective study (Soleimanpour *et al.*, 2014) both demonstrated that laser therapy reduces pain and is an effective treatment for human patients suffering from painful osteoarthritis. A recent prospective, randomized, cohort study further demonstrated that chondroprotective injections, together with laser therapy, should be incorporated into the standard conservative (non-surgical) treatment protocol for symptomatic arthritis in human patients (Ip, 2015). Doses for Toby's treatment ranged from 10 to 14J/cm^2, depending on the joint being treated (Box 25.1).

Once Toby's pain was under control, we began underwater treadmill sessions, which helped to strengthen and build muscle mass. Several weeks after therapy was initiated, it was discovered that Toby had started to experience pain in his left shoulder. After consulting with the referring veterinarian, we revised his laser treatment to include delivery of 12J/cm^2 to the joint, which seemed to provide additional relief and continued mobility.

Outcome

After several months, the referring veterinarian diagnosed Toby with degenerative myelopathy. The frequency of Toby's maintenance laser treatments increased from monthly to weekly. He was given additional pain medication in the low-to-medium dose range for his advancing osteoarthritis. Toby also continued with weekly underwater treadmill sessions. At age 14, he is still able to ascend and descend the stairs at home.

Box 25.1 Laser therapy protocol for Toby, a 12-year-old Rottweiler with multiple-joint osteoarthritis.

14J/cm^2 to each of the dorsal aspects of the coxofemoral joints
12J/cm^2 to each of the elbows
11J/cm^2 to the left tarsus
11J/cm^2 to the right stifle
10J/cm^2 to each to three sections of the spine from T13 to L5

Terrier Mix with Degenerative Joint Disease of the Tarsus

Signalment

"Ira," 14 years old, terrier mix, NM, 14.5 kg.

Client Complaint

Ira was presented to the rehabilitation center with obvious lameness in the left hind limb. The referring veterinarian advised he had palpated mild crepitus in the left tarsus.

Current Medications

Ira had been prescribed carprofen and gabapentin for inflammation and pain. He had also been prescribed oral and injectable chondroprotective agents. Ira had a history of elevated liver enzymes and was taking an S-Adenosylmethionine with silybin–phosphatidylcholine complex.

Physical Examination

Upon initial evaluation, Ira was grade 2/4 lame in the left hind limb at a walk. Left hind-limb weight-bearing muscles were atrophied. Hind-limb girth measurements were 20 cm on the left and 22 cm on the right, taken at 70% of the distance from the greater trochanter to the patella. There was no pain on palpation of the spine or any joints with the exception of the left tarsus, which was thickened medially and laterally. Range-of-motion movement of the left tarsus elicited moderate crepitus.

Diagnostic Imaging

Radiographs of the left hock showed advanced degenerative joint disease and swelling in the soft tissues around the joint (Figure 25.1).

Treatment Plan

Our goal was to reduce pain and inflammation and eliminate or at least reduce his dependence on medications, especially NSAIDs. Laser therapy has been demonstrated to reduce pain and inflammation, decrease stiffness, and increase range of motion and walking duration in humans with osteoarthritis, offering a safe and side effect-free alternative to heavy reliance on NSAIDs (Mokmeli *et al.*, 2006). Ira was the perfect candidate for laser therapy treatments (see Box 25.2).

Ira was given an induction phase series of six laser treatments to the left tarsus over a 3-week period. His owner reported an increase in his activity level after the fourth treatment. Immediately following Ira's fifth laser treatment, we started exercising him in the underwater treadmill twice weekly in order to strengthen and build the left hind-limb muscle mass. His owner was instructed to gradually increase the length of his walks and his activity levels at home.

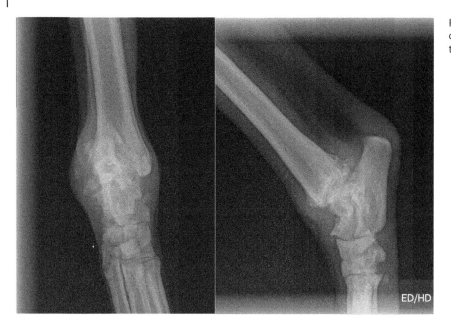

Figure 25.1 Radiographs of advanced degenerative joint disease in a 14-year-old terrier mix.

Box 25.2 Laser therapy protocol for Ira, a 14-year-old terrier mix with degenerative joint disease of the tarsus.

6 J/cm^2 to the left tarsus

Box 25.3 Laser therapy protocol for Sashka, a 13-year-old husky mix with multiple-joint osteoarthritis.

10 J/cm^2 to dorsal surface of hips bilaterally
10 J/cm^2 to shoulders bilaterally

Outcome

Now aged 15, Ira comes to the rehabilitation center for weekly laser therapy treatments to the left tarsus. He no longer takes gabapentin and his carprofen has been reduced to one dose every other day. He remains very active. The referring veterinarian regularly monitors his liver enzymes and is comfortable with this regimen.

Husky Mix with Multiple-Joint Osteoarthritis

Signalment

"Sashka," 13 years old, husky mix, FS, 29.5 kg.

Client Complaint

Sashka was initially presented to the rehabilitation center at 13 years of age, with grade 2/4 lameness in the left fore limb and both hind limbs at a walk. Sashka was not on any NSAID or pain medication and her owners were interested in alternative treatments for her pain.

Physical Examination

The patient appeared slightly more lame in the right hind limb than the left, but this could have been due to compensation from pain in the left fore limb. Her gait was rigid and extension was limited in both hips. A head bob was noted repeatedly down on the right fore limb at a walk. Hind-limb girth was measured at 26 cm bilaterally, taken at 70% distance from the greater trochanter to the patella. Fore-limb girth was measured at 21.5 cm on the left and 20.5 cm on the right, taken at one finger's width above the elbows. There was no pain found on palpation of the spine. The patient was grade 3/5 pain on extension of the hips bilaterally. She did not give a pain response on palpation of the shoulders, but there was limited shoulder extension, with less extension of the left than the right.

Treatment Plan

The owners' expectations of rehabilitation were for the patient to have continued mobility and a better quality of life for as long as possible. Our goals were to control her pain and inflammation, strengthen her overall muscle mass, and give her increased flexibility. Our plan was to administer laser therapy treatments to her hips and shoulders twice weekly for 3 weeks (Box 25.3, Figure 25.2), to exercise her over the Cavaletti rails, and eventually to place her in the underwater treadmill when her pain was better controlled. We also recommended the referring veterinarian prescribe injectable and oral chondroprotective agents.

Outcome

Sashka's rehabilitation started right away and her owners reported seeing increased activity after just the third laser treatment. We then began working her in the underwater treadmill for strengthening. The owners gradually increased the length of her walks at

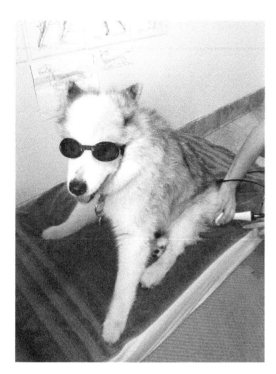

Figure 25.2 Laser therapy treatment of Sashka, a geriatric 15-year-old canine with multiple-joint osteoarthritis.

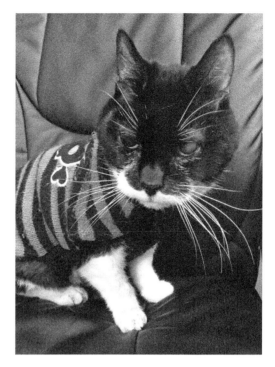

Figure 25.4 Kit10, a 13-year-old feline with multiple-joint osteoarthritis.

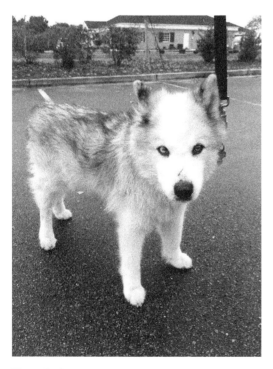

Figure 25.3 Sashka, a 15-year-old canine with multiple-joint osteoarthritis, mobile and weight bearing after rehabilitation, which included laser therapy.

home. At age 14, she required no pain medication and her owners saw her more mobile and comfortable than she had been in years (Figure 25.3). As her osteoarthritis progressed, the referring veterinarian prescribed

tramadol for her increasing pain. Now, at age 15, Sashka continues to visit the rehabilitation center monthly for a laser treatment and her injection.

Feline (13 Years Old) with Multiple-Joint Osteoarthritis

Signalment
"Kit10," 13 years old, domestic shorthair, MN.

Client Complaint
Kit10 was presented to the rehabilitation center with a diagnosis of spondylosis of the thoracolumbar spine and advanced osteoarthritis of the bilateral hips, stifles, shoulders and elbows. The owners had noted he was no longer able to jump up on chairs and he seemed unhappy and restless (Figure 25.4).

Current Medications
The referring veterinarian had started the patient on an oral chondroprotectant.

Physical Examination
Kit10 was extremely reluctant to be manipulated and was gauged at grade 3/5 pain upon palpation of the spine in multiple areas and grade 5/5 upon range of motion of the hips and stifles. Crepitus was apparent in both stifles.

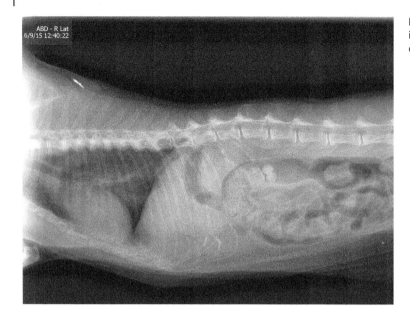

Figure 25.5 Spondylosis of the thoracolumbar spine in a 13-year-old feline with multiple-joint osteoarthritis.

> **Box 25.4 Laser therapy protocol for Kit10, a 13-year-old feline with multiple-joint osteoarthritis.**
>
> $6 \, J/cm^2$ to thoracic spine
> $6 \, J/cm^2$ to lumbar spine
> $6 \, J/cm^2$ to coxofemoral joints bilaterally
> $12 \, J/cm^2$ to stifles bilaterally
> $12 \, J/cm^2$ to shoulders bilaterally
> $12 \, J/cm^2$ to elbows bilaterally

Diagnostic Imaging

Radiographs showed spondylosis of the thoracolumbar spine and advanced osteoarthritis of the bilateral hips, stifles, shoulders, and elbows (Figure 25.5).

Treatment Plan

We immediately started a laser therapy regimen to treat all of the affected areas, three times weekly for 2 weeks, followed by laser maintenance every 2 weeks (Box 25.4). We recommended Kit10 be prescribed an injectable chondroprotective agent with an appropriate feline dosing schedule, which we administered during his rehabilitation treatments. We were successful in getting the patient to follow a laser pointer over the bottom rungs of a chair and other obstacles, creating "kitty Cavaletti rails" exercises to help strengthen his muscles. We advised the owners to provide a warm rice sock in Kit10's bed, which he snuggled at his discretion.

Outcome

Within 2 months, it was obvious Kit10 was more comfortable and the owners occasionally found him lounging on furniture again. As time passed, the patient was prescribed buprenorphine for his advancing osteoarthritis and he required more frequent laser therapy treatments to maintain his comfort. At age 16, he visits the rehabilitation center weekly for his treatment.

Feline (21 Years Old) with Multiple-Joint Osteoarthritis

Signalment

"Chloe," 21 years old, domestic shorthair, FS.

Client Complaint

Chloe was presented to the rehabilitation center with a complaint of increasing lameness, reduced activity, and inability to jump on and off furniture.

Current Medications

Chloe was on buprenorphine for pain and an antibiotic for recurring urinary tract infections. The owner was administering subcutaneous fluids daily, as directed by the referring veterinarian. Chloe had been put on an injectable chondroprotectant 2 years earlier, but the owner did not see any difference in her mobility, so the injections had been discontinued.

Physical Examination

A physical examination showed Chloe to be grade 2/4 lame bilaterally in the hind limbs, with the right more affected than the left. All of her joints were manipulated and pain responses were elicited upon extension of the shoulders and hips on both sides. No pain responses were elicited on palpation of the spine or with range-of-motion movements of any other joints.

Box 25.5 Laser therapy protocol for Chloe, a 21-year-old feline with multiple-joint osteoarthritis.

9 J/cm^2 to shoulders bilaterally
4 J/cm^2 to hips bilaterally

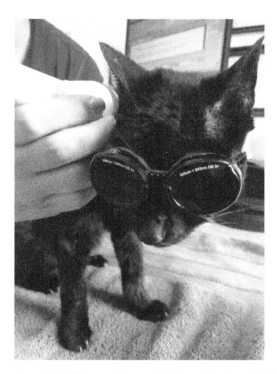

Figure 25.6 Chloe, a 21-year-old feline with osteoarthritis of the hips and shoulders, being treated with the therapy laser.

Treatment Plan

The owner's expectations for rehabilitation were for Chloe to have decreased pain and to be able to maintain, or possibly increase, her mobility. We started laser therapy treatments to Chloe's shoulders and hips immediately (Box 25.5, Figure 25.6).

Outcome

After the third treatment, the owner advised that Chloe had jumped on the bed, which was something she had not done in months. Chloe continued with her induction phase of six laser treatments over a 3-week period, and then treatment frequency was gradually decreased. The long-term goal will be to administer treatments as frequently as required to maintain her increased mobility.

Guinea Pig with Multiple-Joint Osteoarthritis

Signalment

"Cinderella," 6 years old, guinea pig, FS, 864 g.

Client Complaint

Cinderella was presented to the rehabilitation center having been non-ambulatory for several months. She was experiencing fecal incontinence.

Current Medications

Cinderella had been prescribed meloxicam, but the owner had not been giving it because she felt Cinderella was not in pain. During the examination, the owner could appreciate that the patient was experiencing pain, so she agreed to administer the NSAID as prescribed.

Physical Examination

During Cinderella's initial evaluation, it was noted that both stifles were experiencing grade 3/5 pain on flexion and extension and the right front limb was experiencing grade 2/5 pain on palpation. Goniometry of both stifles was performed with the following results: right flexion/extension 50/132°, left 54/138°; both with empty end feels secondary to pain. Goniometry of the front limbs was not performed due to their small size and the difficulty in obtaining an accurate reading.

Diagnostic Imaging

Radiographs confirmed severe degenerative joint disease of the stifles and shoulders (Figure 25.7).

Treatment Plan

Our goals were to reduce Cinderella's pain and to strengthen her muscles to afford mobility. We began therapeutic exercises of passive range of motion to all four limbs several times daily. We also performed assisted stands, which we accomplished by placing rolled paper towels lengthwise under her abdomen. This allowed her to stand with less body weight carried by her joints. We initiated a laser therapy regimen of three treatments the first week, two treatments the second week, and one treatment the third week (Box 25.6). Treatment was administered to Cinderella's stifles and shoulders bilaterally. We instructed the owner to apply heat therapy to the affected joints twice daily for a period of 10 minutes at a time, using rice socks warmed in the microwave oven.

Outcome

With a compliant owner and this multimodal approach, Cinderella was able to stand and take three unassisted steps after her second laser treatment. We then showed the owner how to perform weight-shifting exercises by gently tapping the patient's side to effect muscle contractions in order to correct her stance. Cinderella's mobility had returned but, unfortunately, she died of an acute abdominal crisis before further treatment and was lost to case monitoring.

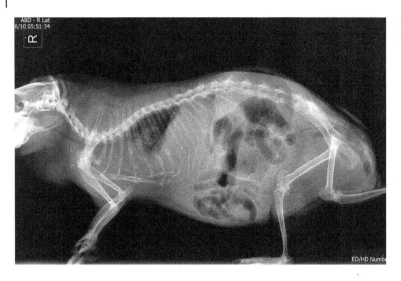

Figure 25.7 Degenerative joint disease affecting the stifles and shoulders of a 6-year-old guinea pig.

Box 25.6 Laser therapy protocol for Cinderella, a 6-year-old guinea pig with multiple-joint osteoarthritis.

20 J/cm² to shoulders bilaterally
14 J/cm² to stifles bilaterally

Conclusion

With devoted owners and attentive veterinary care, many pets live long lives; however, with advancing age comes a myriad of geriatric health problems. Practitioners should help owners avoid the mindset that "old age" is a medical condition rather than a stage of life during which some common medical conditions may occur.

It is possible for many geriatric patients to maintain active and mobile lifestyles. Physical rehabilitation, with its multiple modalities, can help geriatric patients maintain mobility and function. As the cases in this chapter demonstrate, laser therapy can play an important role as part of comprehensive physical therapy management plans.

References

Gallagher, B. *et al.* (2015) Chondroprotection and the prevention of osteoarthritis progression of the knee: a systematic review of treatment agents. *Am J Sports Med.* **43**(3):734–744.

Hegedűs, B. *et al.* (2009) The effect of low-level laser in knee osteoarthritis: a double-blind, randomized, placebo-controlled trial. *Photomed Laser Surg.* **27**(4):577–584.

Impellizeri, J.A. *et al.* (2000) Effect of weight reduction on clinical signs of lameness in dogs with hip osteoarthritis. *J Am Vet Med Assoc.* **216**(7):1089–1091.

Ip, D. (2015) Does addition of low-level laser therapy (LLLT) in conservative care of knee arthritis successfully postpone the need for joint replacement? *Lasers Med Sci.* **30**(9):2335–2339.

Ip, D. and Fu, N.Y. (2015) Can combined use of low-level lasers and hyaluronic acid injections prolong the longevity of degenerative knee joints? *Clin Interv Aging.* **10**:1255–1258.

Marshall, W.G. *et al.* (2010) The effect of weight loss on lameness in obese dogs with osteoarthritis. *Vet Res Commun.* **34**(3):241–253.

Millis, D.L. and Ciuperca, I.A. (2015) Evidence for canine rehabilitation and physical therapy. *Vet Clin North Am Small Anim Pract.* **45**(1):1–27.

Mlacnik, E. *et al.* (2006) Effects of caloric restriction and a moderate or intense physiotherapy program for treatment of lameness in overweight dogs with osteoarthritis. *J Am Vet Med Assoc.* **229**(11):1756–1760.

Mokmeli, S. *et al.* (2006). Low level laser therapy (LLLT) for knee osteoarthritis: a clinical study on 386 patients. *Proceedings of the 6th International Congress of the World Association of Laser Therapy.* October 25–28, 2006. Limassol.

Pryor, B. and Millis, D.L. (2015) Therapeutic laser in veterinary medicine. *Vet Clin North Am Small Anim Pract.* **45**(1):45–56.

Saunders, D.G. and Millis, D. (2014). Laser therapy in canine rehabilitation. In: *Canine Rehabilitation and Physical Therapy*, 2 edn., pp. 359–380. Elsevier, Amsterdam.

Soleimanpour, H. *et al.* (2014) The effect of low-level laser therapy on knee osteoarthritis: prospective, descriptive study. *Lasers Med Sci.* **29**(5):1695–1700.

Taylor, R.A. *et al.* (2004) Physical rehabilitation for geriatric and arthritis patients. In: *Canine Rehabilitation & Physical Therapy*, p. 412. Saunders, Philadelphia, PA.

Verbruggen, G. (2006) Chondroprotective drugs in degenerative joint diseases. *Rheumatology (Oxford).* **45**(2):129–138.

Part VII

Clinical Applications of Laser Therapy in Exotic Animals

26

Laser Therapy for Exotic Small Mammals

Jörg Mayer[1] and Robert D. Ness[2]

[1] *Department of Small Animal Medicine and Surgery, University of Georgia, Athens, GA, USA*
[2] *Ness Exotic Wellness Center, Lilse, IL, USA*

Introduction

The body of evidence regarding the efficacy of photobiomodulation therapy (PBMT) in small mammals is staggering, as most of the research in this area usually includes at least one species of small mammal in the early stages of investigation. It is beyond the scope of this chapter to list all scientific publications that are currently available. The authors will focus on the most clinically applicable publications and on the applications of laser therapy that are most commonly used in clinical daily practice. The body of knowledge in this area will continue to grow. The reader is encouraged to update their database frequently by searching for novel applications of PBMT in small mammals.

Precautions and Contraindications

Safety precautions must be observed for all species when utilizing PBMT, as with any form of medical therapy. Most of the precautions and contraindications regarding exotic small mammals discussed in this chapter are extrapolated from recommendations for other species.

Due to the near-infrared wavelength of therapeutic lasers, regulatory agencies require that protective eyewear, calibrated to the proper wavelength, be worn to prevent injury to the retina. Everyone in the room, including the patient, must have their eyes protected during laser therapy, since there is risk of retinal damage from direct exposure to the laser beam, as well as from reflection of the laser light. The patient's eyes are protected simply by covering them with a dark cloth or towel.

Due to the inherent power of some therapy lasers relative to the small size of many of the exotic small-mammal species, extra care should be exercised when using these devices with these patients. Smaller patients require a lower therapeutic dose, which is accomplished by adjusting the laser settings (Table 26.1). This can involve modifying the delivery mode, power, or time. A pulsed delivery can be utilized instead of a continuous delivery, thereby reducing the rate of delivery by 50% (assuming a 50% duty cycle). Similarly, a lower energy dose can be delivered by decreasing the treatment time or the laser power.

Overheating of the skin and fur is a potential risk of improper operator technique. Darkly pigmented skin and dark hair absorbs photons, increasing the chances of overheating, and thus require caution in the dosing and administration of PBMT. Running a finger behind the laser beam over the animal is encouraged, as the operator will immediately feel the temperature of the skin and hair as the laser handpiece is moved. If anything other than a pleasant, gentle warming is noted, the handpiece should be moved more quickly, the power reduced, or the spot size enlarged.

Contraindications to PBMT are generally a result of prudence rather than clinical data. A current recommendation is that treatment over malignancy sites be considered contraindicated, but some studies suggest PBMT may have an inhibitory effect on some cancerous tissue in mammals (Myakishev-Rempel *et al.*, 2012; Santana-Blank *et al.*, 2012). The risk/benefit ratio has to be considered for each case, because the analgesic and anti-inflammatory effects of the treatment may be of greater benefit than the risk of stimulating a cancerous growth (e.g., the benefit of the analgesic property might outweigh the risk of complicating a case of osteosarcoma).

It is recommended that prolonged treatment be avoided over certain endocrine organs, such as the thyroid gland and gonads, even though there are minimal and contradictory data suggesting an adverse effect to these tissues.

Metal implants do not absorb photons, but they do reflect them back into tissues that are more superficial, so the dose of energy applied to tissue directly over metallic implants, such as bone plates or screws, should be reduced.

Laser Therapy in Veterinary Medicine: Photobiomodulation, First Edition. Edited by Ronald J. Riegel and John C. Godbold, Jr.
© 2017 John Wiley & Sons, Inc. Published 2017 by John Wiley & Sons, Inc.

Table 26.1 Laser therapy dose recommendations for exotic small mammals.

Disorder	Recommended dosage (J/cm²)
Integumentary disorders	
Abscesses	4–6
Cuturebra larvae	2–4
Deep wounds	8–10
Edema	4–5
Hair loss	8–10
Lacerations	1–2
Pododermatitis	2–6
Superficial wounds	2–4
Surgical incisions (for skin)	1
Surgical incisions (for deep)	2–3
Musculoskeletal disorders	
Arthritis	8–10
Fractures	8–10
Muscular sprain and strain	2–4
Scurvy	1–8
Spondylosis	10
Neurologic disorders	8–10
Head and neck disorders	
Dental disease	2–4
Otitis	10
Otorhinolaryngological conditions	6–8
Temporomandibular disorders	6–8
Abdominal disorders	
Ascites	7–10
Gastrointestinal disorders	7–10
Urinary disorders	6–8
Thoracic and respiratory disorders	
Laryngitis	6–8
Bronchitis and pneumonia	8
Pulmonary congestion	6–8
Pulmonary ischemia	6–8

Since PBMT increases microcirculation in tissues, treatment of actively hemorrhaging tissue is discouraged.

The effect of PBMT on a developing fetus or on parturition is unknown, but prudent care suggests avoiding application of PBMT directly over a gravid uterus. In one study, the hemodynamic changes and variations in liver and kidney function in pregnant rats with pre-eclampsia were observed after treatment with low-energy laser irradiation. In the treatment groups, laser irradiation of the chest was carried out after day 16 of gestation. Blood pressure, urine protein, liver and kidney function, and hemodynamic

changes were observed in order to assess the systemic effects of the treatment and its potential side effects. The study concluded that low-energy laser irradiation in the chest area may improve the hemodynamic indices, decrease blood pressure and urine protein, and ameliorate liver and kidney functions in pregnant rats with pre-eclampsia (Sun *et al.*, 2010). This may suggest that the use of laser in pregnant rats with pre-eclampsia is of benefit for the animal.

In human medicine, the CO_2 laser has the most evidence supporting its use during pregnancy. It is considered safe for the treatment of genital condylomas during pregnancy (Lee *et al.*, 2013). It has also been demonstrated that the use of laser therapy after a human cesarean section does not compromise blood prolactin levels or lactation status (Mokmeli *et al.*, 2009). This study concluded that PBMT after cesarean section had no serious deleterious effects on lactation, and that it helped to modulate metabolic processes and promote wound healing post-surgery.

Clinical Indications

Integumentary Disorders

Abscesses
Abscesses tend to heal more rapidly when treated with PBMT. A deep wound setting of $4–6 J/cm^2$ can expedite recovery when used in conjunction with appropriate antimicrobial therapy. As expected, smaller and more superficial abscesses can be treated at lower therapeutic doses than deeper lesions that penetrate beyond the skin and immediate superficial tissues.

Cuterebra Larvae
Cuterebra infestation in rabbits and other small mammals is a common example of a condition that responds well to PBMT. The lesions are caused by the development of Cuterebra larvae under the skin after deposition of eggs by the Cuterebra fly (Figure 26.1). The standard treatment is careful removal of the infested Cuturebra larvae and standard management of the resulting wound. PBMT at $2–4 J/cm^2$ reduces the severe inflammation around the wound, reduces the pain, accelerates the healing response, and accentuates resolution of tissue infection.

Deep Wounds
Deep wounds in exotic small mammals are treated similarly to those in dogs and cats, at a starting dosage range of $8–10 J/cm^2$. Minimal adjustment of treatment parameters is necessary for the size of the patients, since the therapeutic dosage is dependent of the size of the lesion, which is relatively smaller in smaller patients. Higher dosages have been used in exotic small mammals without untoward effects.

Al-Watban and Zhang (1999) conducted a study to define the ideal dose of laser light in the treatment of skin

(a)

(b)

(c)

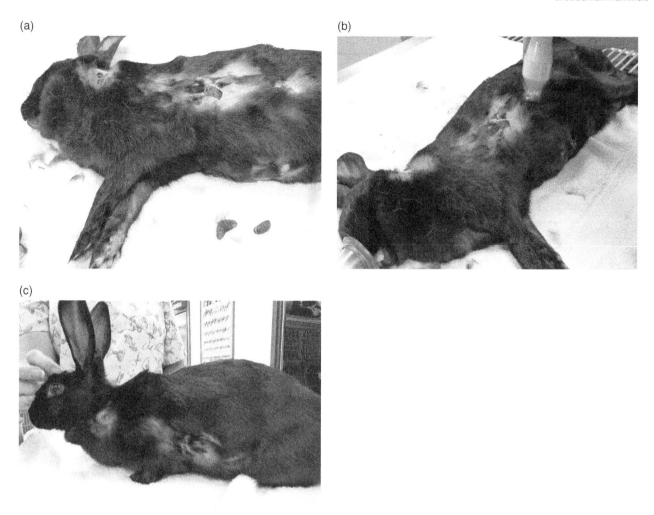

Figure 26.1 Cuterebra larva infestation in a rabbit kept outdoors. (a) The rabbit is sedated for removal of the larvae. (b) Laser therapy is aplied to the resultant wounds using a deep-wound target dose. The rabbit healed rapidly following removal of the larvae and a single laser therapy session. (c) Healing and hair regrowth around the lesions after 5 days. Images courtesy of Dr. Robert D. Ness.

wounds on the backs of rats. In a comparison of fluencies of 10, 20, and $30\,J/cm^2$ applied three times weekly, the best results were obtained with $20\,J/cm^2$. Another analysis showed that the combination of 685 and 830 nm wavelengths ($10\,J/cm^2$ each; total $20\,J/cm^2$) promoted the best skin wound healing at the end of the experimental period (Mendez *et al.*, 2004). Because of the large number of studies involving wound healing in small mammals in the laboratory, using widely varying parameters, there is no consensus about the ideal parameters for the application of PBMT for tissue repair and pain relief (Enwemeka, 2009). The parameters recommended in this chapter have produced positive clinical results; other parameters may do so as well.

Edema

Edema and swelling are normal responses of the body to inflammation and insult, leading to increased fluid in the tissues (Figure 26.2). Common causes include direct trauma, allergic response, circulatory compromise, cardiac disease, and metabolic disorders. PBMT relieves swelling by improving local circulation and stimulating the anti-inflammatory cascade. The higher end of recommended superficial tissue target dosage, at $4–5\,J/cm^2$, is usually effective in a single to a few laser therapy sessions.

Hair Loss

Hair loss in small mammals ranges from slight patchy thinning of the fur to complete alopecia. Many etiologies exist for each species, including ectoparasites, psychogenic barbering, endocrine disorders, metabolic diseases, chemical irritation, thermal burns, bite wounds, and other topical trauma. Regardless of the underlying cause, many of these patients will show hair coat improvement with the use of PBMT if their hair follicles are viable. PBMT addresses the outward clinical manifestation. The underlying etiology should be determined and treated appropriately, as well. Initial target doses range from 8 to $10\,J/cm^2$, depending on the severity of the alopecia, with some recommendations as high as $20\,J/cm^2$. Superficial traumatic or direct physical insult may respond within one or two sessions of PBMT, while systemic conditions may require multiple sessions, with a plan for long-term maintenance treatments. It is interesting to note that the first report of what we now know as PBMT was of its effect on hair follicles in mice: Mester *et al.* (1968) noticed a more rapid hair growth on shaven mice that were treated with therapeutic lasers than on non-treated control animals.

Lacerations

Laceration and skin tears are common in exotic small mammals, due to their inquisitive nature getting them into trouble or to bite wounds among housemates (Figure 26.3). These types of injury respond well to PBMT,

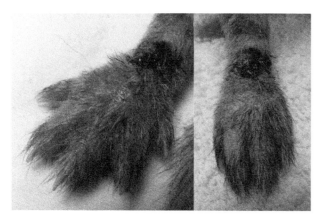

Figure 26.2 Cellulitis of the front paw of a ferret after surgical removal of a mast cell tumor over the carpus. Note the improvement seen 2 days after a single laser therapy session. Image courtesy of Dr. Robert D. Ness.

healing much more rapidly, and with fewer complications, than with conventional therapy alone. A superficial PBMT target dose of $1–2\,J/cm^2$ is usually sufficient in just a few sessions repeated every few days until healed.

A study showing the benefits of PBMT was conducted in rabbits, where full-thickness wounds $(3 \times 3\,cm)$ were artificially created and then treated with laser exposure $(4\,J/cm^2)$ on days 0, 3, and 6 post-wounding with a 808 nm diode laser. In the control group, a moist wound dressing was applied. The wound-healing process was evaluated by both gross and pathological assessment, and it was found that PBMT accelerates wound healing in some phases of the healing process (Hodjati *et al.*, 2014).

Pododermatitis

Pododermatitis is a common foot lesion encountered in clinical practice, resulting from improper cage flooring and substrate, and is often complicated by obesity and improper hygiene (Figure 26.4). A recent publication noted that laser therapy has been used to encourage wound healing in a rabbit with pododermatitis (Blair, 2013). In the reported case, the treatments were performed twice weekly for six treatments, in conjunction with topical medications, bandages, and improvements in the rabbit's husbandry. Because PBMT is very often used in conjunction with other therapies, the significance of its role in the resolution of these cases is difficult to determine, but clinicians often report positive results.

Osteoarthritis is a common sequela to pododermatitis, especially in guinea pigs and rabbits. A study in which osteoarthritis was induced in rabbits and then treated with PBMT showed a significant improvement in the treated animals. In the study, two different lasers were used. One used 808 nm, with a continuous delivery and an output of 1 W. The other used 904 nm, with an intermittent superpulsed delivery and an average output of 1 W.

(a)

(b)

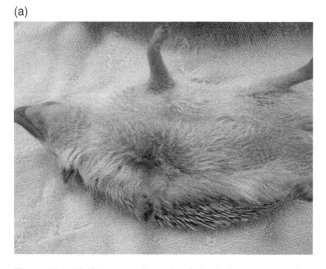

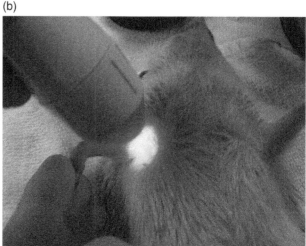

Figure 26.3 (a) Skin tear in the axilla of a hedgehog. (b) Laser therapy of the tear using a superficial wound setting of $2\,J/cm^2$. Images courtesy of Dr. Robert D. Ness.

(a)

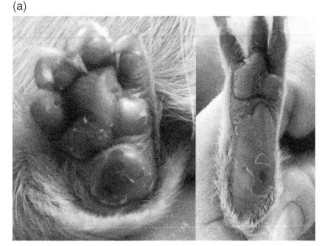

(b)

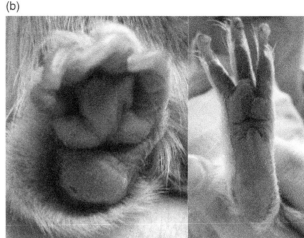

Figure 26.4 (a) Pododermatitis in a guinea pig, which presented with swelling and superficial abrasion of both front and hind foot pads. No siginificant ulcerations or bony involvment were detected in this case. (b) Full resolution of pododermatitis lesions on both front and hind feet within 1 week of single laser therapy session at a superficial lesion dose of 2 J/cm^2. Images courtesy of Dr. Robert D. Ness.

The study concluded that PBMT is effective in treating induced osteoarthritis based on superoxide dismutase (SOD) activity, computed tomography (CT), gross observation, and histopathology. In addition, the study mentioned that no significant difference was seen between the two different laser irradiation methods, but that a significant improvement was seen in both PBMT groups compared to the osteoarthritis control group (Lee *et al.*, 2014).

Superficial Wounds

In varying animal models, *in vitro*, and clinically, wound healing is improved using a variety of different wavelengths and powers. As already discussed with regard to lacerations, Hodjati *et al.* (2014) demonstrated that PBMT accelerates wound healing in rabbits at a dose 4 J/cm^2. This dose is representative of what is commonly used clinically. However, no optimal set of parameters has yet been identified (Kuffler, 2016), and in the literature evidence is readily available for both improved wound healing and a lack of an observable effect on wound healing.

In cases where the results of a study do not indicate a significant difference in wound healing with the use of PBMT, it is important to verify the methodology. In many wound-healing studies, the a single animal is used as both case and control. Multiple lesions are created on the same animal, only one of which is treated with laser therapy, with the others serving as controls or receiving other treatment modalities. Studies have clearly indicated that PBMT has additional systemic effects besides the local effects on the treated tissues. Rodrigo *et al.* (2009) describe a study in which rats were treated with PBM and healing was more advanced in the wound located furthest from the point of laser application.

Another study evaluated the systemic effects of local PBMT, using rats with injuries in the peripheral and central nervous system (CNS), skin wounds, and burns. These animals were irradiated with a 632.8 nm laser at a power of 16 mW and different energy densities for 21 days (Gal *et al.*, 2006). The laser was applied only to the right side of the animals, after bilateral skin wounds were produced. At the end of the study, the authors observed better healing of both wounds than in the control group, which did not receive any irradiation. Statistical analysis showed a significant difference between the group treated with laser and the control group. The authors concluded that the laser application had a marked systemic effect on the skin and adjacent tissues, as well as on the severely damaged peripheral nerves and the corresponding regions of the marrow. According to the authors, the effects persisted for a long time after laser irradiation. They suggest that these systemic effects are relevant for the clinical application of laser therapy and for basic research into its possible mechanisms of action.

PBMT appears to accelerate healing of third-degree burns. Ezzati *et al.* (2009) found that irradiation of a third-degree burn model with 11.7 J/cm^2 (890 nm) significantly increased wound closure rate compared with control burns in rats. In addition, their data showed that the incidence of *Staphylococcus epidermidis*, Lactobacillus, and diphtheria decreased significantly in laser-treated groups compared with other groups.

Surgical Incisions

As with other superficial wounds, incisions appear to heal more rapidly, with less inflammation and minimal scarring, when treated with PBMT at the conclusion of a surgical procedure. Most elective-surgery, minor wound-closure, and basic dental-procedure patients require a single treatment at 1 J/cm^2 immediately after the procedure. Surgical patients with procedures causing more extensive tissue disruption, such as orthopedic and laparotomy cases, should receive additional treatments at 2–3 J/cm^2, administered every second to third day until healed.

Musculoskeletal Disorders

Arthritis

Arthritis is a common consequence of aging in all species. In human medicine, Ip (1015) evaluated the use of PBMT in the conservative care of knee arthritis and found it helped postpone the need for joint replacement. In this longitudinal study, which included follow-ups after 6 years, it was concluded that PBMT should be incorporated into standard conservative treatment protocols for symptomatic knee arthritis.

Strong evidence from a systematic review and meta-analysis of the effectiveness of PBMT for non-specific chronic low back pain in humans indicated that PBMT is an effective method for relieving pain (Huang *et al.*, 2015). Similarly, it has been demonstrated in a comparative evaluation of laser and systemic steroid therapy in adjuvant-enhanced arthritis of rat temperomandibular joints that PBMT has a long-term promising effect on the severity of inflammation of temperomandibular joint syndrome (similar to that of betamethasone) in its earlier stages (Khozeimeh *et al.*, 2015).

When rats were used as models to evaluate PBMT in different stages of rheumatoid arthritis, it was shown that the therapy could modulate inflammatory response in both early and late progression stages (Alves *et al.*, 2013). It has also been shown that PBMT has significant beneficial effects on joint pain, synovitis, and anabolic and catabolic factors in a progressive osteoarthritis rabbit model (Wang *et al.*, 2014). Similar effects have been shown in osteoarthropathy induced in the rabbit (Cho *et al.*, 2004).

In the clinical setting, PBMT is used to control pain and reduce inflammation of this degenerative condition in exotic small mammals. The initial starting dosage in most cases is 8–10 J/cm^2, depending on severity and chronicity.

Fracture

Fracture healing is stimulated by the use of PBMT at deep-tissue settings of 8–10 J/cm^2. Patients have healed in 25–50% less time compared to those without PBMT. However, the laser light is scattered by bandage material, so fractures cannot be treated through splint or casting material. To overcome this obstacle, practitioners can design the splint or cast with a small window or fenestration over the fracture site that can be accessed during PBMT.

It is interesting to note that in the research setting, much higher doses have been used with good success.

A study showed that 830 nm laser irradiation, at 120 J/cm^2, was able to increase the biomechanical properties and bone mineral density of osteopenic rats without causing side effects (Renno *et al.*, 2006). Thus, current dose recommendations may be adjusted in the near future.

The reported effects of PBMT on bone regeneration depend not only on the total dose of irradiation, but also on the irradiation time and the irradiation model (Saito and Shimizu, 1997). As early as 1987, evidence existed that PBMT produced an increased osteoblastic activity, increased the number of blood vessels, and increased the amount of mineralized bone (speeding up early bone repair) when used on fractures (Trelles and Mayayo, 1987). Currently, multiple scientific publications show a significant benefit of using PBMT on fracture healing. Studies demonstrate that a variety of wavelengths and doses provide a variety of beneficial effects, so it is difficult to recommend the perfect dose.

In one publication, a 790 nm laser demonstrated a 10% increase in the amount of mineralized bone present in irradiated animals at day 7 (Silva Júnior *et al.*, 2002). This study reported a more positive effect of 830 nm laser light in comparison to 632.8 or 790 nm. This is most likely due to a higher penetration of laser light with a longer wavelength.

Besides wavelength, the energy delivered to the tissue is also of importance when treating fractures. The influence of the power delivered to the area of interest has clearly been identified in a variety of studies (Gomes *et al.*, 2015; Silva Júnior *et al.*, 2002). In one experiment, rabbits received a dental implant and were treated with 5, 10, or 20 J/cm^2. The results clearly indicated a significant improvement in the stability of the bone implant in the 20 J/cm^2 group (Gomes *et al.*, 2015).

High doses were used in another study, and it is interesting to note that there appears to be a ceiling effect, as the healing benefits in rat fractures were not significantly different with 60 versus 120 J/cm^2 at 830 nm (Bossini *et al.*, 2012). The results of this study do support the notion that laser therapy improves bone repair in the tibia of osteoporotic rats through the stimulation of newly formed bone, fibrovascularization, and angiogenesis.

Another study showed the benefit of using laser therapy as an adjuvant in combination with calcitonin (Ribeiro *et al.*, 2012). It found that PBMT using 830 nm light combined with calcitonin improved bone repair and reduced the duration of the bone-repair process.

Another study looked at the synergy of using laser therapy and an anti-cyclooxygenase 2 (COX-2)-selective drug (celecoxib) in the tibia of rats (Ribeiro and Matsumoto, 2008). The results showed that PBMT improved bone repair as a result of up-regulation of COX-2 expression in bone cells. The group that received celecoxib and PBMT showed better results than the group that received just celecoxib alone, which was better than the control group.

Muscular Sprain and Strain

Muscular sprains and strains in exotic small mammals are treated with PBMT in a similar manner to dogs and cats. A target dose of $2–4\,J/cm^2$ is typically sufficient, with only a few sessions repeated over a couple weeks. The underlying causes of lesions within the muscles and connective tissue are also similar to those in other companion animals, and must be appropriately treated.

Scurvy

Scurvy in guinea pigs is caused by hypovitaminosis C and is characterized by inflammation in the temporomandibular joints, limb joints, costochondral joints of ribs, and spine. Clinical signs include swelling of the limbs, lameness, weakness, poor appetite, loose teeth, hemorrhage, and death. Treatment includes vitamin C supplementation and supportive therapy, as indicated by presenting clinical signs. PBMT is useful in treating the resultant inflammation in the body, presenting as swollen and painful joints. The dosage ranges from $1\,J/cm^2$ for the temperomandibular joint to $8\,J/cm^2$ in the spine or pelvis, repeated as needed according to the severity of inflammation.

Spondylosis

Spondylosis is common in rabbits, due to their inherent biomechanics. Spinal arthritis is typically age-related, but can also be initiated by spinal trauma or irritation. As with any case of arthritis, analgesia and anti-inflammation can be achieved with PBMT. A higher therapeutic dosage of $10\,J/cm^2$ is often necessary to obtain a consistent therapeutic effect, especially in chronic or advanced cases.

Neurologic Disorders

Evidence of the beneficial effects of laser therapy for spinal cord injury and other neurological conditions in small mammals are accumulating in the scientific literature. In one study, rat spinal cords were injured and the lesion sites were directly irradiated with an 808 nm diode laser positioned either perpendicular or parallel to the spine immediately after the injury and daily for five consecutive days (Ando *et al.*, 2013). The authors found that regardless of the polarization direction, the functional scores of rats with spinal cord injury that were treated with the 808 nm laser were significantly higher than those of the untreated group from day 5 after injury. However, the locomotive function of spinal cord injury rats irradiated parallel to the spinal column was significantly improved from day 10 after injury, compared to spinal cord injury rats treated with linear polarization perpendicular to the spinal column (Ando *et al.*, 2013).

Two different rat models of spinal cord injury, one hemisection and one contusion, were used in two different studies (Byrnes *et al.*, 2005; Wu *et al.*, 2009). In both studies, the authors transcutaneously applied an 810 nm laser, which penetrated to the depth of the injured spinal cord and promoted axonal regeneration and functional recovery.

Together, these studies demonstrate that laser irradiation significantly suppresses immune cell activation and cytokine and chemokine expression, suggesting that a decrease in the inflammatory response is one of the recovery mechanisms in PBMT for spinal cord repair (Ando *et al.*, 2013).

Selecting the right wavelength and power settings is most likely of clinical importance when treating a small mammal for a neurological problem. A study specifically addressing this point measured the *in vivo* penetration of infrared light applied to the skin of anesthetized rabbits. An average of 2.45% of the light reached the depth of the peroneal nerve (Anders *et al.*, 2014). This pilot study revealed that 4 W treatment inhibited nerve regeneration, while 2 W treatment significantly improved axonal regrowth, despite the fact that both groups received a total energy dose of 65 J. Overall, the irradiated group performed significantly better in the toe-spread reflex test than the control group from week 7 post-injury.

Head and Neck Disorders

Dental Disease

PBMT has been shown to enhance tissue regeneration and tissue growth, with effects on fibroblastic (Almeida-Lopes *et al.*, 2001) and chondral (Schultz *et al.*, 1985) proliferation, collagen synthesis (Majaron *et al.*, 2000), wound healing (Lowe *et al.*, 1998), bone regeneration (Ekizer *et al.*, 2015; Saito and Shimizu, 1997), and nerve regeneration (Anders *et al.*, 2004). These effects mean that PBMT can be used to treat a variety of dental diseases in the exotic small-mammal patient.

Dental malocclusion is common in rabbits and rodents, ranging from incisor malocclusion with elongation to molar root deviation and abscessation. This disorder results in oral lesions and anorexia in these species. PBMT is beneficial in controlling the pain and inflammation associated with the trimming and extraction of affected teeth, as well as in healing of the oral soft tissues and subsequent jaw and temporomandibular lesions. A single PBMT session administered at a setting of $2\,J/cm^2$ can facilitate healing of the mouth following incisor extraction in rabbits and rodents. Therapeutic dosages for molar malocclusion with jaw lesions range from 2 to $4\,J/cm^2$ and should be administered at least twice times weekly until appetite returns. Higher dosages and increased intervals may be indicated in chronic or more severe cases.

Otitis

Otitis and torticollis respond to PBMT when treated at higher therapeutic dosages of at least $10\,J/cm^2$. The clinical improvement is thought to be the result of reduced inflammation within the vestibular apparatus and healing of deeper tissues within the ear canal. Though the benefit of PBMT on otitis has been demonstrated in humans and companion animals, further evaluation is warranted to assess the clinical effects in torticollis, since current information is based on only a few clinical cases.

Otorhinolaryngol Disorders

The positive effect of PBMT on a variety of otorhinolaryngol problems has been documented in human medicine. Treatment of pollinosis, adenoiditis and rhino-sinusitis, tonsillitis, and otitis with infrared and red laser irradiation resulted in positive results in 85% of patients (Gogeliia *et al.*, 2006; Nikitin *et al.*, 2008). Similar effects could be expected in comparable otorhinolaryngol disorders in exotic small mammals.

Temporomandibular Disorder

Temporomandibular disorder (TMD) is characterized by pain. It is sometimes a sequela to primary dental disease in small mammals such as guinea pigs. PBMT was performed for 10 minutes daily in rats with experimentally induced TMD, starting the day after the confirmation of osteoarthritis. Treatment was at the right side of the temporomandibular joint (TMJ), using an 880 nm laser with 100 mW of power (Peimani and Sardary, 2014). After 7 days of therapy, the grade of cartilage defects, number of inflammatory cells, number of cell layers, and severity of arthritis improved compared to controls.

Abdominal Disorders

Ascites

Ascites is the accumulation of fluid in the abdominal cavity as a result of a metabolic imbalance causing changes in osmotic pressure and hemodynamic permeability. Classic etiologies in exotic small mammals include hepatic disorders, cardiovascular disease (CVD), and cancer. PBMT is appropriate for the treatment of ascites resulting from hepatic and cardiac diseases. It should be avoided in cases of suspected neoplasia. PBMT has the potential to decrease fluid accumulation by improving the cellular integrity of the vessels and lymphatics, affecting the cell membrane potential and sodium ion exchange in the abdomen, and reducing inflammation of the tissues. A dose of $7–10\,J/cm^2$ is recommended.

Gastrointestinal Disorders

Gastrointestinal disorders are common in many exotic small mammals kept as pets. Conditions ranging from gastrointestinal stasis to gastritis and inflammatory bowel disease (IBD) are commonly seen. Malnutrition, gastrointestinal foreign bodies, and trichobezoars can all lead to slowing of gastrointestinal transit and, ultimately, stasis. PBMT should be included with other appropriate medical therapies in the management of these cases. In one study using rats with experimental chronic atrophic gastritis, laser treatment showed a good adjuvant therapeutic effect on the rats' gastric mucosa (Yang *et al.*, 2005).

In practice, utilizing PBMT in cases of gastrointestinal disorder at around $7–10\,J/cm^2$ has greatly improved the recovery of these patients by reducing inflammation and providing similar abdominal pain relief to that seen in other deep conditions in companion small animals (Ness, 2016).

Urinary Disorders

Urinary disorders of exotic small mammals include cystitis and cystic calculi. They can be positively affected by PBMT through a reduction of inflammation of the bladder and management of pain. The target dosage is calculated by approximating the entire three-dimensional area that the bladder and other affected tissues occupy in the abdomen. Certain laser therapy units have specific preset parameters determined for the treatment of the urinary tract, while others may have abdominal settings calculated for the entire abdominal cavity. Therefore, it is prudent to estimate one's own starting target dose of approximately $6–8\,J/cm^2$ until one is confident with the laser device and its software. Depending on the degree of inflammation, the effective dose may be significantly higher or lower than the device's proposed dosage or preset. In addition, the frequency of PBMT treatments will depend on the case, ranging from daily in severe acute cases to possibly weekly in chronic low-grade conditions.

Older rats often suffer from glomerulonephritis. PBMT has the potential to be used for direct treatment of glomerulonephritis. It has been demonstrated that externally directed PBMT suppresses the activity of rat anti-glomerular basement membrane (GBM) crescentic glomerulonephritis (Yamato *et al.*, 2013).

Thoracic and Respiratory Disorders

Laryngitis

Intubation can be challenging in some exotic small-mammal patients. Often, blind intubation is performed, which carries a risk of laryngeal damage and inflammation. The placement of a nasogastric tube is often associated with laryngitis in humans (Lima-Rodrigues *et al.*, 2008). Multiple studies in rats with experimentally induced laryngitis followed by laser therapy treatment have demonstrated that PBMT is potentially useful in controling reflux laryngitis secondary to nasogastric intubation. PBMT reduces the influx of neutrophils to the injured area and improves the reparative collagenization of the laryngeal tissues (Marinho *et al.*, 2013a, 2013b).

Bronchitis and Pneumonia

Pneumonia and bronchitis cases in any species can benefit from PBMT through a reduction in inflammation, increase in leucocyte activity, and improvement in fluid resorption. Rats with mycoplasma pneumonia develop poor compliance in the chest from dramatically increased inflammation and congestion in their lungs. These patients are difficult to manage with standard treatments alone, but can show clinical improvement with the addition of PBMT at approximately $8\,J/cm^2$. The same results are seen in rabbits with *Pasteurella multocida* and guinea pigs with *Bordetella bronchiseptica*.

Pulmonary Congestion and Pleural Edema

Pulmonary congestion and pleural effusion occur in respiratory cases involving excess fluid accumulation within (pulmonary congestion) or around (pleural effusion) the lungs. PBMT helps with resorption of excess fluid by providing improved circulation and osmotic pressure changes. Target dosing for pulmonary congestion starts at $6-8\,J/cm^2$, and for pleural effusion at $10\,J/cm^2$.

Pulmonary Ischemia

A study evaluated the effect of PBMT on lung remote-organ injury induced by skeletal-muscle ischemia and reperfusion. Animals were treated with laser therapy over the skin above the right upper bronchus at varying intervals after hind limbs were subjected to ischemia induced by femoral artery occlusion followed by reperfu-sion. This study found that PBMT alleviated the lung-tissue injuries following skeletal muscle ischemia and reperfusion (Ashrafzadeh Takhtfooladi *et al.*, 2015).

Conclusion

A wealth of information is available about the use of PBMT in mammals. Knowledge continues to grow as practitioners in both the human and the veterinary realms realize the potential of this phenomenal modality. Much of the information available in the literature regarding PBMT in the exotic small-mammal species comes from research for human and companion-animal applications. As with all other species, virtually any condition affecting an exotic small mammal that benefits from analgesia, anti-inflammation, and increased rate of healing can improve with PBM.

The information provided here is intended as a starting point from which to expand the use of PBMT in exotic small mammals. Though many of the common disorders treated in exotic-pet practice have been presented, this is not an exhaustive list. The authors hope the information provided here will encourage and stimulate the use of this treatment modality in exotic-pet practice.

Practitioners are also encouraged to add to this practical knowledge base by documenting and reporting the application of PBMT, the use of which is constrained only by one's imagination and ingenuity. When applying this modality, the authors encourage detailed documentation of treatment parameters, including the wavelength and dose (J/cm^2), in order to standardize treatment and facilitate communication with other clinicians.

References

Almeida-Lopes, L. *et al.* (2001) Comparison of the low level laser therapy effects on cultured human gingival fibroblasts proliferation using different irradiance and same fluence. *Lasers Surg Med.* **29**(2):179–184.

Alves, A.C. *et al.* (2013) Low-level laser therapy in different stages of rheumatoid arthritis: a histological study. *Lasers Med Sci.* **28**(2):529–536.

Al-Watban, F.A.H. and Zhang, X.Y. (1999) The acceleration of wound healing is not attributed to laser skin transmission. *Laser Therapy.* **11**(1):6–10

Anders, J.J. *et al.* (2004) Phototherapy promotes regeneration and functional recovery of injured peripheral nerve. *Neurol Res.* **26**(2):233–239.

Anders, J.J. *et al.* (2014) In vitro and in vivo optimization of infrared laser treatment for injured peripheral nerves. *Lasers Surg Med.* **46**(1):34–45.

Ando, T. *et al.* (2013) Low-level laser therapy for spinal cord injury in rats: effects of polarization. *J Biomed Opt.* **18**(9):098002.

Ashrafzadeh Takhtfooladi, M. *et al.* (2015) Effect of low-level laser therapy on lung injury induced by hindlimb ischemia/reperfusion in rats. *Lasers Med Sci.* **30**(6):1757–1762.

Blair, J. (2013) Bumblefoot: a comparison of clinical presentation and treatment of pododermatitis in rabbits, rodents, and birds. *Vet Clin North Am Exot Anim Pract.* **16**(3):715–735.

Bossini, P.S. (2012). Low level laser therapy (830nm) improves bone repair in osteoporotic rats: similar outcomes at two different dosages. *Exp Gerontol.* **47**(2):136–142.

Byrnes, K.R. *et al.* (2005) Light promotes regeneration and functional recovery and alters the immune response after spinal cord injury. *Lasers Surg Med.* **36**(3):171–185.

Cho, H.J. *et al.* (2004) Effect of low-level laser therapy on osteoarthropathy in rabbit. *In Vivo.* **18**(5):585–591.

Ekizer, A. *et al.* (2015) Effect of LED-mediated-photobiomodulation therapy on orthodontic tooth movement and root resorption in rats. *Lasers Med Sci.* **30**(2):779–785.

Enwemeka, C.S. (2009) Intricacies of dose in laser phototherapy for tissue repair and pain relief. *Photomed Laser Surg.* **27**(3):387–393.

Ezzati, A. *et al.* (2009) Low-level laser therapy with pulsed infrared laser accelerates third-degree burn healing process in rats. *J Rehab Res Dev.* **46**(4):543–554.

Gal, P. *et al.* (2006) Histological assessment of the effect of laser irradiation on skin wound healing in rats. *Photomed Laser Surg.* **24**(4):480–488.

Gogeliia, A. *et al.* (2006) Experience on treatment of children with otorhinolaryngological diseases by low intensity laser irradiation. *Georgian Med News.* **130**:84–86.

Gomes, F.V. *et al.* (2015) Low-level laser therapy improves peri-implant bone formation: resonance frequency, electron microscopy, and stereology findings in a rabbit model. *Int J Oral Maxillofac Surg.* **44**(2):245–251.

Hodjati, H. *et al.* (2014) Low-level laser therapy: an experimental design for wound management: a case-controlled study in rabbit model. *J Cutan Aesthet Surg.* **7**(1):14–17.

Huang, Z. *et al.* (2015) The effectiveness of low-level laser therapy for nonspecific chronic low back pain: a systematic review and meta-analysis. *Arthritis Res Ther.* **17**:360.

Ip, D. (2015) Does addition of low-level laser therapy (LLLT) in conservative care of knee arthritis successfully postpone the need for joint replacement? *Lasers Med Sci.* **30**(9):2335–2339.

Khozeimeh, F. *et al.* (2015) Comparative evaluation of low-level laser and systemic steroid therapy in adjuvant-enhanced arthritis of rat temporomandibular joint: a histological study. *Dent Res J (Isfahan).* **12**(3):215–223.

Kuffler, D.P. (2016) Photobiomodulation in promoting wound healing: a review. *Regen Med.* **11**(1):107–122.

Lee, K.C. *et al.* (2013) Safety of cosmetic dermatologic procedures during pregnancy. *Dermatol Surg.* **39**(11):1573–1586.

Lee, J.Y. *et al.* (2014) Healing effects and superoxide dismutase activity of diode/Ga-As lasers in a rabbit model of osteoarthritis. *In Vivo.* **28**(6):1101–1106.

Lima-Rodrigues, M. *et al.* (2008) A new model of laryngitis: neuropeptide, cyclooxygenase, and cytokine profile. *Laryngoscope.* **118**(1):78–86.

Lowe, A.S. *et al.* (1998) Effect of low intensity monochromatic light therapy (890 nm) on a radiation-impaired, wound-healing model in murine skin. *Lasers Surg Med.* **23**(5):291–298.

Majaron, B. *et al.* (2000) Deep coagulation of dermal collagen with repetitive Er:YAG laser irradiation. *Lasers Surg Med.* **26**(2):215–222.

Marinho, R.R. *et al.* (2013a) Potentiated anti-inflammatory effect of combined 780 nm and 660 nm low level laser therapy on the experimental laryngitis. *J Photochem Photobiol B.* **121**:86–93.

Marinho, R.R. *et al.* (2013b) Potential anti-inflammatory effect of low-level laser therapy on the experimental reflux laryngitis: a preliminary study. *Lasers Med Sci.* **29**(1):239–243.

Mendez, T.M. *et al.* (2004) Dose and wavelength of laser light have influence on the repair of cutaneous wounds. *J Clin Laser Med Surg.* **22**(1):19–25.

Mester, E. *et al.* (1968) The effect of laser beams on the growth of hair in mice. *Radiobiol Radiother (Berl).* **9**(5):621–626.

Mokmeli, S. *et al.* (2009) The application of low-level laser therapy after cesarean section does not compromise blood prolactin levels and lactation status. *Photomed Laser Surg.* **27**(3):509–512.

Myakishev-Rempel, M. *et al.* (2012). A preliminary study of the safety of red light phototherapy of tissues harboring cancer. *Photomed Laser Surg.* **30**(9):551–558.

Ness, R.D. (2016) Photobiomodulation in exotic pet practice. *Proceedings CE at SEA: Raising the Standard of Veterinary Care with Laser Therapy.* The American Institute of Medical Laser Applications. February 22–26, 2016. Fort Lauderdale, FL.

Nikitin, A.V. *et al.* (2008). Effectiveness of laser puncture in elderly patients with bronchial asthma accompanied by chronic rhinosinusitis. *Adv Gerontol.* **21**(3):424–426.

Peimani, A. and Sardary, F. (2014) Effect of low-level laser on healing of temporomandibular joint osteoarthritis in rats. *J Dent (Tehran).* **11**(3):319–327.

Renno, A.C. *et al.* (2006) Effects of 830-nm laser, used in two doses, on biomechanical properties of osteopenic rat femora. *Photomed Laser Surg.* **24**(2):202–206.

Ribeiro, D.A. and Matsumoto, M.A. (2008) Low-level laser therapy improves bone repair in rats treated with anti-inflammatory drugs. *J Oral Rehabil.* **35**(12):925–933.

Ribeiro, T.P. *et al.* (2012) Low-level laser therapy and calcitonin in bone repair: densitometric analysis. *Int J Photoenergy.* **28**(1):45–49.

Rodrigo, S.M. *et al.* (2009) Analysis of the systemic effect of red and infrared laser therapy on wound repair. *Photomed Laser Surg.* **27**(6):929–935.

Saito, S. and Shimizu, N. (1997). Stimulatory effects of low-power laser irradiation on bone regeneration in midpalatal suture during expansion in the rat. *Am J Orthod Dentofacial Orthop.* **111**(5):525–532.

Santana-Blank L. *et al.* (2012) Concurrence of emerging developments in photobiomodulation and cancer. *Photomed Laser Surg.* **30**(11):615–616.

Schultz, R.J. *et al.* (1985). Effects of varying intensities of laser energy on articular cartilage: a preliminary study. *Lasers Surg Med.* **5**(6):577–588.

Silva Júnior, A.N. *et al.* (2002). Computerized morphometric assessment of the effect of low-level laser therapy on bone repair: an experimental animal study. *J Clin Laser Med Surg.* **20**(2):83–87.

Sun, L. *et al.* (2010) Hemodynamic changes of pregnant rats with pre-eclampsia after treatment with low-energy laser irradiation of the chest. *Nan Fang Yi Ke Da Xue Xue Bao.* **30**(10):2259–2262.

Trelles, M.A. and Mayayo, E. (1987). Bone fracture consolidates faster with low-power laser. *Lasers Surg Med.* **7**(1):36–45.

Wang, P. *et al.* (2014) Effects of low-level laser therapy on joint pain, synovitis, anabolic, and catabolic factors in a progressive osteoarthritis rabbit model. *Lasers Med Sci.* **29**(6):1875–1885.

Wu, X. *et al.* (2009) 810 nm wavelength light: an effective therapy for transected or contused rat spinal cord. *Lasers Surg Med.* **41**(1):36–41.

Yamato, M. *et al.* (2013) Low-level laser therapy improves crescentic glomerulonephritis in rats. *Lasers Med Sci.* **28**(4):1189–1196.

Yang, Y. *et al.* (2005). Effects of He-Ne laser on gastric mucosa in rat with chronic atrophic gastritis. *Sheng Wu Yi Xue Gong Cheng Xue Za Zhi.* **22**(5):926–929.

27

Laser Therapy for Birds

Robert D. Ness[1] and Jörg Mayer[2]

[1] Ness Exotic Wellness Center, Lilse, IL, USA
[2] Department of Small Animal Medicine and Surgery, University of Georgia, Athens, GA, USA

Introduction

To date, very little scientific information is available on the effect of laser therapy on the avian patient in the clinical setting. This chapter accumulates the information currently available from a variety of experimental studies, and looks at how it might apply in the clinical setting. In addition, the authors share their clinical experience on the use of laser therapy. A 2015 publication of a roundtable discussion shared the clinical experience of the authors and other practitioners using laser therapy in exotic patients (Ritzman *et al.*, 2015). Undoubtedly, the knowledge of how this treatment modality can affect the avian patient will continue to grow. While the general effects of photobiomodulation (PBM) on the avian system will be the same as for other species, anatomical and physiological differences in the avian patient dictate certain adjustments, as outlined in this chapter.

Photobiomodulation therapy (PBMT) has shown well-documented benefits in many species. The purpose of this chapter is to define the science behind this new treatment modality in avian medicine, and to elucidate its practical uses and applications in the clinical setting.

Precautions and Contraindications

Certain safety precautions must be observed for all species when utilizing PBMT, as with any form of medical therapy. This is especially true with birds, due to their high metabolism and thin skin. Most of the precautions and contraindications discussed regarding the avian species are extrapolated from recommendations for other species.

Due to the near-infrared wavelength of therapeutic lasers, regulatory agencies require that protective eyewear be worn, calibrated to the proper laser light wavelength. Everyone in the room, including the patient, must have their eyes protected when the laser is in use, since there is risk of retinal damage from direct exposure to the laser beam, as well as from reflective scatter of the laser light. The bird's eyes can be protected by covering them with a dark cloth or towel. Raptor hoods can be effective eye shields for patients that tolerate them.

Due to the inherent power of some therapy lasers and the relatively thin skin of birds, special considerations should be taken when treating avian species. Adjustments can be made to lower the power density and dose by modifying the delivery mode, power, or time. A pulsed delivery can be utilized instead of a continuous one, reducing the rate of delivery by 50% (assuming a 50% duty cycle). Similarly, a lower energy dose can be delivered by decreasing the treatment time or the laser power. Overheating of the skin and feathers is a potential risk from improper operator technique. The pigments in darkly pigmented skin or dark feathers absorb near-infrared photons, and thus overheat easily, requiring caution and adjustment in dosing and administration of laser therapy. Running a finger over the animal behind the laser beam is encouraged, as the temperature of the skin and feathers will immediately be felt as the laser handpiece is moved. If anything other than a pleasant, gentle warming is noted, the handpiece should be moved more quickly, the power reduced, or the spot size enlarged.

Contraindications to PBMT are generally a result of prudence rather than clinical data. A current recommendation is that treatment over malignancy sites is usually considered contraindicated, though some studies suggest PBMT may have an inhibitory effect on some cancerous tissue. A number of published studies confirm that, under certain parameters, PBMT might indeed be safe for use in cancer patients, despite decades of controversy (Myakishev-Rempel *et al.*, 2012; Santana-Blank *et al.*, 2012). The risk/benefit ratio has to be considered on a case-by-case basis, because the analgesic and anti-inflammatory effects of treatment may outweigh the risk of stimulating a cancerous growth.

It is recommended that prolonged treatment be avoided over certain endocrine organs, such as the thyroid gland and gonads, even though there is minimal suggestion of an adverse effect on these tissues, and the data that are available are contradictory. The effect of PBMT on a developing egg in the oviduct is unknown. Thus, one should avoid PBMT in the breeding hen while gravid. However, as discussed later, there is some suggestion that PBMT may be of benefit to the normally developing avian embryo. It has been shown to decrease third-week mortality rates during the developmental phase when fertile chicken eggs are treated once per day on embryonic days 0–20 (Yeager *et al.*, 2006).

Metal implants do not absorb photons, but they do reflect them back into tissues that are more superficial.

The dose of energy delivered to tissue directly over metallic implants, such as bone plates or screws, should thus be decreased.

Since PBMT increases microcirculation in tissue, treatment of actively hemorrhaging tissue is discouraged.

Clinical Indications

Integumentary Disorders

The skin and feathers of birds are vastly different from the skin and fur of mammals, but many of the same conditions treated by laser therapy in companion mammals can also be treated in birds. In addition, several unique opportunities exist for PBMT of the integument of birds (see Figure 27.1).

(a)
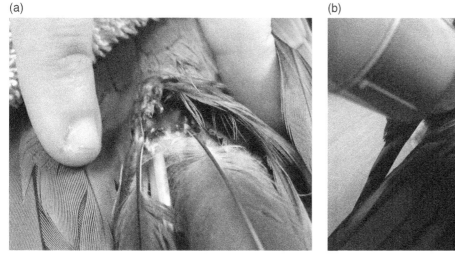

(b)
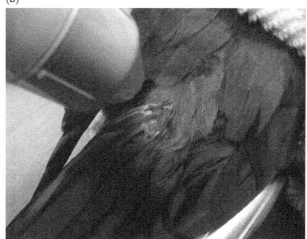

(c)
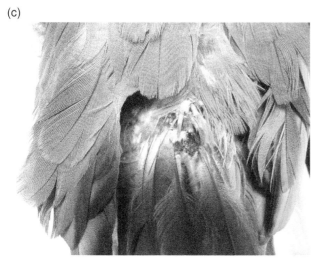

Figure 27.1 (a) Chronic self-mutilation of an impacted uropygial gland in a severe Macaw. (b) Application of laser therapy to the area of the traumatized, impacted uropygial gland. (c) Reduced inflammation and initial healing after laser therapy. Continued application of PBMT is indicated to further the healing process. Images courtesy of Dr. Robert D. Ness.

Deep Wounds

Deep wounds are treated with PBMT in the same manner as in mammals, but at relatively lower target dosages (Figure 27.2). A typical target dose of $4\,J/cm^2$ is often effective, rather than the $6–8\,J/cm^2$ for a similar lesion in mammals (see Table 27.1). In addition, fewer treatment sessions are necessary to obtain a positive response.

Feather Disorders

Feather disorders are very common in birds, and the underlying causes are numerous and varied (Figure 27.3). This may range from snipped or chewed feathers due to over-grooming to complete feather loss due to psychotic feather plucking or underlying metabolic disease. Regardless of the underlying cause, PBMT can benefit patients that still possess some degree of follicular activity. It helps by reducing the inflammation of folliculitis and stimulating feather regrowth in quiescent follicles. As for most superficial conditions in birds, the target dose is generally between 2 and $3\,J/cm^2$. The frequency of treatment can vary greatly, from every once every 1–2 days to as little as once a week, depending on the severity of the feather loss or damage and the level of inactivity of the feather follicles (Ness, 2015). Some clinical cases have shown limited response with sessions as infrequent as once a month.

Lacerations

Lacerations and skin tears in birds are treated with PBMT in a similar manner to how they are in mammals, except that the target dose is typically lower because of the thinner and more delicate skin (see Table 27.1). A superficial target dose of $2\,J/cm^2$ is typically sufficient, with only one to two sessions normally required.

Patagium Restriction

Patagium restriction is one of the unique conditions in birds for which PBMT is among the more promising therapies. The patagium often becomes limited in its range of motion due to fibrous tissue constriction following trauma to the tissue itself, or secondary to decreased range of motion of the wing due to arthritis or trauma. The authors' personal experience with clinical cases of patagium restriction indicates that laser therapy can help reduce fibrous tissue and improve the elasticity of soft tissue, aiding in restoring a wider range of motion with treatment. We recommend a superficial target dose of $4–6\,J/cm^2$. This appears to be effective in just a few sessions, scheduled at several-day intervals. Though the response may be limited in severe cases, some birds can regain flight after successful therapy.

Pododermatitis

Pododermatitis is commonly referred to as "bumble foot" in birds, particularly in birds of prey. It can be quite severe and is often a challenge to treat. However, it often responds favorably to PBMT as an adjunctive therapy. A dose of $3–4\,J/cm^2$ is usually sufficient in even the more complicated cases (Blair, 2013). Several laser therapy sessions may be necessary over a few weeks to elicit a successful outcome.

(a)

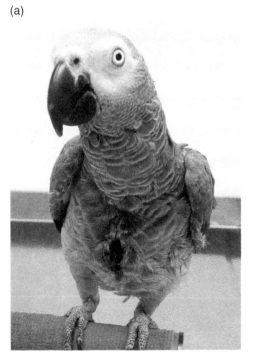

(b)

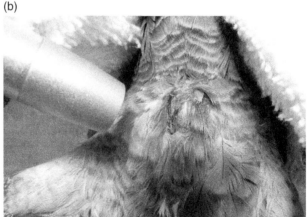

Figure 27.2 (a) African grey parrots are known for keel trauma from falling after over-trimming of their wings. (b) PBMT of the keel wound promotes healing of the lesion and helps minimize scar-tissue formation. Image courtesy of Dr. Robert D. Ness.

Table 27.1 Laser therapy dose recommendations for birds.

Disorders	Recommended dosage (J/cm²)
Integumentary disorders	
Deep wounds	4
Feather disorders	2–3
Lacerations	2
Patagium restriction	4–6
Pododermatitis	3–4
Self-mutilation	2–4
Surgical incisions	1
Thermal burns	1
Musculoskeletal disorders	
Arthritis	4–8
Articular gout	6–8
Edema	1–3
Fractures	4–8
Muscular sprain and strain	4–8
Splayed legs	4–8
Wing tip trauma	1–2
Coelomic cavity disorders	
Ascites	4–6
Gastrointestinal disorders	4–6
Renal disease	4
Miscellaneous	
Neuropathic pain	2

Self-Mutilation

Self-mutilation is a common condition in certain species of bird, and is usually related to underlying stress and other psychological issues. These cases are often aggravated by secondary infections and complications. PBMT can serve as an adjunctive therapy by reducing inflammation and pain at the trauma site and so deterring the patient from further mutilation, as well as by reducing the healing time and minimizing scar-tissue formation. Depending on the depth of the lesions and the severity of mutilation, these cases typically require a moderate target dose of 2–4 J/cm². Self-mutilation cases usually require a minimum of twice-weekly treatment sessions until the healing is complete.

Surgical Incisions

Surgical incisions can be treated postoperatively in birds, as in other species. A single brief PBMT session of approximately 1 J/cm² is usually effective in reducing postoperative pain and speeding the healing process of the surgical wound. Be cautions when hemorrhage is possible, since PBMT increases microcirculation in

tissues, and do not treat over the surgical site from which a malignancy has been removed.

Thermal Burns

Though presentations of thermal burns in avian species will only rarely be seen, such injuries are indications for PBMT being a part of the overall management protocol. A case of extensive skin wound management from burn injuries was treated with 1 J/cm², and a dramatic improvement was noted in the first 48 hours (Zehnder, 2007).

Musculoskeletal Disorders

Arthritis

Arthritis in avian species can develop as a result of age as well as of metabolic dysfunction or trauma. Regardless of the predisposing factors, the pain and inflammation associated with arthritic joints can be managed with appropriate use of laser therapy. A target dose of 4–8 J/cm² is administered as often as once a day in acute cases. Chronic cases may initially be treated several times a week, followed by long-term maintenance treatments every 10–14 days. Most avian cases of arthritis are treated on an as-needed basis once the initial pain and joint restriction are reduced. The ultimate therapeutic goal is management of the arthritic symptoms, but significant improvement in joint function and stability is possible with PBMT.

Articular Gout

Articular gout is a painful and debilitating condition associated with uric acid deposition in the joints of birds. PBMT reduces the pain and inflammation of affected joints, as in other arthritic conditions. In response to treatment, some cases can have a significant decrease in the swelling of joints from uric acid deposition. The target dose for articular gout is generally at the higher end of the arthritic setting recommendations, typically around 6–8 J/cm².

Edema

Edematous swelling is a normal response of the body to injury or inflammation leading to increased fluid in the tissues. Common causes in birds, as in other species, include direct trauma, circulatory constriction, allergy, metabolic disease, and cardiac disease. PBMT relieves the swelling by improving circulation and stimulating anti-inflammatory cascades. Utilizing superficial target doses of 1–3 J/cm² is usually effective in a single or a few PBMT sessions.

Fractures

Fractures in birds tend to heal more rapidly than comparable injuries in mammals, but they can heal quicker still, with less inflammation and pain, when PBMT is incorporated in their treatment (Figure 27.4). Avian practitioners have reported fractures healing in half the expected time when laser therapy was added to the overall fracture-management plan.

(a)

(b)

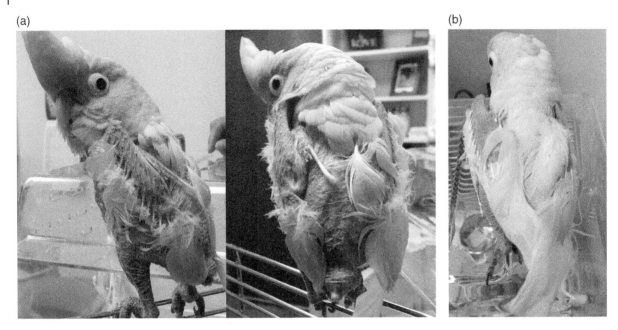

Figure 27.3 (a) Chronic feather plucking in a Goffins cockatoo. Self-induced feather trauma is common in many parrot species. Feather plucking stems from behavioral, homornal, metabolic, and infectious etiologies, which must be addressed to enable a successful resolution. (b) Feather regrowth after several laser therapy sessions. PBMT stimuates feather growth by increasing follicular activity and reducing inflammation of feather follicles. Images courtesy of Dr. Robert D. Ness.

Tibia-tarsal fractures in cockatiels heal within 2–3 weeks when using a laser at $4–6 J/cm^2$ twice weekly for 2 weeks, along with proper splinting of the fracture site. Lower target dosages can be administered more frequently to elicit similar results.

Fractures of the carpus or radius and ulna heal similarly in small to medium-sized birds, while larger parrots and raptors may take an additional week. Depending on the size of the patient and the bone that is fractured, a higher dose of $4–8 J/cm^2$ may be required in some larger birds.

A bill fracture in a duck was managed with a dose of $1 J/cm^2$ administered once daily for 4–5 days. The clinicians reported an increased rate of granulation and overall wound healing during the course of treatment (Zehnder, 2007). A pilot study evaluating the use of PBMT in addition to traditional treatment of bone fractures in wild birds noted that preliminary observations suggested PBMT might be beneficial in promoting bone healing in birds (Desprez *et al.*, 2015).

Muscular Strain and Sprain

Muscular strains or sprains in birds are treated with PBMT as in other mammals, but at a lower target dose. A target dose of $4–8 J/cm^2$ is used. Usually, a single PBMT session will result in significant improvement when administered acutely.

Splayed Legs

Splayed legs can develop in chicks as developmental tendon and ligament deformities from a number of underlying etiologies, including improper nesting material or nest box size, certain mineral deficiencies, and congenital deformities. Many cases also involve bowing and deformity of the long bones in the legs. The addition of PBMT to the treatment plan aids in tendon and ligament stability and function, which in turn aids in realignment of the deviated limbs.

Wing-Tip Trauma

Wing-tip trauma and inflammation are often the result of a startled bird or the consequence of "night fright," when the bird traumatizes its wings by flapping against the bars and cage accessories. The usual soft-tissue trauma of the carpus leads to swelling and inflammation, which are classic indications for PBMT. Many of these cases respond well to just one or two treatments at $1–2 J/cm^2$.

Coelomic Cavity Disorders

Ascites

Ascites is the retention of fluid within the coelomic cavity of a bird when faced with a variety of metabolic conditions. The avian coelom is comparable to the abdomen in mammals, with the distinction that birds do not possess a diaphragm to separate the thorax from the abdomen. Conditions that can lead to ascites in birds include hepatic disease, cardiac disease, and reproductive disorders. Reproductive disorders include egg binding, egg yolk peritonitis, cystic ovary, and ovarian or oviduct neoplasia. Neoplastic disease of any coelomic organ may

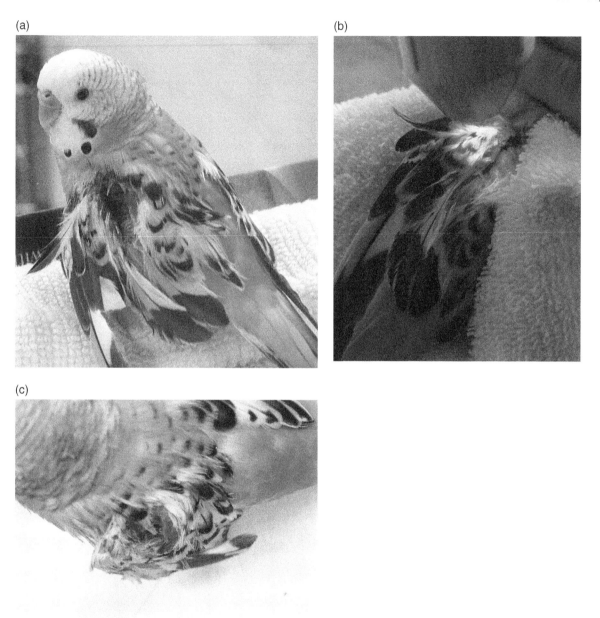

Figure 27.4 (a) Open-wing fracture in a budgerigar, caused by getting its wing caught in the cage bars. This client declined surgery to close the open fracture or amputate the wing. Instead, PBMT, bandaging, and oral medications were chosen for treatment. (b) Application of laser therapy to stimulate fracture repair and wound healing of the injured wing. The wing bandage was removed for laser therapy and reapplied after each session. Another option for bandaged or casted lesions is to leave access windows in the bandage, through which laser therapy can be applied. (c) Good healing response of the fractured wing was present after 1 week and three PBMT sessions. The injury was fully healed and the final bandage was removed in less than 3 weeks after the injury. Images courtesy of Dr. Robert D. Ness.

lead to ascites within the coelom, in which case PBMT may be contraindicated. PBMT is an effective means of aiding fluid resorption in cases of non-neoplastic origin when dosed at 4–6 J/cm². The use of laser therapy on the coelomic cavity highlights the need to establish an appropriate diagnosis prior to treatment. The differentiation between an inflammatory, infectious, or neoplastic process should be established prior to treating coelomic pathology.

Gastrointestinal Disorders

Gastrointestinal disorders in birds often lead to inflammation and distention of digestive organs, particularly the proventriculus, intestines, and cloaca. Conditions that cause dilation of the proventriculus and intestine in birds include food or foreign-body impaction, heavy-metal toxicity, avian gastric yeast, avian bornavirus disease (Piepenbring *et al.*, 2012), and bacterial proventriculitis. Though each of these has different etiologies and treatment plans, they can all potentially benefit from the use of PBMT, especially if inflammation is part of the pathological process. The precise target dose varies depending on the severity and underlying etiology, but typically is 4–6 J/cm^2.

Renal Disease

Little is known about the use of PBMT in cases involving renal disease. However, in an experimental study in which chicken kidney tissue was insulted with the potent toxin 2,3,7,8-tetrachlorodibenzo-p-dioxin (TCDD), PBMT treatment with 670 nm light at 4 J/cm^2 resulted in a significant benefit in the renal tissue. The results of this study suggest that 670 nm PBMT may be useful as a non-invasive treatment for renal injury resulting from chemically induced cellular oxidative and energy stress (Lim *et al.*, 2008).

Similarly, in another toxicity study (dioxin and TCDD) conducted on developing chicks in the egg, it was shown that embryonic growth and hatching of the chicks was positively influenced in the 670 nm phototherapy treatment group. The therapy resulted in earlier pip times (a small hole created 12–24 hours prior to hatch) and an increased hatchling size and weight in the 200 parts per thousand dioxin dose group (Yeager *et al.*, 2006). While these studies explore the effects of PBMT in an experimental setting, knowledge of these data might be valuable when confronted with a clinical case of renal toxicity.

While the beneficial effect of PBMT is of value in the developing chick exposed to a variety of toxins, evidence also exists of its benefit in the normally developing avian embryo. Third-week mortality rates were decreased during the developmental phase when fertile chicken eggs were treated once a day from embryonic days 0 to 20 with 670 nm LED light at a fluence of 4 J/cm^2 (Yeager *et al.*, 2006). This study might be of interest to avian breeders, especially when dealing with endangered species. It found that there was a 41.5% decrease in mortality rate in the light-treated chickens overall. In addition, body weight, crown–rump length, and liver weight increased as a result of the 670 nm phototherapy. Light-treated chickens pipped earlier and had a shorter time between pip and hatch (Yeager *et al.*, 2006).

Miscellaneous

Neuropathic Pain

The importance to the efficacy of treatment of using the appropriate dose and wavelength was recently demonstrated in a clinical case involving the management of suspected neuropathic pain in a prairie falcon, using a multimodal approach (Shaver *et al.*, 2009). Initially, the falcon was treated with a very low dose (<5 mW, 630–680 nm, 5-second application per site) directed to the skin wounds and healed metacarpus once daily. The falcon failed to improve, and changes to the overall management plan were made. One adjustment was to increase the treatment parameters to a higher dose and longer wavelength (1040 mW, 830 nm, 2 J/cm^2). Clinical signs improved immediately. While in this case the changes in treatment were multimodal (medications were changed as well), the role of the increased and more appropriate laser dose may have been part of the more effective treatment.

One author reported improvement in multiple avian patients affected with multiple inflammatory conditions (Gordon, 2011). Unfortunately, the specific settings of the treatment regimens were not provided. It is important to be precise when recording treatment settings in order to duplicate findings in future patients.

Conclusion

This chapter has summarized the current knowledge on the use of PBMT in the avian patient. Many disorders common in avian medicine have been presented; however, this is not an exhaustive list of conditions that may benefit from PBMT. In fact, virtually any condition that benefits from analgesia, anti-inflammation, and accelerated rate of healing may show improvement with PBMT. The authors hope the information provided here will encourage and stimulate the use of PBMT in avian patients. When applying this modality, the authors encourage detailed documentation of treatment parameters, including the wavelength and dose (J/cm^2), in order to standardize treatment and facilitate communication between clinicians. With proper documentation, evaluation of effectiveness and meaningful recommendations can continue to be made.

References

Blair, J. (2013) Bumblefoot: a comparison of clinical presentation and treatment of pododermatitis in rabbits, rodents, and birds. *Vet Clin North Am Exot Anim Pract.* **16**(3):715–735.

Desprez, I. *et al.* (2015) Potential benefit of low level laser in fracture healing in birds an initial assessment.

Proceedings of the I-CARE Conference. April 18–23. Paris.

Gordon J. (2011) Cold laser therapy (3LT) in the management of avian inflammatory conditions. *Proceedings of the Association of Avian Veterinarians Conference.* August 6–12. Seattle, WA.

Lim, J. *et al.* (2008) Attenuation of TCDD-induced oxidative stress by 670 nm photobiomodulation in developmental chicken kidney. *J Biochem Mol Toxicol.* **22**(4):230–239.

Myakishev-Rempel, M. *et al.* (2012) A preliminary study of the safety of red light phototherapy of tissues harboring cancer. *Photomed Laser Surg.* **30**(9):551–558.

Ness, R.D. (2015) Laser therapy in avian patients. *Proceedings of the Association of Avian Veterinarians Conference.* August 29–September 2. San Antonio, TX.

Piepenbring, A.K. *et al.* (2012) Pathogenesis of avian bornavirus in experimentally infected cockatiels. *Emerg Infect Dis.* **18**(2):234–241.

Ritzman, T.K. *et al.* (2015) Therapeutic laser treatment for exotic animal patients. *J Avian Med Surg.* **29**(1):69–73.

Santana-Blank, L. *et al.* (2012) Concurrence of emerging developments in photobiomodulation and cancer. *Photomed Laser Surg.* **30**(11):615–616.

Shaver, S.L. *et al.* (2009) A multimodal approach to management of suspected neuropathic pain in a prairie falcon (*Falco mexicanus*). *J Avian Med Surg.* **23**(3):209–213.

Yeager, R.L. *et al.* (2006) Brief report: embryonic growth and hatching implications of developmental 670-nm phototherapy and dioxin co-exposure. *Photomed Laser Surg.* **24**(3):410–413.

Zehnder, A. *et al.* (2007) Physical rehabilitation in exotic species. *Proceedings of the Association of Avian Veterinarians Conference.* August 5. Providence, RI.

28

Laser Therapy for Reptiles

Jörg Mayer[1] and Robert D. Ness[2]

[1] *Department of Small Animal Medicine and Surgery, University of Georgia, Athens, GA, USA*
[2] *Ness Exotic Wellness Center, Lilse, IL, USA*

Introduction

Very little is documented scientifically concerning the effect and efficacy of photobiomodulation therapy (PBMT) in reptiles. Most of the evidence in this subset of the exotic patient population comes from personal experience, which is shared at conferences or in Internet forums. At first glance, this may seem to devalue a clinician's expertise and reasoning, but "... evidence-based medicine (EBM) requires the integration of the best research evidence with our clinical expertise and our patient's unique values and circumstances" (Straus *et al.*, 2005). Veterinarians have modified this definition slightly to describe evidence-based veterinary medicine (EBVM), since animal patients cannot communicate their values to us: "EBVM is a process of clinical decision-making that allows veterinarians to find, appraise, and integrate current best evidence with individual clinical expertise, clients' wishes, and patients' needs" (Schmidt, 2007). A good understanding of the basic treatment principles and laser mechanics is valuable when starting to treat reptiles, as very little scientific and peer-reviewed material is currently available.

Nardini and Bielle (2011) point out that the wavelength used during treatment has significant implications. In their opinion, 685 nm light is very helpful for treating superficial and fresh wounds of the skin, exposed organs following carapacial fractures in chelonians, and lesions on the oral and cloacal mucosa. By contrast, 830 nm light can be employed to reach deeper tissues, such as pericloacal tissues in chelonians, in order to reduce swelling after bite trauma or, in the case of granuloma, before surgery.

Precautions and Contraindications

Safety precautions must be observed for all species when utilizing therapeutic lasers, as with any form of medical therapy. Most of the precautions and contraindications discussed regarding reptiles are extrapolated from dog and cat recommendations, with modifications for skin characteristics and general metabolic differences. In general, the frequency of treatment in reptiles is lower than in mammals due to their relatively slower metabolic rate.

Because of the near-infrared wavelength of therapeutic lasers, regulatory agencies require that protective eyewear, calibrated to the proper wavelength, be worn during treatment to prevent injury to the retina. Everyone in the room, including the patient, must have their eyes protected, since there is a risk of retinal damage both from direct exposure to the laser beam and from reflective scatter of the laser light. The patient's eyes are protected simply by covering them with a dark cloth or towel.

Due to the inherent power of some therapy lasers relative to the small size of many reptile species, extra care should be exercised when using these devices in these patients. Smaller patients require a lower therapeutic dosage, which is accomplished by modifying the delivery mode, power, or time (Table 28.1). A pulsed delivery can be utilized instead of a continuous one to reduce the rate of delivery by 50% (assuming a 50% duty cycle). Similarly, a lower energy dose can be delivered by decreasing the treatment time or the laser power.

Overheating of the skin is a potential risk of improper operator technique. The pigments in darkly pigmented skin and shells absorb photons, increasing the chances of

Table 28.1 Laser therapy dose recommendations for reptiles.

Disorders	Recommended dosage (J/cm^2)
Integumentary disorders	
Abscesses	6
Blister disease	1–2
Deep wounds	6–10
Lacerations	5–10
Rodent bites	10
Pododermatitis – superficial	1–2
Pododermatitis – deep	4
Surgical incisions	5
Thermal burns – superficial	1–2
Thermal burns – deep	8–10
Oral disorders	
Stomatitis	0.5–1.0
Musculoskeletal disorders	
Arthritis	6
Fibrous osteodystrophy	8–10
Fractures	8–10
Muscular sprain and strain	4–8
Spondylosis	7–10
Coelomic cavity disorders	
Ascites	6–8
Egg binding or retention	4–6
Constipation and regurgitation	4–10
Inappetence	4–6

overheating, and thus require caution in the dosing and administration of PBMT. Running a finger behind the laser beam over the animal is encouraged, as the operator will immediately feel the temperature of the skin and scales as the laser handpiece is moved. If anything other than a pleasant, gentle warming is noted, the handpiece should be moved more quickly, the power reduced, or the spot size enlarged.

Contraindications to PBMT are generally a result of prudence rather than clinical data. A current recommendation is that treatment over malignancy sites be considered contraindicated, but some studies suggest PBMT may have an inhibitory effect on some cancerous tissue in mammals (Myakishev-Rempel *et al.*, 2012; Santana-Blank *et al.*, 2012). The risk/benefit ratio has to be considered for each case, because the analgesic and anti-inflammatory effects of the treatment may be of greater benefit than the risk of stimulating a cancerous growth (e.g., the benefit of the analgesic property might outweigh the risk of complicating a case of osteosarcoma).

It is recommended that prolonged treatment be avoided over certain endocrine organs, such as the thyroid gland and gonads, even though there are minimal and contradictory data suggesting an adverse effect to these tissues.

Metal implants do not absorb photons, but they do reflect them back into tissues that are more superficial, so the dose of energy applied to tissue directly over metallic implants, such as bone plates or screws, should be reduced.

Since PBMT increases microcirculation in tissues, treatment of actively hemorrhaging tissue is discouraged.

For an in-depth discussion of contraindications, see Chapter 7.

Clinical Indications

Integumentary Disorders

Abscesses
Abscesses heal more rapidly when treated with PBMT, which is important in reptiles, where infections generally take longer to heal then in other species. A deep wound setting of approximately 6 J/cm^2 can expedite recovery when used in conjunction with appropriate antimicrobial therapy. As expected, smaller and more superficial abscesses can be treated at lower therapeutic doses than deeper lesions, which may penetrate beyond the skin and immediate superficial tissues.

Blister Disease
Blister disease is a form of dermatitis caused by poor hygiene and humidity. It is often complicated by secondary infection of the skin lesions if not addressed early. This condition can be resolved with PBMT at superficial wound settings of 1–2 J/cm^2 if treated in the early stages, or as high as 6 J/cm^2 with complicated deep lesions. With correction of the causative environmental issues and prompt attention using PBMT, these cases may resolve within three sessions.

Deep Wounds
In a recent publication, the use of laser therapy was described in a soft-shelled tortoise with deep severe dermal ulceration (Kraut *et al.*, 2013). Some of the cutaneous lesions were locally treated with laser therapy every fourth day (with a wavelength of 980 nm, continuous wave (CW), using a non-contact delivery at a power of 2.0–2.5 W). Laser therapy was performed starting at three applications of 10 seconds per lesion, with a break of a few seconds to avoid heating the tissue and a power of 2 W. It continued with a power of 2.5 W and 40 seconds (two applications of 20 seconds) per lesion. These power levels were used with a defocusing handpiece held 10 cm from the irradiated surface. The authors refrained from any topical treatment of the lesions to avoid falsification of the results of laser therapy. They concluded that on comparing the healing processes by inspection, the irradiated lesions of the carapace, leg, and plastron

showed a subjectively better and faster improvement than the untreated ones.

Lacerations

Skin lacerations from traumatic injuries can be effectively addressed with PBMT. The successful treatment of two skin lacerations in turtles has been reported (Pelizzone *et al.*, 2014), where treatments were applied by means of a diode laser with a wavelength of 808 nm CW. In both patients, the healing was complete, without any side effects. The authors conclude that the use of lasers has contributed to a 25% reduction in their reptile patients' recovery time.

Rodent Bites

Rodent bites are the result of clients feeding live prey to their snakes (Figure 28.1). The bites can lead to severe damage of the skin and musculature. These patients are treated with PBMT as deep wounds with settings up to 10 J/cm². Recovery is more rapid and complete with the use of PBMT in conjunction with appropriate antibiotic therapy and wound dressing.

Pododermatitis

Pododermatitis in lizards and tortoises can be addressed using PBMT, as in other species. Superficial lesions can be treated with target doses of 1–2 J/cm², while deeper, contaminated wounds may require at least 4 J/cm² for effectiveness.

Surgical Incisions

A study was recently conducted in ball pythons (*Python regius*) to determine the effects of a therapeutic laser on first-intention incisional wound healing (Cole *et al.*, 2015). It looked at whether incisions treated with PBMT would heal more rapidly and with less histologic reaction (reduced inflammation, necrosis, and edema) than untreated control incisions. The results showed no significant difference in wound healing between incisions treated with a therapeutic laser and controls; however, there were lower gross wound scores and an increase in collagen deposition in the laser-treated incisions on day 14. In this study, treatment consisted of a power output of 0.5 W for 90 seconds once daily for seven consecutive days. The dose delivered to each incision was 5 J/cm², with a wavelength of 980 nm CW. The authors acknowledge that it is possible that the protocol used in this study was insufficient because of a possible greater reflection or absorption of photons by reptilian scales. A problem with this study is that each animal was treated and no true controls were used to assess the healing effects.

With laser treatment, it has been shown that if an area is treated locally, certain systemic effects can be observed in distant areas. A study in rats showed that the application of laser directly to standardized skin wounds stimulated their healing, as well as the healing of wounds distant from the point of application (Rodrigo *et al.*, 2009). The authors noted that wounds located where the laser was applied had the worst mean ranks of healing, while those in the intermediate position had the best. In conclusion, a systemic effect of laser was found in the wounds located most distal from the point of laser application on the third postoperative day.

One of the authors of this chapter (Mayer) has been conducting a study on wound healing in iguanas, which uses a true control group (i.e., instead of using each animal as its own control) because of the previously mentioned systemic effects on local laser therapy. At the end of the study, it was noted that wounds treated with laser at 10 J/cm² were significantly smaller than those treated at 5 J/cm². On day 14, wounds treated at 10 J/cm² were significantly smaller than those treated with a topical ointment. Based on these results, it may be suitable to treat skin wounds in iguanas with a laser at 10 J/cm².

Thermal Burns

Thermal burns are commonly encountered in reptiles, particularly snakes, resulting from direct contact with

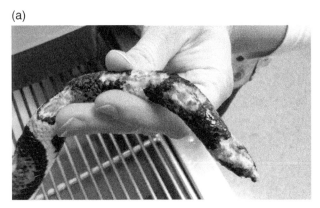
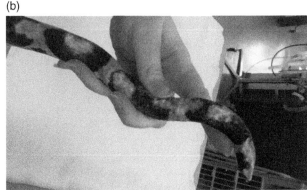

(a)   (b)

Figure 28.1 (a) Rat bite wounds on the tail of a boa constrictor, caused by leaving a live rat in the snake's enclosure. (b) Relatively rapid healing of the rat-bite lesions after three sessions of laser therapy administered over 2 weeks.

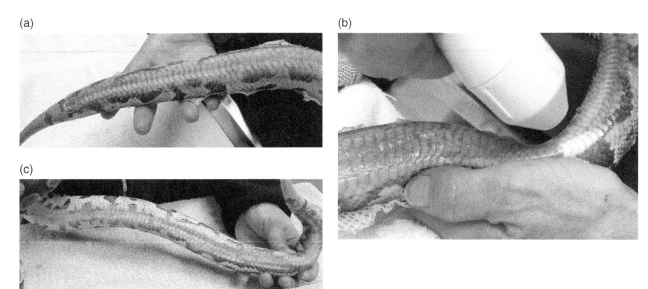

Figure 28.2 (a) Thermal burns on the ventral aspect of a ball python, caused by contact with an exposed healing element in its cage. (b) Laser therapy being administered at 2 J/cm² to the burn area. (c) Resolution of the thermal burns after two laser therapy sessions administered 1 week apart.

heating elements or uncovered flooring with under-tank heating (Figure 28.2). These lesions can vary from superficial discoloration to full-thickness third-degree burns. PBMT is quite useful in speeding the healing process and reducing inflammation when administered at from 1–2 J/cm² for superficial lesions to 8–10 J/cm² for deep, extensive wounds. These cases normally take months to resolve with standard treatment protocols; when PBMT is added to the regimen, they may resolve within several weeks, with a typical 25–30% decrease in overall healing time.

Oral Disorders

Stomatitis

Stomatitis can be a symptom of a simple localized infection or an indication of a much more serious systemic illness in reptiles. Therefore, proper diagnostics and systemic therapy are indicated in these cases. However, most instances of stomatitis can be positively affected by PBMT, which reduces the inflammation and relieves the painful effects of the gingival lesions, leading to more rapid return to eating. A superficial therapeutic dose of 0.5–1.0 J/cm² is usually effective in reducing inflammation and healing the gingiva.

Musculoskeletal Disorders

Arthritis

Arthritis occurs in reptiles, just as in other species, but it often manifests itself more slowly and at a later stage in life. PBMT at around 6 J/cm² can reduce swelling and inflammation in the reptile's joints, thereby increasing its mobility. Pain management in reptiles is difficult to assess and treat by conventional means, so PBMT offers an additional way

of addressing this problem. Though research is lacking concerning the analgesic effects of PBMT in reptile species, there is extensive data indicating that PBMT can reduce the pain and inflammation in arthritic joints in other species (Brosseau *et al.*, 2000; Carlos *et al.*, 2014; Fukuda *et al.*, 2015; Peimani and Sardary, 2014; Wang *et al.*, 2014).

Fibrous Osteodystrophy

Fibrous osteodystrophy in reptiles is commonly referred to as "metabolic bone disease." The typical cause is a deficiency of calcium or vitamin D3, or both, in the diet, or a lack of proper UV-B lighting, leading to nutritional secondary hyperparathyroidism. A related condition is renal secondary hyperparathyroidism caused by underlying renal disease, which typically occurs in older reptiles. Common clinical signs include osteomalacia of the jaw and long bones, angular limb deformities, pathologic fractures, and seizures. Addition of PBMT at fracture settings of at least 8–10 J/cm² can help strengthen bone integrity and speed recovery in these patients.

Fractures

As in other species, fracture repair in reptiles is augmented by PBMT. Reptiles heal more slowly than their avian or mammalian counterparts, but typically their fractures heal 25–30% quicker with PBMT than without. A target dose of 8–10 J/cm² is a good starting point for fracture repair, but this depends on the general health status of the patient and the severity and characteristics of the fracture. Pathologic fractures should be treated with higher target doses then traumatic fractures, since the body must overcome the deficiency in integrity and bony foundation.

Muscular Strain or Sprain

Muscular sprains and tendon and ligament strains can be a challenge to diagnose effectively in reptiles. Since they are poikilothermic, they do not elicit the characteristic elevation in temperature with inflammation within the strained or sprained soft tissue. PBMT can be utilized at approximately $4J/cm^2$ in cases where the clinical maniestation suggests sprain or strain.

A box turtle presented to one of the authors (Ness) with the inability to extend her left hind leg to ambulate (Figure 28.3). She was evaluated radiographically to rule out a fracture, a dislocation, or a mass. Since the problem appeared to be of soft-tissue origin, a presumptive diagnosis of a sprain was made. The client declined PBMT at initial evaluation. The patient was treated with an injection of buprenorphine for analgesia, followed by daily administration of meloxicam as an anti-inflammatory for 10 days. Upon re-check examination, minimal improvement was seen in the use of the left hind leg. PBMT was then permitted by the owner, and administered at $8J/cm^2$. Significant improvement in the turtle's mobility was reported 3 days later, with normal extension of the hind limb. Some persistent limping then resolved over the next few days.

Spondylosis

Spondylosis and spondylitis are described in reptiles as spinal arthritis caused by a number of contributing factors. Applying PBMT at similar target dosages to other forms of arthritis can elicit clinical results. A rainbow boa diagnosed with spondylitis was given treatment starting with meloxicam and tramadol, which had limited positive effects on the animal. The snake did not start to eat or move around normally, and it would strike when touched in the affected area. Laser therapy (1500 J)

was applied to the affected area. There was an 80–90% improvement within just three treatments, and the animal began moving more normally the following week and eating normally again. In addition, the animal could be handled without striking or biting. Once the laser treatment was stopped, the patient relapsed to the original clinical signs. Medical therapy was started again, but it was noticed that the animal was only about 50% better. Laser treatment was initiated again, which completely restored its behavior to normal. The patient has been managed for a long time without any negative side effects (Stremme, 2012).

Coelomic Cavity Disorders

The coelom in reptiles, like birds, is equivalent to the combined thoracic and abdominal cavity of mammals, in that reptiles lack a diaphragm to separate these two regions. In addition, the reptile's organs are modified to accommodate the longer and narrower body cavity. Therefore, PBMT of the body cavity of reptiles is different from that of mammals. Calculation of the therapeutic laser dosage for a general coelomic disorder would include measurement of the entire body cavity. Similarly, PBMT of a gastrointestinal issue might include the entire coelom, whereas a specific lung or urinary bladder condition might only involve laser treatment of that particular portion of the coelom. This differentiation must be considered when utilizing therapy laser software protocols that are designed to treat the entire coelomic cavity, in order to calculate an accurate dosage (Figure 28.4).

Ascites

Ascites is a consequence of osmotic difference caused by a circulatory disorder, hepatic disease, neoplasia, or other metabolic imbalance. PBMT can assist in the

(a)

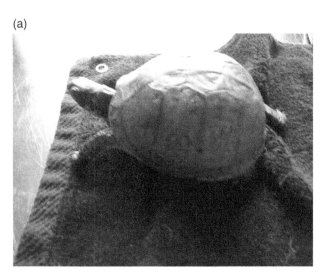

(b)

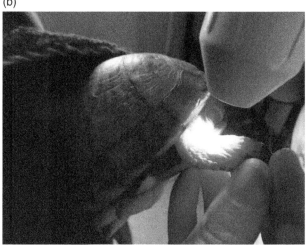

Figure 28.3 (a) Sprained leg in a box turtle exhibiting lameness of unknown origin. (b) Laser therapy was administered to the lame leg at $8J/cm^2$. The lameness resolved after treatment and the turtle resumed normal function within 1 week of the application of PBMT.

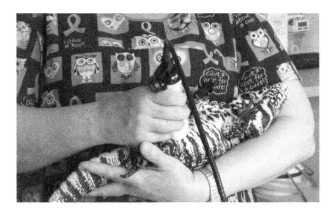

Figure 28.4 Calculation of the therapeutic laser dosage for a general coelomic disorder would include measurement of the entire body cavity. A lung or urinary bladder condition might involve laser treatment only of that particular portion of the coelom, and the therapeutic laser dosage would thus be lower than for the entire coelomic cavity.

dispersal of excess intracoelomic fluid in most of these disorders, except neoplasia. Therefore, if neoplasia has been ruled out, instituting a PBMT protocol is indicated. Typical target dose settings of at least $6\,J/cm^2$ can facilitate the resorption of fluid. Further diagnostic and theraeutic regimens must be employed to address the etiologic component.

Egg Binding or Retention

Egg binding or retention is seen in certain reptile species, including various lizards, terrapins, and snakes. Extrapolating from studies on the effects of PBMT on fertilized bird eggs, there would appear to be no ill effect on the reptile egg when PBMT is used on the gravid female. By reducing inflammation, the gravid patient may more successfully lay her eggs after a PBMT session at $4-6\,J/cm^2$.

Gastrointestinal Disorders

Gastrointestinal disorders such as vomiting, maldigestion, and constipation may improve with PBMT application, depending on the underlying cause. If inflammation is a factor in the clinical presentation, then PBMT is likely to be beneficial. Target dosages of $4-10\,J/cm^2$ have been implemented with positive results in patients with constipation and regurgitation. In addition, snakes and lizards with inappetence have shown increased appetite after a single session of PBMT at $4-6\,J/cm^2$, though other cases have showed no response. Of course, identification and treatment of the underlying medical factors and environmental issues are vital in eliciting a positive outcome.

Miscellaneous

In the scientific literature, multiple studies have reported the use of therapeutic laser therapy for the treatment of a variety of inflammatory responses, including to snake venom (Aranha de Sousa *et al.*, 2013; Nadur-Andrade *et al.*, 2012). Dourado *et al.* (2003) showed that laser therapy was effective in the reduction of myonecrosis after injection of *Bothrops moojeni* snake venom, while Barbosa *et al.* (2008) reported that laser therapy significantly reduced the edema and leukocyte influx induced by *B. jararacussu* snake venom when the muscle was irradiated with a dose of $4.2\,J/cm^2$ from a semiconductor laser operating at 685 nm. This anti-edematogenic action was magnified when laser and antivenin therapies were used together. For an in-depth discussion of publications concerning the effect of PBMT on snake envenomation and current recommendations for treating snakebites, see Chapter 12.

Conclusion

As with all other species, virtually any reptile condition that benefits from analgesia, reduced inflammation, and increased speed of healing can improve with PBMT. The information provided here is intended as a starting point from which to expand the use of PBMT in reptilian patients. When applying this modality, the authors encourage detailed documentation of treatment parameters, including the wavelength and the dose (J/cm^2), in order to standardize treatment and to facilitate communication between clinicians. As with much of reptile medicine, further research about the use of PBMT in reptiles and clinical documentation of results is needed if we are to better serve these patients.

References

Aranha de Sousa, E. *et al.* (2013) Effects of a low-level semiconductor gallium arsenide laser on local pathological alterations induced by *Bothrops moojeni* snake venom. *Photochem Photobiol Sci.* **12**(10):1895–1902.

Barbosa, A.M. *et al.* (2008) Effect of low-level laser therapy in the inflammatory response induced by Bothrops jararacussu snake venom. *Toxicon.* **51**(7):1236–1244.

Brosseau, L. *et al.* (2000) Low level PBMT for osteoarthritis and rheumatoid arthritis: a metaanalysis. *J Rheumatol.* **27**(8):1961–1969.

Carlos, F.P. *et al.* (2014) Protective effect of low-level PBMT (LLLT) on acute zymosan-induced arthritis. *Lasers Med Sci.* **29**(2):757–763.

Cole, G.L. *et al.* (2015) Effect of laser treatment on first-intention incisional wound healing in ball pythons (*Python regius*). *Am J Vet Res.* **76**(10):904–912.

Dourado, D.M. *et al.* (2003) Effects of the Ga-As laser irradiation on myonecrosis caused by *Bothrops moojeni* snake venom. *Lasers Surg Med.* **33**(5):352–357.

Fukuda, V.O. *et al.* (2015) Short term efficacy of low level PBMT in patients with knee osteoarthritis: a randomized, placebo-controlled, double-blind clinical trial. *Revista Brasileira de Ortopedia.* **46**(5):526–533.

Kraut, S. *et al.* (2013) Laser therapy in a soft-shelled turtle (*Pelodiscus sinensis*) for the treatment of skin and shell ulceration. A case report. *Tierarztl Prax Ausg K Kleintiere Heimtiere.* **41**(4):261–266.

Myakishev-Rempel, M. *et al.* (2012) A preliminary study of the safety of red light phototherapy of tissues harboring cancer. *Photomed Laser Surg.* **30**(9):551–558.

Nadur-Andrade, N. *et al.* (2012) Effects of photobiostimulation on edema and hemorrhage induced by *Bothrops moojeni* venom. *Lasers Med Sci.* **27**(1):65–70.

Nardini, G. and Bielli, M. (2011) Low Level Laser Therapy (LLLT) in Reptile Medicine. *Association of Reptilian and Amphibian Veterinarians.* August 6–12. Seattle, WA.

Peimani, A. and Sardary, F. (2014) Effect of low-level laser on healing of temporomandibular joint osteoarthritis in rats. *J Dent (Tehran).* **11**(3):319–327.

Pelizzone, I. *et al.* (2014) Laser therapy for wound healing in chelonians: two case reports. *Veterinaria (Cremona).* **28**(5):33–38.

Rodrigo, S.M. *et al.* (2009) Analysis of the systemic effect of red and infrared laser therapy on wound repair. *Photomed Laser Surg.* **27**(6):929–935.

Santana-Blank, L. *et al.* (2012) Concurrence of emerging developments in photobiomodulation and cancer. *Photomed Laser Surg.* **30**(11):615–616.

Schmidt, P.L. (2007) Preface. *Vet Clin North Am Small Anim Pract.* **37**(3):xi–xii.

Straus, S.E. *et al.* (2005) *Evidence-Based Medicine: How to Practice and Teach EBM*, 3 edn. Elsevier, Philadelphia, PA.

Stremme, D.W. (2012) Confessions of a therapy laser neophyte. *Vet Practice News.* **24**(3):20.

Wang, P. *et al.* (2014) Effects of low-level PBMT on joint pain, synovitis, anabolic, and catabolic factors in a progressive osteoarthritis rabbit model. *Lasers Med Sci.* **29**(6):1875–1885.

29

Laser Therapy for Aquatic Species

Donald W. Stremme

Academy of Natural Sciences of Drexel University and AQUAVET & Cornell University College of Veterinary Medicine, Cape May Beach, NJ, USA

Introduction

How does one define an aquatic species? As an organism that lives in water all or most of its life. This includes fish (teleosts and chondrichthyes), aquatic invertebrates (e.g., cephalopods, sea stars, jellies, sea cumbers), aquatic reptiles (e.g., turtles, sea snakes, marine iguanas), aquatic birds (e.g., penguins, ducks, other anseriformes), amphibians (e.g., frogs, salamanders), and aquatic mammals (e.g., cetaceans, beavers, pinnipeds).

There are almost unending possibilities for the administration of laser therapy to aquatic species.

Utilizing laser therapy as a part of standard veterinary care in aquatic practice has generated notable clinical results for me. The most noteworthy include:

- Improvement in chronic conditions such as osteoarthritis and degenerative joint disease in older penguins.
- Commencement of free movement, cessation of striking of the handler, and resumed eating 24 hours after administration of laser therapy to a rainbow boa (*Epicrates cenchria*) with severe spondylitis.
- Good response in traditionally non-responsive disorders such as head and lateral line erosion (HLLE) when laser therapy is applied either alone or in conjunction with a traditional pharmacological treatment plan.

Safety Concerns and General Treatment Guidelines

Safety

The treatment guidelines and safety procedures of importance in the treatment of aquatic species are very similar to those of importance in the treatment of domestic and companion animals. General safety guidelines are discussed in depth in Chapter 4. However, there are several unique challenges when applying laser therapy to fish, and safety procedures are more difficult to accomplish.

Eye protection is a challenge, since aquatic species are often treated in a water environment. When treating any patient in or around water, you must provide eye protection for both the patient and all other people and animals within the nominal ocular hazard zone.

When treating a fish at the surface of a tank, consideration should be given to the reflection of light both from the surface and from the bottom of the tank. Both of these reflective surfaces endanger the aquarist's and the therapist's eyes, as well as the patient's opposite eye.

Aquatic animals are often kept in group situations and are often difficult to isolate for treatment. Inadvertent ocular exposure to the others in the group is a concern; therefore, isolate the patient whenever possible.

The safety of treating the gonads is discussed in Chapter 7. Current information suggests that excessively high doses should not be applied directly into the gonads. In some aquatic species, the gonads take up a lot of the coelomic cavity, and care must be taken to avoid prolonged exposure during treatment of nearby tissues.

General Treatment Guidelines

Application of laser therapy can be achieved using either a point-to-point or a scanning technique, depending on the equipment being used. Point-to-point application is self-explanatory. Therapy is applied in one area, and then the handpiece is moved to another and the therapy repeated. Scanning is normally at a rate of 6 cm/sec or faster, depending on the settings. Irrespective of the equipment being used, ensure that the correct dosage is administered during each treatment. Modify the administration technique to facilitate this goal.

More laser energy is absorbed in pigmented areas, resulting in more tissue warming. When you apply laser therapy over these areas, it is prudent to utilize a slightly different technique. With both application techniques, it is easy to have one of your fingers remain in direct contact with the skin, feathers, or scales at all times, serving as a constant temperature monitor to ensure patient comfort. If more than comfortable warming is noted while scanning, move the handpiece at a faster rate, reduce the power output, or use a pulsed delivery. The same principles apply when using a point-to-point technique.

An example of the adaptation required when treating aquatic species is the treatment of a penguin with black and white feathers. The feathers cannot be removed, yet sufficient energy must pass through them to obtain the desired clinical result in the target tissues. A faster scanning speed should be utilized over the black feathers than over the white. If the scanning speed is not sufficient, the patient will "feel" the treatment and move. The administration parameters must be adjusted to nullify this sensation (Figure 29.1).

Many patients react to treatment when they recognize the new sensory stimulus of tissue warming, even if it is not painful. For this reason, many patients seem to be more comfortable and more receptive when the handpiece is placed in contact with the skin, feathers, or scales, which creates a more familiar sensation. This may not always be possible, and some species, such as snakes, seem to be more comfortable when they are not being touched. Though at first patients may move or twitch due to the sensory sensation of heat or of being touched, they learn to recognize these sensations and relax.

When treating either fish or snakes, it is important consider the scales. There are issues regarding light reflection and penetration with these structures. Though it is normally important to administer the laser therapy beam perpendicular to the tissue, you often have to change the angle of administration to achieve the best penetration under and around the scales. The thicker the scale, the less penetration can be achieved through it; also, there will be more light reflection when scales are lighter in color. Increase dosages to balance for incidental losses of photonic energy when treating patients with scales.

When treating regular skin (no scales), administer the appropriate dosage at different angles and in a perpendicular fashion to the target tissues. Visualize the anatomy of the target tissue during administration. Administer horizontally and vertically at right angles, then diagonally, and end with a circular motion. Visualize where the light is going in the tissue to facilitate accurate administration and photon permeation of the target tissue.

When handling fish and amphibians, care must be taken not to inflict any damage to their delicate skin, or to the mucus ("slime") layer present on most fish. Efficient and successful treatment can often be accomplished while the patient is partially immersed in water within a shallow container. In some cases, treatment is facilitated by sedation. These patients tend to have thinner skin, so consider a reduction in the dosage needed to penetrate to deeper target tissue.

Always protect the laser therapy equipment from potentially damaging moisture. It is prudent to use a cover over the delivery handpiece. This must be cleaned immediately after each use. The bigger issue is splashing water reaching and thus possibly damaging the laser unit itself. A solution is to use large, very clear plastic bags to cover the unit very loosely. This will keep the device dry while still allowing the air circulation that prevents overheating. These covers can be used several times and replaced when necessary (Figure 29.2).

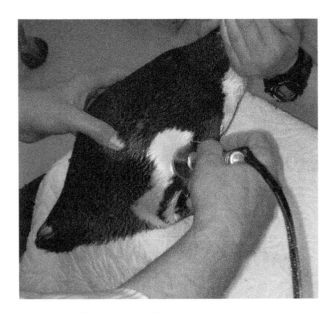

Figure 29.1 Administration of laser therapy to a penguin.

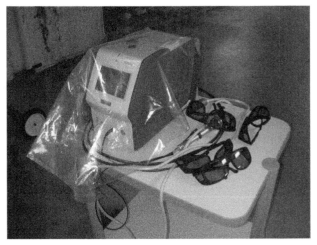

Figure 29.2 Protective plastic cover to prevent water splashing on the laser.

Expect the Unexpected When Treating Aquatic Species

Some species of trematode parasitize the superficial tissue of stingrays. Infected stingrays rub against the substrate, resulting in lesions, which often require antibiotic treatment. Of course, removing the parasites is the main treatment goal (usually with a treatment bath). It is usually not possible to remove them permanently, as eggs in the main system are practically impossible to destroy. Since laser therapy accelerates wound healing (Avci *et al.*, 2013; Peplow *et al.*, 2010), it has been applied to these lesions in an attempt to stimulate the healing process. I have noted an added benefit: a large number of the parasites will move into the treated areas. Logic suggests that this is because of the increase in local blood circulation stemming from the laser therapy (Larkin *et al.*, 2012). This is an unexpected bonus, as it leaves the parasites localized and thus more easy to remove after therapy.

As with domestic animal patients, a physical examination should be completed and a diagnosis reached before initiating laser therapy. An aquarist once presented an emperor angelfish (*Pomacanthus imperator*) with obvious HLLE lesions to me, but balked at the request to do a physical exam (which would require sedation), believing it an unnecessary procedure. When permission was finally granted, I found masses on the gills. Needle aspirates showed acid-fast rods, making this a likely diagnosis of mycobacterial granulomas, a non-treatable condition. This fish had an underlying disease, which may or may not have been the cause of the HLLE lesions (a discussion beyond the scope of this chapter). In any case, it was not likely it would respond to laser treatment, since it had a chronic untreatable condition. The decision was made to not treat this patient.

Dosage and Frequency of Administration

General Dosage Guidelines

Use species-specific software protocols if they are available in the therapy laser equipment being used. Alternatively, since software protocols are not available for all aquatic species, use easy-to-adjust formulas to deliver appropriate doses.

For superficial lesions the size of the palm of your hand, set the power at 3 W, use continuous-wave (CW) emission, and apply for 2.5 minutes. This will deliver a dose of 450 J to an area approximately 100 cm², resulting in an appropriate superficial-condition dose of 4.5 J/cm². If the area is twice that size, double the time and apply evenly over the entire target area.

If the lesion extends deeper (e.g., 2–3 cm) into the tissue, set the power output at 4–5 W, use CW emission, and apply for 3 minutes to an area of approximately 100 cm². This results in an appropriate deeper tissue-condition dose of 7–8 J/cm².

To allow the shortest possible treatment time when treating larger aquatic species, place the laser unit in CW and administer the treatment at the highest appropriate power. Do not hesitate to use lasers that have average power outputs of 15 W or more. Utilizing higher average power outputs will shorten the treatment time. This is a real benefit in larger aquatic patients exhibiting larger lesions, given the difficulties in handling that arise with such patients.

Frequency of Treatment

Acute lesions are initially treated more aggressively. When clinical progress is noted, treatments can be gradually spaced further apart until the lesion is resolved. Treat daily for three to nine treatments, then administer therapy every other day or twice a week until resolved.

Chronic lesions are treated in a similar manner to acute conditions, with the difference that after the treatment goal is reached, treatments are administered periodically to maintain the level of response. Treat three times a week for six to fifteen treatments. Once progress is noted, reduce treatment to twice a week for 2 weeks, then to once a week for 2–3 weeks, then to every other week. Ideally, treatments can then be spaced out to once every 2–3 months, or whatever schedule is necessary to maintain the desired level of clinical response.

Case Studies

Degenerative Joint Disease in an African Penguin

An 18-year-old female African penguin (*Spheniscus demersus*) presented with a chronic limp persisting for nearly a year. A period of trial-and-error treatment was administered, utilizing numerous pharmacological plans. The best response was to a combination of meloxicam, omega-3 fatty acid, and tramadol. Despite these efforts, a significant limp persisted. I referred the penguin for a computed tomography (CT) scan and radiographs, which demonstrated degenerative joint disease of the stifle.

Laser therapy was initiated. Initial treatment was administered cautiously to the stifle area at a low energy level (5 W, CW, 60 seconds, 300 J). No clinical improvement was noted after several treatments. The number of joules and the size of the area treated were increased (proximally and distally to the stifle). After just 2 weeks (four treatments) of treating a larger area at a higher energy level (5 W, CW, 240 seconds, 1200 J), the penguin was walking almost normally for the first time in nearly a year. This case provides an example of the importance of applying laser therapy beyond the focal area of concern.

After responding to laser therapy, the penguin was transitioned to a maintenance phase of treatment about once a month. Medications were gradually reduced: first tramadol, then omega-3, and then meloxicam. As these were removed, there was no increase in limping. The penguin was maintained on laser treatments about once every month or two, without medications.

HLLE

HLLE is a multifactorial condition that produces erosions around a fish's head and lateral line, generally on both sides of the body. The lesions cause disfigurement and make fish less suitable for public display. Many possible causes have been theorized, but treatment is elusive. Moving the animal to a different ecosystem is recommended.

Work has been done to treat HLLE using becaplermin (Adams and Michalkiewiz, 2005; Fleming *et al.*, 2008; Roberts, 2009). Most treatment plans with becaplermin are a one-treatment process and call for topical application and for holding the fish (or the affected part of the fish) out of water for a few minutes. Sometimes, aquarium fish have long-term lesions that do not heal for weeks or months. In order to avoid handling fish, aquarists frequently want to wait to see if they heal on their own.

Before laser therapy was available, I used becaplermin on these lesions when a determination was made to treat such patients. When laser therapy became available, I began treating HLLE with the laser first (treatment based on wound size and depth), and then becaplermin if it was available. My anecdotal observation is that these wounds heal more quickly with a combination of laser therapy and becaplermin than with becaplermin alone.

After my initial successful experience treating HLLE with laser therapy, I conducted a small, informal trial with two purple tangs (*Zebrasoma xanthurum*) with long-term HLLE lesions. One received laser therapy and one served as a control. Nothing was changed about their husbandry conditions or tank mates during the trial. The initial plan was to treat three times a week for 2 weeks, then twice a week for 2–3 weeks, and then to re-evaluate.

These tangs were approximately 12 cm long (fork length: V of the tail to the rostrum). The lesions were on the face, around the eyes and extending down to the mouth, and caudally along the whole side of the fish to the tail on both sides. The HLLE lesions were more narrow (2–6 mm) away from the head.

HLLE is a superficial lesion; therefore, the laser was set at 4 W, CW for 90 seconds, delivering 360 J to the entire target area on the fish. Therapy was administered for 20 seconds per side on the lateral line lesions and another 25 seconds per side on the face, around the eyes

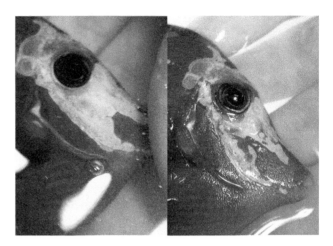

Figure 29.3 HLLE lesions in a purple tang before and after multiple laser therapy treatments.

and mouth, for a total of 45 seconds, or 180 J per side. Treating the face required care, since the dark cloth protecting the eyes had to be repositioned to expose areas to be treated while continuing to protect the eye.

The initial plan was to treat three times a week; however, due to staffing issues, the fish only received treatment twice a week. The control animal was handled the same as the treated fish (timing of anesthesia, physical handling including eye covering, use of a laser handpiece that emitted only a red directional light for the same amount of time, recovery period). There was little to no change on the control animal, but the treated animal had noticeable improvement (HLLE lesions shrinking and becoming pigmented) after just four treatments (Figure 29.3). The staffing issues became critical and I was asked to stop treatment. However, I was able to do a few more treatments and doubled the time to 4 W for 180 seconds, or 720 J for the whole fish. The conclusion was that the lesion would heal completely with laser alone, but due to the staff shortages, therapy was discontinued before this was accomplished.

Non-Healing Wound in a Stingray

A similar protocol was utilized in a case involving a freshwater stingray (*Potamotrygon motoro*). It had a "chronic" wound that was not healing after 2 months. The aquarist only allowed one handling episode, for an exam and treatment under anesthesia. Though it was not ideal to be limited to one treatment opportunity, laser therapy was administered, followed by becaplermin injections. The wound began healing very quickly and was completely healed in 4 weeks (Figure 29.4).

Stomatitis in a Savannah Monitor Lizard

Successful treatment of stomatitis in a savannah monitor lizard (*Varanus exanthematicus*) was accomplished by

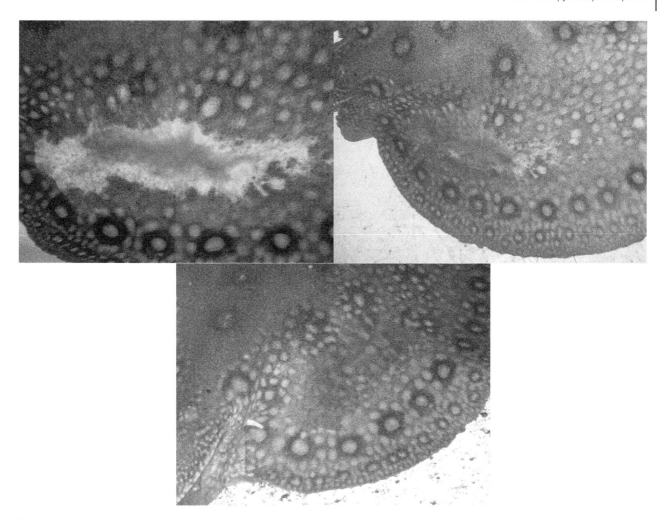

Figure 29.4 Chronic, non-healing wound in a stingray. Clockwise from upper left: before laser treatment, after 5 days, after 1 month.

applying laser therapy externally to the oral cavity. Like a domestic cat with stomatitis, the patient was reluctant to have its mouth opened for an exam, let alone for treatment. It was also not eating. I elected to start laser therapy before other treatment modalities because of the difficulty in administering oral medications. Treatment was accomplished externally utilizing minimal restraint. This resulted in no apparent discomfort or stress to the patient. Soon after treatment, the patient began to eat. This response allowed the deduction that the laser treatment was alleviating pain, as has been documented in other species (Chow *et al.*, 2011).

Initially, only the laser was used (no antibiotics or other medications). It was set at 5 W, CW, 180 seconds, and 900 J, and treatment was administered every other day. After just two treatments, a 40% improvement was observed. At this point, the patient allowed gentle opening of the mouth to administer oral antibiotics. After ten treatments, an 80% clinical improvement was noted. Both the laser and the antibiotics were discontinued and the patient continued to heal to resolution.

Spondylitis in a Rainbow Boa

Aquatic snakes are common species in aquarium displays. As with other species, arthritic changes can occur in their spinal joints, and laser therapy is a viable option in such cases.

As an example, laser therapy was very effective in the treatment of a terrestrial rainbow boa (*Epicrates cenchria*) I diagnosed with severe spondylitis. Previously, this patient had been only minimally responsive to oral and injectable meloxicam and enrofloxacin. The animal presented with a history of striking and biting (something new) and inappetence for several months. It had a firm 20 cm-long, 4–5 cm-thick cylindrical swelling about one-third of the body length from the rostrum. The animal was in so much pain that it was tensing, and the area of interest felt like a solid mass. Radiographs showed this area had extensive spondylitis and ruled out a mass. The remainder of the snake's spine had no significant lesions (Figure 29.5).

The patient refused to eat and handling was apparently painful, so oral medications were almost impossible to

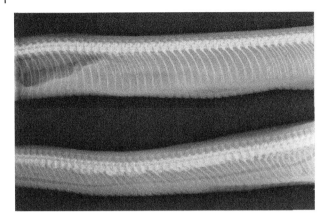

Figure 29.5 Normal spine (top) and spondylitis (bottom) in a rainbow boa.

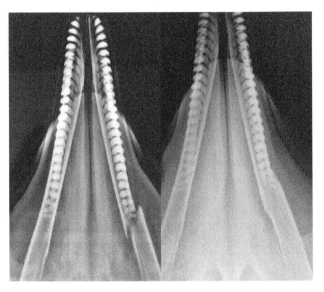

Figure 29.6 Radiographs of a fractured dolphin mandible (left) depicting a small, solid, homogenous callus after laser therapy and healing (right).

administer. The injections of meloxicam and enrofloxacin were also minimally helpful and continued to make the behavior worse. I made the decision to initiate laser therapy.

The target area on the boa was about 20 cm in length, extended down the sides of the snake from the dorsum to the lateral processes (4–5 cm), and was approximately 1 cm deep. Taking the scales into consideration, treatment of the spine was accomplished from the dorsal aspect, then from side to side (180° in an arc) at an angle to the skin matching the direction of the scales. The laser was set at 5 W CW, and therapy was administered for 5 minutes (300 seconds). This resulted in 1500 J being administered to the entire area. The handpiece was angled from 90 to 30° in reference to the skin, with particular attention paid to applying the laser beam nearly parallel to the alignment of the scales along the skin.

The snake would strike when handled due to apparent pain, so therapy was applied with no restraint. A black cloth was positioned over the head to provide protection to the eyes. The patient immediately sensed the application of the photonic energy and started to move away from the stimulation. The head was held to protect the therapist from being bitten and to allow accurate delivery of the therapy. There was a significant and immediate clinical improvement. The keeper estimated there was about a 60% improvement in the way the snake moved immediately after treatment. The patient stopped striking and began eating the very next day.

The client was advised to repeat this treatment three times a week, but could only comply with a twice-a-week schedule. The second treatment required no restraint. Treatment was accomplished with the patient lying in its large carrier, with only a black cloth over the head to provide eye protection. The client reported an 80% improvement after the second treatment, and 90% after the third. Therapy was continued twice a week for two more weeks.

At that point, the patient was eating, allowing handling, and not striking at all.

The patient started striking again 2 months later. Treatment was resumed twice a week. Again, the patient responded and returned to a comfortable level after six treatments. The maintenance treatment plan involved monthly treatments in an effort to avoid any relapses. This plan was successful, and the animal continued to eat, not strike, and readily allow handling.

Mandible Fracture in a Dolphin

Dr. Leonardo Ibarra reported by personal communication the results he had when using laser therapy to treat a dolphin that suffered from a traumatic jaw fracture (Figure 29.6). The fracture was where the bone of the body of the mandible is thinnest, just distal to the angle. Historically, these types of fracture do not heal well, and they usually develop huge callouses.

Treatment of the fracture followed reduction of the fracture by hand. There was no stabilization other than repositioning. Laser therapy was initiated with a treatment every other day for four sessions. The laser was set at 4 W CW for 180 seconds, which resulted in a delivery of 720 J. Application to the fracture site was accomplished using a non-contact technique circumferentially around the mandible, with a portion of the energy being applied from the buccal side. After the initial four sessions, the power was increased to 6 W and the same target area was re-treated for 2–3-minute sessions (720–1080 J) every other day. This fracture healed better than expected, with a small homogenous callus.

Oral SCC in Cetaceans

Cetaceans (whales, dolphins, and porpoises) occasionally present with oral squamous cell carcinoma (SCC) or other cancerous lesions. These malignancies can sometimes be resected, but the animals then stop eating due to pain. My experience with other animals suggests that laser therapy may provide these patients with much needed palliative pain management during healing.

Conclusion

Laser therapy has a diverse range of applications within the aquatic practice. Though little has been published concerning laser therapy treatment of aquatic species, anecdotal reports and the evidence and experience from treating other species indicate that treatment is appropriate. Recording clinical results – both successes and failures – and comparing these findings throughout our profession is essential to the expansion of knowledge about how best to use laser therapy in treating aquatic species.

References

Adams, L. and Michalkiewiz J. (2005) Effect of Regranex Gel concentration or post application contact time on the healing rate of head and lateral line erosions in marine tropical fish. *IAAAM 36th Annual Conference Proceedings*. International Association for Aquatic Animal Medicine. May 14–18. Seward, AK.

Avci, P. *et al.* (2013) Low-level laser (light) therapy (LLLT) in skin: stimulating, healing, restoring. *Semin Cutan Med Surg.* **32**(1):41–52.

Chow, R. *et al.* (2011) Inhibitory effects of laser irradiation on peripheral mammalian nerves and relevance to analgesic effects: a systematic review. *Photomed Laser Surg.* **29**(6):365–381.

Fleming, G. *et al.* (2008) Treatment factors influencing the use of recombinant platelet-derived growth factor (Regranex®) for head and lateral line erosion syndrome in ocean surgeon fish (*Acanthurus bahianus*). *J Zoo Wildl Med.* **39**(2):155–160.

Larkin, K. *et al.* (2012) Limb blood flow after class 4 laser therapy. *J Athl Train.* **47**(2):178–183.

Peplow, P.V. *et al.* (2010) Laser photobiomodulation of wound healing: a review of experimental studies in mouse and rat animal models. *Photomed Laser Surg.* **28**(3):291–325.

Roberts, H. (2009) *Fundamentals of Ornamental Fish Health*. John Wiley and Sons, New York.

30

Zoological Applications of Laser Therapy

Liza Dadone[1] and Tara Harrison[2]

[1] *Cheyenne Mountain Zoo, Colorado Springs, CO, USA*
[2] *North Carolina State College of Veterinary Medicine, Raleigh, NC, USA*

Introduction

While laser therapy is increasingly utilized in domestic species and in private practice (Saunders and Millis, 2014), most zoo veterinarians have not yet started to use this treatment modality. As of March 2016, at least 10 of the 233 Association of Zoos and Aquariums (AZA) (www.aza.org) accredited zoos and aquariums in North America owned Class 4 therapeutic lasers (R.J. Riegel, pers. comm.). This is less than 2% of all North American zoos (if non-AZA zoos and sanctuaries are excluded). In comparison, close to 20% of veterinary hospitals in North America were estimated to be using therapeutic lasers in 2015 (Pryor and Millis, 2015). It is unknown how many other types of non-surgical laser devices are currently used in AZA zoos and by non-AZA zoos and sanctuaries. While zoo veterinarians may have less access to therapy lasers, many zoos could collaborate with local veterinarians to utilize both this equipment and their local expertise.

Laser therapy, also known as photobiomodulation therapy (PBMT), has been shown to reduce inflammation, reduce pain, and promote healing in humans (Pryor, 2009), in laboratory animals, and in some domestic species (Draper *et al.*, 2012; Pryor and Millis, 2015). Currently, there are only a small number of peer-reviewed studies on the efficacy of laser therapy in non-domestic species.

Reports describing the medical benefits of laser therapy in zoo animals are generally anecdotal or difficult to interpret. Due to the complexity of the cases and the high profile of some patients, most receive other treatments concurrently. Sometimes, the underlying cause is undiagnosed and clinicians must focus on treating symptoms. When laser therapy cases appear to be clinically successful, reports do not always publish dosing information.

This makes it challenging to determine whether treatment effects are repeatable. As zoos house a wide variety of species (many of which are endangered), it is impractical, cost-prohibitive, and potentially unethical to perform controlled studies to determine treatment protocols for each medical condition in each species.

Laser therapy is a non-invasive and generally safe treatment modality that might help manage some medical conditions in zoo animals. In some cases, the high conservation value of zoo animals warrants trying off-label treatments. This is similar to how drug doses are often extrapolated across species, as pharmacokinetic studies in zoo species are uncommon. Instead, many drug dosages are based on perceived clinical response, clinical experience, and lack of observable toxicity (KuKanich, 2011). Similarly, the potential benefits of reduced pain and faster healing time may mean that with the incorporation of laser therapy, patients need to be off display for less time and require shorter treatment times with other medications. This benefits the animal's overall welfare and may reduce costs and staff time for the zoo.

As in any species and with any treatment, clinicians should use equipment appropriately and should modify treatments as needed for the case. Safety precautions include always wearing appropriate eye protection when operating the laser and taking care around reflective surfaces. Additional safety measures may be needed to work in close proximity with some zoo species, especially venomous snakes, primates, carnivores, and megavertebrates. Therapy lasers should be used according to manufacturer instructions and treatments should not be directed at eyes or potential sites of cancer, and are generally not recommended for use in pregnant or neonatal animals. For additional information on safety and contraindications, see Chapters 4 and 7.

Special Considerations

The wide range of anatomic difference in zoo species will make it challenging to determine appropriate laser therapy settings for effective tissue penetration. The variability in patient size, skin thickness, coloration, pellage, and depth of target tissues means that species-specific protocols may be needed and that an effective treatment in one species might not be universally therapeutic. In general, longer wavelengths are needed to reach deeper tissues. In human patients, up to 66% of percutaneous laser light energy is absorbed or scattered in the first 2 mm of skin (Esnouf *et al.*, 2007). For a mid-sized dog, the therapeutic window of wavelengths is generally from 600 to 1100 nm; a wavelength of 635 nm might be appropriate for treating superficial wounds, and a longer wavelength of 800 nm would reach most musculoskeletal conditions (Pryor and Millis, 2015). Above a certain wavelength, treatments will not be therapeutic and may inhibit the desired tissue response (Sims *et al.*, 2015). The safety and penetration of laser light through the thick epidermis of reptiles and fish is currently unknown (Rychel, 2011), as is the ability of the therapy laser to penetrate the thick skin of megavertebrates such as elephants.

Similarly, the wide range of anatomical differences may make it challenging to determine appropriate dosing of energy to target tissues. Therapy laser software protocols quantify dosages delivered at the skin surface but cannot measure how much energy is absorbed when deeper tissues are targeted. In humans, superficial tissues with lower protein levels (dermis, epidermis) are typically dosed with $1-4 \text{J/cm}^2$ and deeper tissues or tissues with higher protein content are often dosed with $8-12 \text{J/cm}^2$ (Sims *et al.*, 2015). For a mid-sized dog, a surface contusion would be treated with $2-3 \text{J/cm}^2$, while a deep musculoskeletal condition might require $8-10 \text{J/cm}^2$. Based on what is currently known, when treating zoo animals similar treatment doses will probably be more applicable to treating superficial tissues (e.g., dermal wounds) or when patient size is relatively small (in other words, not an elephant).

Zoos are increasingly using operant conditioning to train for husbandry and medical behaviors. This training could make laser treatment sessions easier to perform, less stressful to the animal, and less time-consuming for zoo staff. For clinical effects, most laser treatments require repeat dosing that decreases in frequency over time. In certain situations, this could require multiple sedations or weekly general anesthesia procedures. Operant conditioning is especially beneficial for patients that are too large or dangerous to restrain manually. It is strongly recommended that zoos invest in staff time to train the animals under their care for stationing or holding near where laser therapy could be used before a medical condition develops, as ill patients and patients in pain may be slower to learn trained behaviors (Dadone *et al.*, 2016).

Management of Cutaneous Wounds

Superficial wounds are relatively accessible for laser therapy treatments and are not limited by challenges related to deep-tissue penetration. In a small study of the effects of laser therapy in multiple cases at one zoo, it was found to be helpful in wound management, more consistently than in the management of lameness or joint pain (Howard *et al.*, 2014). While there are few systematic studies verifying the effectiveness of laser therapy, wound management is likely one of the best clinical applications.

Based on findings in humans and companion and laboratory animals (Kuffler, 2016), it is strongly recommended that surgical wounds in any species be treated with a single laser treatment after they have been closed, both to promote wound healing and to minimize postoperative pain. As always, this would not be recommended for ocular or skin cancer surgeries. One of the authors (Harrison) has instituted the use of laser therapy postoperatively for every surgical procedure in exotic pet species, including rabbits, guinea pigs, and birds. The therapy seems to have subjectively improved healing in these species. Similarly, accelerated wound healing and analgesic benefits have been appreciated when managing a range of trauma cases in zoo patients (E. Lipanovich, pers. comm.).

Birds

Pododermatitis (bumblefoot) in Magellanic penguins (*Spheniscus magellanicus*) showed clinical improvement with multimodal treatments that included photodynamic therapy (laser therapy plus a photosensitizer, PDT). Magellanic penguins with pre-existing advanced pododermatitis underwent surgical debridement of the lesions and were then treated either medically (topical and systemic antibiotics, plus anti-inflammatory medications) or with PDT but no medications (Nascimento, 2015). For the PDT group, the wound was first instilled with an aqueous solution of methylene blue (the photosensitizer) for 5 minutes, then irradiated every 1 cm, with the number of treatment sites varying based on wound size. The wound was treated using a wavelength of 660 nm at a dosage of 133.3J/cm^2 every 3 days for 84 days. Using this protocol, healing rates and average healing times were significantly better for penguins treated with PDT than for those that received medical management. In another study, five Magellanic penguins with previous pododermatitis lesions on their foot pads were treated with PDT. All of the treated lesions regressed and no recurrence was noted during a 6-month follow-up (Sellera *et al.*, 2014).

Chronic pododermatitis in ducks showed similar clinical improvement when treated with laser therapy (Harrison, unpublished results). Clinically, the wounds showed improvement, though the calluses appeared to show slower improvement.

Chronic pododermatitis in a red-tailed hawk (*Buteo jamaicensis*) improved with laser therapy (L. Wright, pers. comm.). After managing chronic non-healing footpad scabs for over 6 months, laser therapy was started. Within a couple months, the wounds had healed enough that the hawk no longer needed bandages on its feet.

A variety of other injuries may heal better when treated with laser therapy. In some raptors with wing-tip lesions associated with edema, avascular necrosis, and dry gangrene, laser therapy may assist in tissue recovery (Lacasse, 2015). Similarly, in a case of a keel wound in a bald eagle (*Haliaeetus leucocephalus*), a faster healing time than expected was seen when laser therapy treatments were incorporated (Cushing *et al.*, 2013).

A distal wing-tip fracture in a dove was initially treated with laser therapy but ultimately required amputation (Harrison, unpublished results). In this case, the fracture site was treated twice weekly for 3 weeks and then weekly thereafter. After the fracture site was surgically removed, laser therapy treatments of the wound were continued, and the wound appeared nearly healed within a week.

Mammals

Pododermatitis in rabbits has been managed with aggressive multimodal therapies, which can include medical and surgical management, bandaging, correction of underlying causes, and laser therapy (Blair, 2015). In one case, a rabbit was dosed with 150 J for each foot lesion. Laser treatments were carried out twice weekly for six doses, in conjunction with topical medications, bandages, and husbandry changes.

A non-resolving scab on the front leg of a hedgehog became markedly worse after a single laser treatment and was then diagnosed as a squamous cell carcinoma (SCC) (L. Wright, pers. comm.). This case highlights the potential risks of treating a chronic wound prior to biopsy, especially in species that may be prone to developing certain types of neoplasia.

Complications from declaw surgeries in both a caracal (*Caracal caracal*) and a serval (*Leptailurus serval*) healed well when management included laser therapy (E. Lipanovich, pers. comm.). Both cats were housed at a sanctuary and had chronic complications and granulomas at the declaw sites. While declaws of large cats is strongly not recommended, in this case surgical removal of third phalangeal bone remnants combined with medical management and laser therapy helped both cats heal superficial wounds and have improved long-term comfort.

Hygromas in three 2-year-old Amur tigers (*Panthera tigris altaica*) were successfully managed using laser therapy (Harrison, unpublished results). All hygromas were present to varying degrees on the elbows bilaterally for each animal (Figure 30.1a). When the hygromas were first seen, husbandry changes were made, but there was no obvious clinical improvement after 1 month. The tigers were target-trained to station in a squeeze chute for laser therapy. They would position themselves between 2 and 4 inches from the side of the squeeze chute and the laser was placed outside of the chute (Figure 30.1b). The laser was used twice a week for 2 months. Application was centered on the hygromas, as

(a)

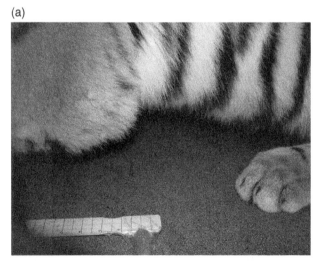

(b)

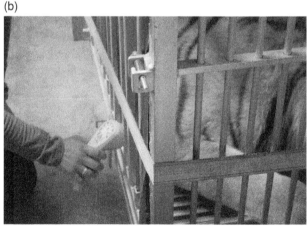

Figure 30.1 (a) Amur tiger hygroma of the elbow prior to laser therapy. (b) Amur tiger in a squeeze chute receiving laser therapy for a hygroma of the elbow. Through operant conditioning and training, it was possible to position the tiger within inches of the squeeze chute bars for closer laser access to the hygroma.

well as acupuncture points LI-11 and SI-9. After starting laser therapy, the hygromas noticeably decreased in size, and they resolved within 2 months.

Elephants

There have been a number of attempts to facilitate wound healing in elephants by using PBMT. In several cases, PBMT has helped with wound healing benefits and has resulted in faster wound healing than expected. At other times, no clinical improvement has been seen. To avoid damaging the optics of the laser unit and maximize the chances for treatment success, it is strongly recommended to avoid using a contact handpiece in a scanning application on elephants (R.J. Riegel, pers. comm.).

Before the increased availability of Class 3 and 4 lasers, pressure sores on the hips of a 58-year-old female Asian elephant (*Elaphas maximus*) were managed using direct-contact infrared irradiation, which was associated with clinical improvement (Gage *et al.*, 1997). Initially, the wounds appeared in areas of devitalized tissue near the ischial tuberosity. Prior to each treatment, the wounds were debrided and gently cleaned. They were treated for 30–45 minutes daily for 60 days, then every other day until the end of the experimental period. Infrared light-therapy pads were applied over cleaned wounds each treatment, and kept moist between treatments using isotonic saline gel. In this case, irradiation of pressure sores seemed to result in faster wound healing than expected, and the clinicians reported that the treatment was notably associated with no wound infections and with a good bed of granulation tissue.

Cheek-patch dermatitis in an Asian elephant (*Elaphas maximus*) improved with therapy laser treatments (Cushing *et al.*, 2013). A schedule of three treatments in the first week, two in the second week, and one weekly thereafter was used in this case. The clinicians reported that this treatment was associated with reduced healing time and inflammation compared with clinical expectations. When a similar protocol was attempted for an African elephant (*Loxodonta Africana*) with cheek-pad dermatitis, no clinical improvement was appreciated (Dadone, unpublished results).

A trunk laceration in an elephant healed rapidly when treated with laser therapy (E. Lipanovich, pers. comm.). A 31-year-old female Asian elephant (*Elaphus maximus*) presented with a large laceration to the distal third of her trunk, possibly caused by another elephant (Figure 30.2). Under standing sedation, the wound was debrided and sutured closed twice in the first week, but dehisced each time and showed signs of infection despite routine wound care and antibiotics. The elephant was sedated again 10 days after the initial injury, the wound was debrided, and laser therapy was started. Bandages were not tolerated by the patient. The laceration was dosed with a mixed wavelength of 808 and 905 nm and $1.2 \, J/cm^2$. Treatments were carried out three times the first week, then twice weekly for 3 weeks, and once weekly for 3 weeks. During the first 3 weeks of treatment, the elephant was also sedated weekly for wound debridement. Within 2 weeks of starting the laser therapy, the wound had excellent granulation and reduced infection, and seemed less sensitive during wound care. About 7 weeks after starting treatment, the laceration had healed and medical management was discontinued. The site of the wound appeared to be slightly lighter in coloration than the other side and had no obvious nerve damage.

Reptiles

Wound healing in bearded dragons (*Pogona vitticeps*) did not show histologic evidence of epithelialization after a single laser therapy treatment (Gustavsen *et al.*, 2013). Two full-thickness 4 mm-diameter punch biopsies were created on the dorsum of each dragon and splinted open to minimize dermal contact. In the study group (n = 5), one wound in each dragon received a single treatment of 4 J of 670 nm light. The wounds from all the study animals were resected *en bloc* for histologic evaluation 4 days after the initial biopsy. Compared with the control group (n = 4), the wound margins were not correlated with epithelialization. While lack of histologic evidence of wound healing may suggest that laser therapy is not a useful treatment modality in bearded dragons, further study could help determine whether faster wound healing occurs closer to the time of a normal shed or with repeat applications of laser therapy.

Septicemic ulcerative dermatitis in a soft-shelled turtle (*Pelodiscus sinensis*) was effectively treated using laser therapy and medical management (Kraut *et al.*, 2013). In this case, the laser therapy treatments were associated with good clinical outcomes for both the skin and the shell lesions.

Shell lesions in a western pond turtle (*Actinemys marmorata*) resolved with laser therapy treatment (Harrison, unpublished results). In this case, chronic shell lesions were associated with excessive algal growth. Laser therapy was performed twice a week for 2 months and then once a week for 2 months. Improvements were noticed in the shell within 1 month, and continued over the 4 months of treatment.

Skin lesions in two mata mata turtles (*Chelus fimbriata*) seemed to heal more quickly than expected when treated with laser therapy (L. Wright, pers. comm.). Both turtles had full-thickness skin lesions in the dorsal skin around the tail and back legs, caused by bite wounds from a pleco fish in the same aquarium. The turtles were moved off exhibit (away from the fish) and medically managed for over 1.5 months, with no clinical change. Laser treatments were then started, and rapid wound

(a)

(b)

(c)

(d)

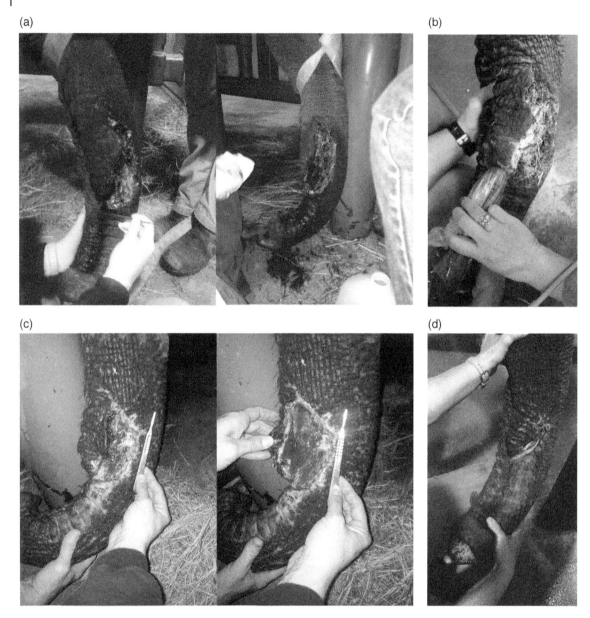

Figure 30.2 Laser therapy helped with wound healing and provided analgesia in an elephant with a trunk laceration. The wound was surgically repaired twice in the first week, but dehisced both times and became infected. Laser therapy began 10 days after initial injury and resulted in complete wound closure within about 6 weeks. (a) Trunk laceration before (left) and after (right) wound debridement on day 10 when laser therapy treatments began. (b) Laser therapy treatment of the contaminated trunk wound on day 19 after injury. Despite contamination, the wound shows some contraction. (c) Wound healing of the laceration on day 26 after injury. (d) Trunk laceration on the final day of laser therapy treatment, 54 days after initial injury. Images courtesy of Dr. Erica Lipanovich.

healing was seen within 2 weeks, but this then slowed and the final stages of wound healing took some time.

Extensive thermal burns in a savannah monitor (*Varanus exanthematicus*) were treated with laser therapy and showed clinical improvement (Cushing *et al.*, 2013). Minimal wound healing was seen in 11 months of routine wound care. The monitor was then treated with laser therapy three times in week 1, twice in week 2, and weekly thereafter. The wound showed considerable improvement to full healing over the next 4 months. No adverse effects were reported.

Management of Neurologic Injuries

Birds

Trauma-induced torticollis in raptors was more likely to resolve in birds treated with physical therapy, sometimes including laser therapy, than with medical management alone (Nevitt *et al.*, 2015). In three cases, laser therapy ($1-2\,\mathrm{J/cm^2}$) was applied to the soft-tissue restrictions to promote muscle relation and improve circulation. The beam of the laser was also focused on the caudal calvarium overlying the cerebellar and vestibular regions of the nervous system. This was done in conjunction with passive range of motion, soft-tissue therapy, and sometimes acupuncture. In this study, all five raptors treated with physical therapy improved clinically to the point that they could be released to the wild, while none of the birds that were not treated with physical therapy were releasable.

Lameness in an ostrich (*Struthio camelus*) was not successfully managed with laser therapy (Harrison unpublished results). Acupuncture and laser therapy were used at Bai hui, BL-40, GB-21, BL-23, and BL-10. The ostrich tolerated the laser therapy well, and no adverse effects were seen. However, it did not show improvement and was euthanized. Post mortem, a femoral fracture was diagnosed.

Mammals

Acute-onset torticollis in a a 2-year-old male reticulated giraffe (*Giraffa camelopardalis reticulata*) showed marked clinical improvement using a combination of medical management, chiropractic adjustments, laser therapy, and range-of-motion exercises (Dadone *et al.*, 2013). During transport between zoos, the giraffe developed a severe mid-cervical segmental torticollis that progressed to focal muscle spasms of the neck, marked neck sensitivity, and decreased range of motion. With the help of operant training, laser therapy was used to manage soft-tissue pain and hypertonicity (Figure 30.3). Laser therapy was applied twice weekly for 4 weeks, with treatments focused over sites of muscle contracture. Sites were treated with a blended wavelength of both 810 and 980 nm, and each treatment site received a total dose of 4800 J. The cervical range of motion was significantly improved in left lateral bending, muscle hypertonicity and contracture were reduced, and the left side of the neck was less sensitive to palpation 1 month after initiation of laser therapy. Therapy was continued once weekly for 9 months. The giraffe continues to be maintained with daily range-of-motion exercises 6 years later, and has sired two calves.

Nutritional metabolic bone disease and subsequent fractures in a 5-year-old spayed striped skunk (*Mephitis mephitis*) were effectively managed with laser therapy (Dadone and Marsden, unpublished results). This former pet developed bilateral femoral fractures and suspected microfractures around the spine, with subsequent hind-leg paresis. Management included analgesics, laser therapy of the lumbar spine region, diet change, and supplemental vitamin D3. The skunk was treated with a blended wavelength of 810 and 980 nm, and was dosed with 8–10 J/cm^2 administered to the lower back, the hips, and the left rear leg. Over several months, the skunk had marked improvement in her gait, radiographic evidence of fracture healing, and improved bone density.

Reptiles

Acute-onset paresis in a Komodo dragon (*Varanus komodoensis*) showed short-term marked clinical improvement with laser therapy treatments to the cervical spine when used with medical management (Dadone, Marsden, and Johnston, unpublished results). A 17-year-old female Komodo dragon presented with mild dragging of a front leg. Within 1 week, she was severely ataxic on all four legs, had difficulty eating, had a visible bend in the proximal neck (Figure 30.4), and had a distended gullar pouch area. Management included broad-spectrum antibiotics, anti-inflammatories, analgesics, heat therapy to the neck, and laser therapy to the neck. Laser treatments were dosed at 25 J/cm^2. Within about 1 week of starting laser therapy, the dragon showed marked

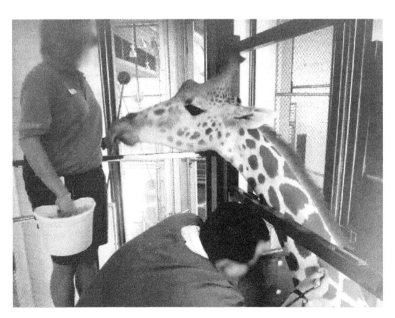

Figure 30.3 A 3-year-old male reticulated giraffe with acute-onset torticollis being treated with laser therapy. In combination with medical management, chiropractic adjustment, and range-of-motion exercises, this giraffe made a full clinical recovery and has since sired two calves. Image courtesy of Raymond Romero, CVT.

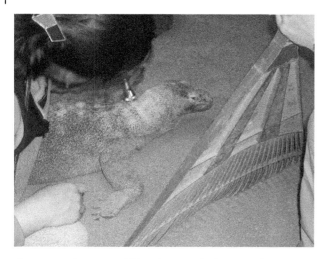

Figure 30.4 A 17-year-old female Komodo dragon with proprioceptive deficits and neck pain being treated with laser therapy for a spinal cord injury associated with cervical instability. The dragon showed marked clinical improvement within 1 week of starting therapy. Prior to this injury, this animal had been managed full contact with the keeper staff, who would carry a rake for protection. Note the dragon's knuckled-over front foot. Image courtesy of Raymond Romero, CVT.

improvement in strength, coordination, and ability to eat, and reduced neck-guarding behaviors. She was found dead 54 days after presentation. Histopathology indicated the cause of death was an egg yolk embolus, potentially unrelated to the suspect spinal cord injury. This case resembles past reports of cervical subluxation and compressive myelopathy in Komodo dragons, which thus far have not been successfully managed with either supportive care or surgical decompression (Zimmerman *et al.*, 2009). The clinical improvement suggests that laser therapy may help manage pain and reduce inflammation in other cases of suspected compressive myelopathy in Komodo dragons.

Laser therapy was attempted on a case of acute-onset torticollis in an Aldabra tortoise (*Centrochelys sulcata*), but treatment was not tolerated by this patient (Johnston, Klaphake, and Dadone, unpublished results). Treatments were targeted to lateral neck muscles that appeared contracted, but the tortoise immediately tried to bite the clinician, so laser treatments were discontinued. Instead, the tortoise was managed with non-steroidal anti-inflammatory drugs (NSAIDs) and range-of-motion exercises. Clinical signs resolved. This highlights the potential significance of anatomic variation in species: in this case, the skin on the lateral and ventral neck palpates thinner than dorsally, and may require a lower dose than a dorsal midline neck lesion.

A spinal cord injury in a bearded dragon (*Pogona vitticeps*) showed clinical improvement with multimodal treatments that included laser therapy (Dadone and Klaphake, unpublished results). A male bearded dragon, estimated to be 11 years old, presented with a lateral

bend in the lumbar spine caused by nutritional secondary hyperparathyroidism and associated hind-leg proprioceptive deficits and constipation. The dragon was started on diet and lighting changes, supervised warm-water soaks, and laser treatments. After starting the laser therapy treatments, the dragon had less constipation, and used his hind legs more normally. After about a year, laser treatment was discontinued, but the dragon became clinically worse so treatments were resumed. Ultimately, the dragon lived three more years from the time laser therapy was started.

Management of Acute and Subacute Musculoskeletal Injuries

Laser therapy has provided inconsistent results when managing lameness and soft-tissue injuries in giraffe (Dadone, unpublished results). In one giraffe with hoof overgrowth, pedal osteitis, and suspected laminitis, laser treatments around the coronary band were not associated with any clinical effect. However, in a different giraffe with front-hoof overgrowth, suspect laminitis, and partial tears of the deep digital flexor tendons, a laser treatment was administered one time to the swollen region below the fetlock during general anesthesia, in conjunction with a corrective hoof trim and digital perfusion of medications. That giraffe had an excellent anesthetic recovery and lameness resolved within days of the anesthesia. During the same anesthesia, the giraffe developed muscle inflammation in one region of the neck. This resolved during anesthesia after repositioning the neck, doing focal tissue massage, administering laser therapy to the site, applying ice, and administering a systemic NSAID.

A closed distal metacarpal fracture in an orphaned newborn mountain bongo (antelope, *Tragelaphus eurycerus isaaci*) was successfully managed with stall rest and laser therapy (Reillo and Clubb, 2015). About 1 week after presentation, laser therapy was applied circumferentially to the fracture site using a wavelength of 635 nm at a dosage of $0.68\,J/cm^2$, daily for 3 weeks. Follow-up radiographs at about 6 weeks and 6 months showed excellent remodeling and lengthening of the metacarpus. Normal walking was observed by day 65, and the calf continued to have no long-term health issues about 1 year later. The authors concluded that these non-invasive management techniques were warranted and effective for this antelope with such high conservation value.

An acute presentation of severe front-leg lameness in an African elephant (*Loxodonta Africana*) was managed with multimodal therapies that included laser therapy, and showed some improvement (L. Wright, pers. comm.). The elephant presented acutely not wanting to bend its elbow and walking with the leg locked ("peg leg"). A wide variety of treatments were utilized, so it is undetermined how significant the laser therapy was in

undetermined how significant the laser therapy was in subsequent improvements to the soft-tissue swelling and the gait.

Laser Therapy and Dental Disease

While laser therapy is increasingly utilized to accelerate healing in human dentistry and is frequently applied in laboratory animal studies (Aoki *et al.*, 2015; Massotti *et al.*, 2015; Matos *et al.*, 2016; Tang and Arany, 2013), it is rarely used to help manage dental diseases in zoos.

Mammals

Necrobacillosis (lumpy jaw) in a Parma wallaby (*Macropus parma*) was effectively treated using a combination of comprehensive endodontic therapy, apicoectomy, and laser therapy (Kilgallon *et al.*, 2010). In this case, an apicoectomy was performed on the mandibular incisor, and laser treatment was applied to the site to decontaminate the pulp cavity and provide anti-inflammatory and biostimulatory effects. Using a wavelength of 810 nm, the pulp cavity and alveolar bone defect were treated with 15 J before starting dental restoration.

In rabbits, photobiostimulation at a site of incisor extraction and dental implant placement promoted new bone formation around the implant (Massotti *et al.*, 2015). In this study, 24 male New Zealand rabbits were randomly divided into four groups, then each had a mandibular incisor extracted and a titanium dental implant immediately inserted. Except for the control group, all rabbits were treated with laser therapy every 48 hours for seven treatments, and then the mandibles were evaluated histologically. Significantly more collagen fibers and bone-to-implant contact were seen in the treatment group that received 20 J/cm^2 each treatment. This helps validate the potential accelerated wound healing but does not quantify any possible analgesic benefits from this treatment. A study in humans did validate a significant reduction in pain, trismus, and swelling in human patients receiving PBMT immediately following mandibular third molar-removal surgery and on the third postoperative day (Abdel-Alim *et al.*, 2015).

Laser Therapy for Chronic Musculoskeletal Injuries

Birds

Chronic leg swelling and fusion ("peg leg") in a Victoria crowned pigeon (*Goura victoria*) improved when treated with laser therapy (L. Wright, pers. comm.). The pigeon had a chronic non-union fracture above the foot with a large fibrous callous and severe osteomyelitis involving the joint. The fracture was over a year old when laser therapy was tried. Laser therapy was associated with reduced swelling of the foot and a return of some range of motion that had not been seen in over a year, but the use of the foot remained limited.

Mammals

Laser therapy has been recommended as a management tool for chronic pain in geriatric mammals (Figure 30.5). In a small trial across multiple species at one zoo, managing lameness or joint pain had inconsistent and sometimes ineffective results (Howard *et al.*, 2014). In geriatric primates, laser therapy is recommended as a treatment option for pain management of osteoarthritis and degenerative disk disease (Boesch, 2012).

Osteoarthritis pain management in a koala was very successful at another institution (P. Bapodra pers. comm.). In this case, medical management was subsequently reduced and laser therapy continued long-term. Lameness in a geriatric goat showed temporary clinical improvement for a couple hours after each laser therapy treatment, but no long-term improvement (L. Wright, pers. comm.). In this case, the goat was treated for osteoarthritis in both front legs for several months, with dosing as recommended by the laser company representative.

Lameness caused by osteoarthritis in a Sicilian burro showed dramatic improvement when treated with laser therapy (Harrison, unpublished results). The burro was diagnosed with severe osteoarthritis of the coxofemoral joint and presented with a marked lameness. The lameness remained severe despite medical management, which included gabapentin and firocoxib. Laser therapy and acupuncture were started. The acupuncture points used were GB-21, BL-23, Bai-hui, Shen Shu, Shen Jiaco, BL-54, ST-31, and SP-11. The laser treatments

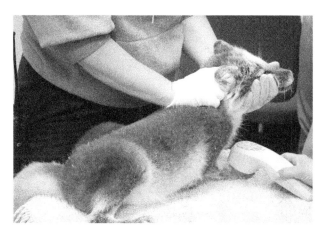

Figure 30.5 Arctic fox receiving laser therapy for chronic osteoarthritis.

were applied at Shen-jiao, BI-23, and BL-54, with aqua-acupuncture with vitamin B12 at Bai-hui, BL-23, BL-18, and BL-54. After two treatments, the burro's lameness was much less severe, so the firocoxib dose was decreased. Additional treatments included hyaluronic acid joint injection and a methylprednisolone acetate injection in the affected coxofemoral joint. With 1 month of all therapies, the burro was off all medications and the lameness had clinically resolved. Though laser therapy was one of multiple therapies, the use of non-steroidal medication could be decreased after only two treatments.

Laser therapy appeared to be ineffective for the management of osteoarthritis of the lumbosacral spine and femoral heads in an Amur tiger (*Panthera tigris altaica*). Based on its gait and radiographs, the tiger was trained to position itself against a fence for treatments, and the laser was angled between wire mesh. The lack of clinical improvement may partly be attributable to the excessive distance between the laser handpiece and the target tissue, inappropriate settings, or the targeting of anatomy that was not causing the most pain. Later, on necropsy, the tiger's osteoarthritis was much more severe than expected, most notably in the cervical and thoracic spine regions. These sites had neither been radiographed pre mortem nor treated with laser therapy. This highlights the importance of a thorough exam and work-up, in order to better localize pathology and sources of pain.

Four adult or geriatric gorillas (*Gorilla gorilla*) were treated with laser therapy for arthritis pain and flare-ups, but it was undetermined if the treatments were beneficial or appropriately dosed (Dave and Leach, 2014). Based on the individual case, treatments targeted arthritis of the hands, elbows, knees, feet, or hips. Treatments were voluntary and depended on trained behaviors to position the gorilla appropriately next to the mesh. Using a non-contact delivery, laser treatments were dosed by extrapolating from domestic species and were administered two to three times the first week, then one to two times weekly to biweekly, and then variably for maintenance (K. Leach, pers. comm.). Variation was seen, with females generally tolerating lower power (5–6 W) and one silverback comfortable with a higher power (8–9 W); this could be related to differences in patient size or sex, or to differences in skin color. Individual gorilla compliance was highly variable, and for some individuals limited mobility related to the joint that the treatment was targeting actually interfered with the ability to position themselves effectively for treatments.

Elephants

Based on an analgesia survey in megavertebrates, a fair clinical response was reported in two Asian elephants treated with laser therapy (Kottwitz *et al.*, 2016). The elephants were dosed at 80 J across four to eight points, administered 3 times weekly for three weeks, then weekly, then every 2 weeks. No additional details were recorded in the survey concerning anatomic location or possible diagnosis in each case.

Laser therapy for soft-tissue swelling and decreased joint mobility in the carpus of an Asian elephant (*Elaphas maximus*) seemed to help more with reducing soft-tissue swelling than with improving range of motion in the leg (L. Wright, pers. comm.). The geriatric elephant had decreased motion of the carpus and generalized swelling of the leg for several years. As part of multimodal treatment, the lower third of the leg was treated twice weekly until a marked decrease in swelling was seen; laser therapy was continued weekly thereafter.

Lameness associated with osteoarthritis of the stifle in an African elephant (*Loxodonta africana*) showed no clinical improvement with laser therapy (Dadone, unpublished results). This was likely due to both an insufficiently low dose and scuffing of the end of the massage ball-type handpiece, caused by the abrasive skin of the elephant. Because of the limited maximum power of the therapy laser used, each stifle treatment for an elephant took about 30 minutes, which could be time-limiting. With newer and more powerful units available, it is possible laser therapy could be an effective treatment for elephant osteoarthritis management, but for now it is unproven.

Reptiles

Limited mobility attributed to extensive spondylosis in a geriatric rosy boa (*Lichanura trivirgata*) was managed with laser therapy, which resulted in improved mobility (L. Wright, pers. comm.). Concurrently, the snake had an anal gland swelling. Laser therapy was targeted to the whole spine and the anal gland swelling. Following laser treatment, the snake resumed climbing and moved better, and the anal gland swelling resolved.

Future Role for Thermography-Assisted Laser Therapy

Ongoing challenges to validating the effectiveness of laser therapy in a zoo setting include accurately localizing the affected anatomy. Thermography aids in localizing surface temperature asymmetries, which may be physiologically significant to the patient. These temperature asymmetries may be related to localized inflammation, poor perfusion, nerve injuries, or other potential abnormalities.

(a)

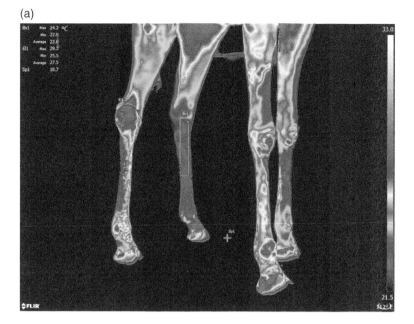

(b)

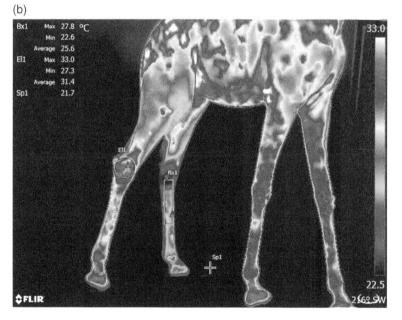

Figure 30.6 Digital thermography can help identify physiologically significant areas of inflammation and help quantify whether laser therapy or other treatments are effective. A 30-year-old female reticulated giraffe presented with a 1.5-year history of soft-tissue swelling of the right lateral hock and severe front-foot hoof overgrowth with intermittent lameness. The giraffe was uncooperative for awake hoof trims and showed minimal improvement with oral medications. (a) Digital thermography imaging confirmed increased heat of the right lateral tarsal joint and decreased heat in the left hind distal limb. (b,c) 3 months later, the giraffe was clinically lame on the front feet; the thermograph shows increased heat in the front legs and more severe temperature asymmetry in the hind legs.

To help assess and quantify the potential benefits of using thermography with laser therapy, a geriatric giraffe with chronic lameness was imaged and then treated with laser therapy (Dadone, unpublished results). A 30-year-old female reticulated giraffe (*Giraffa camelopardalis reticulata*) presented with a 1.5-year history of chronic soft-tissue swelling and an open wound on the lateral tarsal joint (Figure 30.6). Concurrently, this giraffe had chronic hoof overgrowth and intermittent front-foot lameness. Despite an established hoof-work training program, the giraffe stopped participating in any training that involved handling the feet. A range of antibiotics and analgesics were given, but the giraffe stopped cooperating with any hoof work for several months.

(c)

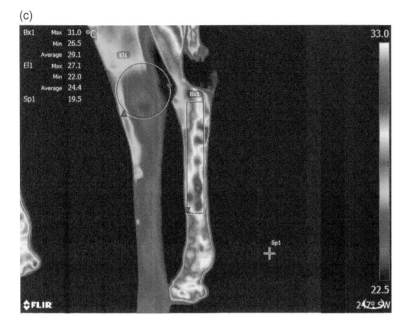

Figure 30.6 (Continued)

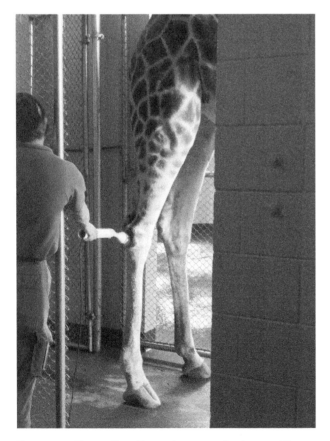

Figure 30.7 The giraffe in Figures 30.6 was trained to stand in a hallway and receive laser therapy to the right lateral hock, with the laser head on a polyvinyl chloride (PVC) pipe extension for staff safety. Within 2 days of starting treatment, the giraffe started cooperating with awake hoof trims.

Voluntary radiographs of the swollen joint suggested cellulitis and only relatively mild arthritis. Thermal imaging showed increased surface temperatures in the right lateral hock, right medial metatarsus, and front feet, plus a marked relative decrease in surface temperatures in the left hind leg (about 6 °C cooler than the inflamed side and cooler than the other legs). These results suggest inflammation of the right hock, laminitis of the front feet, and abnormal circulation or nerve injury to the left hind leg, potentially caused by asymmetric weight distribution at the pelvis.

In addition to continuing medical management, grain was removed from the giraffe's diet and laser therapy was initiated to the lateral right hock. Using a polyvinyl chloride (PVC) pipe extension on the laser unit and maintaining protected contact, the wound and surrounding lateral hock inflammation were treated with about 8000 J three times weekly for 1 month (Figure 30.7). Within 48 hours of the first treatment (only 4000 J), the giraffe started voluntarily participating in corrective hoof trims, suggesting that she was in less pain and possibly weight bearing across her feet more normally. Within several weeks of starting treatment, not only had she cooperated for multiple major hoof trims, but the inflammation pattern was consistently improved on the right hind leg (Figure 30.8). This case suggests that laser therapy can have almost immediate analgesic effects, which may result in more compliant behaviors, and that thermography may help zoo veterinarians better target and quantify the effectiveness of therapy laser treatments.

(a)

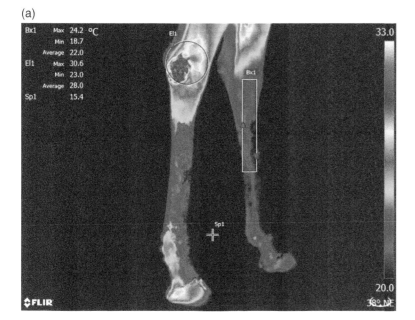

(b)

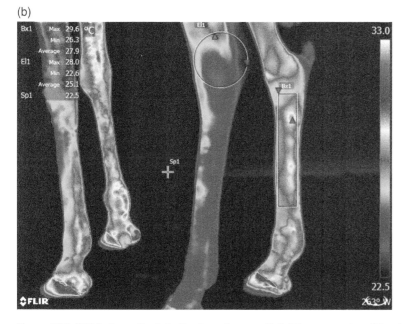

Figure 30.8 Within 1 month of starting laser therapy, digital thermographs of the giraffe in Figure 30.6 showed reduced temperature asymmetries to the hind legs, most notably the right medial metatarsus. At the time of press, treatment was ongoing.

Conclusion

To date, laser therapy has been used relatively infrequently in zoo medicine, but it has helped improve clinical outcomes in some cases that were refractory to medical management. To help improve the efficacy of laser therapy, more studies and widespread reporting of cases are needed. Thermography may also help localize abnormalities, especially in patients that cannot be readily handled or are too large for other types of imaging, and it can help quantify whether clinical improvements are seen with laser therapy and other treatments.

Acknowledgments

Thanks to Drs. Melanie Marsden, Matthew Johnston, Eric Klaphake, and Ron Riegel for helping create zoo laser protocols at Cheyenne Mountain Zoo, to the dedicated zookeepers for training essential medical behaviors, and to the veterinary staff and Raymond Romano for performing laser treatments. Thanks also to the many colleagues who shared cases and advice for this chapter, including Drs. Erica Lipanovich, Lewis Wright, Kate Leach, Priya Bapodra, and Kim Henneman.

References

Abdel-Alim, H.M. *et al.* (2015) A comparative study of the effectiveness of immediate versus delayed photobiomodulation therapy in reducing the severity of postoperative inflammatory complications. *Photomed Laser Surg.* **33**(9):447–451.

Aoki, A. *et al.* (2015) Periodontal and peri-implant wound healing following laser therapy. *Periodontol 2000.* **68**(1):217–269.

Blair, J. (2013) Bumblefoot: a comparison of clinical presentation and treatment of pododermatitis in rabbits, rodents, and birds. *Vet Clin North Am Exot Anim Pract.* **16**(3):715–735.

Boesch, J.M. (2012) Update on primate analgesia. *Proceedings of the Annual Conference of the AAZV.* Oct 21–26. Oakland, CA.

Cushing, A.C. *et al.* (2013) Abstract: The use of class IV laser therapy in zoo and wildlife medicine. *Proceedings of the Annual Conference of the AAZV.* September 28–October 4. Salt Lake City, UT.

Dadone, L.I. *et al.* (2013) Successful management of acute-onset torticollis in a giraffe (*Giraffa camelopardalis reticulata*). *J Zoo Wildl Med.* **44**(1):181–185.

Dadone, L.I. *et al.* (2016) Training giraffe (*Giraffa camelopardalis reticulata*) for front foot radiographs and hoof care. *Zoo Biol.* **35**(3):228–236.

Dave, M. and Leach, K. (2014) Poster: May the Force be With You: Laser Treatment in Gorillas. *2014 International Gorilla Workshop.* June 9–13. Atlanta, GA.

Draper, W.E. *et al.* (2012) Low-level laser therapy reduces time to ambulation in dogs after hemilaminectomy: a preliminary study. *J Small Anim Pract.* **53**(8):465–469.

Esnouf, A. *et al.* (2007) Depth of penetration of an 850nm wave-length low level laser in human skin. *Acupunct Electrother Res.* **32**(1–2):81–86.

Gage, L.J. *et al.* (1997) The use of direct contact infrared irriadiation to aid the healing of pressure sores in elephants (*Elaphus maximus*). *Proceedings of the Annual Conference of the AAZV.* October 26–30. Houston, TX.

Gustavsen, K. *et al.* (2013) Evaluation of low-level laser therapy in a model of cutaneous wound healing in bearded dragons (*Pogona vitticeps*). *Proceedings of the Annual Conference of the AAZV.* September 28–October 4. Salt Lake City, UT.

Howard, L.L. *et al.* (2014). Abstract: Functional assessment and multi-modal approach to pain management in zoo patients. *Proceedings of the Annual Conference of the AAZV.* October 18–24. Orlando, FL.

Kuffler, D.P. (2016) Photobiomodulation in promoting wound healing: a review. *Regen Med.* **11**(1):107–122.

Kilgallon, C.P. *et al.* (2010). Successful treatment of chronic periapical osteomyelitis in a Parma wallaby (*Macropus parma*) using comprehensive endodontic therapy with apicoectomy. *J Zoo Wildlife Med.* **41**(4):703–709.

Kottwitz, J. *et al.* (2016) Results of the megavertebrate analgesia survey: elephants and rhino. *J Zoo Wildlife Med.* **47**(1):301–310.

Kraut, S. *et al.* (2013) Laser therapy in a soft-shelled turtle (*Pelodiscus sinensis*) for the treatment of skin and shell ulceration. A case report. *Tierarztl Prax Ausg K Kleintiere Heimtiere.* **41**(4):261–266.

KuKanich, B. (2011) Clinical interpretation of pharmacokinetic and pharmacodynamic data in zoologic companion animal species. *Vet Clin North Am Exot Anim Pract.* **14**(1):1–20.

Lacasse, C. (2015) Falconiformes (falcons, hawks, eagles, kites, harriers, buzzards, ospreys, caracaras, secretary birds, old world and new world vultures). In: *Zoo and Wild Animal Medicine*, Vol. 8, pp. 127–142. St. Louis, MO.

Massotti, F.P. *et al.* (2015) Histomorphometric assessment of the influence of low-level laser therapy on peri-implant tissue healing in the rabbit mandible. *Photomed Laser Surg.* **33**(3):123–128.

Matos, F.S. *et al.* (2016) Effect of laser photobiomodulation on the periodontal repair process of replanted teeth. *Dent Traumatol.* **32**(5):402–408.

Nascimento, C.L. *et al.* (2015). Comparative study between photodynamic and antibiotic therapies for treatment of footpad dermatitis (bumblefoot) in Magellanic penguins (*Spheniscus magellanicus*). *Photodiagnosis Photodyn Ther.* **12**(1):36–44.

Nevitt, B.N. *et al.* (2015) Effectiveness of physical therapy as an adjunctive treatment for trauma-induced chronic torticollis in a raptor. *J Avian Med Surg.* **29**(1):30–39.

Pryor, B. (2009) *Class IV Laser Therapy Interventional and Case Reports Confirm Positive Therapeutic Outcomes in Multiple Clinical Indications.* LiteCure, LLC, Newark, DE.

Pryor, B. and Millis, D.L. (2015) Therapeutic laser in veterinary medicine. *Vet Clin North Am Small Anim Pract.* **45**(1):45–56.

Reillo, P.R. and Clubb, S.L. 2015. Natural metacarpus fracture remodeling in a bottle-reared mountain bongo antelope calf (*Tragelaphus eurycerus isaaci*) with presumed failure of passive transfer. *Int J Appl Res Vet Med.* **13**(2):89–92.

Rychel, J.K. *et al.* (2011) Zoologic companion animal rehabilitation and physical medicine. *Vet Clin North Am Exot Anim Pract.* **14**(1):131–140.

Saunders, D.G. and Millis, D. (2014). Laser therapy in canine rehabilitation. In: *Canine Rehabilitation and Physical Therapy*, 2 edn., pp. 359–380. Elsevier, Amsterdam.

Sellera, F.P. *et al.* (2014) Photodynamic therapy for pododermatitis in penguins. *Zoo Biol.* **33**(4):353–356.

Sims, C. *et al.* (2015) Rehabilitation and physical therapy for the neurologic veterinary patient. *Vet Clin North Am Small Anim Pract.* **45**(1):123–143.

Tang, E. and Arany, P. (2013) Photobiomodulation and implants: implications for dentistry. *J Periodontal Implant Sci.* **43**(6):262–268.

Zimmerman, D.M. *et al.* (2009) Compressive myelopathy of the cervical spine in Komodo dragons (*Varanus komodoensis*). *J Zoo Wildl Med.* **40**(1):207–210.

Part VIII

Clinical Applications of Laser Therapy in Equine Practice

31

Fundamentals of Equine Laser Therapy

Ronald J. Riegel

American Institute of Medical Laser Applications, Marysville, OH, USA

Introduction

Therapeutic lasers have been utilized in the equine industry for over 35 years. This modality has evolved from the first 1 mW laser of the late 1970's to the ≥30 W equipment available today. New information is being discovered weekly providing a greater insight into broader clinical and regenerative medical applications of laser therapy, or as it now commonly known, photobiomodulation therapy (PBMT). This chapter will address dosages and general application techniques for the treatment of a localized area, its corresponding acupuncture points, and all of its associated compensatory and tertiary areas. It will also look at how this modality can be used in a holistic approach to obtain a consistent clinical response. Fundamental information about the physics, physiological and biochemical events, and general principals of PBMT can be found in the first few introductory chapters of this text.

Patient Preparation

There should be open communication with the owner and trainer. They should understand why you are recommending laser therapy and have realistic expectations as to the clinical outcome. Several important points should always be discussed: there are no side effects, cells that are functioning normally are not affected, and there is no withdrawal time before competition. Realistic therapeutic goals and a treatment plan should be outlined. This will encourage client compliance and understanding.

When laser treatment is administered, the surrounding environment should be relaxed, tranquil, and free of distracting noise. An area that is confined on most or all sides with materials impenetrable to light (e.g., a wash stall) is ideal. This enclosed environment complies completely with laser safety standards. The patient should be hand-held by a person familiar with their mannerisms and behavior. Cross ties are not ideal, but are often necessary when assistance is not available.

The skin must be clean and free of any photo-absorbing materials. Microfiber cloths are useful in removing dirt, sand, and dust. Washing may be required if the animal is particularly dirty or when leg paints, poultices, or ointments have been applied. Ideally, the animal should be dry when applying PBMT, but damp skin has little effect on photonic penetration. Wounds should be cleaned and debrided before the application of PBMT, as these materials will become incidental absorbers of the applied energy.

Safety recommendations should be followed when using any laser system. This is exceedingly important when utilizing any Class 3 or 4 therapeutic system (any therapeutic laser emitting over 0.5 W). Appropriate eye protection should be worn by the therapist, the handler, and the patient before the laser is turned on. Eye protection for the patient is extremely easy: simply use a thick black towel or piece of black felt, folded or doubled over several times. These material eye shields are both simple and very comfortable for the patient. They can be washed or easily discarded and replaced when soiled. Always have assistance when working around the head area so that accidental eye exposure is minimized. Laser safety signage should be in a visible place.

Calming and Sedation

Equines are innately flight-response creatures. The application of laser therapy is a new stimulus in their immediate environment and may evoke nervousness and anxiety. Calm patients by applying a dosage of 50–150 J to the acupuncture relaxation points (Table 31.1, Figure 31.1) (Fuchtenbusch and Rosen, 2006). Each patient responds to this technique differently: some will respond after stimulation of the first few points; others will require administration within the higher range of dosing; still others will not respond at all. This technique is effective about 80% of the time. Good horsemanship is always expected.

Laser Therapy in Veterinary Medicine: Photobiomodulation, First Edition. Edited by Ronald J. Riegel and John C. Godbold, Jr.
© 2017 John Wiley & Sons, Inc. Published 2017 by John Wiley & Sons, Inc.

Table 31.1 Acupuncture points for calming and sedation.

Acupuncture points	Yin Tang, GV 26, CV 24, KI 1, BL 23, LV 3, BL 18, BL 19, SP 6, BL 20, LU 1, LU 11, BL 13

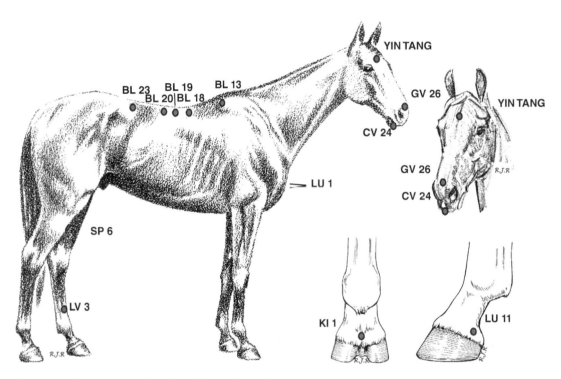

Figure 31.1 Acupuncture points for calming and sedation.

Therapeutic Dosage Considerations

Treatment of a Specific Localized Area

The key to proper dosing is the application of a sufficient number of joules (J) at a therapeutic penetrating wavelength over a specific anatomical area (cm²) to give a sufficient amount of energy at the target tissue to elicit a clinical response. (An in-depth discussion of the terminology and concepts used in PBMT dosing can be found in Chapter 2.)

In review, the formula used to calculate dosage is:

$$\text{dose} = \text{power (watts)} \times \text{time (seconds)} /$$
$$\text{area of treatment (square centimeters)}$$
$$= \text{joules per square centimeter} \left(\text{J/cm}^2 \right)$$

As more research has been published, recommended dosage levels have gradually increased. Table 31.2 gives the current recommended dosages for the treatment of equine species.

Many current therapeutic lasers have highly advanced software that can aid in properly dosing the patient. Considerations are given to the color of both the skin and the hair coat, the length of the hair coat, the body weight, and the anatomical area being treated. Some software even has preset protocols for various specific conditions within each anatomical area. Once the correct data are entered, the software will calculate a dosage, how this dosage should be emitted, the treatment time, and in some instances the correct handpiece to use. Such programs do not cover every disorder, but similar conditions can easily be extrapolated to match the diagnosis. They give you a place to initiate therapy, which can be modified according to the re-evaluation examination before each therapy session.

Treatment of Trigger and Acupuncture Points

Acute myofascial trigger points are areas within the fascia surrounding skeletal muscle that exhibit a painful response upon palpation. They present as palpable nodules within taut bands of skeletal muscle fibers (Travel and Simons, 1999). Pain radiates out from these points and usually follows the orientation of the surrounding muscle fibers.

The ideal therapeutic laser protocol for these points is to treat on-contact with sufficient pressure to release the spasm of muscle surrounding the point and all affected adjoining local areas. The application of

Table 31.2 Equine dosage guidelines.

Application	Dose
Wounds/dermal lesions (lacerations, abrasions, post-op incisions)	$6 \pm 4\,\text{J/cm}^2$
Superficial structures (DDF, SDF, suspensory tendons)	$12 \pm 5\,\text{J/cm}^2$
Deep musculature (thoracolumbar spine, cervical and gluteal muscles)	$25 \pm 10\,\text{J/cm}^2$
Joints (tarsal, carpal, metacarpal, metatarsalphalangeal joints)	$20 \pm 5\,\text{J/cm}^2$
Large joints (femoropatellar and femorotibial joints)	$25 \pm 5\,\text{J/cm}^2$
Unique applications (lumbosacral area, L/S joint, SI joint, and surrounding musculature)	$30 \pm 10\,\text{J/cm}^2$
Trigger points	$4 \pm 2\,\text{J/cm}^2$
Acupuncture points	Superficial 80–200 J/point
	Deep 125–200 J/point

2–$6\,\text{J/cm}^2$ combined with a massage technique yields excellent resolution (Airaksinen *et al.*, 1989).

Performing acupuncture with the stimulatory power of a laser is a patient-friendly and painless alternative to the classic needle. The use of lasers to stimulate acupuncture points is termed "laserpuncture" or "laser acupuncture" (Lorenzini *et al.*, 2010). Laser acupuncture possesses several advantages when compared to classic needle acupuncture (Martin and Klide, 1987; Schoen and Wynn, 1998):

- painless application;
- complication-free;
- short treatment time;
- non-invasive;
- minimal restraint.

Acupuncture will greatly contribute to any rehabilitation protocol by providing relief of pain and an increase in circulation throughout the muscled tissues (le Jeune *et al.*, 2016).

Photonic stimulation of the average-depth needle acupuncture point requires the administration of an irradiated dose of 80–200 J/point. Deeper points – those surrounded by large muscle masses and bone, such as Bai Hue – should be stimulated with a dose of 125–200 J/point (Fuchtenbusch and Rosin, 2006). These dosages should be administered slowly, using wavelengths within the therapeutic window at a low wattage (0.5 W), utilizing a pulsed mode of emission.

The total treatment time per point depends on the average output power setting of the equipment and the depth of the point. Therapy lasers that emit a higher average power output will require less treatment time when treating any point or area than will lower average-power lasers.

When solely using laser acupuncture techniques, versus a localized therapy and complementary acupuncture-point stimulation, the frequency of treatment varies with the severity of the disorder and the compliance of the client. Ideally, treatment frequency would be twice weekly until the therapeutic goal is reached.

A meta-analysis of the human literature on the use of laser acupuncture for the treatment of musculoskeletal pain was carried out by Law *et al.* (2015) and published in the *Journal of Acupuncture and Meridian Studies.* Two-thirds of the studies reviewed (31/49) reported positive effects when dosages were properly reported and the study was of methodological quality. The remaining studies were poorly designed and used much lower dosages. Consistent positive clinical outcomes were achieved after long-term follow-up, rather than immediately after treatment.

Despite the loss of energy as the laser beam passes deeper into the tissue, the stimulatory effect is sufficient even when the acupuncture point is difficult to locate. Precise location of the point is ideal. This will ensure that sufficient energy is applied to the point. Administration on-contact with a circular massage motion and slight pressure is ideal for thorough penetration. A list of important equine acupuncture points, described using Western nomenclature, can be found in Chapter 33.

More data are needed to refine these applications. Parameters such as wavelength, type of emission, and frequency of treatment should be examined to optimize and refine results (Jagger, 1984).

Treatment of Secondary, Tertiary, and Compensatory Areas

Laser therapy should always be applied to the localized area of the diagnosed disorder. When PBMT is also applied to any compensatory secondary or tertiary areas, the clinical results are even more rewarding. This is a holistic approach to these cases, allowing for a quicker recovery or even achievement of a higher or more consistent level of performance. Each secondary or tertiary area has to be identified and then treated as an individual area utilizing a proper dosage, technique, and number of sessions to relieve any lameness or soreness.

General Treatment Techniques

Diagnosis

An accurate diagnosis is essential before initiating PBMT. When treating lameness issues, this diagnosis should include all secondary and tertiary compensatory concerns and all corresponding acupuncture and trigger

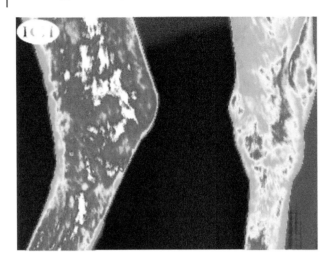

Figure 31.2 Digital thermograph of a right tarsus with an APMLO view. Increased thermal gradients (white and red) should receive special attention while applying PBMT.

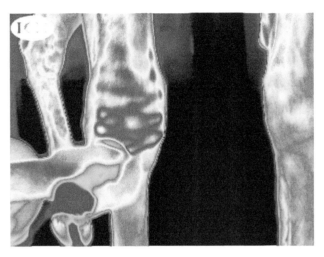

Figure 31.4 Digital thermograph, showing how the application of PBMT can be visualized during administration. The path of increased thermal gradient corresponds to the PBMT application using a scanning technique.

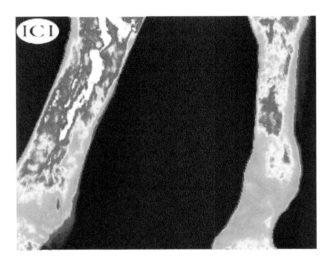

Figure 31.3 Oblique thermographic view of right and left metatarsals. Areas of increased thermal gradient (white and red) should receive thorough examination and be considered for special attention when applying PBMT.

points involved. Utilizing this comprehensive holistic treatment technique will maximize the clinical response. This is also true when treating wounds: compensatory secondary and tertiary areas and wide margins surrounding the area should be identified and included in the therapeutic protocol.

Digital thermal imaging, or infrared thermography, identifies primary, secondary, and tertiary areas of concern, monitors the therapist's technique, and provides a quantitative measurement of the progress of the therapy (Turner, 2001). Before initiating therapy, record a baseline set of images to provide a guide for the application of PBMT. These baseline images are a "road map" of all of the areas that should be considered for treatment (Figures 31.2 and 31.3).

Digital thermographic images can be taken during the therapeutic application (Figure 31.4). This will provide a visual guide that ensures all areas in need of therapy are addressed. These images can also provide a picture of the saturation of the tissues. If the therapy is completed and there is not a sufficient increase or decrease in the circulatory pattern, additional therapy should be administered.

Re-evaluations should be made before the initiation of any subsequent therapeutic laser session. Clinical signs should be noted, such as a decrease in swelling, a lesser degree of lameness, and other indicators of progress or regression. Digital thermal imaging aids in the evaluation of the progression of the case (Figure 31.5). This is not a subjective observation; it is an objective measurement. Subsequent images, when quantitatively compared to the initial images, provide a very accurate guideline for additional therapy. This technology also provides visualization to the owner and trainer of the extent and progression of the case. This is an ideal client communication tool that should be utilized until the issue is resolved.

General Application Techniques

When applying PBMT to any area of the horse, a few key points should be noted:

- Always have complete control of the handpiece.
- Keep the handpiece perpendicular to the skin at all times. Any inclination of the beam will result in an increase in the reflection of the energy.
- Whether the equipment uses a point-to-point or scanning treatment technique, treat on-contact whenever possible. This eliminates a great deal of the reflective loss of energy from the skin, allowing more energy

(a)

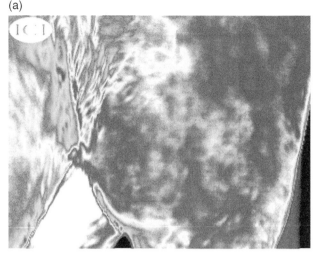

(b)

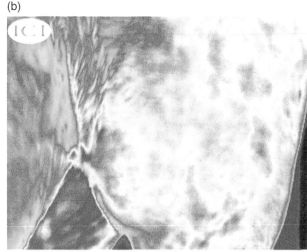

Figure 31.5 (a) Oblique thermographic view of the left stifle before the application of PBMT. Increased thermal gradients throughout the femoropatellar and femoraltibial joints and surrounding soft tissues are present. (b) Oblique thermographic view of the left stifle 24 hours after the last laser treatment. Three treatments were administered: initial, at ~24 hours, and at ~48 hours. The progress of the PBMT can be objectively measured. The increased thermal gradients have resolved and the horse is clinically sound.

to enter the tissues. There is also a blanching of the tissue, which removes some of the blood supply. This removes a percentage of the hemoglobin and oxyhemoglobin that would cause an incidental absorption of energy. The actual amount of this has yet to be determined through research.

- When using point-to-point or scanning application, always drag or place your finger next to the handpiece. This provides an easy temperature monitor of the tissue you are treating.
- Apply therapy at right angles in opposite directions. This allows the energy to be applied evenly throughout the area.
- Your medical records should note the clinical progress of the case, the total number of joules administered to each anatomical area, the specific application technique, and the plan for the following therapy session.

Frequency of Administration

The frequency of administration of laser therapy is unique to each case. It will depend on the patient, client compliance, and the patient's response to the therapy. PBMT is normally applied in three phases:

1) **Induction phase:** An aggressive phase in which therapy is administered on consecutive days or every other day until a significant clinical response is noted.
2) **Transition phase:** Therapy is applied less often until the treatment goal is reached (e.g., twice a week).
3) **Maintenance phase:** Therapy is administered as frequently as needed to maintain the treatment goal or quality of life over a long period.

How these phases are specifically scheduled will depend on whether the condition being treated is acute or chronic:

- **Acute condition:** Treat daily until a significant clinical response is noted. Then, treat at a lesser frequency until the case is resolved.
- **Chronic condition:** Treat every other day for several sessions until a clinical response is noted. Then, treat at a lesser frequency until the therapeutic goal is reached. Thereafter, treat periodically to maintain this therapeutic goal.

Case Study: A Holistic Approach to the Treatment of Cunean Tendonitis/Bursitis – Distal Tarsitis Syndrome

Each laser therapy treatment session should include a localized application over the area of primary concern, treatment of all secondary and tertiary involvements, plus treatment of all trigger points and acupuncture points that are associated with these areas.

Localized Treatment

The entire tarsal area is treated circumferentially with a dosage of $12\,J/cm^2$. Particular attention and individualized therapy are applied to the distal tarsal joint, the cunean tendon, and its corresponding bursa. Even though the hock is a very boney area, contact administration should be utilized whenever possible. This can be given

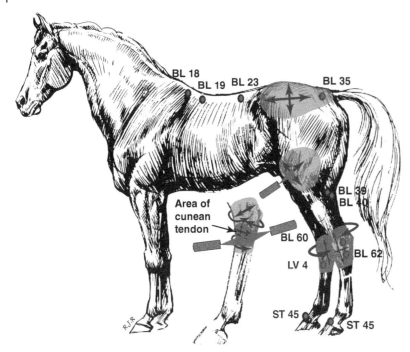

Figure 31.6 Administer PBMT circumferentially and at right angles on-contact throughout all of the anatomical structures of the hock. Address every possible angle to saturate each soft-tissue structure and intra-articular area. Administer a higher dosage to all of the areas of the distal tarsal joint, the cunean tendon, and the cunean bursa lying beneath (darker shaded area on insert). Treatment of all compensatory secondary and tertiary structures, the lumbosacral area, the sacroliliac areas, both hips, both stifles, and the opposite hock should then be accomplished using appropriate dosages for each. Lastly, apply photonic energy to stimulate all complementary trigger and acupuncture points.

Table 31.3 Trigger and acupuncture points for the treatment of cunean tendonitis/bursitis – distal tarsitis.

Trigger points	BL 35 and BL 40
Acupuncture points	BL 18, BL 19, BL 23, BL35, BL 39, BL 60, BL 62, ST 45, LV 4

using either a scanning or a point-to-point treatment technique. If the area is extremely painful, treat off-contact initially, until the immediate analgesic effect allows contact administration.

Therapy should be directed from all angles on the medial side to ensure saturation of the distal tarsal joint and the length of the cunean tendon (see Figure 31.6, and note the darker shaded area on the illustration of the medial hock). It is often easier to administer this from the opposite side of the horse, depending on their temperament. Certain patients will require one of their front legs to be lifted and held off the ground to keep them bearing weight on the hind limb being treated.

Secondary and Tertiary Treatment

If there is an issue with the cunean tendon, there will be a biomechanical strain on at least the unilateral stifle structures. Both stifles should be examined by digital palpation to detect any soreness or swelling within the joints and the surrounding soft-tissue structures. Administer a dosage of $20\,J/cm^2$ on-contact to all identified areas of soreness.

Consider treatment of both hips, the gluteal areas, and the lumbosacral area; essentially, all areas that palpate sore or are identified by other clinical signs should be treated. These deeper target tissues require higher dosages, and a range of $25–30\,J/cm^2$ utilizing on-contact administration should be considered. When possible, utilize digital thermal imaging to identify all anatomical areas that will benefit from therapy.

The ideal treatment would also include all of the tarsal structures on the opposite leg. This joint and the associated soft-tissue structures will be under more weight-bearing stress as the patient compensates for the opposite painful cunean tendon, bursa, and arthritic condition.

Trigger Points and Laser Acupuncture

A dosage of $125–200\,J$ should be administered to all associated acupuncture and trigger points. Typically, these cases involve the points listed in Table 31.3 (Xie and Preast, 2007). Each individual case will have to be assessed, and the proper points chosen.

Conclusion

Fundamental information and application techniques are crucial to consistent clinical results. Consideration of dosages, application techniques, areas of treatment (not just localized areas, but all compensatory areas), and frequency of administration should be given to each individual case. The only explanations for an inconsistent or unsuccessful clinical outcome are that the diagnosis was incorrect, all secondary and tertiary compensatory areas were not identified and included in the treatment, the photonic energy did not reach the target tissues with a significant therapeutic dose, or the therapy was not administered frequently enough.

References

Airaksinen, O. *et al.* (1989) Effects of infra-red laser irradiation on the treated and non-treated trigger points. *Acupunct Electrother Res.* **14**:9.

Fuchtenbusch, A. and Rosin, P. (2006) *Laser Therapy and Acupuncture on Horses: Treatment Protocols.* Fuchtenbusch.

Jagger, D.H. (1984). Alternative veterinary medicine. *Vet Rec.* **114**(17):435.

Law, D. *et al.* (2015) Laser acupuncture for treating musculoskeletal pain: a systematic review with meta-analysis. *J Acupunct Meridian Stud.* **8**(1):2–16.

Le Jeune, S. (2016) Acupuncture and equine rehabilitation. *Vet Clinics North Amer Equine Pract.* **32**(1):73–85.

Lorenzini, L. *et al.* (2010) Laser acupuncture for acute inflammatory, visceral and neuropathic pain relief: an experimental study in the laboratory rat. *Res Vet Sci.* **88**(1):159–165.

Martin, B.B. and Klide, A.M. (1987) Treatment of chronic back pain in horses. Stimulation of acupuncture points with a low powered infrared laser. *Vet Surg.* **16**(1):106–110.

Schoen, A.M. and Wynn, S.G. (1998) *Complementary and Alternative Veterinary Medicine Principles and Practice*, 1 edn. Mosby, Maryland Heights, MO.

Travel, J.G. and Simons, L.S. (1999) *Myofascial Pain and Dysfunction: The Trigger Point Manual*, 2 edn. Lippincott Williams and Williams, Philadelphia, PA.

Turner, T.A. (2001) Diagnostic thermography. *Vet Clinics North Amer Equine Pract.* **17**(1):95–113.

Xie, H. and Preast, V. (2007) *Xie's Veterinary Acupuncture*, 1 edn. Blackwell, Hoboken, NJ.

32

Administering Laser Therapy to the Equine Patient

Ronald J. Riegel

American Institute of Medical Laser Applications, Marysville, OH, USA

Introduction

The application of laser therapy (or photobiomodulation therapy, PBMT) to the equine patient has evolved into both a scientific and clinical evidence-based therapy since its early use in the 1970's. This evolution has occurred with the development of new therapeutic laser equipment capable of delivering photonic energy deep into target tissues, the development of new software providing consistent therapy and current suggested dosages, and better understanding of the importance of power, wavelength, treatment technique, and frequency of application in obtaining consistent clinical results.

In this chapter, we provide an overview of the various anatomical areas, outlining several optimal treatment techniques for each. Current suggested dosages for application to several of the common disorders within each area will be presented, along with suggestions on treatment of the primary, compensatory secondary, and tertiary areas, and the corresponding acupuncture points. (A list of important equine acupuncture points described using Western nomenclature can be found in Chapter 33.) The goal of this chapter is to provide guidance in order to maximize the relief of pain, modulation of inflammation, and the acceleration of the healing processes for our equine patients.

The Head

The number-one concern when applying photobiomodulation therapy (PBMT) to the head is protection of the patient's eyes. This is easily accomplished with thick black cloth or felt. These fabrics can be doubled over to provide excellent protection while still being very comfortable to the horse. Even with this cloth barrier or other protective shielding in place, never expose the eye to the direct beam.

Lacerations in this area are treated as a superficial wound. A dosage of $2-3 \text{J/cm}^2$ is applied over the wound itself and to a good margin of healthy tissue surrounding it. This same protocol would be followed when treating the aftermath of any minor procedure (e.g., a cheek tooth extraction).

Venomous snakebites are one of the most traumatic injuries to the muzzle and face. These respond well to laser therapy (see Chapter 12). A dosage of $8-10 \text{J/cm}^2$ should be administered as soon as possible after the bite. Though only a few conditions benefit from twice-a-day therapy, multiple treatments in the same day are recommended for snakebites. Aggressively treat until the case is resolved. In all of these cases, laser therapy should be used as an addendum to normal standard-of-care procedures.

Sinusitis is an inflammation of the sinus cavities. PBMT provides a modulation of this inflammatory reaction and provides an added benefit to traditional care. Precautions must be taken to protect the eyes, since PBMT is applied to the sinus cavity of primary concern and to all adjacent sinus structures. Drainage through the nostrils often occurs within the first 5 minutes of therapy. Higher dosages than might be expected are employed to treat sinusitis, since you want to penetrate not only the skin and bone, but also the photoabsorbing exudate within the sinus cavity. Dosages of $15-20 \text{J/cm}^2$ are a suitable starting point, applied daily for three or four sessions, followed by every other day until resolved.

Within the disciplines that require natural balance and self-carriage, with the head and neck positioned sufficiently high to facilitate "working uphill" as the center of gravity moves backwards (e.g., dressage), there is often stress to the anatomical area at the base of the skull and the first few cervical vertebrae and the adjacent musculature. PBMT will accomplish two goals when applied to this area: there will be a relief of any inflammation and soreness and, with application before the event, there will be more flexibility in the area. Comfort and

Laser Therapy in Veterinary Medicine: Photobiomodulation, First Edition. Edited by Ronald J. Riegel and John C. Godbold, Jr.
© 2017 John Wiley & Sons, Inc. Published 2017 by John Wiley & Sons, Inc.

suppleness in this area will allow better balance for both the horse and the rider. This assists in freeing up the front end of the horse off the ground, creating a more uphill, airborne movement. Dosages of $10-12\,J/cm^2$ should be administered on-contact from all areas surrounding the base of the skull and adjacent musculature to the level of C2–3. Passive range of motion during application can be achieved by having an assistant flex and extend the head during therapy.

Numerous conditions within the oral cavity respond well to the application of laser therapy. Traumatized tissue of any nature will respond, including lesions produced by improper fitting of the bit, lacerations to the tongue, inflammation of the mucous membranes, periodontal disease, and fractures. PBMT should be included in the post-op care following dental extraction. Frequently, the target tissue in this area is superficial and requires only a dosage of $2-4\,J/cm^2$ to accelerate the healing process. Deeper target tissues require a higher dosage.

Ensure that the oral cavity is opened with a full mouth speculum or a mouth gag and that the patient is under control at all times. These two pieces of equipment always have reflective characteristics and will reflect the laser beam, so protective eyewear is required. Clean and sanitize the handpiece between application procedures.

Tempomandibular joint syndrome (dysfunction) responds well to laser therapy in experimental conditions (Lemos *et al.*, 2016) and clinically in human medicine (Ayyildiz *et al.*, 2015; Machado *et al.*, 2016). Administer on-contact to the area highlighted in Figure 32.1. Therapy should be provided at $8-12\,J/cm^2$ while the joint is going through passive range of motion. Passive range of motion during therapy is easily accomplished by offering a carrot or other treat and applying PBMT while the patient is chewing.

There are many superficial acupuncture points located on the head and ears that are complementary to the tempomandibular joint (Sutherland *et al.*, 1994). These include those listed in Table 32.1 and illustrated in Figure 32.1. Stimulate these points with a dose of 100–150 J/point.

The Throat

Numerous disorders of the upper respiratory system respond well to laser therapy. Two of the primary functions of laser therapy are the reduction of pain and modulation of the inflammatory reaction. Both are present in every disorder within this anatomical region. Therapy is provided to these structures from outside the skin of the horse. The handpiece should be on-contact with the skin, with a slight amount of pressure applied. Therapy should be applied bilaterally as shown in Figure 32.2, at $10-15\,J/cm^2$.

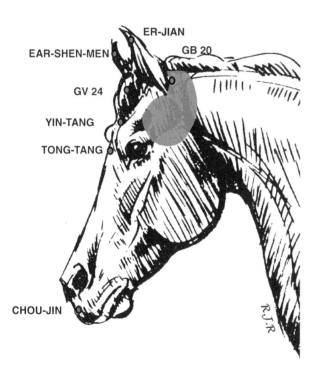

Figure 32.1 Acupuncture points for the temporomandibular joint.

Table 32.1 Acupuncture points for the temporomandibular joint.

Condition/disorder	Corresponding acupuncture points
Temperomandibular joint	Yin-Tang, Tong-Tang, Chou-Jin, ER-Jian, Ear Shen-Men, GB 20, and GV 24

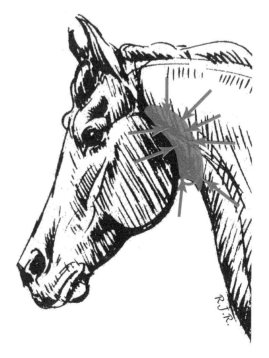

Figure 32.2 Application of PBMT to the throat: bilaterally on-contact from all directions.

It has been this author's experience that pharyngeal lymphoid hyperplasia responds extremely well to PBMT when combined with traditional therapy. Treatment is applied through the skin at a dosage of $15–20\,J/cm^2$. Swelling, inflammation, and a reduction in the size and number of lymphoid follicles are usually seen within the first three therapy sessions. Re-evaluate with an endoscopic exam after the third session. If little improvement is seen, increase the dosage. PBMT should be used as an adjunct to traditional care, such as nebulization and systemic approaches.

There are three significant disorders involving the guttural pouches: tympany, mycosis, and emphysema. This structure is difficult to reach with a sufficient amount of photonic energy to achieve significant clinical success. PBMT can be utilized as an addendum in the traditional treatment of mycosis and emphysema, but is of little use in the treatment of tympany.

There have been only anecdotal reports of the use of PBMT for the entrapment of the epiglottis. CO_2 lasers are a very efficient instrument for surgical repair of this condition. The only efficacious benefit of laser therapy in these cases has been in its postoperative application after surgical correction. Standard postoperative protocols are used with a dosage of $4–8\,J/cm^2$.

The cause of laryngeal hemiplegia is an irritation or damage to the left recurrent laryngeal nerve. Theoretically, PMBT would be of great benefit in the re-establishment of this neural pathway (Anders *et al.*, 2004). There have been no reports of consistent clinical success utilizing only laser therapy. This could be due to the difficulty of reaching the target tissues with the energy or a matter of proper dosing. Utilizing laser therapy on the surgical incision from a laryngoplasty combined with a ventriculectomy surgical correction greatly accelerates the healing process (Calisto *et al.*, 2015).

"Strangles" is a highly contagious disease. PBMT would be beneficial in reducing the pain and inflammation associated with this disorder, but one must weigh the possibility of spreading this disease before initiating treatment. If therapy is administered to one of these patients, strict sanitary procedures should be followed with the handpiece, the fiber-optic cable, the equipment, and the therapist. Merely placing the therapy unit inside a sealed plastic bag is not a guarantee of sterility.

The Cervical Spine and Soft Tissues of the Neck

Numerous disorders within the neck region respond to PBMT. These include trauma because of a fall or injection-site myositis, secondary or tertiary muscle soreness arising from distal primary lameness disorders, phlebitis,

Table 32.2 Acupuncture points for cervical pain.

Condition/disorder	Corresponding acupuncture points
Cervical pain	GB 20, BL 10, TH 16, SI 16, LI 16, BL 11, GB 21

and transient neurological disorders. Large areas are treated with each disorder, administering a dosage of $8–20\,J/cm^2$ on-contact. The deeper the target tissue resides, the higher the dosage required to saturate it. The frequency of treatment varies with each individual, but aggressive treatment of acute cases should always be considered. Treatment of cervical vertebral compression and instability has been clinically non-rewarding with the exception of providing analgesia.

Combining PBMT and chiropractic adjustment allows many equine athletes to maintain their level of performance. Protocols vary, but in many instances a dosage of $5\,J/cm^2$ is given to all target muscles before any adjustment is made. This usually results in a relaxed state, allowing an easier adjustment. After all chiropractic corrections are made, PBMT is applied to all compensatory and secondary areas as needed. Often, additional treatment of the target musculature within the neck can deliver another $10–15\,J/cm^2$ to supply additional relief of pain and inflammation.

Stimulation of the acupuncture points with dosages of $120–200\,J/point$ provides an additional relief of pain and increased circulation. Table 32.2 and Figure 32.3 list and illustrate the acupuncture points that are important for the relief of cervical pain (Fleming, 1998).

The Shoulder Region

This region includes the scapula, the scapulohumeral joint, and the musculature of the shoulder girdle. Several disorders within this anatomical area respond well to laser therapy. These include bicipital bursitis, sweeny, myositis, some scapular fractures, and disorders within the scapulohumeral joint.

The bicipital bursa is located between the biceps brachii tendon and the bicipital groove of the humerus. Pain and inflammation within this structure results from trauma or occurs as a secondary compensatory lameness issue. Penetration and saturation of this bursa with photonic energy has been difficult because of its location, but utilization of higher-powered lasers has made treatment of this area a reality. On-contact therapy should be applied throughout the entire area at a dosage of $8–10\,J/cm^2$. This is an acute condition and should be treated as frequently as possible; daily and then every-other-day treatment is recommended until resolution. PBMT is a viable addition to systemic treatment with anti-inflammatories and intrabursal injection.

Figure 32.3 Acupuncture points for cervical pain.

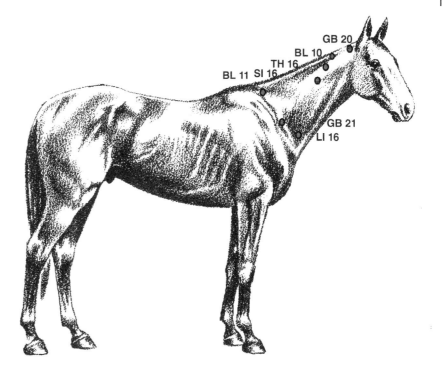

Trauma to the suprascapular nerve results in an atrophy of both the supraspinatus and infraspinatus muscles. PBMT provides increased circulation within these atrophied muscles. There have been anecdotal reports of benefit to the damaged nerve. Dosages should be administered on-contact at a rate of 8–10 J/cm². Concurrent physical therapy utilizing massage and stretching exercises has yielded occasional resolution. Often, these cases appear to improve immediately but then plateau at a point where the patient is still unusable due to lameness. The administration of laser therapy can do no harm in these cases, so consideration of this modality is warranted.

Laser therapy has been proved to accelerate the healing of fractures in numerous studies (Chang *et al.*, 2014; Kazem *et al.*, 2010). Most fractures of the scapula are readily accessible to photonic stimulation. This will provide pain relief, a modulation of the inflammatory reaction, and acceleration of the healing of these lesions. Utilize a dosage of 10–15 J/cm², administered on-contact.

The muscles of the shoulder girdle are composed of aponeuroses and ligamentous attachments. These attachments differ slightly from other species to allow for a maximum range of motion in the locomotion of the equine. The muscles can become inflamed for a variety of reasons and respond extremely well to laser therapy. When possible, the application of PBMT should be distributed throughout the entire muscle structure, from origin to insertion. Administer higher dosages to the large muscle masses to ensure complete saturation of the tissues. This dosage can range from 10 to 20 J/cm², administered on-contact in conjunction with massage. More superficial muscle structures will respond to lower doses. An administration to these structures before an

Table 32.3 Acupuncture points for shoulder pain.

Condition/disorder	Corresponding acupuncture points
Shoulder pain	SI 9, 10, TH 13, SI 3, LI 11, 4, 1, SI 1, LU 1

event serves as a "warm–up," allowing for maximum flexibility and function (Levine *et al.*, 2015).

In addition to the localized treatment, it is beneficial to stimulate corresponding acupuncture points by administering 80–200 J/point depending on the depth of the point (Table 32.3) (Fleming, 1998). This will result in a further relief of pain.

Case Studies

History

A 4-year-old thoroughbred filly exhibited a left front-limb lameness after a collision with another horse, which ran directly into its shoulder approximately 3 days before presentation.

Signalment

Short stride on left front. Grade 3/5 lame.

Work-up and Diagnostics

Manual palpation revealed only a slight tenderness within and around the origin of the supraspinatus muscles and along the anterior boarder of the scapula cartilage.

Radiographs were negative for the scpulohumeral joint and all boney tissues of the shoulder. Ultrasound examination of soft tissues was within normal limits. Scintigraphic images were within normal limits. A complete series of nerve blocks to the limb did not alleviate the lameness.

Management

Initially, the animal was rested in a stall for 30 days while being administered a normal systemic regimen of analgesics and non-steroidal anti-inflammatories. This resulted in no change in the lameness status.

PBMT

PBMT was initiated 34 days after the onset of the lameness. The animal had been off all pharmaceuticals for the previous 72 hours. Laser therapy was applied to all of the soft tissues surrounding the shoulder: both the trapezius cervicalis and thoracis muscles from the midline to their involvement with the scapula, the deltoideus, both the long and lateral head of the triceps brachii, and the brachiocephalicus. These were dosed at $40\,J/cm^2$ on-contact using a scanning administration technique. The goal of this high dosage was to allow sufficient photon penetration to the deeper musculature. The scapulohumeral joint was treated in its entirety at a dosage of $25\,J/cm^2$.

Laserpuncture Administration
After treatment of the tissues, a dose of $125\,J/point$ was administered to the following acupuncture points in the following order: SI 9, 10, TH 13, SI 3, LI 11, 4, 1, SI 1, LU 1.

Frequency of Therapy
Three therapy sessions were conducted in the first week, each separated by 48 hours. Therapy was then administered twice a week for the next 3 weeks.

Rehabilitation
Following the first three treatments, the animal was massaged for 30 minutes over the shoulder musculature and then lightly across the whole body. The left front leg was brought forward in a controlled stretch, but only at about 30°. The animal was then hand walked for at least 30 minutes under complete control.

As the therapy sessions progressed, the massage method remained the same, but the stretching of the limb became more aggressive. Hand walking was increased to an hour twice a day. In the last week of treatment, the patient was placed on a walker for 1 hour three times a day.

Resolution
A slight improvement in the walk was noticed after the first week of therapy. At the conclusion of the second week (five therapy sessions), the animal was only slightly off (grade 1/5 lame). Clinically, the patient was brighter

and much more energetic. After the fourth week, the animal was completely sound and exhibited no sign of lameness and full range of motion of this front limb.

Recommendations and Conclusion

Light training was initiated and progressed normally over the next 5 weeks. When ready for competition, the animal proceeded to win over $3,000,000 in purse money before retiring. While this is a successful case, no solid conclusions can be deducted from an N_1. Further data should be collected to evaluate this therapy protocol versus others.

The scapulohumeral joint is a simple spheroidal joint that has both extension and flexion as its major movements. A myriad of disorders occur within the joint, including osteochondritis dessicans and osteoarthritis. Applying PBMT to the structures within this joint is very difficult. There are similar challenges when treating the same joint in a human patient. However, we can accomplish a thorough treatment in the human patient due to the ability to flex and extend this joint and perform abduction and adduction range-of-motion movements, allowing better access to the joint during administration. These movements cannot be accomplished in the equine species. Therefore, penetration is very limited due to the accessibility of this joint, and often these disorders are clinically non-responsive.

The Upper Arm and Forearm

The humerus and its associated structures constitute the anatomy of the upper arm, while the radius and ulna with the corresponding humeroradial or elbow joint make up the forearm. Consideration should be given to utilization of laser therapy for the following disorders in this area: fractures, radial nerve paralysis, hygroma of the elbow, superior check ligament strain, and epiphysitis.

Fractures in this region are usually a result of external trauma. Stress fractures, fractures of the deltoid tuberosity, olecranon, and greater and lesser tubercles of the humerus all respond to laser therapy. Fractures of the radius and ulna are quite rare and normally require surgical intervention. Do not be afraid to apply PBMT over surgical implants such as plates or screws. These are merely reflective and do not heat up from the application of laser therapy. Manage these like any post-op case, with application to the incision line and over the entire area of the fracture. Those fractures that are treated conservatively should receive therapy over the entire area, with large surrounding margins, using aggressive on-contact treatment at a dosage of $12–20\,J/cm^2$. Diaphyseal fractures of the humerus are often accompanied by radial nerve paralysis, and the prognosis is very poor.

The radial nerve is the largest branch of the brachial plexus. Along the humerus, the radial nerve travels within the musculospiral groove. This is where it is most vulnerable to trauma. Laser therapy should be applied to this area not only in a perpendicular fashion, but also angling the handpiece in every direction to ensure saturation of the target tissues. Nerve tissue responds well to laser therapy (Wang, C.Z. *et al.*, 2014) and dosages as high as $25-30\,J/cm^2$ should be considered.

A hygroma is a fluid-filled sac or cyst that forms over the point of the olecranon tuberosity. It results from trauma and is usually neither painful nor inflamed. If it becomes chronic, surgical removal is the ideal treatment plan. This incision is treated just like any other, using an off-contact technique with a dose of $2-5\,J/cm^2$, starting immediately after surgery.

The radial head of the superficial digital flexor tendon originates from the distal caudomedial surface of the radius. It merges with the main tendon of the superficial digital flexor at the level of the carpus. This, by definition, is a ligament, since no muscle tissue is involved in its structure. A strain (trauma) of this ligament results from two distinct concurrent hyperextensions of the carpus and fetlock. It is painful and inflamed, and therefore very responsive to PBMT.

Injection of this ligament with steroids has been the classical approach to the management of this disorder. Though it usually yields immediate results, this drastically impedes the healing process. Management of these cases with applications of PBMT combined with physical therapy and controlled exercises yields excellent clinical outcomes. Apply laser therapy before physical therapy exercises and, ideally, again several hours later. Only a few clinical conditions benefit from twice-a-day treatment; this one does. Since this ligamentous tissue is quite dense, utilize dosages of $10-15\,J/cm^2$ with an on-contact application technique. Initially, be as aggressive as possible until clinical results are visualized, and then transition through less frequent administration of treatments until the disorder is completed resolved.

Epiphysitis is a condition seen in yearlings and 2-year-olds and is characterized by swelling and pain. Lameness is uncommon, and the condition is self-resolving with proper diet and rest. However, it results in a blemish that affects the value of the animal when sold at auction. There has always been a precautionary statement regarding the application of laser therapy to this area. The theoretical concern is an abnormal growth of the bone, resulting in an angular limb deformity. This would be extremely difficult to cause with PBMT. Caution should be exercised during administration, but administering PBMT circumferentially to the growth plate in an even distribution will aid in the alleviation of pain and inflammation. Administer dosages of $10-12\,J/cm^2$ on-contact, daily or every other day, until resolution.

The Carpus

PBMT provides a relief of pain, a modulation of the inflammatory reaction, and an increase in circulation (Jang and Lee, 2012). These physiological events make this an ideal therapy for disorders of the carpus, such as degenerative joint disease, carpitis and synovitis, hygroma of the carpus, carpal tunnel syndrome, osteoarthritis, and postoperative care.

Animals such as jumpers, 3-day eventers, and thoroughbred racehorses benefit from routine therapy sessions to this anatomical area intended to maintain their performance at the highest level. After a hard workout or event, recovery time is accelerated by PBMT, allowing a rapid return to training.

Administration of PBMT to the three carpal joints is extremely easy. Therapy can be administered circumferentially, while the joints are flexed and very open, while the joints are being placed through passive range of motion, and at rest, bearing weight on the limb. Administer PBMT with the laser handpiece perpendicular to the target tissues in one direction circumferentially, and then repeat circumferentially at a right angle to the first direction (Figure 32.4). During passive range-of-motion exercises, the beam should be directed toward all parts of the joint capsule and every possible joint surface.

Consider treating the animal holistically by first treating the entire carpal area and then providing stimulation of the corresponding acupuncture points (Table 32.4, Figure 32.5). Depending on the depth of the point, dosages range from 80 to 200 J/point (Fleming, 1994; Xie and Preast, 2007).

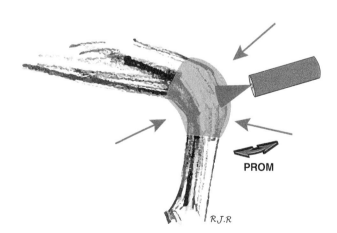

Figure 32.4 Application of PBMT for carpal pain. ~30% of the dose should be applied circumferentially at right angles while the animal is bearing weight on the limb. The remainder should be applied as illustrated while placing the joints and tissues through a passive range-of-motion (PROM) exercise. The handpiece should be kept perpendicular to the skin at all times. Note the margins receiving therapy above and below the carpus.

Consideration should be given to all secondary, tertiary, and compensatory anatomical areas as well. These areas should be identified and then treated during each therapy session. Digital thermal imaging is a useful tool for identifying all areas that require further investigation and therapy. Digital thermal images taken during therapy will illustrate the path of the application by delineating an increased thermal gradient that corresponds to changes in tissue temperature during PBMT application (Figure 32.6).

The Metacarpus

This anatomical area manifests numerous conditions responsive to PBMT. These may be injuries to the soft tissues, the boney structures, or, often, both. Common soft-tissue injuries include dorsal metacarpal disease, inflammation of the interosseous ligament, suspensory desmitis, tendonitis, tendosynovitis, bowed tendons,

Table 32.4 Acupuncture points for carpal pain.

Condition/disorder	Corresponding acupuncture points
Degenerative joint disease	LI 6, TH 5, LU 7, LI 4, SI 3
Carpal pain	LI 17, BL 13,BL14, BL 22, BL 25
Carpitis, synovitis, hygroma, carpal tunnel syndrome	BL 11, BL 23, SI 9, TH 5, PC 6, SI 3, TH 1, LI 1, LU 11
Performance maintenance	BL 11, TH 1, LI 1, LU 11

and inferior check ligament desmitis. The primary applications of PBMT to hard tissues in the metacarpus are stress fractures and postoperative care after major orthopedic surgery.

Application of laser therapy to this anatomical area should not only accomplish a stimulation of the target cells but also stimulation of all of the surrounding tissues. Treatment of soft-tissue disorders such as injuries to either the superficial or deep digital flexor tendons should include administration of photonic energy along these structures from just distal to the carpus and concluding proximal to the metacarpalphalangeal joint. Administration should be delivered both at right angles and circumferentially while the animal is bearing weight and while the carpus is flexed and these structures are in a relaxed posture. Slight passive range of motion can be accomplished by manually flexing and extending the fetlock while the carpus is in a flexed posture.

Metacarpal structures seem to be superficial, so logically one assumes a lower dosage can be utilized for treatment. However, the extensor, flexor, and suspensory tendons are extremely thick and fibrous and warrant higher dosages on the skin in order to achieve therapeutic levels of photonic energy at the target tissues. Dosages of $12–20 \, J/cm^2$, or even higher, are warranted for consistent clinical success.

Stress fractures are common within the third metacarpal bone. Dosages of $10–12 \, J/cm^2$, administered on-contact, with good margins, are efficacious. Other fractures requiring surgery are treated postoperatively with similar doses. Laser therapy can be applied over any orthopedic appliance.

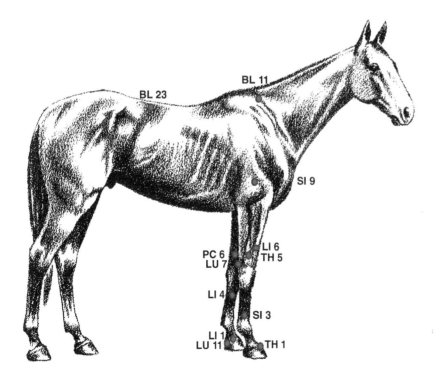

Figure 32.5 Acupuncture points for carpal pain.

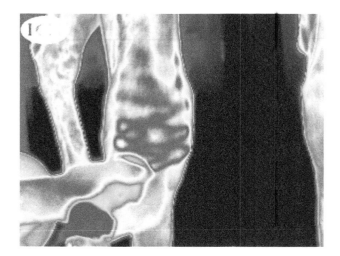

Figure 32.6 Digital thermal image of a carpus. The path of increased thermal gradient corresponds to the PBMT application using a scanning technique.

Table 32.5 Acupuncture points for metacarpal pain.

Condition/disorder	Corresponding acupuncture points
Dorsal metacarpal disease	TH 1 SI 1, SI 3, SI 4, SI 9, GB 21, BL 11, BL 23, HT 8,
Interosseous ligament tear, fracture of 2nd and 4th metacarpal	TH 1, SI 1, SI 3, LU 1, LU 10, LU 11, LI 4, LI 11, LI 15, LU 1, PC 8, GB 21, BL 11, BL 23
Suspensory desmitis; superficial and deep flexor tendons, subacute, acute, and chronic bowed tendons, inferior check ligament desmitis	BL 18, BL 19, GB 34, KI 3, LV, 3, LI 4, TH 1, PC 9

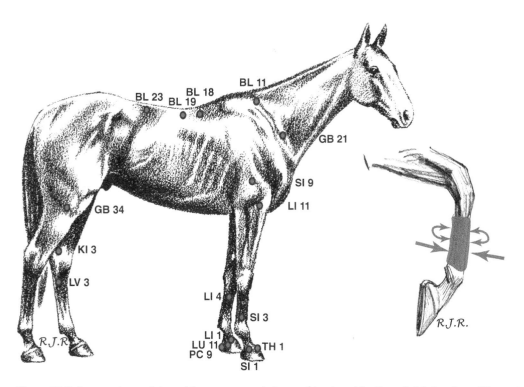

Figure 32.7 Acupuncture points and the recommended area of treatment for the painful disorders of the metacarpus.

Consider concurrent administration of PBMT to both the corresponding acupuncture points and any secondary, tertiary, and compensatory areas associated with the diagnosed disorder (Table 32.5, Figure 32.7) (Fleming, 1994; Xie and Preast, 2007). Even inflammation of the interosseous ligament will usually have a secondary inflamed area within the shoulder areas and possibly even the opposite front limb. Treat holistically for consistent optimal clinical results.

The Fetlock and Pastern

The metacarpalphalangeal joint, sesamoids, and the first and second distal phalanx areas are also susceptible to numerous lameness disorders that are very responsive to laser therapy. These include degenerative joint disease, sesamoiditis, fractures of the sesamoids, chronic proliferative synovitis, osslets, osteochrondosis, ringbone (all four classifications), and palmar annular ligament constriction.

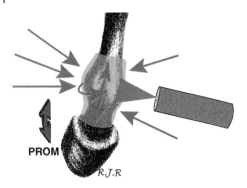

Figure 32.8 Recommended area of treatment for fetlock disorders.

Laser therapy should be administered circumferentially throughout this entire anatomical area (Figure 32.8). The therapy session could be initiated while the patient is bearing full weight on the limb. When the patient is acclimated to the procedure, proceed by picking up the foot and placing the joint through passive range-of-motion exercises during circumferential administration. An effort should be made to direct the beam inside the joint, targeting the joint surfaces, the synovial membrane, and all areas surrounding the sesamoids. Dosages range from 8 to $12\,J/cm^2$. On-contact administration, utilizing either a scanning method or a point-to-point method, is preferred to non-contact administration.

When treating a case of degenerative joint disease (osteoarthritis) or osteochrondrosis, target the joint surfaces. If PBMT is used as the sole treatment, treat aggressively for several days and then every other day until a clinical response is noted. Laser therapy applied to this disorder can also be a complement to an intra-articular administration of platelet-rich plasma (PRP) or hyaluronic acid (HA). The general rule is to wait 3–7 days post-injection before initiating laser therapy. The determination of when to initiate PBMT should be made on an individual case basis.

The etiology for sesamoiditis, fractures of the sesamoid bones, and chronic proliferative synovitis, as well as for the majority of the lameness disorders in this anatomical area, is constant, repetitive, concussive force. These disorders begin with an inflammatory response to this trauma. PBMT modulates this inflammatory reaction, slowing or in certain instances stopping the deleterious process (Assis *et al.*, 2016). Direct the laser energy to encompass all of the synovial membrane, joint capsule, surrounding ligaments, and sesamoid bones. Dosages of $10–12\,J/cm^2$ are required to penetrate and saturate these structures. In the acute phase, administer as often as the client will allow (e.g., several consecutive days, followed by a longer transitional phase between each therapy session, based on the clinical response). Always place the target structures through passive range of motion during administration.

Table 32.6 Acupuncture points for fetlock pain.

Condition/disorder	Corresponding acupuncture points
Degerate joint disease, osslets, ringbone, sesamoinditis	BL 11, 23, 26, SI 9, LI 4, SI 3, TH 1, LI 1
Fetlock pain	LI 1, 16, BL 25, BL 23, LU 1, SI 9

Osslets and all four classifications of ringbone are difficult to manage with PBMT. Osslets form from repetitive concussive trauma to the metacarpophalangeal joint. They are accompanied by a joint capsulitis and simultaneous synovitis. The result is a traumatic arthritic condition with the formation of calcium deposits. When this becomes chronic, an ossification will develop within the joint capsule. Ringbone is very similar in the formation of new bone growth on the dorsal, dorsolateral, and dorsomedial surfaces of the first and second phalanges and the extensor process of the third phalanx. These deposits of calcium will not be resolved with the administration of PBMT. Laser therapy will alleviate the inflammation and pain, but will only decelerate this deleterious sequence. Aggressively treat these cases with daily administrations and then transition to a maintenance level of administration individualized to each patient. Dosages should be administered on-contact and during passive range-of-motion exercise with a dose of $10–12\,J/cm^2$.

Encircling the synovial-lined joints are the tough, fibrous continuations of the fascial sheath called the annular ligaments. When these ligaments become strained or traumatized, they become inflamed, which leads to a thickening of this structure, resulting in constriction. Administer PBMT to these cases to prevent the initial thickening of these structures (Figure 32.8). Once this thickening occurs, the application of PBMT reduces the inflammation and slows this vicious cycle. Provide performance-maintenance applications during both training and athletic endeavors.

After localized treatment of the fetlock is completed, treat all of the corresponding acupuncture points and any additional compensatory secondary or tertiary inflamed areas (Table 32.6, Figure 32.9) (Fleming, 1998; Xie and Preast, 2007).

The Hoof

The conformation or shape of the foot, with regard to the height of the heel, the length of the toe, and the overall angulation, determines which anatomical structures are accessible to the application of PBMT. The hoof is the interface between the musculoskeletal system and the

Figure 32.9 Acupuncture points for fetlock pain.

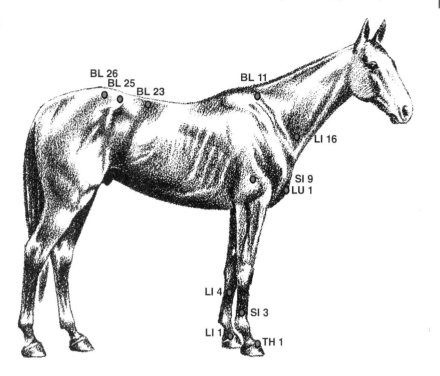

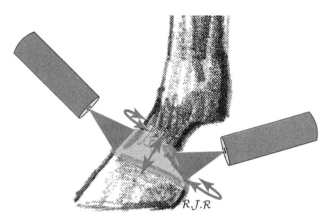

Figure 32.10 Application of PBMT to the hoof.

ground. This structure is composed of the epidermal hoof itself (which is often pigmented), the connective tissue or dermal layer, the digital cushion, the distal phalanx, the lateral cartilages of the digital phalanx, the distal interphalangeal joint, the distal extremity of the short pastern bone, the navicular bone, the navicular bursa, several ligaments, and the tendons of insertion of the common digital extensor and deep digital flexor tendons. All of these parts differ in density and structure. To some degree, all inhibit the passage of photonic energy. The pigmented hoof wall displays almost 100% inhibition. Therefore, the efficacy of laser therapy is limited to those structures that can be irradiated through the dermal areas surrounding the coronary band and throughout the heels.

The higher the heel and the shorter the toe, the fewer are the targets that can receive PBMT. When considering the average foot, disorders of the following structures will respond to treatment:

- attachment of the common digital extensor tendon;
- insertion of the superficial digital flexor tendon;
- portions of the deep digital flexor tendon;
- portions of the lateral cartilages;
- portions of the lateral and medial ligaments;
- portions of the medial and lateral collateral ligaments;
- portions of the "T" ligament;
- portions of the navicular bursa;
- portions of the navicular bone;
- portions of the coffin joint.

Additionally, laser therapy applied to both the coronary band and corresponding acupuncture points will serve as a supplement to traditional care for both navicular syndrome and laminitis.

Techniques for the Application of Laser Therapy to the Foot

Localized treatment consists of administering 8–10 J/cm^2 on-contact, using a point-to-point or scanning technique. Therapy is applied from the middle of the first phalanx to the coronary band circumferentially, including the heels and pastern cavity (Figures 32.10 and 32.11). Administer a portion (~30%) of the energy while the patient is bearing weight on the limb, and the remainder while the foot is picked up and placed through passive range-of-motion exercise.

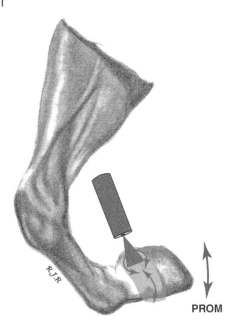

PROM

Figure 32.11 Application of PBMT to the heel.

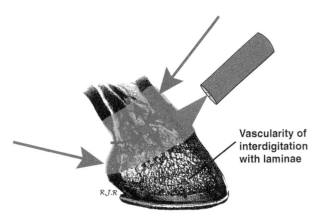

Vascularity of interdigitation with laminae

Figure 32.12 Application of PMBT throughout the coronary band.

PBMT has the ability to influence both the vascular and the neurologic supply to the hoof (Chow *et al.*, 2011). This is significant, since a large number of the disorders of the foot involve pain and inflammation and are vasoconstrictive. Visualizing the location of these structures aids the therapist in guiding the application of PBMT.

The neurovascular supply originates both medially and laterally from the digital artery, vein, and nerve. Arterial branches that arise at the level of the coronet supply the periople and coronary dermis. Those that originate opposite the pastern joint supply branches to the digital cushion and the dermis of the caudal aspect of hoof, including the frog. The third branch of arterial supply arises from the dorsal and palmar terminal branches and supplies the laminella and sole. This is the only anatomical area of the body where the venous supply does not correspond to the arterial supply. The venous supply forms an extensive interlocking network in the dermis

Table 32.7 Acupuncture points for hoof pain.

Condition/disorder	Corresponding acupuncture points
Hoof pain	LI 18, PC 1, BL 13, BL 25, BL 15, BL 27, BL 14, SI 9
Ting points forefoot	LI 1, HT 9, SI 1, LU 11, P 9, TH 1
Ting points hindfoot	LV 1, SP 1, BL 67, GB 44, ST 45, KI 1

and underlying subcutis, continuous with the coronary band (Riegel and Hakola, 1996, pp. 26–40).

At the level of the fetlock, descending both medially and laterally, the medial and lateral palmar nerve gives rise to the medial and lateral palmar digital nerves. Almost immediately, these nerves give off a dorsal branch. The dorsal branches supply sensory and vasomotor innervation of the skin, a portion of the fetlock joint, dorsal portions of the interphalangeal joints, the coronary corium, dorsal parts of the laminar and solar coria, and the dorsal part of the cartilage of the distal phalanx. As the palmar digital nerves continue distally, they innervate the palmar structures of the digit: the skin, pastern joint capsule, digital synovial sheath, flexor tendons, distal sesamoidean ligaments, coffin joint capsule, navicular bone (and its ligaments and bursa), laminar corium, coria of the sole and frog, and digital cushion (Stashak, 1976). Often, there are branches of communication between the lateral and medial palmar nerves; these are important areas to include during the focal administration of photonic energy.

Knowledge of these structures is extremely important, since numerous disorders of the foot, laminitis, podotrochleosis, and degenerative joint benefit from the relief of pain and the vasodilatory effect of PBMT (Maegawa *et al.*, 2000; Nakamura *et al.*, 2014). Area administration that uses these vascular and neurological structures as a road map will result in an improved clinical outcome (Figure 32.12).

Stimulation with photonic energy of the acupuncture points for the disorders within the foot yields more consistent clinical outcomes (Table 32.7). The advantages of this technique are that it is non-invasive in a very high vascular area, it is aseptic, it requires minimal restraint, and it can be accomplished in a very short time. This is done in addition to localized treatment utilizing dosages of 150–200 J/point administered on-contact (Xie and Preast, 2007). The Ting points are all located on the coronary band and should receive special attention to ensure their stimulation when applying PBMT (Figures 32.13 and 32.14). The Ting points are the beginning or end points of the meridian, where energy is exchanged with the exterior (Rathgeber, 2001). Stimulate each Ting point separately with at least 50 J.

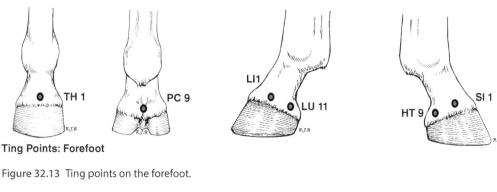

Ting Points: Forefoot

Figure 32.13 Ting points on the forefoot.

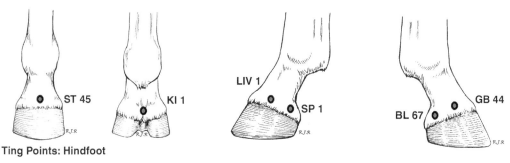

Ting Points: Hindfoot

Figure 32.14 Ting points on the hindfoot.

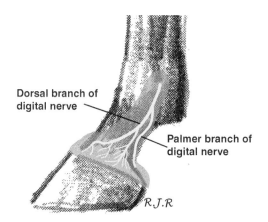

Figure 32.15 Application of PBMT to relieve foot pain.

Treatment of Specific Disorders of the Foot

Foot Pain

The distal aspect of the horse's lower limb, from the middle of the cannon bone to the sole of the foot, has an extremely complex anatomy, with each of the structures subject to a myriad of injuries and disorders. Whether it is a common disorder such as laminitis or podotrochleosis, or one of the many disorders that are all classified as "palmar foot pain," the two common symptoms are pain and inflammation. Therefore, the application of PBMT, resulting in the release of a biochemical cascade of events causing relief of pain and modulation of inflammation to those structures that can be irradiated,

is a great supplemental therapy to the classical treatment of these disorders.

Relief of pain and inflammation is accomplished utilizing the following treatment technique (Figure 32.15). Palpate both the lateral and medial palmar nerves, located just above the fetlock. Initiate therapy at 6–8 J/ cm^2 along both the medial and the lateral palmar nerves, following the nerve pathway distally (including the dorsal branches of each) to the coronary band. Circumferentially, using the same dosage, treat the entire foot, including the entire heel, along the coronary band. This includes all areas from the middle of the second phalanx to the coronary band. Always consider where your target tissues are anatomically, and focus the energy as perpendicular as possible to these. Finally, apply 150–180 J to each corresponding acupuncture point.

Laminitis

Even with all of our current technology, some aspects of laminitis remain an enigma. In brief, irrespective of the etiology, the patient experiences a lactic acidosis and systemic endotoxemia, which results in an inflammatory response. During this response, there is a release of catecholamines, prostaglandins, histamine, serotonin, cachectin, and interleukin 1 (IL1). These inflammatory mediators have a profound effect on the foot. They produce an initial increase in arterial blood flow, coupled with a systemic hypertension, resulting in arteriovenous shunting within the microvasculature and decreased capillary perfusion within the laminae. Ultimately, there is an ischemic necrosis at the laminar level (Riegel and Hakola, 1996, pp. 54–80). Recently, studies utilizing high-carbohydrate feeding to induce laminitis concluded that inflammation may not be the only factor involved in the pathophysiology of laminitis (Burns *et al.*, 2015).

Recent scientific evidence suggests a deformation of the lamellar attachment apparatus. This begins during the developmental phase of laminitis. Compromise of the basement membrane zone occurs when the production of constituent lamellar enzymes, metalloproteinase-9, membrane-type metalloproteinase, and aggrecanase is increased to a point where they destroy key components of the lamellar suspensory apparatus (Budak *et al.*, 2009; Coyne *et al.*, 2009; Loftus *et al.*, 2008).

The level of pain experienced by laminitis patients is directly proportional to the amount of ischemic necrosis and deterioration of the lamellar attachment apparatus. This pain stimulus causes a release of catecholamines from the adrenal glands, which potentiate further vasoconstriction of the arteriovenous anastomoses within the laminae. This causes additional ischemic necrosis to the laminar tissue, which perpetuates this destructive vicious cycle, eventually allowing the rotation of the distal phalanx (Riegel and Hakola, 1996, pp. 104–108).

In summary, the pathophysiology of laminitis involves inflammation, increased production of lamellar enzymes, and pain. PBMT, used as an addendum to classical treatment, provides a relief of pain (Enwemeka, 2009), and more importantly, when applied to the coronary band,

has a significant influence on the circulatory pattern of the entire foot (Maegawa *et al.*, 2000).

PBMT should be administered, preferably on-contact if the patient allows, throughout the region of the coronary band and heels, utilizing a dose of 4–6 J/cm^2 (Figure 32.16). Each Ting point should receive a total of no less than 120 J. All corresponding acupuncture points should also receive laser puncture stimulation in the range of 150–200 J. In the acute phase, this could initially be administered twice a day, with the frequency tapering off as the laminitis condition is resolved.

Podotrochleosis

Podotrochleosis encompasses a broad spectrum of conditions that affect the navicular bone, its bursa, and the flexor tendons. The navicular bone, or distal sesamoid, is located palmar to the middle and distal phalanges and their corresponding joint space. It lies between the deep digital flexor tendon and is palmar to the distal interphalangeal joint. About 30% of its surface comprises the distal articular surface, which is covered in hyaline cartilage.

Early clinical signs of this disorder include an intermittent, progressive lameness that subsides with rest. Pressure applied to the middle of the frog will reveal pain in only 30–40% of the patients. A phalangeal and fetlock flexion test for a few minutes aggravates this condition about 80% of the time.

Due to their location, it is often difficult to deliver sufficient photonic energy to the target tissues to elicit a clinical

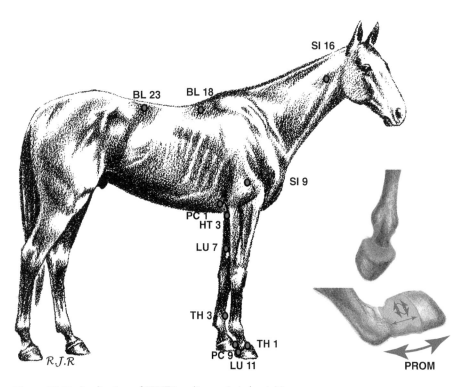

Figure 32.16 Application of PBMT to relieve pain in laminitis.

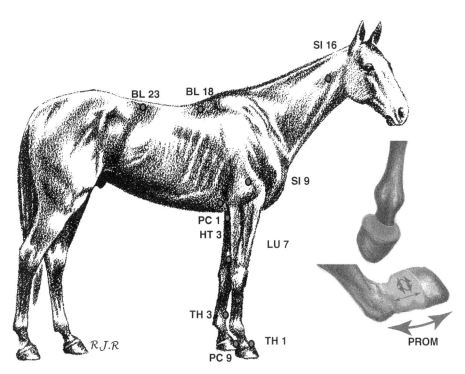

Figure 32.17 Application of PBMT to relieve pain in podotrochleosis.

response. Accessibility of these target tissues is dependent on the conformation of the foot. Even with ideal conformation, only portions of the deep digital flexor tendon, the navicular bursa, and the navicular bone will receive treatment. These cases should be handled utilizing a multimodal approach of proper shoeing, systemic medications, and PBMT, the latter used to aid in the reduction of local pain and inflammation common with this syndrome.

The treatment protocol for PBMT is as follows (Figure 32.17). Apply $10–15 \text{J/cm}^2$ on-contact in a safe manner to the entire area of the heel. Place both the fetlock and the phalangeal joints through passive range of motion while attempting to keep the handpiece pointed perpendicular to the target tissues. Treat all corresponding acupuncture points. Treat aggressively for four to six therapy sessions and then re-evaluate to determine when to transition to treatments spaced further apart. If successful, a program of less frequent maintenance therapy can be formulated.

Some of these cases will show a certain degree of response, and some will show very little. Application of PBMT can do no harm and should be considered on a case-by-case basis.

The Back (Thoracolumbar Spine)

Back disorders are one of the major causes of diminishing performance levels in the equine athlete. Studies published in the United Kingdom indicate the incidence

of thoracolumbar spine problems rangs from 0.9% in general practice to 94% in specialty referral practices (Anon., 1965; Jeffcoat, 1980a). The incidence of throracolumbar problems is even higher in competitive jumpers, both show and eventing, and dressage (Jeffcoat, 1980b). All of these disorders manifest themselves as pain and a change in performance level.

The thoracolumbar spine is defined by those areas of the axial skeleton from the withers (T3–7) to the lumbosacral joint (L6–S1), the bilateral sacroiliac joints, and the sacrum (S5). It includes the intervertebral disks, the overlying large thick muscles, fascia, ligamentous structures, and all of their associated nervous and circulatory systems. All can be the cause of a painful disorder (Dyce *et al.*, 2002). It is the complex nature of this large anatomical area, the variable clinical signs, and the distinctive, unique requirements for each discipline that often makes a definitive diagnosis difficult to obtain.

It is easy to visually identify and manually palpate those patients experiencing back pain and diminishing performance, but very difficult to get a definitive diagnosis. Even with the use of the advanced diagnostic equipment at our disposal (digital radiography, sharper imaging ultrasounds, nuclear scintigraphy, and digital thermal imaging), it is difficult to identify and localize the exact problematic disorder or its origin. Consequently, large areas will require PBMT to achieve a clinical response.

Back pain is categorized as primary or secondary. Primary back pain is the clinical response to a direct insult to the anatomical structures, such as fractures,

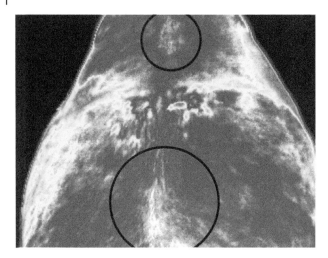

Figure 32.18 Digital thermal image, indicating inflamed areas of the patient's back. Note the increased thermal gradients (white and red) within the areas of the circles. When compared symmetrically, the areas laterally on the right side of the thoracolumbar spine have a higher thermal gradient than those on the left. These areas require closer examination and warrant thorough PBMT treatment.

decompressions, subluxations, the sacroiliac joint, scoliosis, lordosis, arthritis, and myositis. There are many patients in which a combination of these etiologies occurs simultaneously. Secondary back pain is commonly a secondary or tertiary result of lower limb lameness, dental problems, poor-fitting saddles and bits, and, more often than is admitted, poor riding technique and skill.

The goal is to identify all of the areas that would benefit from therapy. Secondary back disorders will not be alleviated if the etiology has not been identified and managed. Digital thermal images can help identify all affected areas (Figure 32.18).

The crucial element in the application of PBMT to this anatomical area is the ability to deliver enough photonic energy to the skin safely so as to penetrate and saturate the target tissues, using a wavelength that the target chromophores can absorb. Correct dosages, the frequency of therapy, and the administration technique are all paramount to successful clinical outcomes.

Dosages of photonic energy administered to this area have increased from as low as $0.6\,J/cm^2$ in the late 1970's to $25–40\,J/cm^2$ today. Clinical results were realized when low dosages such as $5\,J/cm^2$ were utilized just a few years ago. However, treatment outcomes to this anatomical area were very inconsistent. Logically, these results could have resulted from the stimulation of the key acupuncture points that occur within this treatment area. When laser therapy technology allowed a safe administration of higher dosages, treatment outcomes became more consistent and were achieved in less time.

Table 32.8 Acupuncture points for back pain.

Condition/disorder	Corresponding acupuncture points
Back pain	Bai Hui, BL 18, BL 23, BL 25, BL 27, BL 28, BL 32, BL 40, BL 60, SI 3

Therapy should be administered to the entire thoracolumbar area from the withers to the last sacral vertebrae, including all nine pairs of lumbosacral muscles. Administration of the energy should be done on-contact when possible, and combined with therapeutic massage. This combination of massage and PBMT allows a passive range of motion within the target tissues – the muscle tissues – during administration. Additional benefits include an increase in the circulation and a reduction in the spasticity and tenderness within the muscles and trigger points.

Each patient should be treated to effect. Each is a unique individual and has specific physiognomies depending on the breed and disciple. The anatomy should be constantly digitally palpated during administration, and treated until the tissues are as pain-free as possible.

The frequency of administration will depend on the patient, the compliance of the client, and the amount of preparation time available before the next competitive event. For simplicity, equine back cases are classified as either acute or chronic.

When managing an acute case, treatment should be administered as aggressively as possible. Several daily treatment sessions are ideal, for two to four treatments, or at least every other day for the first week. When a significant clinical improvement is noted, a transition is made to less frequent treatment by spacing more time between sessions. These cases are treated to resolution. At least one additional treatment should always be administered after the issue is resolved, and the patient should be re-checked periodically to see if a maintenance therapy regime is warranted.

Initially, chronic cases should also be handled aggressively, with therapy sessions at least every other day until clinical improvement is noted. Sessions can then be spaced further apart until the pre-established therapeutic goal is reached. The last stage is to determine a maintenance program in order to prevent reoccurrence, or at least maintain as high a level of performance or quality of life as possible.

Acupuncture is well established as an important part of the multimodal management of back pain in the equine (Ridgway, 1999; Rogers, 1999; Xie *et al.*, 1997). After applying therapy to all localized areas requiring it, stimulate the corresponding acupuncture points with 150–200 J/point (Table 32.8, Figure 32.19) (Xie and Preast, 2007). Several of these points will be stimulated

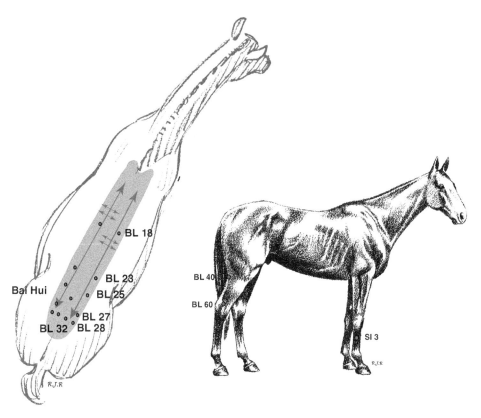

Figure 32.19 Acupuncture points and the recommended area of treatment for the painful disorders of the thoracolumbar spine and surrounding musculature.

during the administration to the localized area. Repeat the stimulation of these points with an approximate 50% reduction in the number of joules compared to the other points not receiving energy during the localized treatment.

The Hip, Pelvis, and Upper Hind Limb

This anatomical area includes the pelvis (which is part of the axial skeleton), the pelvic girdle, the coxofemoral joint, the sacroiliac joint, the femur, and all the sublumbar, cranial, lateral, and medial layers of musculature and their corresponding neurovascular supplies. It is the focal point for the transfer of supportive, locomotive, and propulsive forces from the hind limb to the trunk. PBMT is an excellent addendum to traditional standard-of-care treatment for many of the maladies originating here.

Historically, this area has been both a conundrum and an enigma. Injuries and lameness issues were thought to be a very uncommon finding, and mostly the result of external trauma. New technologies in the development of digital radiography, nuclear scintigraphy, and diagnostic ultrasonography have expanded our ability to diagnose and appreciate the complexity of the disorders within this

area. A prospective study, over a period of 2 years, performed in Newmarket, England, revealed 245 pelvic fractures in young racing thoroughbreds (Bathe, 1994).

The two universal clinical manifestations of all the disorders within this area are pain and inflammation. Though there is still a great deal of research to be completed on the efficacy of PBMT in managing several of these disorders (e.g., sacroiliac joint injuries), there are numerous disorders that have a great deal of supportive clinical evidence for the use of PBMT. Those disorders involving primary or secondary myositis, trochanteric bursitis, several tendon and ligament injuries, the coxofemoral joint, and fibrotic and ossifying myopathies all respond to PBMT. The technology will soon evolve to allow the safe penetration of photonic energy into deep-tissue targets such as the structures surrounding the sacroiliac joint.

A physiological–biochemical cascade of events can only occur if photonic energy reaches the cellular photoreceptor cytochrome c oxidase (CCO) in the inner lining of the mitochondria (Poyton and Ball, 2011). Realization of the difficulty in efficiently delivering the energy required to produce effective PBM within these cells requires an understanding of the light's loss of irradiance as it penetrates from the outer epidermis, through the epidermis, dermis, fat, and the very large muscle masses, to the target tissue (L. De Taboala, pers. comm.). Due to this loss, PBMT is commonly used in addition to both systemic and intra-articular pharmacological treatments. With a pharmacological or regenerative intra-articular administration to the coxofemoral joint, the cause of the disorder is then addressed, and PBMT can be administered to the inflamed, painful compensatory surrounding musculature and portions of the joint. The goal is always an accelerated recovery from the disorder. The stimulation of these structures will allow a holistic or multimodal approach, by decreasing the pain, increasing the circulation, and modulating the inflammatory cycle (Bjordal *et al.*, 2006).

Dosages administered on-contact range from 20 to $40 J/cm^2$. Such higher doses, administered to all of the localized areas utilizing a massage technique, are required when treating any myositis. These areas include the psoas major and minor, the iliacus, the quadratus lumboram, the gluteals, the biceps femoris, and the semimebranosus and semitendinosus muscles.

When the patient suffers an acute injury, it should initially be treated as frequently as possible until a clinical response is recognized. Areas of inflammation within these muscles are present in all the racing thoroughbreds and sport horses. A maintenance therapy program should be developed to minimize this and allow these athletes to compete pain-free at a high level.

Table 32.9 Acupuncture points for hip pain.

Condition/disorder	Corresponding acupuncture points
Hip pain	Bai Hui, BL 27, BL 28, BL 35, BL 40, GB 28, GB 29, GB 30

Trochanteric bursitis is a localized inflammation of the bursa beneath the tendon of the middle gluteal muscle as it passes over the greater trochanter of the femur. This issue is usually a compensatory secondary result of a lameness issue within the tarsal structures. This is a common finding in standardbreds, as they are trained many miles in the same direction on an inclined track. Acutely, therapy should be administered daily or at least every other day until this area is not painful upon palpation. The area can then usually be kept pain-free with weekly maintenance therapy sessions.

The coxofemoral joint is a ball-and-socket joint capable of abduction, adduction, rotation, and circumduction movements. Even with a high dosage at an ideal wavelength, penetration to this joint is very limited. Doses of $35–40 J/cm^2$ should be used, with the on-contact handpiece angled in all possible directions toward the target tissues. The benefit of PBMT in this disorder is the relief of pain and inflammation within the surrounding tissues and portions of the joint.

Fibrotic and ossifying myopathies are the result of traumatic insult to the semitendinosus, semimembranosus, biceps femoris, and gracilis muscles. These injuries are usually the result of an intramuscular injection or of the slide-to-a-stop movements frequently made in reining and rodeo events. They are very responsive to PBMT. The relief of pain and inflammation, coupled with the increase in circulation, allows an increased rate of cellular remodeling.

After administering localized treatment slowly at a high dose over the entire involved area, 150–200 J/point should be applied to all complementary acupuncture points (Table 32.9, Figure 32.20) (Fleming, 1998).

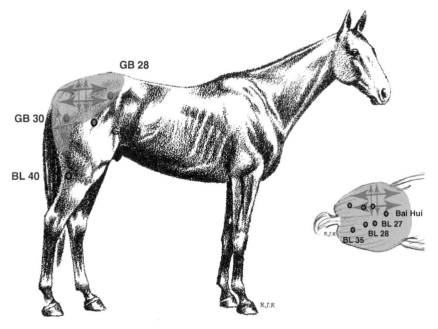

Figure 32.20 Acupuncture points and the recommended area of treatment for the painful disorders of the hip.

The Stifle

This is the largest and most intricate articulation in the equine. It consists of two joints, the femoropatellar and the femorotibial, which connect the femur, patella, and tibia, yet it contains three, sometimes communicating synovial compartments. It is stabilized by numerous ligaments: lateral and medial femoropatellar ligaments; lateral, middle, and medial patellar ligaments; anterior and posterior cruciate ligaments; and medial and lateral collateral ligaments. The stifle joint extends through 150° range of motion, and it is often subjected to uneven stress loads during locomotion. In summary, this is the weakest joint in the horse. It is predisposed to numerous hard- and soft-tissue conditions, which result in a diminished level of performance or lameness.

A majority of the lameness disorders of the stifle originate from the soft-tissue structures surrounding the joint. Numerous times, lameness is a combination of disorders within the joint itself and in the surrounding soft tissues. Both the joint and these adjacent ligaments are very responsive to PBMT. These structures are not obscured by massive amounts of muscle tissue and are therefore easier to saturate with photonic energy than some other anatomical areas. PBMT combined with traditional standard of care (e.g. intra-articular injection of an anti-inflammatory or regenerative substance) provides an accelerated route to recovery and return to competition.

There is a lack of double-blind scientific studies utilizing the equine as the research model, yet there are an abundant number of documented clinical cases supporting a 90% efficacy rate. Scientific findings and techniques utilized in human medicine can be extrapolated to the equine athlete. An excellent example of this is a double-blind study by Ip and Fu (2015), in which they examined whether a combination of intra-articular HA injection and PBMT in addition to standard conventional physical therapy could successfully postpone the need for joint-replacement surgery in elderly patients with bilateral symptomatic tricompartmental knee arthritis. They randomly divided 140 elderly patients into one of two treatment protocols. The first group received conventional physical therapy, a sham light source, and intra-articular saline. The second group received conventional physical therapy, PBMT (810 nm wavelength, 20 mW/cm^2 power density, therapy administered three times per week for 6 weeks), and an intra-articular injection of HA. Treatment failure was defined as breakthrough pain requiring joint replacement. Of the 70 subjects in the group receiving HA and PBMT, only 1 required joint replacement, compared to 15 of the 70 subjects in the control group.

One example alone is not the foundation of scientific evidence, but from January 2015 to June 2016 16 papers have been published, all using PBMT and the knee as the model, and all concluding efficacious results. During this time, one study was published that did not show efficacy, but it used very low dosages and the Achilles tendon as its model (de Jesus *et al.*, 2016).

Fekrazad *et al.* (2016) presented a paper on the effects of PBMT and mesenchymal stem cells on articular cartilage defects in rabbits. The results of this study showed the improvement of the control group was due to an increase in the bone growth within the deficits. This study utilized 10 subjects with bone marrow-derived stem cells injected into both knees, with one knee receiving PBMT. PBMT was administered at a wavelength of 810 nm, at a dose of 4 J/cm^2, every other day for 3 weeks. Utilization of this dosage on the knee of the rabbit lends credibility to the much higher doses utilized on our equine patients, since equine patients have significantly more difficult-to-reach target cells.

Visual identification of an upward fixation of the patella is a straightforward diagnosis. There is a stress and insult to the medial patellar ligament, which results in inflammation and pain within this structure and all of the surrounding tissues. Mild cases respond well to PBMT administered at 20–25 J/cm^2 on-contact for several consecutive days and then every other day as needed to re-establish normal function. If after three or four treatments there is still inflammation and pain within the medial patellar ligament, a medial patellar desmotomy should be considered. PBMT can then be delivered to the surgical site and surrounding tissues to accelerate healing and reduce scar formation.

Ligamentous strains and sprains of the structures surrounding the stifle joint are commonplace in competitive equine athletes. Uneven stress loads to these structures while training long and hard over unforgiving surfaces are universally unavoidable. These injuries can also be the result of a biomechanical compensation from another primary lameness issue. Rarely do these injuries involve just one structure, so it is imperative to apply PBMT locally to the area of concern and to all adjacent structures. These are thick ligamentous bands of tissue requiring dosages of 20–30 J/cm^2, applied on-contact. It is nearly impossible to place this area through passive range of motion during treatment, so manual massage should be utilized during administration. Often, in the acute stage of these injuries, the patient will be experiencing enough pain to be uncooperative with on-contact treatment. This is easily resolved by treating off-contact for a period of time, or even for several treatment sessions, until the analgesic effect has taken place and the patient allows contact administration. Acute cases benefit from daily or at least every-other-day therapy sessions. These are then spaced out until the case is resolved. Since the training surface seldom changes with these athletes, maintenance therapy sessions administered weekly after a hard work-out will allow them to recover faster and perform at a higher level.

A number of disorders occur within the stifle joint. These include capsulitis, synovitis, osteochondritis dessicans, subchondral bone cysts, and osteoarthritis. Due to the anatomical structure of this joint and its inaccessibility medially and posteriorly, it contains areas that are difficult to reach with photonic stimulation. The fluid within the joint is yet another density for the light to penetrate. Dosages range from 20 to 40 J/cm^2, delivered safely on-contact, with particular attention being paid to applying at all possible angles toward the target tissues. Therapy should be administered daily or at least every other day when an acute condition exists. This will continue until resolution of the case. Chronic disorders benefit from the establishment of a maintenance program of at least one therapy session per week.

PBMT is a beneficial follow-up to post-intra-articular injection. Numerous combinations of intra-articular injection can be performed on this joint, so for simplicity they will be categorized into non-regenerative (HA and cortisone) and regenerative (PRP and stem cells) types. The goal of treatment post intra-articular injection with a non-regenerative substance is to maintain the anti-inflammatory response. It is prudent to wait at least 3 days post injection before initiating a maintenance application of PBMT. This strategy allows for a greater time before repeating the injection. An added benefit is that instead of a continuous cycle of not painful to so painful that another intra-articular injection is needed, the patient is maintained with a minimum of pain and inflammation. This results in an animal that is more comfortable to train and is a sounder competitor.

There is scientific evidence of the benefits of administering PBMT in conjunction with intra-articular regenerative therapies, but a controversy over when it is beneficial to apply PBMT post intra-articular injection of these regenerative substances (Ginani *et al.*, 2015). Initially, due to prudence caused by not knowing how PBMT works, it was advised that therapy not be applied for at least 90 days. The flaws with this advice are evident. There is absolutely a need for scientific studies on which to base sound recommendations for these cases, but through the time-tested trial and error of daily practice, it is safe to say that administration of PBMT at least 10 days post regenerative intra-articular administration is beneficial. This recommendation may change as more information becomes available.

Consistent clinical results are obtained when PBMT is applied to the primary, compensatory secondary, and tertiary areas. As in other anatomical areas, digital thermal imaging can help identify all affected areas (Figure 32.21). Following PBMT of all affected areas, complementary acupuncture points should be stimulated with 150–200 J/point (Table 32.10, Figure 32.22) (Fleming, 1998).

Case Studies

Presentation

A 4-year-old standardbred gelding presented with a history of intermittent left rear leg lameness. Out of the previous five starts, this gelding had finished first and second twice, but in the last two races it had tried to make a break. An intra-articular injection of HA and corticosteroid 3 weeks prior had resulted in no improvement.

Work-up

Digital palpation revealed swelling and soreness over both the medial and the lateral patellar ligaments and

(a)

(b)

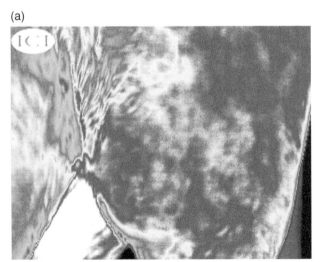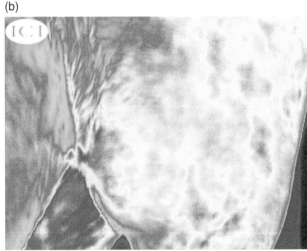

Figure 32.21 (a) Oblique thermographic view of a left stifle before the application of PBMT. Increased thermal gradients can be seen throughout the femoropatellar and femoraltibial joints and surrounding soft tissues. (b) The same stifle 1 day after initial PBMT treatment. The progress of the PBMT can be objectively measured by a reduction in the thermal gradients. Though the horse was sound at this point, two additional treatments were administered at 24-hour intervals.

soreness over the medial patellar collateral ligament. The patient was 2/5 lame. Radiographs revealed only slight osseous change over the medial condyle of the femur. Ultrasound study revealed numerous areas of fluid and swelling within both the medial and the lateral patellar ligaments, with no evidence of tears. All other soft-tissue structures were within normal limits.

Diagnosis

Strain of both the medial and lateral patellar and the medial collateral patellar ligaments.

Treatment Plan

- Systemic non-steroidal anti-inflammatory administration for 10 days.
- Administration of PBMT locally throughout both the medial and the lateral soft-tissue structures surrounding the left stifle joint at a dose of 25 J/cm^2

Table 32.10 Acupuncture points for stifle pain.

Condition/disorder	Corresponding acupuncture points
Stifle Pain	Bai Hui, BL 20, BL 21, BL 27, BL 36, BL 37, BL 38, LV 8, SP 9, KI 10

daily for 3 days, then every other day for six more treatments.
- Administration of PBMT to the left and right hip, the lumbosacral area, and the right stifle at appropriate dosages.
- Stimulation at the end of each session of the following acupuncture points with 150 J/point: Bai Hui, BL 20, BL 21, BL 27, BL 36, BL 37, BL 38, LIV 8, SP 9, and KI 10.
- Hand walking for the first 3 days, followed by jogging for 2 miles on the regular training schedule. Training at speed and paddock turnout were restricted until a re-evaluation could be completed.

Resolution

Re-check revealed no pain or noticeable swelling upon digital palpation. The trainer stated that after the first week of therapy, the patient was sound at the jog. Then, 2 days prior to this follow-up exam, the trainer had a difficult time restricting speed at the jog. Ultrasound exam revealed a resolution of the swelling and fluid previously present on both the medial and the lateral collateral patellar ligaments.

Recommendations

- Increase jogging distance and train normally in 1 week.
- Administer two more PBMT sessions, one in 2 days and one immediately after training.

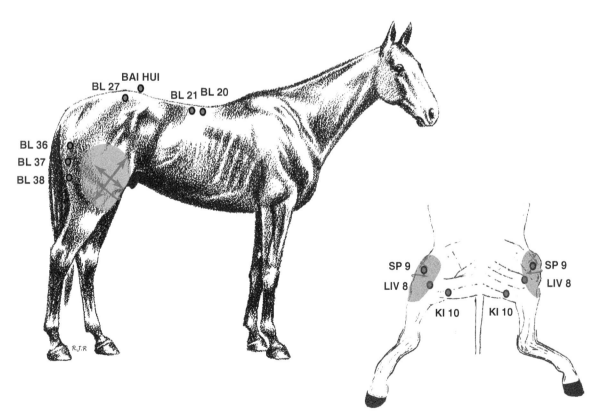

Figure 32.22 Acupuncture points and the recommended area of treatment for the painful disorders of the stifle.

Results

Training sessions went well, with no evidence of lameness. The patient was cleared to race after requalification due to time off. PBMT was administered after the qualifying race. He was trained again the following week, and PBMT was administered after he was cooled. The patient was entered to race and had a PBMT session 2 days prior to the event. He raced at his previous level and finished third. PBMT was administered the day after the race, and the patient was hand walked. The normal training scheduled was followed after the day off. Two more PBMT sessions were administered before the race the following week. The patient finished first and had a personal record of 3/10 seconds faster than its previous lifetime mark (track was fast). This therapy regimen was followed for the next 5 weeks. The total purse money after the initiation of PBMT as a treatment and a maintenance program was approximately $46 000. The total cost of PBMT sessions was $4200. The horse was then sold to another owner for $80 000 and hauled to another track in another state. Over the next few weeks, the performance of the horse gradually declined after it won the first race for the new owner.

The Hock (Tarsus) and Metatarsus

The hock has three functions: it absorbs energy in the early stance phase, provides forward propulsion in the late stance phase, and raises and lowers the height of the hoof during the swing phase. Biomechanical studies, using radiopharmaceutical uptake with nuclear scintigraphy, have shown the greatest amount of compression occurs on the distal medial aspect of the tibia and the proximal lateral aspect of the third metatarsus. This suggests that the force ascending the limb is transferred from medial to lateral through this structure (Badoux *et al.*, 1987; Murray *et al.*, 2004). This area is subjected to a large amount of torque and a large compressive force. These biomechanical forces are the etiology for most of the lameness disorders that clinically transpire here.

The hock is composed of three rows of tarsal bones. The talus and calcaneus make up the proximal row. A central tarsal bone is the main component of the intermediate row, along with portions of the fused first and second tarsal bones. The third row comprises the third and fourth tarsal bones, in addition to the fused first and second tarsals. There are three metatarsal bones, and they have the same general anatomy as the corresponding metacarpal bones, with only a slight difference in angulation and length (Riegel and Hakola, 1996, pp. 134–150).

The hock joint is composed of three areas of articulation: the tarsocrural, intertarsal, and tarsometatatarsal

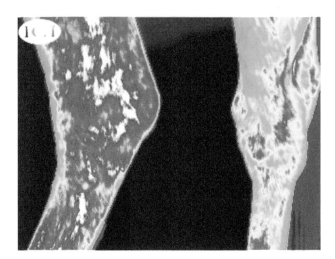

Figure 32.23 Digital thermal image of the right tarsus. In this APMLO view, increased thermal gradients are present. These are areas of increased blood flow and inflammation, and should receive special attention when applying PBMT.

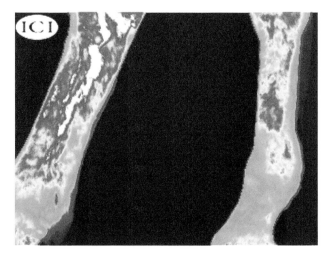

Figure 32.24 Digital thermal image of the right and left metatarsals. Areas of increased thermal gradient require thorough examination and should be considered for special attention when applying PBMT.

articulations. These contain four communicating synovial sacs for lubrication.

There are six common ligaments surrounding the hock joint: laterally, the long and short lateral ligaments; medially, the long and short medial ligaments; the plantar ligament on the plantar surface; and the dorsal ligament on the dorsal surface. Throughout these soft-tissue structures is a very complex neurovascular supply that also supplies the remainder of the distal limb.

This complex anatomical structure, and the amount and direction of biomechanical forces ascending through it, is often the primary source of hind-limb lameness. It is very superficial and is easily accessible to saturation of photonic energy (Figures 32.23 and 32.24).

The disorders in this area that respond well to PBMT are synovitis, joint capsulitis, cunean bursitis, cunean tendonitis, fracture repair, bone spavin (osteoarthritis and osteitis), bog spavin (tarsocrural synovitis), and curbs (tarsal plantar desmitis), and in some cases osteochondrosis, stringhalt, and capped hocks (hygroma). These disorders can occur as a single manifestation, but normally a combination of several maladies occurs simultaneously.

Before initiating any PBMT treatment plan, establish an accurate diagnosis of the primary and all possible secondary disorders. Administer dosages of $20–25 \text{J/cm}^2$ on-contact. On-contact treatment may not be possible if the target area is in too much pain for the patient to tolerate even the slight contact pressure of the handpiece (e.g., acute cunean tendonitis). If this occurs, administer the therapy off-contact until the analgesic effect is initiated, which will allow an on-contact technique.

Treatment of this area is performed while the patient is weight bearing. It is often necessary to pick up a fore limb to keep the hind limb stationary. Apply the therapy to the entire area circumferentially at all angles. It is often easier to administer therapy to the medial structures from the opposite side of the patient. Administer at least 60% of the total dose at all angles directly over the area of concern. Visualize the anatomy beneath the skin and ensure the primary area of concern and all surrounding soft tissues and joint spaces receive adequate amounts of energy.

The frequency of the therapy sessions will depend on the severity of the condition, whether it is acute or chronic, the compliance of the owner and trainer, and the schedule of competitive events. Acute cases should initially be treated very aggressively, daily or every other day, then tapered in frequency once a favorable clinical response is noted until the therapeutic goal is reached and the issue is resolved. When managing chronic issues, the initial therapy sessions should not be as aggressive, and should be administered every other day until a therapeutic goal is reached, at which point a maintenance regime should be initiated to maintain the goal.

The clinical success of the application of PBMT to any of the boney structures within this region relies on the ability of the photonic energy to reach the target. It is difficult to reach many of these structures, since it is difficult, if not impossible, to place this area through passive range of motion during administration.

Bone spavin is common in all breeds of horse, especially the Icelandic horse, where it is thought to be a heritable condition (Axelsson *et al.*, 2001). It is the most common cause of chronic hind-limb lameness. A very painful condition that is not just osteoarthritis, it also includes osteitis, synovitis, and joint capsulitis. The distal intertarsal, tarsometatarsal, and proximal intertrarsal joints can be individually involved, or the condition can occur throughout the entire joint. It often begins on the dorsolateral aspect of these joints, a region of high compression strain (Tranquille *et al.*, 2009). Therefore, even when there is no radiographic evidence of change, ensure that these areas receive a saturating dose of photonic energy from every possible angle.

Osteochondrosis is a condition in which the cartilage at the end of the long bones fails to develop normally. If this condition results in a fragment of the cartilage being displaced, it is defined as osteochondritis dissecans. Wittwer *et al.* (2006) published a study examining 167 South German coldbloods, with a mean age of 14 months. They found an incidence of 61.7% of osteochondrotic lesions in the fetlock or hock joints and 26.9% of osseus fragments. Lesions in racing thoroughbreds and standardbreds are usually seen by age 2, but in warmbloods, which are older when they begin training, clinical signs may not be seen until the age of 5–6 years.

The success of treatment of osteochondrosis with PBMT is contingent upon the location of the lesion. When the lesion can be fully saturated with photonic energy, the clinical results of utilizing PBMT in conjunction with traditional care (both systemic and intra-articular) are very consistent. When the lesion is inaccessible to the light energy, the clinical results will be the same as if the patient were solely on a traditional therapeutic regime.

Even though these lesions seem very superficial, they are covered by the skin, fibrous soft-tissue structures, and the synovial fluid. Therefore, dosages of $25–30 \text{J/cm}^2$ should be administered on-contact, not only directly over the lesion, but also over all surrounding tissues and joint spaces. Therapy should be administered as often as possible, with at least 12 treatments over 30 days, until a follow-up radiographic exam can determine the progress of the case. PBMT should be administered in combination with systemic and intra-articular therapy such as PRP. If intra-articular PRP is administered, the first therapy session should be at least 7 days post injection.

Soft-tissue disorders, tendonitis, desmitis, and any inflammation within the associated bursa respond well to PBMT. These structures usually lie just beneath the dermis and are readily accessible to photonic stimulation. Administer dosages of $15–20 \text{J/cm}^2$ on-contact from the origin to the insertion. Include the bursa sac beneath, any surrounding soft tissues, and the underlying joint. In almost all cases, the general rule is to treat the entire hock circumferentially, with a high percentage of the energy administered directly to the primary and any secondary structures that may also be involved.

Acute tendonitis/desmitis will often respond after the first PBMT session. After the first treatment, it is not unusual for the patient to appear unsound on the opposite hind limb. These conditions are often bilateral, with one limb being more painful than the other. This transformation is not as distinct as a nerve block to the area, but it is visible in the majority of the patients. With the hock being the primary cause of lameness, there will always be compensatory secondary and tertiary areas that would benefit from therapy. Ideally, treatment should be administered to both hocks, stifles, hips, and the lumbosacral areas. Treat as aggressively as possible, daily or every other day for three or four sessions, then less frequently once a clinical response is noted until the treatment goal is reached. These acute cases will often require a maintenance treatment plan to avoid reoccurrence. The maintenance plan will be unique to each patient, depending upon the disciple and the compliance of the client, owner, and trainer, and will be partially determined by the athlete's competition schedule.

The goal when treating a chronic case of tendonitis/desmitis is to maintain the soundness of the animal throughout the competitive season. These cases have a history of systemic and localized pharmaceutical treatment. PBMT sessions should be tailored to each athlete's schedule. Initially, treat aggressively, and then maintain performance at the highest level possible.

The literature states that PBMT plays a protective role in the degradation of cartilage and synovitis in rabbits with progressive osteoarthritis (Wang, P. *et al.*, 2014). Inflammation of the synovial membrane and joint capsule can be caused by direct injury to the joint, constant concussive force resulting from poor conformation, or most disorders within the hock (tarsocrural synovitis, commonly referred to as "bog spavin," is a good example).

Treat these conditions early and aggressively with a dose of 10–15 J/cm^2 on-contact.

Stimulation of the complementary acupuncture points with PBMT should be accomplished after all localized therapy has been administered. Administer 120–150 J/point to the points listed in Table 32.11 and illustrated in Figure 32.25 (Fleming, 1998).

Conclusion

PBMT provides an excellent therapeutic option for a variety of equine disorders. The biochemical cascade of events that occurs upon stimulation results in an alleviation of pain, a modulation of the inflammatory cycle, and an increase in circulation. When administered at the correct dosage, utilizing a good application technique, with a sufficient number of treatments, PBMT will accelerate the healing process, allowing a faster return to competition and an improved quality of life. PBMT has become an integral part of our standard of care for equine patients and should be considered and included in most treatment plans.

Table 32.11 Acupuncture points for hock pain.

Condition/disorder	Corresponding acupuncture points
Hock pain	BL 18, BL 19, BL 23, BL 35, BL 39, BL 60, BL 62, ST 45, LV 4

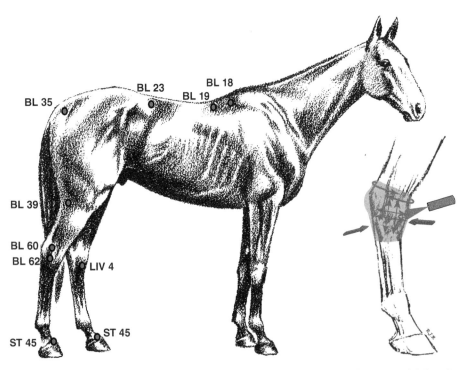

Figure 32.25 Acupuncture points and the recommended area of treatment for the painful disorders of the hock.

References

Anders, J.J. *et al.* (2004) Phototherapy promotes regeneration and functional recovery of injured peripheral nerve. *Neurol Res.* **26**(2):233–239.

Anon. (1965) British Equine Veterinary Association survey of equine disease 1962–1963. *Vet Rec.* **77**:528.

Assis, L. *et al.* (2016) Aerobic exercise training and low-level laser therapy modulate inflammatory response and degenerative process in an experimental model of knee osteoarthritis in rats. *Osteoarthritis Cartilage.* **24**(1):169–177.

Axelsson, M. *et al.* (2001) Risk factors associated with hindlimb lameness and degenerative joint disease in the distal tarsus of Icelandic horses. *Equine Vet J.* **33**(1):84–90.

Ayyildiz, S. *et al.* (2015) Evaluation of low-level laser therapy in TMD patients. *Case Rep Dent.* **2015**:424213.

Badoux, D. (1987) Some biomechanical aspects of the structure of the equine tarsus. *Anat Amz.* **64**(1):53–61.

Bathe, A.P. (1994) 245 fractures in thoroughbred racehorses: results of a 2-year prospective study. *Proc Am Assoc Equine Prac.* **40**:175–178.

Bjordal, J.M. *et al.* (2006) Low-level laser therapy in acute pain: a systematic review of mechanisms of action and clinical effects in randomized placebo-controlled trials. *Photomed Laser Surg.* **24**(2):158–168.

Budak, M.T. *et al.* (2009) Gene expression in the lamellar dermis-epidermis during the developmental phase of carbohydrate overload-induced laminitis in the horse. *Vet Immunol Immunopathol.* **131**(1–2):86–96.

Burns, T.A. *et al.* (2015) Laminar inflammatory events in lean and obese ponies subjected to high carbohydrate feeding: implications for pasture-associated laminitis. *Equine Vet J.* **47**(4):489–493.

Calisto, F.C. *et al.* (2015) Use of low-power laser to assist the healing of traumatic wounds. *Acta Cir Bras.* **30**(3):204–208.

Chang W. *et al.* (2014) Therapeutic outcomes of low-level laser therapy for closed bone fracture in the human wrist and hand. *Photomed Laser Surg.* **32**(4):212–218.

Chow, R. *et al.* (2011) Inhibitory effects of laser irradiation on peripheral mammalian nerves and relevance to analgesic effects: a systematic review. *Photomed Laser Surg.* **29**(6):365–381.

Coyne, M.J. *et al.* (2008) Cloning and expression of ADAM-related metalloproteases in equine laminitis. *Vet Immunol Immunopathol.* **129**(3–4):231–241.

de Jesus, J.F. *et al.* (2016) Low-level laser therapy (780nm) on VEGF modulation at partially injured Achilles tendon. *Photomed Laser Surg.* **34**(8):331–335.

Dyce, K.M. *et al.* (2002) The neck, back, and vertebral column of the horse. In: *Textbook of Veterinary Anatomy*, 3 edn., pp. 598–624. Saunders, Philadelphia, PA.

Enwemeka, C.S. (2009) Intricacies of dose in laser phototherapy for tissue repair and pain relief. *Photomed Laser Surg.* **27**(3):387–393.

Fekrazad, R. *et al.* (2016) Effects of photobiomodulation and mesenchymal stem cells on articular cartilage defects in a rabbit model. *Photomed Laser Surg.* **34**(11):543–549.

Fleming, P. (1994) Acupuncture treatment for musculoskeletal and neurological conditions in horses. In: *Veterinary Acupuncture: Ancient Art to Modern Medicine*, pp. 183–194. Mosby, Maryland Heights, MO.

Fleming, P. (1998) Equine acupuncture. In: *Complementary and Alternative Veterinary Medicine*, 1 edn., pp. 182. Mosby, Maryland Heights, MO.

Ginani, F. *et al.* (2015) Effect of low-level laser therapy on mesenchymal stem cell proliferation: a systemic review. *Lasers Med Sci.* **30**(8):2189–2194.

Ip, D. and Fu, N.Y. (2015) Can combined use of low-level lasers and hyaluronic acid injections prolong the longevity of degenerative knee joints? *Clin Interv Aging.* **10**:1255–1258.

Jang, H. and Lee, H. (2012) Meta-analysis of pain relief effects by laser irradiation on joint areas. *Photomed Laser Surg.* **30**(8):405–417.

Jeffcoat, L.B. (1980a) Disorders of the thoracolumbar spine of the horse – a survey of 443 cases. *Eq Vet J.* **12**(4):197–210.

Jeffcoat, L.B. (1980b) Guidelines for the diagnosis and treatment of back problems in horses. *Proceedings of the 26th Annual Conference of the American Association of Equine Practitioners*. November 30–December 3, 2016. Anaheim, CA.

Kazem, S.S. *et al.* (2010) Effect of low-level laser therapy on the fracture healing process. *Lasers Med Sci.* **25**(1):73–77.

Lemos, G.A. *et al.* (2016) Low-level laser stimulates tissue repair and reduces the extracellular matrix degradation in rats with induced arthritis in the temporomandibular joint. *Lasers Med Sci.* **31**(6):1051–1059.

Levine, D. *et al.* (2015) Effects of laser on endurance of the rotator cuff muscles. *Lasers Surg Med.* **47**(S26):44–45.

Loftus, J.P. *et al* (2008) Leukocyte-derived and endogenous matrix metalloproteinases in the lamellae of horses with naturally acquired and experimentally induced laminitis. *Vet Immunol Immunopathol.* **129**(3–4):221–230.

Machado, B.C. *et al.* (2016) Effects of oral motor exercises and laser therapy on chronic temporomandibular disorders: a randomized study with follow-up. *Lasers Med Sci.* **31**(5):945–954.

Maegawa, Y. *et al.* (2000) Effects of near-infrared low-level laser irradiation on microcirculation. *Lasers Surg Med.* **27**(5):427–437.

Murray, R.M. *et al.* (2004) Nuclear scintigraphic evaluation of the distal tarsal region in normal horses. *Vet Radiol Ultrasound.* **45**(4):345–351.

Nakamura, T. *et al.* (2014) Low level laser therapy for chronic knee joint pain patients. *Laser Ther.* **23**(4):273–277.

Poyton, R.O. and Ball, K.A. (2011) Therapeutic photobiomodulation: nitric oxide and a novel function of mitochondrial cytochrome c oxidase. *Discov Med.* **11**(57):154–159.

Rathgeber, R. (2001) Chapter 4. In: *Understanding Equine Acupuncture*, 1 edn., pp. 36–37. The Blood-Horse, Inc., Lexington, KY.

Riegel, R.J. and Hakola, S. (1996) *Illustrated Atlas of Clinical Equine Anatomy and Common Disorders of the Horse*, 1 edn., pp. 26–40. Primedia Equine Network, Kennett Square, PA.

Ridgway, K. (1999) Acupuncture as a treatment modality for back problems. *Vet Clin North Am Equine Pract.* **15**(1):211–221.

Rogers, P. (1999). Treatment of back pain in the horse and dog by acupuncture. *1st Spanish Inter-University Meeting of Acupuncture and 3rd European Meeting of Acupuncture.* Zaragoza, Spain.

Stashak, T.S. (1976) *Adam's Lameness in Horses*, 3 edn., pp. 15–18. Lea and Febiger, Philadelphia, PA.

Sutherland, E. *et al.* (1994) Cross reference of equine acupuncture points. In: *Veterinary Acupuncture: Ancient Art to Modern Medicine.* Mosby, Maryland Heights, MO.

Tranquille, C. *et al.* (2009) Effect of exercise on thickness of mature hyaline cartilage, calcified cartilage and subchondral bone thickness of equine tarsi. *Am J Vet Res.* **70**(12):1477–1483.

Wang, C.Z. *et al.* (2014) Low-level laser irradiation improves functional recovery and nerve regeneration in sciatic nerve crush rat injury model. *PLoS One.* **9**(8):e103348.

Wang, P. *et al.* (2014) Effects of low-level laser therapy on joint pain, synovitis, anabolic, and catabolic factors in a progressive osteoarthritis rabbit model. *Lasers Med Sci.* **29**(6):1875–1885.

Wittwer, C. *et al.* (2006) Prevalence of osteochondrosis in the limb joints of South German coldblood horses. *J Vet Med A Physiol Pathol Clin Med.* **53**(10):531–539.

Xie, H. and Preast, V. (2007) *Xie's Veterinary Acupuncture*, 1 edn., pp. 254. Blackwell Publishing, Hoboken, NJ.

Xie, H. *et al.* (1997) Equine back pain: a traditional Chinese medical review. *Equine Practice* **19**:2–11.

33

Laserpuncture for the Equine Patient

Ronald J. Riegel

American Institute of Medical Laser Applications, Marysville, OH, USA

Introduction

Acupuncture will greatly contribute to any rehabilitation protocol by providing relief of pain and an increase in circulation throughout the muscled tissues (le Jeune *et al.*, 2016). It is a widely used method of treatment in the multimodal management of a diversity of conditions affecting the horse.

Using the stimulatory power of a laser to perform acupuncture is a patient-friendly and painless alternative to the classic use of needles. The use of lasers to stimulate acupuncture points is termed "laser acupuncture" or "laserpuncture" (Lorenzini *et al.*, 2010). Laser acupuncture possesses several advantages over classic needle acupuncture (Martin and Klide, 1987; Schoen and Wynn, 1998): it is non-invasive, painless, and complication-free, and it requires minimal restraint and a short treatment time.

Use of laser photonic energy to stimulation tissue at the average depth of a needle acupuncture point requires the administration of a dose of 80–200 J/point. Deeper points – those surrounded by large muscle masses and bone – require a higher dose of 125–200 J/point (Fuchtenbusch and Rosin, 2006). Using wavelengths within the therapeutic window, laser acupuncture should be administered slowly, at a low power (0.5 W), utilizing a pulsed mode of emission.

Ideally, laser acupuncture will be used as part of a multimodal management program. If used as the sole therapy, the frequency of treatment will vary with the severity of the disorder and the compliance of the client. Treatment twice weekly until the therapeutic goal is reached is recommended.

Law *et al.* (2015) published a meta-analysis of the human literature utilizing laser acupuncture for the treatment of musculoskeletal pain. Among those studies that were well designed and in which appropriate doses were administered, two-thirds reported consistent positive clinical outcomes after long-term follow-up (versus immediately after treatment).

There is a significant loss of photonic energy as the laser beam passes through superficial tissue into deeper tissue. However, the stimulatory effect is sufficient even when the acupuncture point is difficult to locate. Administration with the laser handpiece on-contact, using a circular massage motion and slight pressure, is ideal for penetration.

Anatomical Locations of Equine Acupuncture Points using Western Nomenclature

All acupuncture point location descriptions in this chapter are given according to the International Veterinary Acupuncture Society (IVAS) (www.ivas.org), unless otherwise indicated. For graphical diagrams of many of these points, refer to the tables and figures in Chapter 32. Additional information about equine acupuncture points is available in Riegel and Hakola (1996), Fleming (1998), Fuchtenbusch and Rosin (2006), Xie and Preast (2007), and Bessent (2011).

In the Western nomenclature system, each point receives a unique combination of letters and numbers to create its name. The prefix, composed of letters, is an abbreviation of the meridian on which the point lies. The numeric suffix represents the sequential position of the point on the meridian. As an example, there are 67 points on the Bladder Meridian (BL). BL 1 would be the first point on this meridian and BL 67 would be the last.

The term "cun" is used to describe a unit of measure relative or proportionate to an individual body. A distance of 1 cun is equal to the width of an individual horse's 18th (last) rib. Many practitioners often use their own fingers to gauge cun measurements: 1 cun is approximately equal to the width of the index and middle fingers, or about 3 cm (1.18 inches), while 2 cun is the width of four fingers (a hand), or about 6 cm.

Laser Therapy in Veterinary Medicine: Photobiomodulation, First Edition. Edited by Ronald J. Riegel and John C. Godbold, Jr.
© 2017 John Wiley & Sons, Inc. Published 2017 by John Wiley & Sons, Inc.

Heart Meridian

HT 7

Superficial location in the depression on the medial surface of the radius, just cranial to the cranial border of the flexor carpi ulnaris muscle, at the level of the dorsal aspect of the accessory carpal bone.

Deeper location between the flexor carpi ulnaris and superficial digital flexor muscle.

HT 8

On the caudolateral aspect of the third metacarpal, half the distance from the carpus to the fetlock, just cranial to the deep digital flexor tendon.

HT 9

On the palmarolateral aspect of the front foot, in the depression just proximal to the coronary band, approximately two-thirds of the distance from the dorsal midline of the coronary band to the palmar border of the lateral bulb of the heel.

Pericardium Meridian

PC 6

In the depression just cranial to the cranial border of the chestnut, midway between the proximal and distal ends of the chestnut.

PC 8

On the fore limb, half the distance from the carpus to the fetlock, on the caudal aspect of the superficial digital flexor tendon.

PC 9

On the palmar midline of the front foot, in the depression between the bulbs of the heel.

Lung Meridian

LU 1

In the depression in the middle of the pectoralis descendens muscle, 1.5 cun lateral to the pectoralis sulcus (in the first intercostal space).

LU 7

In the depression on the medial surface of the radius, 1.5 cun proximal to the most medial prominence of the styloid process, 0.5 cun distal to the level of PC 6.

LU 10

On the medial side of the fore limb, at the halfway junction of the third metacarpal, between the suspensory ligament and the palmar digital vein.

LU 11

On the palmaromedial aspect of the front foot, in the depression just proximal to the coronary band, approximately two-thirds of the distance from the dorsal midline of the coronary band to the palmar border of the medial bulb of the heel.

Stomach Meridian

ST 25

In the depression 1.5 cun lateral to the umbilicus.

ST 34

Approximately 3 cun proximal to the proximal and lateral edge of the patella.

ST 35

In the large depression ventral to the ventral border of the patella, between the middle and lateral patellar ligaments.

ST 36

In the depression just lateral to the tibial crest, in the muscular groove between the tibialis cranialis and long digital extensor muscles, 2 cun distal to the proximal edge of the tibial crest.

ST 45

On the dorsal midline of the rear foot, in the depression just proximal to the coronary band.

Small-Intestine Meridian

SI 1

On the dorsolateral aspect of the front foot, in the depression just proximal to the coronary band, approximately one-third of the distance from the dorsal midline of the coronary band to the palmar border of the lateral bulb of the heel.

SI 3

On the lateral side of the fore limb, in the depression just distal to the end of the 4th metacarpal (lateral splint) bone and proximal to the fetlock, on the palmarolateral border of the 3rd metacarpal bone.

SI 4

On the lateral surface of the fore limb, distal to the carpal joint, upper one-third of the distance from carpus to fetlock, cranial to the suspensory ligament.

SI 6

Distal to the tip of the ulna, over the lateral ulnar muscle.

SI 9

In the large depression caudal to the proximal humerus, along the caudal border of the deltoid muscle and between the long and lateral heads of the triceps brachii muscle.

SI 10
At 2 cun craniodorsal to SI 9.

SI 16
On the dorsal boarder of the brachiocephalicus muscle at the level of the second cervical vertebrae.

Large-Intestine Meridian

LI 1
On the dorsomedial aspect of the front foot, in the depression just proximal to the coronary band, approximately one-third of the distance from the dorsal midline of the coronary band to the palmar border of the medial bulb of the heel.

LI 4
On the medial side of the fore limb, in the depression just palmar to the 2nd metacarpal (medial splint) bone and distal to its base. This would be at the level between the proximal and middle thirds of the 3rd metacarpal (cannon) bone. There are three depressions on the palmar aspect of the 2nd metacarpal bone, and this point is located on the level of the second depression.

LI 6
At 3 cun proximal to the lateral distal tuberositas radii, between the extensor carpi radialis and common digital extensor muscles.

LI 11
In the transverse cubital crease, in the depression just cranial to the lateral epicondyle of the humerus between the extensor carpi radialis and common digital extensor muscles. This point is easily palpated when the elbow is flexed.

LI 15
Just cranial to the point of the shoulder (cranial part of the greater or lateral tuberosity of the humerus).

LI 16
Along the cranial boarder of the scapula, in a depression two-thirds of the distance from TH 15 to the point of the shoulder.

LI 17
At 2 cun craniodorsal to LI 16, on the brachiocephalic muscle.

LI 18
With the head extended, along the line of the ventral mandible to the depression just above the jugular groove.

Liver Meridian

LV 1
On the dorsomedial aspect of the rear foot, in the depression just proximal to the coronary band, approximately

one-third of the distance from the dorsal midline of the coronary band to the plantar border of the medial bulb of the heel.

LV 3
On the medial side of the hind limb, in the depression just plantar to the 2nd metatarsal (medial splint) bone and distal to its base. This would be at the level between the proximal and middle thirds of the 3rd metatarsal (cannon) bone.

LV 4
In the cranial aspect of the hock, on the saphenous vein, medial to the cunean tendon.

LV 8
Posterior to the medial condyle of the femur, in the depression cranial to the insertion of the semitendinosus and semimembranosus muscles and caudal to the saphenous vein.

Gall-Bladder Meridian

GB 20
In the large depression just caudal to the lateral canthus.

GB 21
In the depression cranial to the cranial border of the subclavius muscle, dorsal to the dorsal border of the omotransversarius muscle, and dorsal to the 7th cervical vertebra. Some authors put it at the level of the midpoint of the cranial border of the scapula.

GB 27
At 0.5 cun craniodorsal to the cranial aspect of the iliac spine.

GB 28
In a depression midway between GB 27 and GB 29.

GB 29
In the depression located midway on a line from the ventral aspect of the tuber coxae (coxal tuber) to the palpable middle of the 3rd trochanter of the femur.

GB 30
In the depression caudoventral to the dorsal border of the caudal portion of the greater trochanter, in the biceps femoris muscle.

GB 34
In the interosseous space between the tibia and fibula and between the long and lateral digital extensor muscles, craniodistal to the head of the fibula.

GB 39

In the depression 3 cun proximal to the most lateral prominence of the lateral malleolus of the tibia, caudal to the tibial border, cranial to the deep digital flexor muscle.

GB 44

On the dorsolateral aspect of the rear foot, in the depression just proximal to the coronary band, approximately one-third of the distance from the dorsal midline of the coronary band to the plantar border of the lateral bulb of the heel.

Spleen Meridian

SP 1

On the plantaromedial aspect of the rear foot, in the depression just proximal to the coronary band, approximately two-thirds of the distance from the dorsal midline of the coronary band to the plantar border of the medial bulb of the heel.

SP 6

In the depression 3 cun proximal to the most medial prominence of the medial malleolus of the tibia, just caudal to the caudal border of the tibia and dorsal to the combined heads of the deep digital flexor muscle, tibialis caudalis muscle, and lateral digital flexor muscle. This point is usually located just distal to where the saphenous vein crosses the caudal border of the tibia. Since the fibula does not exist in the horse, SP 06 is located opposite GB 39 on the lateral aspect of the leg.

SP 9

In the depression just ventral to the medial condyle of the tibia, caudal to the caudal border of the tibia, over the popliteus muscle and cranial to the sephenous vein.

SP 13

Directly ventral to the tuber coxae.

Kidney Meridian

KI 1

On the plantar midline of the rear foot, in the depression between the bulbs of the heel.

KI 3

On the medial aspect of the hock area, in the middle of the webbed area cranial to the calcaneal tendon, at the level of the tip of the tuber calcanei (calcanean tuber).

KI 10

On the medial side of the popliteal fossa at the level of BL 40, between the semitendinosis and semimembranosis muscles.

Bladder Meridian

BL 10

In a depression just caudal to the wings of the atlas, 2 cun from the dorsal midline.

BL 11

In the depression just cranial to the craniodorsal border of the scapular cartilage, 1.5 cun lateral to the dorsal midline, over the cervical portion of the trapezius muscle.

BL 13

At the caudal edge of the scapular cartilage (8th intercostal space), 3 cun lateral to the dorsal midline.

BL 14

At the 9th intercostal space, 3 cun lateral to the dorsal midline within the intercostal muscle group.

BL 15

At the 10th intercostal space, 3 cun lateral to the dorsal midline (in the iliocostal muscle groove).

BL 17

In the depression 3 cun lateral to the dorsal midline, in the 12th intercostal space, in the muscular groove between the longissimus thoracis and iliocostalis thoracis muscles.

BL 18

In the depression 3 cun lateral to the dorsal midline. This point has two locations: in the 13th and 14th intercostal spaces, in the muscular groove between the longissimus thoracis and iliocostalis thoracis muscles.

BL 19

In the depression 3 cun lateral to the dorsal midline, in the 15th intercostal space, in the muscular groove between the longissimus thoracis and iliocostalis thoracis muscles.

BL 20

In the depression 3 cun lateral to the dorsal midline, in the 17th (last) intercostal space, in the muscular groove between the longissimus thoracis and iliocostalis thoracis muscles.

BL 21

In the depression 3 cun lateral to the dorsal midline, in the depression caudal to the 18th (last) rib, between T18 and L1 (T–L junction), in the muscular groove between the longissimus lumborum and iliocostalis lumborum muscles.

BL 22

In the first lumbar intervertebral space (L1–L2), 3 cun lateral to the dorsal midline.

BL 23

In the depression 3 cun lateral to the dorsal midline, between the spinous processes of L2 and L3, in the muscular groove between the longissimus lumborum and the iliocostalis lumborum muscles.

BL 25

In the depression 3 cun lateral to the dorsal midline, between the spinous processes of the 5th and 6th lumbar vertebrae (L4 and L5, if L6 is missing). Usually on a line extending from the dorsal midline to the cranial edge of the tuber coxae (coxal tuber).

BL 26

In the depression 3 cun lateral to the dorsal midline, between the spinous processes of the 6th (or 5th, if 6th is missing) lumbar and the 1st sacral vertebrae.

BL 27

In the depression 3 cun lateral to the dorsal midline and 1.5 cun lateral to the 1st sacral foramen.

BL 28

In the depression 3 cun lateral to the dorsal midline and 1.5 cun lateral to the 2nd sacral foramen.

BL 32

In the second sacral intervertebral space, 1.5 cun lateral to the dorsal midline.

BL 35

At the dorsal end of the muscular groove between the biceps femoris and semitendinosus muscles.

BL 36

In the muscular groove between the biceps femoris and semitendinosus muscles, 2 cun distal to the tuber ischii (ischial tuber).

BL 37

In the muscular groove between the biceps femoris and semitendinosus muscles, 5 cun distal to the tuber ischii (ischial tuber).

BL 38

In the muscular groove between the biceps femoris and semitendinosus muscles, 8 cun distal to the tuber ischii (ischial tuber).

BL 39

In the depression just medial to the caudal division of the biceps femoris muscle, at the ventral end of the muscular groove between the biceps femoris and semitendinosus muscles; level with the stifle.

BL 40

In the depression, at the midpoint of the transverse crease of the popliteal fossa, between the caudal division of the biceps femoris and semitendinosus mucles. More easily found with the stifle flexed.

BL 54

In the depression at the intersection of two lines: one from the caudal portion of the greater trochanter to the lumbosacral space, the other from the dorsal aspect of the tuber coxae (coxal tuber) to the tuber ischii (ischial tuber).

BL 60

On the lateral aspect of the hock area, in the middle of the webbed area cranial to the calcaneal tendon, at the level of the tip of the tuber calcanei (calcanean tuber).

BL 62

In the depression just plantardistal to the most lateral prominence of the lateral malleolus of the tibia.

BL 63

In the depression proximal to the base of the 4th metatarsal bone and dorsal to the long plantar ligament.

BL 67

On the plantarolateral aspect of the rear foot, in the depression just proximal to the coronary band, approximately two-thirds of the distance from the dorsal midline of the coronary band to the plantar border of the lateral bulb of the heel.

Triple-Heater Meridian

TH 1

On the dorsal midline of the front foot, in the depression just proximal to the coronary band.

TH 5

In the groove between the tendons of the lateral digital extensor and common digital extensor muscles, at the level of the midportion of the cranial border of the chestnut.

TH 7

On the radial side of the ulna, 3 cun proximal to the carpus.

TH 11

At 1 cun cranial to TH 10.

TH 13

Two-thirds of the distance from TH 11 to TH 14.

TH 14

In the caudal margin of shoulder joint, at the level of the point of the shoulder.

TH 16

At the caudal boarder of the brachiocephalic muscle, between the 1st and 2nd cervical vertebral spaces, cranial and dorsal to SI 16.

TH 17

In the depression between the mandible and the mastoid process, caudoventral to the ear.

Conception-Vessel Meridian

CV 12

On the ventral midline, in the depression halfway between the xiphoid process and the umbilicus.

CV 24

On the ventral midline, 1 cun ventral to the border of the lower lip.

Governing-Vessel Meridian

Bai Hui (Hundred Meetings)

In the depression on the dorsal midline in the lumbosacral space.

GV 14

On the dorsal midline, in the depression between the spinous processes of the 7th cervical and the 1st thoracic vertebrae.

GV 24

On the dorsal midline at the rostral end of the mane.

GV 26

On the midline, between the ventral limits of the nostrils.

Other Points

Yin-Tang

In the depression at the junction of the frontal bones, on the dorsal midline of the face, at the level of the lateral canthi.

Tong-Tang (Communicating Hall)

At the dorsal midline, at the level of the medial canthus of the eye.

Chou-Jin (Pulling Tendon)

On the midline of the upper lip.

ER-Jian (Ear Tip)

At the tip of the ear, on its outer surface, at the junction of the medial, middle, and lateral branches of the auricular vein.

Ear Shen-Men

In the inter-ridge groove 0.5 cun above the distal end of the common cutaneous ridge.

References

Bessent, C. (2011) *Equine Acupuncture Points and Meridians*. Herbsmith, Hartland, WI.

Fleming, P. (1998) Equine acupuncture. In: *Complementary and Alternative Veterinary Medicine*, 1 edn. Mosby, Maryland Heights, MO.

Fuchtenbusch, A. and Rosin, P. (2006) *Laser Therapy and Acupuncture on Horses*. Self-published.

Law, D. *et al.* (2015) Laser acupuncture for treating musculoskeletal pain: a systematic review with meta-analysis. *J Acupunct Meridian Stud.* **8**(1):2–16.

le Jeune, S. *et al.* (2016) Acupuncture and equine rehabilitation. *Vet Clinics North Amer Equine Pract.* **32**(1):73–85.

Lorenzini, L. *et al.* (2010) Laser acupuncture for acute inflammatory, visceral and neuropathic pain relief: an experimental study in the laboratory rat. *Res Vet Sci.* **88**(1):159–165.

Martin, B.B. and Klide, A.M. (1987) Treatment of chronic back pain in horses. Stimulation of acupuncture points with a low powered infrared laser. *Vet Surg.* **16**(1):106–110.

Riegel, R.J. and Hakola, S. (1996) *Illustrated Atlas of Clinical Equine Anatomy and Common Disorders of the Horse*, 1 edn. Primedia Equine Network, Kennett Square, PA.

Schoen, A.M. and Wynn, S.G. (1998) *Complementary and Alternative Veterinary Medicine Principles and Practice*, 1 edn., pp. 173–184. Mosby, Maryland Heights, MO.

Xie, H. and Preast, V. (2007) *Xie's Veterinary Acupuncture*, 1 edn. Blackwell Publishing, Hoboken, NJ.

34

Laser Therapy for the Treatment of Equine Wounds

Ronald J. Riegel

American Institute of Medical Laser Applications, Marysville, OH, USA

Introduction

The basic nature of the "flight response" increases the risk of traumatic injuries to the equine species. Their basic instinct is to flee, often with no regard as to what part of their anatomy is trapped or in close proximity with a sharp object. Cases are presented on a regular basis for lacerations, abrasions, contusions, penetrating, and contaminated wounds. At times, it seems there are only two categories of equine patient in the practice: those that have a wound of some nature, and those that will have a wound. Proper care of these wounds is a long-term, labor–intensive, and sometimes very frustrating activity, with the ultimate goal of restoring these disrupted tissues to normal anatomic activity and leaving little evidence of their initial occurrence. The application of laser therapy (photobiomodulation therapy, PBMT) accelerates the healing proess and restoration of tissues, making it an important addendum to the management of these injuries.

The Influence of PBMT on Wound Healing

Wound healing is the natural, systemic, restorative response to any traumatic insult to the skin or other body tissues, such as muscle or tendon. When a traumatic incident occurs, an orchestrated biochemical cascade of events is set into motion, aimed at repairing the damage (Nguyen *et al.*, 2009). This process is divided into four overlapping phases: hemostasis (clotting), inflammation, tissue growth (proliferation), and maturation (Stadelmann *et al.*, 1998). PBMT has been shown to have a significant stimulating influence on the healing of wounds (AlGhamdi *et al.*, 2012; Mester *et al.*, 1971; Peplow *et al.*, 2010a). Understanding the mechanisms by which PBMT influences each phase allows individualized

modifications to treatment. The result is consistent acceleration of the healing process.

PBMT influences each phase of wound healing, supporting or augmenting the normal progression of physiological events. Photonic energy reaches the electron transport chain embedded in the inner membrane of the mitochondria. The energy is absorbed by chromophores (photoacceptor molecules in fibroblasts and endothelial cells), producing an electronically excited molecular state. This alters primary molecular processes, leading to biological effects at the cellular level via secondary biochemical reactions and cellular signaling (Passarella and Karu 2014). These reactions restore any deficiencies within the respiratory chain, resulting in an improved cellular metabolism (Karu 1998). There is an increase in the production of adenosine triphosphate (ATP), a release of nitric oxide (NO) and reactive oxygen species (ROS), and the advent of numerous biochemical events that normalize cellular functions. Through this biochemical cascade, PBMT has the ability to activate fibroblasts and macrophages, cause the release of growth factors and neurotransmitter substances, cause vasodilation, and influence collagen synthesis. All of these events are important to the healing of wounds (Karu, 1999; Karu and Kolyakov, 2005; Woodruff *et al.*, 2004). (More information on the basic principles of photobiomodulation (PBM) is available in Chapter 5.)

Phases of Wound Healing

Hemostasis Phase

Vasoconstriction occurs within the first few minutes of traumatic insult. This limits blood loss and results in a temporary blanching of the wound, platelet aggregation, and hemostasis. Cytokines, chemokines, and hormones are released, and there is an activation of fibrin, a non-globular protein, which forms a mesh and acts as a "glue" to bind platelets together, forming a clot. This clot plugs the break in the blood vessel, slowing and then preventing further hemorrhage (Versteeg *et al.*, 2013). The chemokines released by platelet activation attract inflammatory cells to the area, leading to the next phase in the healing process.

PBMT should not be applied until a state of hemostasis is reached. If PBMT is applied during active hemorrhage, the resulting vasodilation (Plass *et al.*, 2012) may accelerate the hemorrhaging and prevent normal clot formation. This concept merits more scientific investigation, since some studies have shown that exposure of whole blood to laser irradiation accelerates coagulation and enhances fibrinolysis due to the effect on the vessel wall, and thereby the platelet–wall interaction (Savolainen, 1993).

The vasoconstriction only lasts 5–10 minutes. It is followed by a state of vasodilation, peaking at about 20 minutes post wounding (Stadelmann *et al.*, 1998). This vasodilation is caused by many factors released by platelets and other cells, particularly histamine (Werner and Gross, 2003). Histamine also causes blood vessels to become porous.

Wu *et al.* (2010) showed that laser-irradiated RBL-2H3 mast cells release histamine. Cytochrome c oxidase (CCO), a photoacceptor, absorbs incident photons and initiates mitochondrial signaling. The signals are transferred from the mitochondria to the cytosol. Cytosolic alkalization leads to the opening of Ca^{2+} channels on the membrane (the transient receptor potential vanilloid channels) and an increase of Ca^{2+}, which in turn mediates an enhanced histamine release (Wu *et al.*, 2010; Young *et al.*, 1990).

The increased porosity and release of chemokines by platelet activation attract and facilitate the entry of inflammatory cells (leukocytes) into the wound site, leading to the next phase in the healing process (Gutowska-Owsiak *et al.*, 2014).

Inflammatory Phase

The inflammatory phase prepares the wound for repair. Foreign substances and dead tissue are removed, while vascular and cellular responses prepare the environment to sustain the next two phases of healing. The intensity of these vascular and cellular inflammatory responses correlates with the severity of the trauma to the tissues.

The vascular response includes an initial vasoconstriction, typically only minutes in duration, followed by a more persistent vasodilation mediated by histamine, prostaglandins, kinins, and leukotrienes. Vasodilation is an important means by which the wound can be exposed to increased blood flow, accompanied by the necessary inflammatory cells and factors to fight infection and debride the wound of devitalized tissue. Transdermal application of PBMT modifies vascular endothelial function by increasing its antioxidant and angiogenic potential (Michael *et al.*, 2012; Szymczyszyn *et al.*, 2016).

The cellular aspect of the inflammatory phase occurs within hours of injury, and includes the recruitment of leukocytes from the circulating blood through the various vasoactive mediators, chemoattractants, platelets, and mast cells (Singer and Clark, 1999). Neutrophilic diapedesis, stimulated by vasoactive mediators and chemoattractants, occurs within minutes and peaks several days after the insult. Neutrophils are the first line of defense, destroying cellular debris and bacteria through phagocytosis. They are attracted to the site by fibronectin, growth factors, and substances such as kinins (proteins or polypeptides such as bradykinin). Neutrophils phagocytize debris and kill bacteria by releasing free radicals in what is called a "respiratory burst" (Greenhalgh, 1998). They also cleanse the wound by secreting proteases that break down damaged tissue. Functional neutrophils at the wound site have life spans of only around 2 days, so they usually undergo apoptosis once they have completed their tasks and are engulfed and degraded by macrophages (Martin and Leibovich, 2005). Neutrophilic migration ceases when contaminating substances are cleared from the injury. These cells become entrapped within the clot, which is sloughed during the later phases of repair. Any remaining cells are phagocytosed by the incoming tissue macrophages or modified wound fibroblasts (Leibovich and Ross, 1975; Simpson and Ross, 1972).

Macrophages are essential to wound healing, and perhaps are the most important cells in the early phases of wound healing. Macrophages phagocytose debris and bacteria. They also secrete collagenases and elastases, which break down injured tissue and release cytokines. In addition, macrophages release platelet-derived growth factor (PDGF), an important cytokine that stimulates the chemotaxis and proliferation of fibroblasts and smooth-muscle cells. Finally, they secrete substances that attract endothelial cells to the wound and stimulate their proliferation to promote angiogenesis (Deodhar and Rana, 1997; Newton *et al.*, 2004).

Macrophage-derived growth factors play a pivotal role in new tissue formation, as evidenced by the fact that new tissue formation in macrophage-depleted animal wounds demonstrates defective repair. In studies in which experimental wounds are rendered monocytopenic, subsequent stages of fibroplasia and granulation tissue formation are impaired and the overall rate of wound healing is delayed (Godwin *et al.*, 2013).

T-lymphocytes migrate into the wound during the inflammatory phase, approximately 72 hours following injury. T-lymphocytes are attracted to the wound by the cellular release of interleukin 1 (IL1), which also contributes to the regulation of collagenase. Lymphocytes secrete lymphokines such as heparin-binding epidermal growth factor and basic fibroblast growth factor. Lymphocytes also play a role in cellular immunity and antibody production (de Loura Santana *et al.*, 2016).

The inflammatory phase is a complex sequence of biochemical and physiological events. If these events go astray, the result is suppuration, chronic prolonged inflammation, and excessive fibrosis. The foremost modulation of this inflammatory phase by PBMT is the increased production and release of NO, a potent vasodilator (Chung *et al.*, 2012). This increases the porousness of the blood vessels, which facilitates the entry of leukocytes and macrophages into the wound site.

Mediators, such as cytokines and chemokines, regulate the immunological process of inflammation using complex signaling mechanisms (Viegas *et al.*, 2007). These inflammatory mediators are released when the immune cells are irradiated with certain wavelengths of light (Chung *et al.*, 2012).

PBMT modulates the inflammatory process by regulating inflammatory cytokine IL1β. In male Wistar rats with a cryoinjury, levels of IL1β were decreased in those receiving PBMT (660 nm, 20 mW, 5 J/cm^2) but not in those receiving no PBMT (Fernandes *et al.*, 2013).

Proliferative Phase

The formation of fleshy granulation tissue begins to appear approximately 3–5 days following injury and marks the beginning of the proliferative phase of wound healing. This phase is not distinct and overlaps the last portion of the inflammatory phase. Granulation tissue includes inflammatory cells, fibroblasts, and neovasculature in a matrix of fibronectin, collagen, glycosaminoglycans, and proteoglycans (Falanga *et al.*, 1988).

The proliferative phase can be subdivided into angiogenesis, fibroplasia (collagen deposition and granulation tissue formation), re-epithelialization, and contraction (Clark, 1996).

Angiogenesis

Angiogenesis occurs as microvascular endothelial cells form new capillary blood vessels from pre-existing ones in order to sustain the granulation tissue within the wound bed. Occurring in response to tissue injury and hypoxia, angiogenesis is a complex and dynamic process mediated by diverse soluble factors from both the serum and the surrounding extracellular matrix (ECM) environment. These angiogenic inducers include growth factors, chemokines, angiogenic enzymes, endothelial-specific receptors, and adhesion molecules such as integrins, many of which are released during the inflammatory phase of repair (Li *et al.*, 2003; Liekens *et al.*, 2001).

There have been numerous studies demonstrating that PBMT promotes angiogenesis in a broad spectrum of research models. Hamblin (2008) outlined the beneficial

effects of NO, which include pain relief, resolution of edema, improved lymphatic drainage, and improved wound healing via angiogenesis. Tuby *et al.* (2006) used a laser emitting an 804 nm wavelength to promote cardioprotection and angiogenesis following heart attacks in mice. Utilizing different wavelengths (blue, 470 nm, and red, 629 nm) administered at 50 mW/cm^2, Dungel *et al.* (2014) induced angiogenesis and improved ischemic wound healing in a disturbed rodent flap model. In a crossover study, Larkin *et al.* (2012) used a Class 4 laser to determine a therapeutic dose range for increasing blood flow to the biceps brachii muscle of the forearm. They concluded, using venous occlusion plethysmography, that a setting of 3 W (360 J) was an effective treatment modality.

Fibroplasia

Fibroplasia begins 3–5 days after injury. Fibroblasts and mesenchymal cells migrate, proliferate, and differentiate in response to fibronectin, PDGF, fibroblast growth factor, and transforming growth factors. Fibronectin serves as an anchor for the myofibroblasts as they migrate within the wound. These fibroblasts grow and form a new, provisional ECM by excreting collagen and fibronectin, forming new granulation tissue. This stroma, rich in fibronectin and hyaluronan, replaces the fibrin-containing clot to provide a physical barrier to infection, and importantly, it provides a surface across which mesenchymal cells can migrate (Song *et al.*, 2010).

PBMT has a proliferative effect in a variety of human and animal cell types, including fibroblasts, keratinocytes, endothelial cells, lymphocytes, muscle cells, and stem cells (Basso *et al.*, 2012; Hamblin and Demidova, 2006; Peplow *et al.*, 2010b). The mechanism for this proliferation is not completely understood, but irradiated cells release ROS, resulting in the expression of transcription factors such as nuclear factor kappa B (NF-KB), which then activate a form of nitric oxide synthase (NOS) that leads to proliferation (Alexandratou *et al.*, 2002; Chen *et al.*, 2011; Lubart and Breitbart, 2000).

Mouse fibroblasts and endothelial cells were irradiated with a range of different wavelengths: visible red light from 625 to 675 nm using a potassium titanyl phosphate (KTP)-pumped tunable dye laser and near-infrared light at 810 nm wavelength using a diode laser (power density 5 mW/cm^2; energy density 10 J/cm^2) (Moore, 2005). Cellular proliferation was measured 72 hours post irradiation using a colorimetric assay for viable cells. Compared to control cells, fibroblasts irradiated by the visible red wavelengths had increased proliferation, but cells irradiated with the near-infrared 810 nm wavelength light displayed growth inhibition.

PBMT improved the remodeling of the ECM during the healing process in tendons through activation of matrix metallopeptidase 2 (MMP2) and stimulation of collagen synthesis (Guerra *et al.*, 2013). Light-emitting diode (LED) irradiation emitting a wavelength in the range of 625–635 nm maintained human fibroblast viability and increased collagen synthesis *in vitro* using human fibroblast (HS68) cultures (Huang *et al.*, 2007)

Re-epithelialization

Re-epithelialization of the epidermis occurs alongside fibroplasia. This involves a migration of cells at the wound edges over a distance of <1 mm, from one side to the other. Epithelialization is accelerated in a partial-thickness wound because migrating cells arise not only from the residual epithelium at the wound periphery, but also from remaining epidermal appendages. In this type of injury, the basement membrane is intact, which precludes a lengthy regeneration. Incisional wounds are epithelialized within 48–72 hours after injury.

A large percentage of wounds in equine practice present as full-thickness wounds that undergo second-intention healing. Epithelialization in these cases must await the formation of a bed of granulation tissue to proceed. Wounds in the flank region of a horse epithelialize at a rate of 0.2 mm/day, compared with as low as 0.09 mm/day for wounds in the distal region of the limbs (Jacobs *et al.*, 1984).

PBMT effectively aids in the proliferation of epithelial cells. In a single case study, a patient suffering from thalassemia intermedia with a non-healing ulcer on the ankle was irradiated with a dosage of 17.3 J/cm^2 daily for 2 weeks, followed by an average of 6.5 J/cm^2 for another 2 weeks. There was complete re-epithelialization and no recurrence in a follow-up 6 months later (Dixit *et al.*, 2014). Leite *et al.* (2015) used rats with a 1.5 mm punched dorsum skin wound fed a high-fat diet. They showed that PBMT accelerated cutaneous wound healing by modulating oxidative stress in rats with a metabolic disorder under a high-fat diet.

Contraction

Wound contraction begins concurrently with the synthesis of collagen. It is defined as centripetal movement of the wound edges, which facilitates closure of a wound deficit. Contraction results from the proliferation and action of differentiated fibroblasts (myofibroblasts) in the granulation tissue, which contain filaments of smooth-muscle actin. The filaments in the myofibroblasts connect to other fibroblasts and the ECM and contract, pulling the wound margins toward the center (Darby *et al.*, 1990). This contraction determines the speed of second-intention wound healing and the cosmetic appearance of the scar. Wound contraction is stimulated by certain cytokines but inhibited by inflammation. When the role of the myofibroblasts is close to complete, unneeded cells undergo apoptosis.

PBMT increases the transformation and proliferation of fibroblasts into myofibroblasts, accelerating wound contraction. In 1990, research showed that irradiation by a helium–neon laser increased the transformation of fibroblasts into myofibroblasts (Pourreau-Schneider *et al.*, 1990). Medrado *et al.* (2003) evaluated the effects of PBMT on wound healing by analyzing the role of ECM elements and the proliferation of myofibroblasts. Cutaneous wounds were inflicted on Wistar rats and PBMT was applied at dosages of 4 and 8 J/cm^2. Lesions were analyzed after 24, 48, and 72 hours and 5, 7, and 14 days by histology, immunohistochemistry, and electron microscopy. It was found that the groups receiving PBMT had a reduction in the inflammatory reaction, increased collagen deposition, and a greater proliferation of myofibroblasts (Medrado *et al.*, 2003). The application of PBMT within the immediate postoperative period enhances the tissue repair process in patients with diabetes by modulating the inflammatory process, increasing the synthesis of myofibroblasts, and enhancing collagen organization (de Loura Santana *et al.*, 2015).

Maturation Phase

When the levels of collagen production and degradation equalize, the maturation phase of tissue repair has begun. During maturation, type III collagen, which is prevalent during proliferation, is replaced by type I collagen (Dealey, 2012). Disorganized collagen fibers are rearranged, cross-linked, and aligned along tension lines (Wood *et al.*, 2010).

The onset of the maturation phase can vary extensively depending on the size of the wound and whether it was closed or left open (Lorenz and Longaker, 2008). Deposition of collagen macromolecules peaks within the first week of primary wound care and at between 7 and 14 days in second-intention healing. The deposition of collagen provides the tensile strength of the wound, and though this period corresponds to the most rapid gain in strength, only 20% of the final strength of the wound is achieved in these first 3 weeks of repair (Stashak and Theoret, 2008). At the 3-week point, collagen synthesis is balanced by collagen lysis; this prevents the accumulation of excessive amounts of collagen and the formation of scar tissue.

As the maturation phase progresses, the tensile strength of the wound increases. Collagen will reach approximately 20% of its tensile strength after 3 weeks, increasing gradually to approximately 80% by week 12–14 (Mercandetti and Cohen, 2015).

Stadler *et al.* (2001) used a wavelength of 830 nm at a dosage of 5 J/cm^2 to show that PBMT significantly enhanced wound tensile strength in a murine diabetic mouse model. Vasilenko *et al.* (2010) showed that wavelengths of 635 and 670 nm improved tensile strength on a full-thickness skin incision in rats. Using a wavelength of 635 nm, Kilik *et al.* (2014) measured the effect of equal daily doses of $5\,J/cm^2$ delivered at power densities of 1, 5, and $15\,mW/cm^2$ three times daily on normal and diabetic rats with open skin wounds. All three of these studies demonstrate the value of PBMT in enhancing the tensile strength of a wound during this stage of healing.

Paraguassu *et al.* (2014) examined the effect of PBMT on type I and III collagen expression during wound healing in normal versus hypothyroid rats. PBMT utilizing a GaAIA laser emitting a wavelength of 660 nm, 40 mW, $1\,W/cm^2$, increased the immunoexpression of collagen type I during tissue repair and improved the quality of newly formed tissue in the presence of a hypothyroid condition (Paraguassu *et al.*, 2014).

The tensile strength of the wound is determined by the content and arrangement of collagen fibers. PBMT stimulates a better alignment and normal distribution of type I and III collagen at this phase of healing (Paraguassu *et al.*, 2014; Wood *et al.*, 2010).

Redondo (2015) noted that PBMT increases fibroblast multiplication, differentiation, and motility, and collagen production, all of which result in an earlier wound closure. The collagen generated after PBMT irradiation has a higher percentage of type III collagen, which builds up stronger but less exuberant scars and is important for the cosmetic resolution of wounds in the equine (Oliveira *et al.*, 2009; Peplow *et al.*, 2010a).

Equine PBMT Treatment Techniques

Dosing

Dosages are determined by the anatomical area, whether the wound is open or closed, its age, the tissues involved, the distance to the target tissues, and the presence or absence of infection or contamination. These determining factors must be considered for each individual patient, and there are no universal dosages. Always treat to effect. There is a wide margin of safety, and if too little is administered, there will be no clinical benefit to treatment. The dosages in Table 34.1 are guidelines that can be considered where applicable.

The goal is to safely administer a sufficient quantity of energy on the surface to ensure a saturation of the target tissue with enough energy to elicit a biological and physiological response. This dose, or quantity of energy, should be applied gently. Initially, use a lower power density to acclimate the patient to the procedure. This can be accomplished in several different ways:

- Decrease the power output and increase the treatment time.
- Increase the spot size, which results in a decrease of the power density. This can be readily accomplished by increasing the distance between the handpiece and the tissue.

Table 34.1 Dosages for PBMT of equine wounds.

Wound type	Dose (J/cm²)
Abrasion	4 ± 2
Contusion	4–8
Wheal	2–4
Incisional	4–6
Laceration (sutured)	4–6
Laceration (open)	8–12
Laceration (muscle and tendon involvement)	10–12
Laceration (tendon and hoof involvement)	10–12
Puncture (not infected, minimal muscle damage)	6–8
Puncture (not infected, muscle damage)	8–10
Puncture (not infected, muscle and tendon damage)	8–12
Puncture (infected)	10–12
Chronic	10–12
Chronic (profuse granulation tissue)	10–14

- Use a pulsed rather than a continuous delivery. If a diode therapy laser is set to pulsed delivery, the duty cycle will usually be 50%, meaning the laser is only emitting 50% of the time. For example, a laser set at 10 W pulsed delivery will emit an average of only 5 W over a given period of time relative to continuous delivery.
- Increase the scanning speed over the treatment area. This does not reduce the power density, but it has a similar effect of reducing any potential discomfort in very sensitive tissue.

Software within the therapy laser equipment may provide the therapist with a preset protocol calculated for the area of the wound. These software protocols have to be adapted to the individual case, but serve as an initial guideline for treatment. The total dose can also be manually calculated by measuring the area and multiplying by the dose.

Application Technique

Initially, almost all equine wounds are treated off-contact with either a scanning or a point-to-point administration technique. While keeping the handpiece perpendicular to the target tissue, administer the calculated dosage for the area at 90° angles in a grid-like fashion over the wound. Include a good margin of surrounding healthy tissue (6 cm, if possible). Identify all areas of epithelialization and ensure they receive sufficient therapy

After a few initial treatments, on-contact treatment may be possible. This is ideal for a closed wound and for the areas of epithelialization surrounding an open wound. It is difficult to treat on-contact over an open wound bed because of patient sensitivity and concerns about contamination of the handpiece.

Frequency of Treatment

Acute wounds, open or closed, should receive PBMT daily until a visible clinical response is noted. Therapy sessions can then be spaced out, with a day or more between sessions, until the wound is completely resolved.

PBMT is cumulative in effect, and a clinical response should be witnessed with each treatment. If the diagnosis is correct and there are no conditions preventing the healing process, but no clinical response is seen after the second treatment, then increase the dosage in small increments to ensure a sufficient dosage is reaching the target tissue.

Chronic wounds should receive two to three daily treatments, and then the treatments should be spaced out as needed to correspond with the clinical progress and medical management. Often, these chronic wounds receive an initial debridement, placing them in the acute wound classification. The goal for the treatment of these injuries is complete resolution. However, there will be patients in which a maintenance dose of PBMT is required periodically.

General Wound Management

PBMT is an addendum to the normal standard of care in the management of wounds. A non-invasive therapy, it provides pain relief, modulation of the inflammatory reaction, and increased circulation.

After an initial physical examination and assessment, the treatment plan is determined. Lavage and debridement are completed and a decision is made whether to manage the wound as closed or open. The administration of PBMT then fits within the program for standard wound care, as follows:

- If the wound is closed with sutures, staples, or glue after the initial exam, PBMT can be administered immediately after closure. This is treated as an incision, as described in the next section.
- If the wound is closed after several days of lavage, aimed at removing any contamination or reducing infection, PBMT should be administered after each lavage and before bandaging. The wound is initially treated as an open wound and then managed as a closed wound.
- If the wound is left to heal by second intention and is managed as an open wound during the entire healing process, PBMT should be administered at each bandage change after cleaning, lavage, and debridement, but before the application of any moist dressings or bandages.

Types of Wound

Traumatic wounds can be categorized as open or closed. Closed wounds are those where the skin is not broken through all layers. This is tissue damage without loss of continuity of the skin. These include abrasions, contusions and hematomas, and wheals. Open wounds penetrate through the skin into the subcutaneous and underlying tissues. These include incisions, lacerations and avulsions, and punctures. Chronic wounds require special treatment in horses because of the risk of excessive granulation tissue. Burns, tendon lacerations, and trauma to the hoof also require special consideration.

Closed Wounds

Abrasions

These are friction injuries to the superficial layers of the skin or mucous membrane where the damage does not extend through all of the layers of the skin or mucous membrane. They characteristically ooze serum and have a minimal amount of hemorrhage. They form a scab superficially, which creates a case of second-intention healing. A common example is a rope burn.

Ensure that the hemorrhaging has ceased, and if a scab has formed, do not disturb it by using an on-contact application technique. Abrasions are initially treated off-contact for the comfort of the patient, with transition to on-contact either during the first therapy session or shortly thereafter. Initiate therapy at $2–6\,J/cm^2$, depending on the size of the lesion. Resolution is gained after one to four treatments.

Contusions and Hematomas

Contusions are caused by trauma sufficient to rupture subcutaneous blood vessels and cause localized bruising of the underlying tissues beneath undivided skin. The dorsal surface of the carpus is particularly prone to injury when this structure strikes a fence or stall door. There are three classifications of contusion:

- First-degree contusions display a small amount of hemorrhage beneath and into the skin, with only a very small or no hematoma. Apply PBMT at a dosage of $4–5\,J/cm^2$, on-contact if possible. Typically, these injuries only require one or two treatments to resolve.
- Second-degree contusions involve the formation of a hematoma. They are often the result of a kick or bite from another horse. If the hematoma is small, it will be absorbed, but if large, it could lead to a seroma, scar tissue directly beneath the dermis, and a subsequent blemish (Garvican and Clegg, 2007). A hematoma over the carpal area may form a carpal hygroma. PBMT is a non-invasive way of aiding in the management of second-degree contusions. These lesions should be treated aggressively to resolve the hematoma and minimize the formation of scar tissue. Apply PBMT, off-contact initially, at a dosage of $6–8\,J/cm^2$. When it is comfortable for the patient, move to an on-contact technique. Treat daily for several consecutive days and then every other day until resolved.

- Third-degree contusions are so severe that the damage to the underlying tissue is beyond repair. The skin is not broken from the original blow, but thrombosis of the vasculature occurs, eventually leading to a sloughing of the superficial tissues. PBMT should be applied to all phases of the healing process. Initiate therapy immediately after the injury and apply until both epithelialization and contraction are complete. Initial dosing at $6–8\,J/cm^2$ should be sufficient, but as the structure of the dermis disintegrates, higher dosages may be needed.

Wheals

A wheal is a bulge or serous-filled blister in the skin; no hemorrhagic extravasation is present. If only slightly painful, treat off-contact, then attempt to transition to on-contact after the administration of a few hundred joules. Apply therapy at a dosage of $2–4\,J/cm^2$. Wheals usually resolve after one or two treatments.

Open Wounds

Incisions

These are clean-cut wounds produced by sharp objects, and are characterized by minimal tissue damage. They can be shallow or deep, can hemorrhage profusely or not at all, elicit minimal pain, and may have only a modicum of tissue separation. Incised wounds are sutured, if possible. PBMT administered on-contact at a dosage of $4–6\,J/cm^2$ serves as an adjunct therapy to the standard management. Three or four treatments generally lead to resolution.

Lacerations and Avulsions

Lacerations generally leave rough, jagged edges of skin, and they are characterized by extensive damage to underlying tissues such as tendons and their sheaths, joint capsules, ligaments, muscles, and neurovascular structures. Lacerations are more susceptible to contamination and infection than incisional wounds. They are surgically debrided and sutured or, depending on location and circumstances, managed as second-intention healing or open wounds. Avulsions are partial or complete tearing away of the skin and tissue and are treated as open wounds.

The dosage and frequency of administration of PBMT to lacerations and avulsions are proportional to the severity of the injury. If a laceration involves minimal damage to the underlying tissues and can be easily sutured, administration of $4–6\,J/cm^2$ daily for several days is recommended, followed by treatment as needed to accelerate the healing process. However, when a laceration or avulsion presents with tendon, muscle, ligament, or hoof involvement, higher dosages are warranted.

Administration of PBMT to complex lacerations and avulsions involving multiple tissues should be aggressive. Due to the density of the underlying tendon and muscle tissues, dosages in the range of $10–12\,J/cm^2$ should be administered daily for 3–6 days, and then every other day until resolution. Treatment of lacerations and avulsions deep into the muscle tissues may require even higher dosages to provide enough therapeutic energy.

Bandages, cast materials, splints, and leg wraps all block photonic energy. Laser therapy of lesions must coincide with bandage changes. The other option is to provide a treatment window within the bandage or cast material that allows direct access to the laceration. Care must be taken when considering placement and composition of a therapy window, since immobilization must often be maintained to support the wound and prevent dehiscence.

Punctures

Puncture or penetrating wounds generally look minor at the surface of the skin but can cause significant trauma to the underlying structures. Common causes are horn gores, sharp objects in the stall such as nails, and steel pitchforks. Puncture wounds are commonly complicated by contamination. The skin can heal before the underlying tissues, resulting in abscessation. Punctures are not usually sutured, but managed as an open, draining wound.

Apply only a small portion of the recommended dose to the opening in the skin. Treat all the surrounding structures circumferentially, directing the energy to the deep structures. Encourage healing from the inside of the wound out to the surface. Dose according to the anatomical area and consider the depth of the wound. A range of $6–12\,J/cm^2$ should be considered. If the wound is contaminated, account for the amount of energy that will be absorbed by pus or exudate within the wound, and administer appropriately.

Chronic Wounds

One of the primary goals of wound management is not to allow the wound to become chronic. For a number of reasons, this is not always possible. Factors such as a decreased immune system, age, an endocrine disorder such as Cushing's disease, poor client compliance, and chronic steroid use may contribute to wounds becoming chronic. All chronic wounds are difficult to manage, but infected wounds on the distal limbs present an especially high level of concern.

Exuberant granulation tissue (proud flesh) is a common complication of chronic wounds, particularly if located below the carpus or tarsus. The production of granulation tissue is directly related to the vascular supply and is part of the normal healing process. Contraction of the right amount of granulation tissue moves the skin toward the center of the wound. Excessive granulation tissue impedes contraction and normal epithelialization. Thus, exuberant granulation tissue can enlarge the wound by pushing the edges apart

Treatment of proud flesh often requires surgical intervention. The excess tissue is trimmed to a level just below the dermis. It is highly vascularized, and a significant amount of bleeding occurs. Repeat trimming is sometimes necessary in order to continue to reduce the tissue, but over time, the skin edges will start to pull across the wound. A rule of thumb is that "skin cells don't climb mountains": if there is a protrusion of granulation tissue, the skin edges will not close properly.

Administration of PBMT early in the management of chronic wounds controls the production of proud flesh. The increased rate of epithelialization, coupled with the effect of laser therapy on fibroblasts, leading to contraction, encourages the wound to close normally (Calisto *et al.*, 2015; Hawkins and Abrahamse, 2006; Kuffler, 2016; Reddy, 2004).

Utilize dosages in the range of 10–14 J/cm^2, administered off-contact, on a daily basis for 3–5 days and then every other day until the therapeutic goal is reached. As with other types of wound, treat to effect. Apply the majority of the dose along the epithelial border and the first few centimeters of the tissue margin. Application over granulation tissue should be continued until there is a noticeable leakage of serum or even slight hemorrhage within the tissue. The owner or trainer must be forewarned of this possibility, and the therapist should administer the PBMT with the handpiece in one hand and a gauze sponge in the other. Using this technique will minimize the number of times that granulation tissue has to be surgically removed.

Many chronic wounds must have surgical intervention to encourage healing. The goal is to create a more optimal environment in which for wound healing to continue. A wound in the acute state is created from one that has been chronic. There are many reasons for such surgical intervention, including removal of devitalized tissues or foreign bodies, reduction of excessive granulation tissue, allowance of thorough lavage when the wound is contaminated, and establishment of drainage.

Each chronic wound case will require a unique PBMT treatment plan. Aggressive treatment initiates and promotes the healing process. Frequent treatments at appropriate dosages will change these frustrating cases into positive clinical outcomes.

Wounds Requiring Special Consideration

Burns

Most equine burns are superficial and easily managed. They are commonly caused by friction (rope burns) or improperly used topical agents. Severe burns are uncommon in horses and are usually the result of a barn fire. The more serious burns result in rapid burn shock or hypovolemia, with associated cardiovascular complications. Further complicating the management of serious burns are concurrent smoke inhalation and corneal ulceration (Fox, 1988; Fubini, 1987). Hanson (2005) provides a detailed management plan for burn injuries in horses.

PBMT is a scientific, evidence-based medicine for the treatment of burns. Early research was scarce and showed inconsistent results (Al-Watban *et al.*, 2005; Cambier *et al.*, 1996; Schlager *et al.*, 2000). However, in a study using diabetic rats, Meireles *et al.* (2008) showed improved healing in third-degree burns using 660 and 780 nm wavelengths, 35 mW, a laser beam diameter of 2 mm, and 20 J/cm^2. Ezzati *et al.* (2009) used a pulsed low-level laser with 11.7 J/cm^2 emitting a wavelength of 890 nm on third-degree burns in a rat model and demonstrated a significant increase in the closure of wounds when compared to the control group.

PBMT is a viable addendum to the traditional standard-of-care management of burns. Some of the beneficial clinical physiological responses provided to the burn patient by PBMT are as follows:

- pain management (Chow *et al.*, 2009; Takenori *et al.*, 2016);
- increased cellular metabolism (Yadav *et al.*, 2016);
- increased circulation and angiogenesis (Rhee *et al.*, 2016);
- enhanced nerve regeneration and function (Takhtfooladi *et al.*, 2015);
- increased tissue proliferation and regeneration (Macedo *et al.*, 2015).

PBMT should be administered to burns off-contact, in a gentle manner. Setting the therapy laser to emit at a frequency setting will deliver 50% of the energy over time as compared to continuous-wave (CW). Hold the handpiece perpendicular to the target tissue, but at a distance greater than you would normally use to treat the given anatomical area. In a severe burn, the nerve endings are sometimes non-functional, so the patient will not move voluntarily if the therapy becomes uncomfortable. There is a broad range of possible dosages that can be used to treat these patients. If the burn is superficial, start therapy with the application of 4–6 J/cm^2. If it is severe (second- or third-degree), start with a low initial dose of 4–6 J/cm^2, applied off-contact in a gentle manner, then increase the dosage to correspond to the depth of the target tissue.

Tendon Lacerations

Lacerations of tendons are serious injuries because of the loss of biomechanical function, the loss of tensile strength within the tissues, and the complication of the area filling in with inelastic scar tissue, which predisposes the patient to another injury. PBMT has been demonstrated to have a positive effect on the healing of tendon injuries, stimulating the synthesis and organization of collagen I, MMP9, and MMP2 (Da Ré Guerra *et al.*, 2016).

PBMT dosages in the range of 12–20 J/cm^2 should be administered on-contact to the tendon structures distal to the carpus and tarsus. As soon as the healing progress allows, start to place these structures through passive range-of-motion exercises while administering the therapy. Monitor the healing of the tissues with ultrasonic examinations on a relevant periodic basis and adjust the frequency of treatment accordingly.

Trauma to the Hoof

PBMT will not penetrate the hoof wall. Any therapy laser emitting over a few hundred milliwatts of power will initiate a very small percentage of thermal buildup in the target tissues. Consider the consequences of even a slight buildup of thermal energy within the vasculature of the laminar corium and the stratum internum. However, PBMT can safely be administered to the coronary band and all of the descending neurovascular supply to the foot.

The management of trauma to the hoof has been well described (DeBowes and Yovich, 1989; Stashak, 1989). Addition of PBMT to these time-tested techniques will increase the circulation and provide some degree of pain relief. Initiate therapy at a dosage of 6–8 J/cm^2 in the area of the fetlock and follow all of the neurovascular pathways distal to the coronary band. Apply therapy to the entire coronary band, paying special attention to the area proximal to the injury. All areas not directly involved with the injury should be treated on-contact, if the patient allows it. Painful areas will have to be treated off-contact. Daily application, transitioning to every other day or three sessions per week, is ideal.

Case Study: Treatment of an Open Distal Limb Wound

Presentation

A 19-year-old Paint mare presented with a severe laceration of the left rear leg (Figure 34.1) after trying to jump a smooth-wire electric fence. There was involvement of the tendon sheaths, but the joint capsule and tendon integrity were not compromised. The tissues were contaminated, so a decision was made to treat as an open wound.

Treatment

The wound was cleaned, lavaged with sterile saline, and wrapped with a commercial, semi-occlusive, multi-layer hydrophilic-gel wound product. Sulfamethoxazole and trimethoprim were given orally twice a day for 8 days. Phenylbutazone was administered for 2 days, for pain management. Tetanus antitoxin was administered.

Each day, the bandage was changed, a saline lavage was administered, and the leg was rewrapped with the hydrophilic-gel wound product beneath non-stick gauze pads incorporated into a stout three-layered support bandage.

PBMT was initiated 8 days after injury, applied during bandage changes (Figure 34.2). Dosing was 12 J/cm^2, administered off-contact with a scanning technique

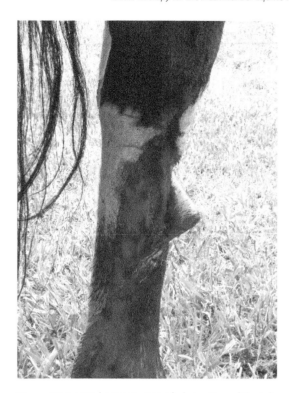

Figure 34.1 Initial presentation of a laceration of the left rear leg of a 19-year-old Paint mare, induced by trying to jump a smooth-wire electric fence. Note the flap of skin, the abrasion extending dorsally through hock, and the slight trauma to the underlying tendons. Image courtesy of Courtenay Marshall, LVT.

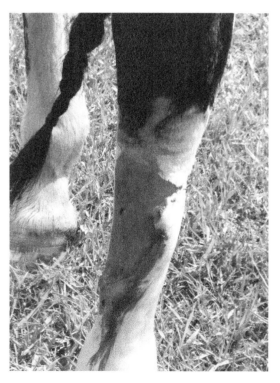

Figure 34.2 Day 8. Picture taken before the first application of PBMT. Image courtesy of Courtenay Marshall, LVT.

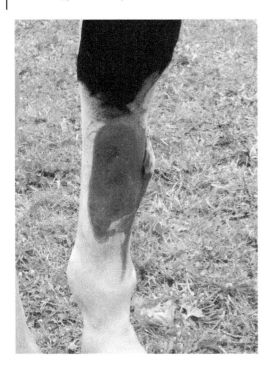

Figure 34.3 Day 12. Picture taken after the first two laser therapy sessions on days 8 and 9. Note the early healing along the epithelial margin, the reduction in swelling and inflammation, and the early adherence of some areas of the skin flap. Image courtesy of Courtenay Marshall, LVT.

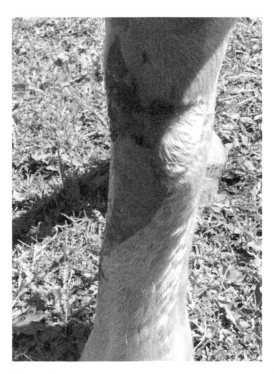

Figure 34.4 Day 18. Appearance of the wound 18 days after the injury and after six therapy laser sessions. The image was taken at a different angle to emphasize the general health of the wound bed, the adherence of the skin flap, the lack of production of exuberant granulation tissue, and the epithelialization of the wound margins. Image courtesy of Courtenay Marshall, LVT.

throughout the wound and a border of skin of about 3 cm around the epithelial margin. The wound was treated proximal to distal at 90° angles, with more energy administered to the epithelial margin and skin border than the wound bed. Several attempts were made to treat the epithelial margin and skin border on-contact, but the patient would not allow it. After each treatment, the wound bed (granulation tissue) oozed serum and a small amount of hemorrhage was visible.

This therapy protocol was repeated daily for two additional days, on days 9 and 10. On day 12, the saline lavage was discontinued and replaced with garden-hose hydrotherapy, with PBMT applied after the therapy and prior to bandaging (Figure 34.3). Treatments were then repeated on days 14, 15, 17, 21, 24, 26, 31, 33, 38, and 43 (Figures 34.4–34.6).

The wound was never scrubbed after the initial cleaning. Moist wraps were applied after each laser therapy session. The wound never required debridement. PBMT was applied aggressively, which avoided the need for debridement of the granulation tissue. The wound contracted very well and the epithelial margin advanced across the wound bed very naturally. On day 43, the animal's range of motion was back to normal, and it was ridden with no sign of lameness. The prognosis is very good for this 19-year-old to return to normal function and resume her career as a trail horse in the Rocky Mountains within a few months (Figure 34.7–34.10).

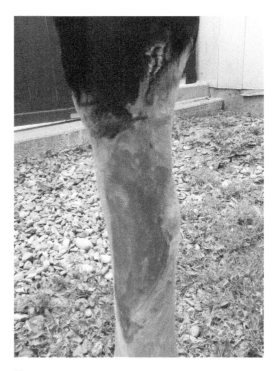

Figure 34.5 Day 26. Progress after eight laser therapy sessions. Note the lack of excessive granulation tissue, the total adherence and healing of the flap, and the advancement of the epithelial margins. Image courtesy of Courtenay Marshall, LVT.

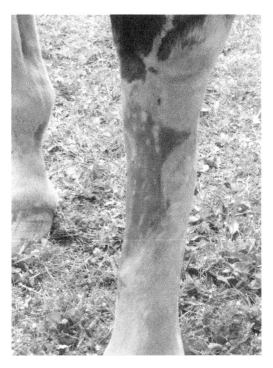

Figure 34.6 Day 32. Progress after 10 laser therapy sessions. Note the degree of contraction of the wound, the health of the wound bed, the almost total healing over the tarsus, and the epithelialization throughout all margins. Image courtesy of Courtenay Marshall, LVT.

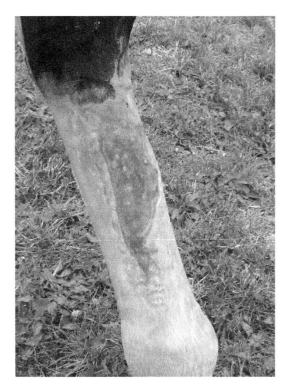

Figure 34.8 Day 46. Continued rapid healing of the wound. At this time, the patient was ridden for a short time, with no sign of lameness. Image courtesy of Courtenay Marshall, LVT.

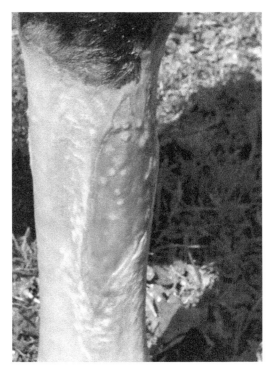

Figure 34.7 Day 44. Progress after 13 laser therapy sessions. Note the continuing progress of epithelialization, the lack of excessive granulation tissue, and the good contraction of the wound. The range of motion was normal and there was no indication of adhesions. Image courtesy of Courtenay Marshall, LVT.

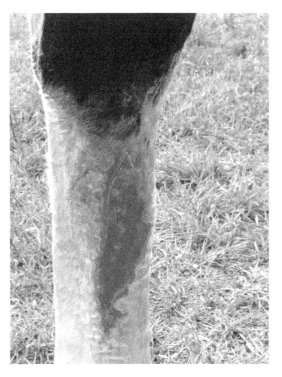

Figure 34.9 Day 52. Progress after 14 therapy laser sessions. Note the continued normal wound healing, without excessive granulation tissue. Image courtesy of Courtenay Marshall, LVT.

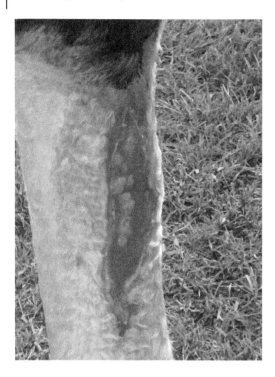

Figure 34.10 Day 55. When this image was taken, the patient was being ridden regularly with the leg wrapped. She will resume her career as a trail horse in the Rocky Mountains within a few months. Image courtesy of Courtenay Marshall, LVT.

Conclusion

PBMT is a scientifically and clinically proven therapy for the treatment of wounds. It provides a relief of pain, a modulation of the inflammatory reaction, and an increase in circulation. All of the physiological effects of PBMT accelerate the healing of any type of wound. All equine patients with wounds will benefit from the addition of this therapy to their wound-management plans.

References

Alexandratou, E. *et al.* (2002) Human fibroblast alterations induced by low power laser irradiation at the single cell level using confocal microscopy. *Photochem Photobiol Sci.* **1**(8):547–552.

AlGhamdi, K.M. *et al.* (2012) Low-level laser therapy: a useful technique for enhancing the proliferation of various cultured cells. *Lasers Med Sci.* **27**(1):237–249.

Al-Watban, F.A. *et al.* (2005) Burn healing with a diode laser: 670 nm at different doses as compared to a placebo group. *Photomed Laser Surg.* **23**(3):245–250.

Basso, F.G. *et al.* (2012) Biostimulatory effect of low-level laser therapy on keratinocytes in vitro. *Lasers Med Sci.* **28**(2):367–374.

Calisto, F.C. *et al.* (2015) Use of low-power laser to assist the healing of traumatic wounds. *Acta Cir Bras.* **30**(3):204–208.

Cambier, D.C. *et al.* (1996) Low-power laser and healing of burns: a preliminary assay. *Plast Reconstr Surg.* **97**(3):555–558.

Chen, A.C. *et al.* (2011) Low-level laser therapy activates NF-kB via generation of reactive oxygen species in mouse embryonic fibroblasts. *PLoS ONE.* **6**(7):e22453.

Chow, R.T. *et al.* (2009) Efficacy of low-level laser therapy in the management of neck pain: a systemic review and meta-analysis of randomized placebo or active-treatment controlled trials. *Lancet.* **374**(9705):1897–1908.

Chung, H. *et al.* (2012) The nuts and bolts of low-level laser (light) therapy. *Ann Biomed Eng.* **40**(2):516–533.

Clark, R.A.F. (1996) Overview and general considerations of wound repair. In: *The Molecular and Cellular Biology of Wound Repair*, 2 edn., pp. 3–33. Plenum Press, New York.

Darby, I. *et al.* (1990) α-smooth muscle actinis transiently expressed by myofibroblasts during experimental wound healing. *Lab Invest.* **63**(1):21–29.

Da Ré Guerra, F. *et al.* (2016) Low-level PBMT modulates pro-inflammatory cytokines after partial tenotomy. *Lasers Med Sci.* **31**(4):759–766.

Dealey, C. (2012) The physiology of wound healing. In: *The Care of Wounds: A Guide for Nurses*, 4 edn., pp. 3–12. Wiley-Blackwell, Hoboken, NJ.

Debowes, R.M. and Yovich, J.V. (1989) Penetrating wounds, abscesses, gravel, and bruising of the equine foot. *Vet Clin North Am Eq Pract.* **5**(1):179–194.

de Loura Santana, C. *et al.* (2015) Tissue reponses to postoperative laser therapy in diabetic rats submitted to excisional wounds. *PLoS One.* **10**(4):e0122042.

de Loura Santana, C *et al.* (2016) Effect of laser therapy on immune cells infiltrate after excisional wounds in diabetic rats. *Lasers Surg Med.* **48**(1):45–51.

Deodhar, A.K. and Rana, R.E. (1997). Surgical physiology of wound healing: a review. *J Postgrad Med.* **43**(2):52–56.

Dixit, S. *et al.* (2014) Closure of chronic non healing ankle ulcer with low level laser therapy in a patient presenting with thalassemia intermedia: case report. *Indian J Plast Surg.* **47**(3):432–435.

Dungel, P. *et al.* (2014) Low level light therapy by LED of different wavelength induces angiogenesis and improves ischemic wound healing. *Lasers Surg Med.* **46**(10):773–780.

Ezzati, A. *et al.* (2009) Low-level laser therapy with pulsed infrared laser accelerates third-degree burn healing process in rats. *J Rehab Res Dev.* **46**(4):543–554.

Falanga, V. *et al.* (1988) Wound healing. *J Am Acad Dermatol.* **19**(3):559–563.

Fernandes, K.P. *et al.* (2013) Effect of photobiomodulation on expression of IL-1beta in skeletal muscle following acute injury. *Lasers Med Sci.* **28**(3):1043–1046.

Fox, S.M. (1988) Management of a large thermal burn in a horse. *Compend Contin Educ Pract Vet.* **10**:88–95.

Fubini, S.L. (1987) Burns. In: *Current therapy In Equine Medicine*, 2 edn., pp. 639–641. Saunders, Philadelphia, PA.

Garvican, E. and Clegg, P. (2007) Clinical aspects of equine carpal joints. *UK Vet Comp Anim.* **12**(1):5–12.

Godwin, J.W. *et al.* (2013) Macrophages are required for adult salamander limb regeneration. *Proc Natl Acad Sci U S A.* **110**(23):9415–9420.

Greenhalgh, D.G. (1998). The role of apoptosis in wound healing. *Int J Biochem Cell Biol.* **30**(9):1019–1030.

Guerra, F.R. *et al.* (2013) LLLT improves tendon healing through increase in MMP activity and collagen synthesis. *Lasers Med Sci.* **28**(5):1281–1288.

Gutowska-Owsiak, D. *et al.* (2014) Histamine enhances keratinocyte-mediated resolution of inflammation by promoting wound healing and response to infection. *Clin Exp Dermatol.* **39**(2):187–195.

Hamblin, M.R. (2008) The role of nitric oxide in low level light therapy. *Proc of SPIE.* **6846**(684602).

Hamblin, M.R. and Demidova, T.N. (2006) Mechanisms of low level light therapy. *Proc of SPIE.* **6140**(612001):1–12.

Hanson, R.R. (2005) Management of burn injuries in the horse. *Vet Clinics North Am Equine Pract.* **21**(1):105–123.

Hawkins, D. and Abrahamse, H. (2006) The role of laser fluence in cell viability, proliferation, and membrane integrity of wounded human skin fibroblasts following helium-neon laser irradiation. *Lasers Surg Med.* **38**(1):74–83.

Huang, P.J. *et al.* (2007) In vitro observations on the influence of copper peptide aids for the LED photoirradiation of fibroblast collagen synthesis. *Photomed Laser Surg.* **25**(3):183–190.

Jacobs, K.A. *et al.* (1984) Comparative aspects of the healing of excisional wounds on the leg and body of horses. *Vet Surg.* **13**(2):83–90.

Karu, T. (1998) Primary and secondary mechanisms of the action of monochromatic visible and near infrared radiation on cells. In: *The Science of Low Power Laser Therapy*, pp. 53–94. Gordon and Breach Science Publishers, London.

Karu, T. (1999) Primary and secondary mechanisms of action of visible to near-IR radiation on cells. *J Photochem Photobiol B.* **49**(1):1–17.

Karu, T. and Kolyakov S.F. (2005) Exact action spectra for cellular responses relevant to phototherapy. *Photomed Laser Surg.* **23**(4):355–361.

Kilik, R. *et al.* (2014) Effect of equal doses achieved by different power densities of low-level laser therapy at 635 nm on open skin wound healing in normal and diabetic rats. *Biomed Res Int.* **2014**:269253.

Kuffler, D.P. (2016) Photobiomodulation in promoting wound healing: a review. *Regen Med.* **11**(1):107–122.

Larkin, K.A. *et al.* (2012) Limb blood flow after class 4 laser therapy. *J Athl Train.* **47**(2):178–183.

Leibovich, S.J. and Ross, R. (1975) The role of macrophage in wound repair: a study with hydrocortisone and antimacrophage serum. *Am J Pathol.* **78**(1):71–100.

Leite, S. N. *et al.* (2015) Phototherapy improves wound healing in rats subjected to high-fat diet. *Lasers Med Sci.* **30**(5):1481–1488.

Li, J. *et al.* (2003) Angiogenesis in wound repair: angiogenic growth factors and the extracellular matrix. *Microsc Res Tech.* **60**(1):107–114.

Liekens, S. *et al.* (2001) Angiogenesis: regulators and clinical applications. *Biochem Pharmacol.* **61**(3):253–270.

Lorenz, H.P. and Longaker M.T. (2008). Wounds: biology, pathology, and management. In: *Surgery – Basic Science and Clinical Evidence*, pp. 191–208. Springer, New York.

Lubart, R. and Breitbart, H. (2000) Biostimulative effects of low-energy lasers and their implications for medicine. *Int J Drug Dev Res.* **50**(3–4):471–475.

Macedo, A.B. *et al.* (2015) Low-level laser therapy (LLLT) in dystrophin-deficient muscle cells: effects on regeneration capacity, inflammation response and oxidative stress. *PLoS One.* **10**(6):e0128567.

Martin, P. and Leibovich, S.J. (2005). Inflammatory cells during wound repair: the good, the bad and the ugly. *Trends Cell Biol.* **15**(11):599–607.

Medrado, A.R. *et al.* (2003) Influence of low level laser therapy on wound healing and its biological action upon myofibroblasts. *Lasers Surg Med.* **32**(3):239–244.

Meireles, G.C. *et al.* (2008) Effectiveness of laser photobiomodulation at 660 or 780 nm on the repair of third-degree burns in diabetic rats. *Photomed Laser Surg.* **26**(1):47–54.

Mercandetti, M. and Cohen, A.J. (2015). Wound healing and repair. Medscape. Available from: http://emedicine. medscape.com/article/1298129-overview (accessed November 30, 2016).

Mester, E. *et al.* (1971) Effect of laser rays on wound healing. *Am J Surg.* **122**(4):532–535.

Michael, C.H. *et al.* (2012) Immediate effects of monochromatic infrared energy on microcirculation in healthy subjects. *Photomed Laser Surg.* **30**(4):193–199.

Moore, P. (2005) Effect of wavelength on low-intensity laser irradiation-stimulated cell proliferation in vitro. *Lasers Surg Med.* **36**(1):8–12.

Newton, P. M. *et al.* (2004). Macrophages restrain contraction of an in vitro wound healing model. *Inflammation* **28**(4):207–214.

Nguyen, D.T. *et al.* (2009) The pathophysiological basis for wound healing and cutaneous regeneration. In: *Biomaterials for Treating Skin Loss*, pp. 25–57. Elsevier, Philadelphia, PA.

Oliveira, F.S. *et al.* (2009) Effect of low level laser therapy (830nm) with different therapy regimes on the process of tissue repair in partial lesion calcaneous tendon. *Lasers Surg Med.* **41**(4):271–276.

Paraguassu, G. *et al.* (2014) Effect of laser phototherapy (660nm) on type I and III collagen expression during wound healing in hypothyroid rats: an immunohistochemical Study in a rodent model. *Photomed Laser Surg.* **32**(5):281–288.

Passarella, S. and Karu, T. (2014) Absorption of monochromatic and narrow band radiation in the visible and near IR by both mitochondrial and non-mitochondrial photoacceptors results in photobiomodulation. *J Photochem Photobiol B.* **140**:344–358.

Peplow, P.V. *et al.* (2010a) Laser photobiomodulation of wound healing: a review of experimental studies in mouse and rat animal models. *Photomed Laser Surg.* **28**(3):291–325.

Peplow, P.V. *et al.* (2010b) Laser photobiomodulation of proliferation of cells in culture: a review of human and animal studies. *Photomed Laser Surg.* **28**(Suppl. 1): S3–S40.

Plass, C.A. *et al.* (2012) Light-induced vasodilation of coronary arteries and its possible clinical implication. *Ann Thorac Surg.* **93**(4):1181–1186.

Pourreau-Schneider, N. *et al.* (1990) Helium-neon laser treatment transforms fibroblasts into myofibroblasts. *Am J Pathol.* **137**(1):171–178.

Reddy, G.K. (2004) Photobiological basis and clinical role of low-intensity lasers in biology and medicine. *J Clin Laser Med Surg.* **22**(2):141–150.

Redondo, M.S. (2015) Laser therapy approach to wound healing in dogs. Vet Times. Available from: http://www. vettimes.co.uk/article/laser-therapy-approach-to-wound-healing-in-dogs/(accessed November 30, 2016).

Rhee, Y.H. *et al.* (2016) Low-level laser therapy promoted aggressive proliferation and angiogensis through decreasing of transforming growth factor-β1 and increasing of AKT/hypoxia inducible factor-1α in anaplasti thyroid cancer. *Photomed Laser Surg.* **34**(6):229–235.

Savolainen, H.O. (1993) Effects of continuous wave and pulsed laser on blood coagulation. An in-vitro thromboelastographic study. *Ann Chir Gynaecol.* **82**(1):37–41.

Schlager, A. *et al.* (2000) Low-power laser light in the healing of burns: a comparison between two different wavelengths (635 nm and 690 nm) and a placebo group. *Lasers Surg Med.* **27**(1):39–42.

Simpson, D.M. and Ross, R. (1972) The neutrophilic leukocyte in wound repair-a study with antineutorphil serum. *J Clin Invest.* **51**(8):2009–2023.

Singer, A.J. and Clark, R.A.F. (1999) Cutaneous wound healing. *N Engl J Med.* **341**(10):738–746.

Song, G. *et al.* (2010) Use of the parabiotic model in studies of cutaneous wound healing to define the participation of circulating cells. *Wound Repair Regen.* **18**(4):426–432.

Stadelmann, W.K. *et al.* (1998) Physiology and healing dynamics of chronic cutaneous wounds. *Am J Surg.* **176**(2A Suppl.):26S–38S.

Stadler, I. *et al.* (2001) 830-nm irradiation increases the wound tensile strength in a diabetic murine model. *Lasers Surg Med.* **28**(3):220–226.

Stashak, T.S. (1989) Management of lacerations and avulsion injuries of the foot and pastern region and hoof wall cracks. *Vet Clin North Am Equine Pract.* **5**(1):195–220.

Stashak, T.S. and Theoret, C.L. (2008) Physiology of wound healing. In: *Equine Wound Management*, pp. 5–29. Wiley-Blackwell, Ames, IA.

Szymczyszyn, A. *et al.* (2016) Effect of the transdermal low-level laser therapy on endothelial function. *Lasers Med Sci.* **31**(7):1301–1307.

Takenori, A. *et al.* (2016) Immediate pain relief effect of low level laser therapy for sports injuries: Randomized, double-blind placebo clinical trial. *J Sci Med Sport.* **S1440–S2440**(16):30002–30010.

Takhtfooladi, M.A. *et al.* (2015) Effect of low-level laser therapy (685 nm, 3 J/cm^2) on functional recovery of the sciatic nerve in rats following crushing lesion. *Lasers Med. Sci.* **30**(3):1047–1052.

Tuby, H. *et al.* (2006) Modulations of VEGF and iNOS in the rat heart by low level laser therapy are associated with cardioprotection and enhanced angiogenesis. *Lasers Surg Med.* **38**(7):682–688.

Vasilenko, T. *et al.* (2010) The effect of equal daily dose achieved by different power densities of low-level laser therapy at 635 and 670 nm on wound tensile strength in rats: a short report. *Photomed Laser Surg.* **28**(2):281–283.

Versteeg, H.H. *et al.* (2013) New fundamentals in hemostasis. *Physiol Rev.* **93**(1):327–358.

Viegas, V.N. *et al.* (2007) Effect of low-level laser therapy on inflammatory reactions during wound healing: comparison with meloxicam. *Photomed Laser Surg.* **25**(6):467–473.

Werner, S. and Grose, R. (2003) Regulation of wound healing by growth factors and cytokines. *Physiol Rev.* **83**(3):835–870.

Wood, V. T. *et al.* (2010) Collagen changes and realignment induced by low-level laser therapy and low-intensity ultrasound in the calcaneal tendon. *Lasers Surg Med.* **42**(6):559–565.

Woodruff, L.D. *et al.* (2004) The efficacy of laser therapy in wound repair: a meta-analysis of the literature. *Photomed Laser Surg.* **22**(3):241–247.

Wu, Z.H. *et al.* (2010) Mitochondrial signaling for histamine release in laser-irradiated RBL-2H3 mast cells. *Lasers Surg Med.* **42**(6):503–509.

Yadav, A. *et al.* (2016) Photobiomodulation effects of superpulsed 904nm laser therapy on bioenergenetics status in burn would healing. *J Photochem Photobiol B.* **162**:77–85.

Young, S.R. *et al.* (1990) Effect of light on calcium uptake by macrophages. *Laser Ther.* **5**:53–57.

35

Laser Therapy and Equine Performance Maintenance

Sean Redman

Equine Integrated Veterinary Solutions, PLLC, Ocala, FL, USA

Introduction

All horses actively enrolled in training for competition or sport should be considered performance horses, regardless of the discipline. Racing, reining, endurance, eventing, hunting, jumping, and polo are all performance activities. Training a horse to perform at high levels in any of these activities takes a significant investment of time, effort, patience, and resources. As valuable athletes, performance horses should be in a well-managed program that helps maintain their peak condition and performance.

The task of equine performance maintenance can be defined as any treatment carried out on a horse for a condition that has not prevented the horse's activity because of lameness. The performance-maintenance program should include proper environment, nutrition, grooming, exercise, hoof and leg care, dentistry, and attention to overall wellness. Other common components of a performance-management program include physiotherapy, acupuncture, chiropractic treatment, massage therapy, and laser therapy (Buchner and Schildboeck, 2006; Haussler, 2010; McGowan *et al.*, 2007; Paulekas and Haussler, 2009).

Therapeutic lasers have been used on the equine athlete for decades. The first such devices were rudimentary, low-power, and most often did not produce notable clinical results. The lack of success changed with the development of newer, more innovative laser devices, now readily available to the equine practitioner. Sophisticated, portable, higher-power therapy lasers deliver photobiomodulation therapy (PBMT) to performance horses with predictable and reproducible results, making laser therapy an essential tool in the modern equine practice.

Lasers for Therapy of the Performance Horse

Lasers have been used for therapeutic purposes since the early 1970's. Much of the research that was published before 2010 measured the effects of laser therapy devices emitting 500 mW or less. There is a wealth of material measuring the intricacies of these lower-power devices, including wavelength, fluence, pulse structure, power density, and the timing and frequency of treatments. These studies have resulted in a vast array of knowledge about the physics, biochemical interactions, and clinical efficacy of laser therapy. They form the basis of the World Association of Laser Therapy's (WALT) 2010 dosage recommendations for laser therapy application (WALT, 2010).

Going back even further, we know from studies conducted on rats in the 1960's that lasers have a measurable effect on living tissue (Mester *et al.*, 1968), a process since named photobiomodulation (PBM). This effect is the result of three actions that must occur simultaneously: penetration of light photons into the tissue of a living organism, reception of those photons by intracellular chromophores, and stimulation or inhibition of physiological function cascades. If any of these three components is absent when living tissue is irradiated with a laser, then what we know today as PBM will not occur. The complex interaction of photons with living tissue, and the remarkable mechanisms involved in the results of this interaction, are well described in Chapter 5.

As laser technology has advanced through the 5 decades since Mester *et al.* (1968) first described photobiostimulation, many researchers have studied the interaction of lasers with living tissue in an effort to better understand the intricacies of this interaction. It has been established and widely accepted that an optical window for tissue penetration exists from approximately 650 to 1200 nm. Penetration into tissue of light within this wavelength range is maximized (Sabino *et al.*, 2016; Smith *et al.*, 2009).

The general optical properties of skin, subcutaneous tissue, and muscle tissue have been studied. Bashkatov *et al.* (2011) presented an overview of the published absorption and scattering properties of skin and subcutaneous tissues, measured in a wide range of wavelengths. For any given wavelength and tissue, the depth of penetration can be calculated. In general, the depth of penetration from the skin surface increases as the wavelength increases in the visible and near-infrared spectrum (Enwemeka, 2003; Uddhav and Lakshyajit, 2008). General knowledge of tissue optical properties and wavelength-dependent depth of penetration is of particular importance when treating thick-skinned, large-muscled performance horses, many of which have pigmented skin.

General Mechanisms of Action of Therapeutic Lasers

Any consideration of the interaction of a laser beam with living tissue must begin with an understanding of a very simple chemical reaction: the attachment of a photon to a specific cellular chromophore. This basic reaction will be the initial step in the PBM process. From the standpoint of equine performance maintenance, the most important mechanisms of laser therapy are:

- relief of pain (Chow *et al.*, 2009);
- modulation of the inflammatory reaction (Assis *et al.*, 2016);
- calming or sedation (Cramond *et al.*, 1994);
- cellular recovery after strenuous work or mild trauma (Ribeiro *et al.*, 2015);
- assistance in optimal cell and organ response to regular training (Levine *et al.*, 2015).

Several secondary chemical reactions occur in the tissue as a direct result of the binding of photons to the complex integral membrane protein molecules of cytochrome c oxidase (CCO) in a stressed or hypoxic cell:

- increase of nitric oxide (NO) release (Poyton and Ball, 2011).
- increase of cellular adenosine triphosphate (ATP) synthesis (Karu, 2010).
- increase of oxygen binding and cellular respiration (Chung *et al.*, 2012; Hamblin and Demidova, 2006).
- increase of generation of reactive oxygen species (ROS) (Chen *et al.*, 2011).

These secondary processes occur virtually simultaneously to oxygen-binding progresses, resulting in a transient increase in ATP and ROS concentrations. This is due to the displacement of NO and the cancellation of its competitive inhibition of oxygen binding to CCO (Farivar *et al.*, 2014). These processes are accompanied by vasodilation, increased blood circulation in the tissue, and increased oxygenation (Chung *et al.*, 2012; Maegawa *et al.*, 2000; Morimoto *et al.*, 1996).

Pain Relief from Laser Therapy Application

Pain relief is achieved through secondary and tertiary physiological and biochemical reactions. Photoreceptors in mitochondrial membranes absorb the energy from photons. The laser energy is transduced into electrochemical changes, initiating a secondary cascade of intracellular events. In neurons, the result is a decrease in the available ATP required for nerve function, including maintenance of microtubules and the molecular motors responsible for fast axonal flow. Laser therapy-induced neural blockade is a consequence of these changes, which provide a mechanism for a neural basis of laser therapy-induced pain relief (Chow *et al.*, 2007).

NO, which is released as a photon binds to CCO and is replaced by oxygen, causes vasodilation and increased blood flow, resulting in a net decrease in the concentration of inflammatory mediators and edema. The increased rate of oxidative phosphorylation further boosts NO levels and generates ROS molecules (Hancock and Riegger-Krugh, 2008). The transient increase in ROS results in a net decrease in ROS concentrations, along with improved function of the local cell population and improved intercellular communication. The cumulative result of these interactions is a decrease in pain, increased release of beta-endorphins (Hagiwara *et al.*, 2007, 2008; Sprouse-Blum *et al.*, 2010), and increased serotonin levels (Magalhaes *et al.*, 2015).

The resting membrane potential of nerve and muscle cells is stabilized. The threshold of pain perception is increased, and trigger-point activity is reduced as muscle tissue relaxes (Cramond *et al.*, 1994). Inflammatory edema, therefore, is reduced by both vasodilation and improved muscle function (Bjordal *et al.*, 2006).

The behavioral results of these biochemical changes are easily observed during the course of a therapeutic laser treatment for painful conditions. They are usually first seen as an overwhelming stillness and relaxation demonstrated by the horse, followed by a gradual lowering of the head and neck. The eyelids will relax, and often close as the horse falls asleep, or the horse will yawn repeatedly as the laser therapy is applied to the painful area. Tissue texture will also change dramatically throughout the session. Depending on the condition of the patient, the texture will change from the tense, hard feeling of spastic muscle to the soft, spongy feel of edema-filled connective tissue.

Dose Guidelines for Equine Laser Therapy

In the absence of a substantial body of research on specific doses for the equine patient, translation of doses used in other species is applicable. This is appropriate when treating equine conditions in superficial tissue, but in deep tissues, the lack of firmly established doses is challenging.

The dose of therapeutic laser light reaching a target tissue will be affected by the wavelength, by parameters such as power and power density, and by patient-related factors, such as etiology, pathology, target tissue depth, hair length, and skin and hair pigmentation (Enwemeka, 2009). Some evidence exists that the interaction of light with living tissue is characterized by biphasic and triphasic dose responses (Huang *et al.*, 2009).

In practice, this all means that a certain dose of laser light energy must be applied to tissue in order to have a measurable biological effect. Clinically, the dose required for a photobiomodulatory effect depends on the animal being treated, the condition, the tissue, the type and biochemical status of the cells being treated, the rate of dose delivery, and the frequency of reapplication of the dose.

The results of clinical trials in humans give some insight into tissue penetration, dosage, and response to treatment in a variety of conditions (Bjordal *et al.*, 2003, 2008; Chow *et al.*, 2009; Huang *et al.*, 2015). The fact that the equine patient has a hair coat (frequently heavily pigmented) and is larger and more heavily muscled than human subjects suggests that doses for equine deep-tissue conditions should usually be increased beyond those recommended for humans. The best way to accomplish this is to understand the fundamental principles of the interaction of light with cells, to begin with recommended therapeutic doses, and then to carefully observe the effects in the clinical setting, and adjust based on response.

The WALT-established photobiostimulation threshold for humans is 5J/cm^2 (WALT 2010). Horses will often benefit from the administration of a considerably higher dose. A horse with chronic exertion myopathy, for example, might show extreme, immediate relief and long-term clinical improvement from the administration of $10–15 \text{J/cm}^2$ over a large area. The best approach in this scenario is to administer two to three treatments, each with a dose of 5J/cm^2, spaced 24–48 hours apart. Such a horse might also benefit from lower-dose maintenance sessions administered weekly or monthly. The goal in dosing is to achieve as much pain relief as possible

with each treatment session, moving the horse from corrective work to maintenance work as rapidly as possible in order to realize the most efficient return to maximal tissue health and peak performance.

Application of Laser Therapy to the Performance Horse

In a 2007 investigation into the depth of penetration of laser therapy into equine tendons *in vivo*, the results appeared to indicate that clipping the area to be irradiated before laser treatment would increase the depth of penetration of the light. This has the most relevance in the treatment of deeper tissues. The results also indicate that cleaning the skin and hair over the area to be irradiated may have a positive effect on photon penetration (Ryan and Smith, 2007). Clipping is out of the question with many performance horses, but cleaning of the area to be treated can easily be accomplished.

Before commencing treatment, a therapy zone (the area to be treated) should be determined based on history, gait evaluation, and palpation findings during the physical exam. This zone might consist of multiple isolated regions, or it might be one relatively large, contiguous zone, but in either case, it should include the specific points of greatest muscle tension, areas exhibiting a reduced range of motion, or areas that elicit pain sensitivity to digital pressure. Focusing the therapy directly on these "hot points" seems to produce greater efficacy than spreading it over a set of predetermined points.

Start the therapy session by "scanning" the body, administering a low dose over a large surface area, and observing the horse's behavioral response. A distinct endorphin response might help you recognize the need to treat an area that was not recognized on your physical exam. Throughout the treatment session, you should ensure even coverage by fully treating one zone in a cross-hatched right-angled pattern before moving on to the next. Keep in mind the total amount of energy you plan to administer to each zone, but be prepared to adapt your treatment to the needs of each horse according to the behavioral response and tissue texture changes; this will ensure a thorough treatment tailored to the horse's needs. Keeping the target dose in mind will prevent you from lingering in one zone too long, and monitoring the skin and hair for temperature changes will help guide the session as it progresses. Minimal temperature change accompanied by a strong endorphin response indicates the need for more energy to be applied, while a rise in temperature alone or with a concurrent tapering of the endorphin response indicates the need to move on to another zone.

When selecting axial myoskeletal sites to irradiate, the practitioner should ideally use both the motion palpation exam (checking for joint motion according to chiropractic

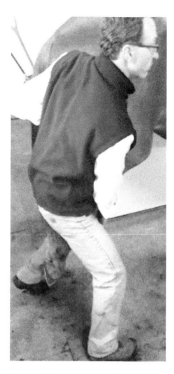

Figure 35.1 Proper patient assessment includes using the motion palpation examination, checking for joint motion according to chiropractic principles, and traditional examination techniques, evaluating tissue texture and response to digital pressure.

principles; Figure 35.1) and traditional examination techniques (evaluating tissue texture and response to digital pressure). All tissue types should be evaluated, including bone, muscle, ligament, and fascia.

When a tense, dysfunctional, or painful site is identified, examine adjacent regions of various tissue types and remote structures and regions with an anatomical or functional link to the primary site. For example, when the poll (atlanto-occipital joint) is the primary site, regional structures to consider are the intercapital ligaments (regional), the nuchal bursa (regional), the proximal and distal insertions of the nuchal ligament (structural remote), and the lower cervical facets (functional remote).

All of these areas should be scanned with the laser, administering a minimum of $1\,J/cm^2$ total dose. Further treatment of up to $5\,J/cm^2$ total dose is justified by the suspicion of primary clinical significance of the area based on a physical and motion-palpation exam, or by the horse's response to treatment (exhibited by the endorphin effect or by changes in tissue texture and the pain response to digital pressure).

If a patient displays even mild skin irritation in response to the laser treatment, the session should be discontinued immediately. In the author's experience, a very small percentage of horses (<1%) are photosensitive and cannot tolerate laser therapy. These horses respond by forming raised plaques (≤1 cm in diameter) that

resolve without treatment within 24 hours. If a horse shows repeated discomfort or aggravation when the laser is applied, treatment in that area should be terminated.

Anything other than minimal restraint should not be applied to the patient. Medical sedation, twitch, lip chain, and any similar restraining techniques should never be necessary during a laser therapy session.

Administration Precautions

When using a laser emitting at a high power (>6 W) and applying the therapy over a rather small area, there is the possibility of a non-therapeutic incidental thermal buildup within the tissues from pigment absorption of photons. If this occurs, several techniques can be used to reduce the power density of the laser beam and thus reduce thermal buildup.

Frequently, the easiest adjustment is simply to move the laser handpiece at a faster rate over the treatment zone. If faster movement is not feasible, the power can be reduced with a proportional increase in treatment time. Likewise, using a pulsed emission instead of continuous wave will increase overall time of delivery.

The laser spot size (the diameter of the laser beam that contacts the tissue) can be increased to reduce power density. Instead of administering the therapy in contact with or just off the tissue, hold the handpiece at increasing distances from, yet perpendicular to, the target tissues. This will increase the spot size and lower the power density. The disadvantage to this technique is an increase in photon reflection from the tissue surface, particularly at the margins of the laser spot.

The treatment zone can also be enlarged. In order to save time when lasering a large treatment zone, the operator can laser a second zone until the first cools sufficiently to accept more irradiation. The purpose of this technique is not to eliminate heating of the tissue but rather to regulate it to the benefit of the patient. Warming of painful, inflamed tissue is not only inherently soothing, it also promotes healing by increasing blood flow, thereby increasing the supply of nutrients and oxygen at the site of injury. Studies have demonstrated that, in humans, a 1 °C increase in core temperature increases metabolic rate 10–13% (Landsberg *et al.*, 2009).

Establishing Optimum Ranges of Motion

Anti-inflammatory laser effects occur as part of the same cascade of reactions responsible for pain reduction. ROS and superoxide dismutase (SOD) production, ion gradient and cell membrane changes, and vasodilation all help to promote beneficial changes in inflammatory mediator concentrations locally, and to establish an improved level of tissue homeostasis (Cotler *et al.*, 2015; Hamblin and Demidova, 2006).

Quieting of nociceptive afferents improves the quality of signal input to the central nervous system (CNS) such that hormone level changes help to create a sense of well-being, but return to normal function may be the most important change from the standpoint of equine performance maintenance (Tsuchiya, 1993). If the back, neck, and pelvis are pain-free, and the soft-tissue structures of each segment are functioning properly, not only should the horse feel better, but so too should it perform better, with fewer training days missed, less lameness, less chance of serious injury, and ultimately a chance at a longer career.

Establishing and maintaining full range of motion in the neck is a very important factor in the athleticism of a sport horse. The neck functions as a unit. It comprises the cervical vertebral column, the cranial thoracic vertebrae T1–T5, the large muscles of the neck and fore limb, core thoracic spinal muscles, and the ligaments on which the head and neck are suspended. Stretched fascia exists throughout the entire neck, with nerves coursing through it.

Every healthy sport horse should be able comfortably to touch its muzzle to its girth if it has proper mechanics (Stubbs and Clayton, 2008). However, just because a horse can do this does not mean that its neck is perfectly healthy. Other factors must also be considered, such as behavior, performance ability as reported by the rider and the trainer and as observed under saddle, tissue texture, and motion palpation.

In facilitating optimal range of motion of the neck, the ultimate goal is to ensure that each individual anatomical structure and tissue type performs its function perfectly, in order to avoid undue stress on adjacent and remote structures and tissues. For instance, complete lateral flexion of the neck originates from proper motion in the joints between the occiput and fifth cervical vertebra. Deficits in the motion of the lower cervical facet joints or core muscle weakness in that region may present only as a range deficit, incoordination, or weakness in the ability to move the muzzle toward the hind fetlock.

Laser therapy is useful along the axial myoskeleton for treating pain and limited range of motion at all levels of the spine and core musculature. Continuous monitoring of the horse's behavior and tissue tension is recommended throughout the course of treatment. The laser will initiate a cascade of biochemical reactions in the patient, which sometimes culminates in a profound endorphin effect. Pain relief and perhaps other aspects of the photobiochemical effect will decrease skin tension, revealing details of the condition of underlying tissue. Soft-tissue edema throughout the neck, usually most apparent in the region of the second and third cervical vertebrae, is a common, painful, performance-limiting condition, which may become apparent to the practitioner through the course of treatment.

Laser Therapy and Equine Athletic Conditioning

Athletic conditioning of the muscles involves breaking down muscle tissue and replacing it with stronger tissue made up of healthier cells. Laser therapy, when used for athletic performance maintenance, can be beneficial both before and after conditioning exercise. The value and importance of laser therapy in conditioning and exercise have been prominent in publications about its application in human and animal models (Antonialli *et al.*, 2014; de Marchi *et al.*, 2012; Ferraresi *et al.*, 2015; Ishide *et al.*, 2008; Larkin-Kaiser *et al.*, 2015; Perini *et al.*, 2016). It is now apparent that PBM can be effective if delivered to normal cells or tissue before the actual insult or trauma, in a pre-conditioning mode. Muscles are protected, nerves feel less pain, and a protective response against subsequent major damage is induced (Agrawal *et al.*, 2014).

Since chromophores located on the mitochondrial membrane are recognized as the principal intracellular photoreceptors, and muscle cells are known to be exceptionally rich in mitochondria, it makes sense that laser therapy has the potential to affect the rate of recovery and the quality of repair in fatigued or damaged muscle tissue.

When to administer laser therapy in relation to conditioning exercise is being explored. Leal Junior *et al.* (2010) determined that laser irradiation immediately before high-intensity exercise inhibited an expected post-exercise increase in creatine kinase levels in human athletes. Borsa *et al.* (2013) demonstrated that PBM from laser therapy administered before resistance exercise affected contractile function, reduced exercise-induced muscle damage, and facilitated post-exercise recovery. The effectiveness demonstrated was dose-dependent, so continuing to establish appropriate treatment variables, such as wavelength and output power, is important. In a 2014 study, laser application before or after fatigue reduced the post-fatigue concentrations of serum lactate and creatine kinase (Dos Reis *et al.*, 2014). The results were more pronounced in the post-fatigue laser group.

Assis *et al.* (2015) applied laser therapy to rats immediately after 1 hour of endurance training, 5 days a week for 8 weeks, and found a significantly reduced lactate level and an increased tibialis anterior fiber cross-sectional area. This suggested that laser therapy could be an effective therapeutic approach for stimulating recovery and improving anabolic response to endurance exercise. Silva *et al.* (2015) demonstrated that pre-exercise laser therapy improves performance and levels of oxidative stress markers in mice subjected to muscle fatigue by high-intensity exercise.

Though no studies have been performed on equine patients, translation of the results from multiple other species seems to indicate that similar effects would be seen in horses. Further research in this area would be helpful in defining how laser therapy could be consistently beneficial in the athletic conditioning of horses involved in speed, power, and endurance sports.

Laser Therapy and Chiropractic Technique

Chiropractic examination and treatment can be hindered by pain, such that a horse will brace and effectively splint the segment of spine that the practitioner is trying to adjust (Figure 35.2). In such cases, the laser can often provide enough immediate pain relief to allow adjustment of a motion unit that would otherwise remain locked. By combining laser therapy with chiropractic, the result of treatment of a patient whose pain level is high may be better than chiropractic alone. This is especially true of neck pain, because nociceptive stimuli emanating from this level of the spine are much less likely to dissipate and thus escape conscious awareness than those originating from the lower back.

Core muscle strength is widely recognized as perhaps the single most important benchmark achievement for an athlete early in training. Establishment of core muscle strength is seen as a prerequisite to heavy training and strenuous athletic endeavors, because of its importance in injury prevention. The primary mover of the joints of the equine spine is the multifidus muscle, and the length of the horse's axial skeleton makes the proper function of this muscle group extremely important.

Momentum is another huge force that moves the horse's back. Mitigation of this force during normal athletic endeavors and during mishaps is important in health maintenance, and relies on core muscle strength, flexibility, tissue integrity, and elasticity of all the structures involved. A chain is only as strong as its weakest link, but in the spine, the joint injured in a slip-and-fall accident may in fact be the one that is functioning the best in the stressed area. The best-moving joint may be the one that is injured, because the others are not doing their fair share of the work. Using the laser to reduce inflammation and maintain joint motion along the entire length of the spine, therefore, may reduce the chance of injury at high-range of motion joints like the lumbosacral joint and at transitional joints like the thoracolumbar junction.

Before initiating laser therapy on the athlete, complete a thorough chiropractic motion-palpation exam. If you are unable to restore motion to a joint of the axial skeleton with a gentle adjustment, use the laser to treat soft-tissue inflammation and muscle spasm, which is the most common cause of a poor response to adjustment. This is most seen around the sacroiliac joints and the atlanto-occipital joint. Often, motion will return to the joint after administration of $2–3\,J/cm^2$ of laser therapy. The horse will concurrently show behavioral evidence of an endorphin effect. The horse's head drops, its eyelids

Figure 35.2 Chiropractic examination and treatment can be hindered by pain. The horse will splint the area that the practitioner is trying to adjust. In such cases, the laser can provide enough immediate pain relief to allow adjustment of a motion unit (lumbosacral joint left, lumbar spine right) that would otherwise remain locked.

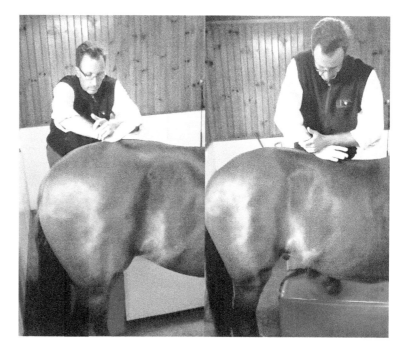

flutter, it shows muscle relaxation, repeated yawning, and a decreased awareness of environmental factors, tissue tension softens, and surface temperature warms. If all of this occurs as expected, you should continue the treatment until the endorphin effect begins to dissipate, as indicated by the horse beginning to show more alertness, or until a total dose of $5\,J/cm^2$ is reached, whichever comes first.

Constantly monitor the surface temperature of the treatment area by digital palpation. Expect the tissue to be warm, but it should never be uncomfortable or affect the patient. If the patient exhibits any discomfort, discontinue treatment in that area immediately, even if the endorphin effect is still present. Move to an adjacent treatment zone and repeat the same process. If you think the original treatment zone requires more irradiation, simply return to it later and treat it again.

The total target dose for each treatment area should be $5\,J/cm^2$. If no endorphin effect is observed by the time $2\,J/cm^2$ has been administered, and if the tissue is warm, then you should discontinue treatment in that zone and move on to another. If you strongly suspect the need for more treatment based on your exam findings, then select an adjacent area or nearby anatomical structure. For example, treat the nuchal bursa as a secondary target structure if the original was the atlanto-occipital joint. Administer 2–$5\,J/cm^2$, then return to the original area for additional irradiation. The reasoning here is that a certain region (your treatment zone) is being braced because of a painful process nearby.

If you have administered $2\,J/cm^2$ with no observable endorphin effect and the surface temperature of the skin in the treatment zone is cold or has increased minimally, then continuing the treatment in the same zone is advisable. Certain horses require a larger dose of irradiation before clinical improvement is observable and pain relief and the endorphin effect are achieved. After $5\,J/cm^2$ of irradiation has been delivered, irradiation of the primary treatment zone should be considered complete.

Laser Therapy and Saddle Fit

The laser can be used to treat inflammation of superficial structures in the withers and upper back caused by pressure points from an ill-fitting saddle. The pain relief for the horse is often dramatic, but it will be short-lived unless the saddle fit problem is corrected.

Even though taking away the saddle is the ultimate solution, laser therapy of the affected tissue is recommended for two reasons. First, return to peak performance is more rapid if the chronic inflammation is treated locally. Second, a certain type of saddle fit problem may result in chiropractic subluxations, and these will often be corrected more completely with concurrent

normalization of cellular function in the affected region. Specifically, nerve-root irritation will interfere with joint motion by causing core muscle spasm, and myofascial pain will cause regional bracing. For both of these conditions, the use of a higher laser power is indicated to maximize the dose delivered to the target tissues.

Case Studies

Left Fore-Limb Lameness

Signalment
"Hoot," 17 years old.

Client Complaint
Presented with a grade 2+/5 left fore-limb lameness of 2 weeks' duration.

History
The owner reported observing a pasture incident in which Hoots was kicked by another horse in the region of the left shoulder. The lameness had been present ever since. The owner also reported the presence of "tension" in the right hip.

Physical and Chiropractic Examination
Evaluation in motion at the walk showed the left hip lower than the right. Evaluation in motion at the trot showed the front fetlocks loaded evenly, but there was a distinct head bob present, consistent with a left fore-limb lameness. No hind-limb lameness was observed. Proper mechanics were observed on lateral neck-bending exercise, with the forehead perpendicular to the ground and the muzzle at shoulder level (Figure 35.3).

Chiropractic findings showed bilateral hip subluxations, right sacrosciatic ligament tension, dorsal rotation of the left sacral base, right poll, and lower cervical subluxations (C5/6 and C6/7). Evaluation in motion after chiropractic adjustments showed an estimated 50–75% improvement in lameness gait deficit at the trot. A mild left fore-limb head bob was still observed intermittently.

Laser Therapy Treatment
Laser therapy was applied at a dose of $5\,J/cm^2$ using $10\,W$ of power. A total dose of $11\,000\,J$ was applied over the right side of neck from the poll to the withers to the base of the neck. Hoot fell asleep during the treatment of the poll and proximal attachment of the nuchal ligament at T4 and T5. He also yawned repeatedly during the treatment of the right lower neck.

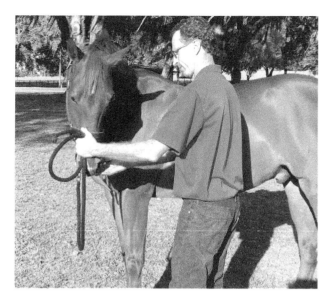

Figure 35.3 "Hoot," 17 years old, demonstrating proper mechanics on lateral neck-bending exercise, with forehead perpendicular to the ground and muzzle at shoulder level.

Outcome

Evaluation in motion immediately after laser therapy showed no lameness present. The horse was shipped from Florida to Kentucky 2 days after treatment, and the lameness did not return, as determined by a phone follow-up 5 weeks after the treatment.

Weakness in the Right Hind Limb, Heaviness on the Left Shoulder, Dull and Depressed

Signalment

"Crunchy," 6 years old, Irish sport horse, MN.

Client Complaint

Crunchy's trainer had noted a weakness in the right hind limb at the canter, worse on the right lead than the left. In addition, the horse felt heavy on the left shoulder and was acting dull and depressed.

History

Crunchy had been imported to United States from Europe in November 2015 as a 1 Star Preliminary Level eventer purchased to be a Novice Level eventer. He was first examined on January 25, 2016.

Chronological Physical and Chiropractic Examination, Laser Therapy, and Response to Treatment

1/25/2016 Chiropractic examination findings and adjustments included bilateral sacroiliac joint and bilateral shoulder subluxations, bilateral atlanto-occipital joint subluxations, right atlanto-axial joint, and left C2/3 and C6/7.

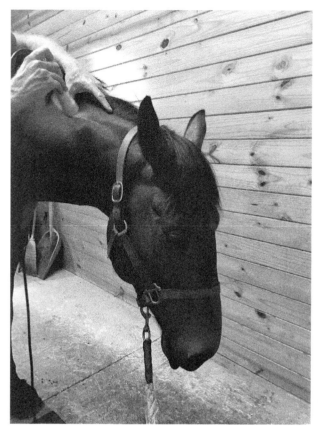

Figure 35.4 Crunchy, 6 years old, displaying typical behavior associated with an endorphin effect during laser treatment of the nuchal ligament near its attachment to C2.

2/9/2016 The trainer reported Crunchy's attitude was brighter and he felt better but was still not right behind and his right lead canter was still very different from his left lead.

Chiropractic examination showed right sacroiliac subluxation, mild left sacroiliac pain, dorsal rotation of the left sacral base, bilateral poll tension, and marked pain on palpation of the supraspinous ligament at L5 and L6.

After chiropractic adjustments, the poll tension remained. Adjustment was unable to restore motion to the intervertebral joints from L1/2 to T12/13 on the left side.

Laser therapy at $5\,\mathrm{J/cm}^2$ was applied to the poll, the sacroiliac joints, L5/6, L2–T13, and the nuchal ligament (Figure 35.4).

The horse fell asleep as soon as the laser session began, and slept through the entire treatment. After the treatment, pain response to digital pressure over L5/6 was absent and very good motion was palpated in all spinal segments.

3/12/16 The trainer reported that Crunchy's personality had changed to very bright and interactive. There had been a dramatic improvement in attitude, and willingness to train had improved greatly. Crunchy's canter was the same in both directions. He was stronger, and was able to train and build muscle.

Chiropractic examination findings and adjustments included right sacroiliac subluxation with mild pain and tension, right ventral thoracolumbar spine subluxations, and mild muscle tension in the right lower neck at C6–T1.

Laser therapy was applied at 5 J/cm^2 over the right sacroiliac joint and L5/6. An excellent behavioral response, with repeated yawning and very good pain dissipation, was noted.

4/12/2016   The trainer reported continued improvement and strengthening in training, with good balance and good attitude, and noted that Crunchy was still pulling like a freight train on the left rein.

Chiropractic examination findings and adjustments included left-side withers subluxations at T5/6–T8/9, bilateral atlanto-occipital joint subluxations with the left side locked and a failure to restore motion, and the right side similarly locked at C7/T1–T3/T4.

Laser therapy was applied at 5 J/cm^2 over the left nuchal ligament (funicular portion), the right base of the neck from C7 to T4, and 3 inches either side of the cranial border of the scapula. A pronounced endorphin effect was noted. The horse dropped his head to shoulder level and appeared very relaxed.

4/14/2016   The trainer reported no significant changes.

Chiropractic examination and adjustments included left-side mid-cervical subluxations at C3/4–C5/6, right atlanto-occipital and atlanto-axial joint, and right

anterior superior ilium. Core-group muscle spasm was present at C6/7 and T1/2 on the left side, and C7/T1 and T1/2 on the right.

Laser therapy was applied at 5 J/cm^2 over the left and right lower cervical regions of muscle spasm, over the funicular nuchal ligament on the right side from the occiput to C6 and T3–T5, and on the left side from C1 to C3. A distinct endorphin response was noted over all treated segments of nuchal ligament. The horse fell asleep as soon as 2 J/cm^2 had been administered over the right poll, and slept throughout treatment of the nuchal ligament.

Conclusion

The mechanisms and far-reaching photobiomodulatory effects of laser therapy have been well established in bench-top laboratory research, *in vivo* and *in vitro* studies, and clinical trials using a wide variety of species, including small mammals and humans. The successful application in other species of what has been learned in research, studies, and trials suggests that PBMT is indicated as a treatment modality for horses. Laser therapy can be an important tool in maintaining performance. Incorporation of laser therapy into an overall management plan for maintaining performance will include using the technology to help establish optimum ranges of motion, help reduce fatigue and hasten recovery during conditioning, and facilitate chiropractic technique.

References

Agrawal, T. *et al.* (2014) Pre-conditioning with low-level laser (light) therapy: light before the storm. *Dose Response.* **12**(4):619–649.

Antonialli, F.C. *et al.* (2014) Phototherapy in skeletal muscle performance and recovery after exercise: effect of combination of super-pulsed laser and light-emitting diodes. *Lasers Med Sci.* **29**(6):1967–1976.

Assis, L. *et al.* (2015) Effect of low-level laser therapy (808 nm) on skeletal muscle after endurance exercise training in rats. *Braz J Phys Ther.* **19**(6):457–465.

Assis, L. *et al.* (2016) Aerobic exercise training and low-level laser therapy modulate inflammatory response and degenerative process in an experimental model of knee osteoarthritis in rats. *Osteoarthritis Cartilage.* **24**(1):169–177.

Bashkatov, A.N. *et al.* (2011) Optical properties of skin, subcutaneous, and muscle tissues: a review. *J Innovative Opt Health Sci.* **4**(9):9–38.

Bjordal, J.M. *et al.* (2003) A systematic review of low level laser therapy with location-specific doses for pain from joint disorders. *Aust J Physiother.* **49**(2):107–116.

Bjordal, J.M. *et al.* (2006) Low-level laser therapy in acute pain: a systematic review of mechanisms of action and clinical effects in randomized placebo-controlled trials. *Photomed Laser Surg.* **24**(2):158–168.

Bjordal, J.M. *et al.* (2008) A systematic review with procedural assessments and meta-analysis of low level laser therapy in lateral elbow tendonopathy (tennis elbow). *BMC Musculoskeletal Disord.* **9**:75.

Borsa, P.A. *et al.* (2013) Does phototherapy enhance skeletal muscle contractile function and postexercise recovery? A systematic review. *J Athl Train.* **48**(1):57–67.

Buchner, H.H. and Schildboeck, U. (2006) Physiotherapy applied to the horse: a review. *Equine Vet J.* **38**(6):574–580.

Chen, A.C. *et al.* (2011) Low-level laser therapy activates NF-kB via generation of reactive oxygen species in mouse embryonic fibroblasts. *PLos One.* **6**(7):e22453.

Chow, R.T. *et al.* (2007) 830 nm laser irradiation induces varicosity formation, reduces mitochondrial membrane potential and blocks fast axonal flow in small and medium diameter rat dorsal root ganglion neurons: implications for the analgesic effects of 830 nm laser. *J Peripher Nerv Syst.* **12**(1):28–39.

Chow, R.T. *et al.* (2009) Efficacy of low-level laser therapy in the management of neck pain: a systematic review and meta-analysis of randomized placebo or active-treatment controlled trials. *Lancet.* **374**(9705):1897–1908.

Chung, H. *et al.* (2012) The nuts and bolts of low-level laser (light) therapy. *Ann Biomed Eng.* **40**(2):516–533.

Cotler, H.B. *et al.* (2015) The use of low level laser therapy (LLLT) for musculoskeletal pain. *MOJ Orthop Rheumatol.* **2**(5):00068.

Cramond, T. *et al.* (1994) ACTH and beta-endorphin levels in response to low level laser therapy for myofascial trigger points. *Laser Ther.* **6**(3):133–142.

de Marchi, T. *et al.* (2012) Low-level laser therapy (LLLT) in human progressive-intensity running: effects on exercise performance, skeletal muscle status, and oxidative stress. *Lasers Med Sci.* **27**(1):231–236.

Dos Reis, F.A. et al (2014) Effects of pre- or post-exercise low-level laser therapy (830 nm) on skeletal muscle fatigue and biochemical markers of recovery in humans: double-blind placebo-controlled trial. *Photomed Laser Surg.* **32**(2):106–112.

Enwemeka, C.S. (2003) Attenuation and penetration of visible 632.8 nm and invisible infra-red 904 nm light in soft tissues. *Laser Ther J.* **13**:16.

Enwemeka, C.S. (2009) Intricacies of dose in laser phototherapy for tissue repair and pain relief. *Photomed Laser Surg.* **3**:387–393.

Farivar, S. *et al.* (2014) Biological effects of low level laser therapy. *J Lasers Med Sci.* **5**(2):58–62.

Ferraresi, C. *et al.* (2015) Muscular pre-conditioning using light-emitting diode therapy (LEDT) for high-intensity exercise: a randomized double-blind placebo-controlled trial with a single elite runner. *Physiother Theory Pract.* **31**(5):354–361.

Hagiwara, S. *et al.* (2007) GaAlAs (830 nm) low-level laser enhances peripheral endogenous opioid analgesia in rats. *Lasers Surg Med.* **39**(10):797–802.

Hagiwara, S. *et al.* (2008) Pre-irradiation of blood by gallium aluminum arsenide (830 nm) low-level laser enhances peripheral endogenous opioid analgesia in rats. *Anesth Analg.* **107**(3):1058–1063.

Hamblin, M.R. and Demidova, T.N. (2006) Mechanisms of low level light therapy. *Proc of SPIE.* **6140**(612001):1–12.

Hancock, C.M. and Riegger-Krugh, C. (2008) Modulation of pain in osteoarthritis: the role of nitric oxide. *Clin J Pain.* **24**(4):353–365.

Haussler, K.K. (2010) The role of manual therapies in equine pain management. *Vet Clin North Am Equine Pract.* **26**(3):579–601.

Huang, Y.Y. *et al.* (2009) Biphasic dose response in low level light therapy. *Dose Response.* **7**(4):358–383.

Huang, Z. *et al.* (2015) The effectiveness of low-level laser therapy for nonspecific chronic low back pain: a systematic review and meta-analysis. *Arthritis Res Ther.* **17**:360.

Ishide, Y. *et al.* (2008) The effect of GaAlA diode laser on pre- sports warming up and post-sports cooling down. *Laser Ther.* **17**(4):187–192.

Karu, T. (2010) Mitochondrial mechanisms of photobiomodulation in context of new data about multiple roles of ATP. *Photomed Laser Surg.* **28**(2):159–160.

Leal Junior, E.C. *et al.* (2010) Effects of low-laser therapy (LLLT) in the development of exercise-induced skeletal muscle fatigue and changes in biochemical markers related to postexercise recovery. *J Orthop Sport Phys Ther.* **40**(8):524–532.

Landsberg, L. *et al.* (2009) Do the obese have lower body temperatures? *A new look at a forgotten variable in energy balance. Trans Am Clin Climatol Assoc.* **120**:287–295.

Larkin-Kaiser, K.A. *et al.* (2015) Near-infrared light therapy to attenuate strength loss after strenuous resistance exercise. *J Athl Train.* **50**(1):45–50.

Levine, D. *et al.* (2015) Effects of laser on endurance of the rotator cuff muscles. *Lasers Surg Med.* **47**(s26):44–45.

Maegawa, Y. *et al.* (2000) Effects of near-infrared low-level laser irradiation on microcirculation. *Lasers in Surgery and Medicine.* **27**(5):427–437.

Magalhaes, M. *et al.* (2015) Light therapy modulates serotonin levels in blood flow in women with headache. A preliminary study. *Exp Bol Med.* **241**(1):40–45.

McGowan, C.M. *et al.* (2007) Equine physiotherapy: a comparative view of the science underlying the profession. *Equine Vet J.* **39**(1):90–94.

Mester, E. *et al.* (1968) The effect of laser beams on the growth of hair in mice. *Radiobiol Radiother (Berl).* **9**(5):621–626.

Morimoto, Y. *et al.* (1996) Low-intensity light induces vasorelaxation: a study for possible mechanism. *Proc of SPIE.* **2681**:126–129.

Paulekas, R. and Hussler, K.K. (2009) Principles and practice of therapeutic exercise for horses. *J Equine Vet Sci.* **29**(12):870–893.

Perini, J.L. *et al.* (2016) Long-term low-level laser therapy promotes an increase in maximal oxygen uptake and exercise performance in a dose-dependent manner in Wistar rats. *Lasers Med Sci.* **31**(2):241–248.

Poyton, R.O. and Ball, K.A. (2011) Therapeutic photobiomodulation: nitric oxide and a novel function of mitochondrial cytochrome c oxidase. *Discov Med.* **11**(57):154–159.

Ribeiro, B.G. *et al.* (2015) The effect of low-level laser therapy (LLLT) applied prior to muscle injury. *Lasers Surg Med.* doi:10.1002/lsm.22381.

Ryan, T. and Smith, R. (2007) An investigation into the depth of penetration of low level laser therapy through the equine tendon in vivo. *Ir Vet J.* **60**(5):295–299.

Sabino, C.P. *et al.* (2016) The optical properties of mouse skin in the visible and near infrared spectral regions. *J Photochem Photobiol B.* **160**:72–78.

Silva, A.A. *et al.* (2015) Pre-exercise low-level laser therapy improves performance and levels of oxidative stress markers in mdx mice subjected to muscle fatigue by high-intensity exercise. *Lasers Med Sci.* **30**(6)1719–1727.

Smith, A.W. *et al.* (2009) Bioimaging: second window for in vivo imaging. *Nature Nanotechnology.* **4**(11): 710–711.

Sprouse-Blum, A.S. *et al.* (2010) Understanding endorphins and their importance in pain management. *Hawaii Med J.* **69**(3):70–71.

Stubbs, N.C. and Clayton, H.M. (2008) *Activate Your Horse's Core.* Xenophon Press, Franktown, VA.

Tsuchiya, K. *et al.* (1993) Diode laser irradiation selectively diminishes slow component of axonal volleys to dorsal roots from the saphenous nerve in the rat. *Neurosci Lett.* **161**(1):65–68.

Uddhav, A.P. and Lakshyajit, D.D. (2008) Overview of lasers. *Indian J Plast Surg.* **41**(Suppl.):S101–S113.

WALT. (2010) WALT dosage recommendations. Available from: http://waltza.co.za/documentation-links/ recommendations/dosage-recommendations (accessed November 30, 2016).

36

Laser Therapy and Multimodal Equine Rehabilitation

Brenda McDuffee

Independent Laser Sales Representative, Ocala, FL, USA

Introduction

Laser therapy, increasingly known as photobiomodulation therapy (PBMT) (Anders *et al.*, 2015; Passarella and Karu, 2014), is one of the most versatile and widely used therapeutic modalities in the equine rehabilitation and equine sports medicine fields. PBMT can be used as the sole approach to the rehabilitation of injuries, but when it is combined with other modalities the recovery time will be shortened and the resolution more complete (Hallstam *et al.*, 2016; Merrick *et al.*, 2012). Applications for PBMT include acute and chronic injuries, the recovery following any surgery, and maintenance of optimal athletic performance.

Like human athletes, equine athletes require not only raw talent, but also a tremendous amount of training and care in order to achieve the highest levels of competition. With the value of equine athletes continuing to increase, it is essential, irrespective of their discipline, to utilize all of the latest technology and all available modalities to prevent injuries, accelerate the healing time for any disorder, improve athletic conditioning, and maintain the highest level of performance.

Until recently, the rehabilitation phase of recovery was primarily a time to rest, with controlled exercise until recovery was achieved. The athlete was then returned to training with the intention of achieving the previous level of competition by slowly increasing the workload. Unfortunately, many times the athlete would re-injure the same area, due to the inferior quality of the tissue formed during the lengthy time off. Alternatively, the athlete might create a new injury because it was so out of condition that the increasing exercise overloaded a compensatory area, which had become predisposed to injury.

As rehabilitation protocols continue to advance in the human field of sports medicine, we realize that these same principals apply to equine athletes. Multimodal therapeutic rehabilitation, utilizing PBMT, has become the standard of care for equine athletes, allowing them to regain strength, restore function, and accelerate their recovery.

Utilizing a multimodal approach by incorporating laser therapy in combination with other therapeutic modalities, veterinarians, owners, and trainers can expect consistent favorable patient outcomes. Patients will have reduced levels of pain and inflammation, better tissue strength and flexibility, a reduction in the loss of bone density, and improved post-injury and post-surgical clinical results (de Jesus *et al.*, 2014, 2015; Williams, 2004).

Fundamental Information

Fundamental information about the physics, physiological and biochemical events, and general principals of PBMT is provided in the first few introductory chapters of this text. Detailed fundamental information about the application of PBMT to horses can be found in Chapter 31. When considering the role of PBMT in multimodal rehabilitation, however, a basic understanding of the physiology of injuries and wounds is also necessary, as is an understanding about the timing and frequency of treatments with the therapy laser.

Acute and Chronic Injuries

Injury, by definition, is damage to the body. Within this broad classification, there exist many different types of injury. Injuries may affect the musculoskeletal system, or they may be confined to other soft tissues.

In the equine rehabilitation field, superficial wounds, deep penetrating and infected wounds, generalized myositis, tendonitis, and desmitis are presented on a daily basis. It is helpful to categorize these injuries as either acute or chronic.

Acute injuries are usually associated with traumatic events that result in damage to bones, muscles, tendons, ligaments, or other soft tissues. Acute musculoskeletal injuries cause sudden, sharp pain that is often severe. Other symptoms are swelling, inability to move a joint through normal range of motion, weakness, and decreased tissue warmth due to loss of circulation in the injured area. Instability while standing or moving, or inability to bear weight, may also be evident.

Chronic injuries usually affect the musculoskeletal system. They are normally caused by overuse during exercise or rigorous competition. Repetitive concussive forces that occur when a 450 kg equine athlete hits the ground result in micro-tears in soft tissues or micro-fractures in bones, or a combination of both. These develop slowly and result in long-standing lameness issues. Symptoms of these types of injury are often mild in comparison to acute injuries, and initially do not cause severe pain. This allows the equine athlete to disregard the injury and continue with the daily training schedule. Understandably, these chronic injuries will never allow optimum performance, and they often result in an acute injury if a compensated anatomical area is pushed past its normal loading capacity.

Wounds

Wounds, by definition, are any injuries that damage the skin and the immediate underlying tissues (Ubbink *et al.*, 2015). These include abrasions, scrapes, cuts, contusions, and surgical incisions. When the epidermis is compromised, the change initiates physiological processes and a biochemical cascade of events aimed at repairing the damage (Nguyen *et al.*, 2009). Utilizing laser therapy within a multimodal rehabilitation approach can modulate these biochemical and physiological events. PBMT induces a rapid analgesia (Chow *et al.*, 2008), a modulation of the inflammatory response (Fabre *et al.*, 2015), and an increase in circulation (Plass *et al.*, 2012). These effects accelerate the overall healing process and allow equine athletes with wounds to return to normal activities more quickly. The biochemical cascade of events within individual cells is highlighted by the release of nitric oxide (NO), an increase in the production of adenosine triphosphate (ATP), and the release of reactive oxygen species (ROS) (Karu *et al.*, 2008). See Chapter 5 for an in-depth explanation of the mechanisms behind the reduction of pain and inflammation and the increase in circulation.

Healing of musculoskeletal injuries occurs in three phases: inflammatory, regeneration, and remodeling (Stadelmann *et al.*, 1998). PBMT affects each of these phases, helping restore the individual cellular structures, organizing tissue repair, and producing an accelerated return to the earlier natural state (Woodruff *et al.*, 2004).

During the initial inflammatory phase, there is a disruption of the circulatory system, creating an insufficient availability of glucose, oxygen, and other components required to produce enough ATP (Versteeg *et al.*, 2013). The body responds with vasodilation, which allows essential cells, antibodies, growth factors, enzymes, and nutrients to reach the wound (Kelly *et al.*, 2012; Michael *et al.*, 2012).

In the regeneration phase, application of photonic energy accelerates angiogenesis (Basso *et al.*, 2012). In fibroplasia and granulation tissue formation, fibroblasts grow and form a new, provisional extracellular matrix (ECM) through the formation of collagen (Midwood *et al.*, 2004). This results in a bridging of disrupted tissues. PBMT delivered to these regenerative cells results in an increased activation rate, which allows tendons, ligaments, bone, muscle, and other tissues to heal at an accelerated rate (Abrahamse and Hawkins, 2006; Basso *et al.*, 2013; Lorenz and Longaker 2003). Concurrently, re-epithelialization of the epidermis occurs, during which epithelial cells proliferate and migrate across the wound bed (Silveira *et al.*, 2013).

When the levels of collagen production and degradation equalize, the remodeling or maturation phase begins. The application of laser therapy during this phase accelerates mitosis and collagen synthesis (Vasilenko *et al.*, 2010; Wood *et al.*, 2010). Throughout maturation, type III collagen, which is prevalent during proliferation, is replaced by type I collagen. Disorganized collagen fibers are rearranged, cross-linked, and aligned along tension lines (Assis *et al.*, 2012). This results in an increase in the tensile strength of the wound and a reduction of scar tissue formation (Karu, 2008).

It is helpful to think of the new fibers created in the regeneration phase as being like a spider's web, unorganized and random. When controlled exercise is introduced during the remodeling phase, the fibers begin to align into a more striated pattern, resulting in a stronger, less fibrous, more flexible and dynamic structure. Even though limited exercise is necessary from the beginning of the regeneration phase, the addition of a more extensive but controlled exercise program should take place during the remodeling phase. This controlled exercise will result in an increase in the tensile strength of the wound and a reduction of scar tissue formation (Karu, 2008). Reducing the pain and inflammation during the initial phases by the application of PBMT allows the patient to move more comfortably into limited controlled exercise earlier in the rehabilitation process. The ability to do some exercise prevents the soft-tissue structures and skeletal framework from losing a significant amount of condition and strength. As the patient progresses in its rehabilitation, it will be able to regain strength, flexibility, and normal function in a shorter period, increasing the possibility of its returning to full functionality and a good quality of life.

By understanding the role PBMT plays in improving the overall healing process, appreciation is gained about the importance of this modality to almost all rehabilitation programs. In conjunction with other modalities, a controlled exercise program, and physical therapy techniques, each patient will have a more beneficial outcome in a shorter period.

Frequency of Laser Therapy Administration

When applying laser therapy, it is helpful to think of the total joules administered per treatment as doses of photonic energy. Just as it is important to administer an appropriate dose of medication to achieve the proper response, it is necessary to treat an injury with the appropriate dose of light energy to achieve the desired therapeutic result.

Each patient requires an individualized laser therapy program. For most acute injuries, two or three consecutive daily treatments are administered. These treatments serve as a loading dose. After the initial loading dose, a transition is made to having more time between laser therapy sessions. Transition-phase treatments are typically administered three times a week for the next few weeks, and then twice a week until resolution. If the patient has a severe injury or wound, or if an infection is present, daily laser therapy treatments are beneficial until the infection is under control, or the injury or wound starts to clinically improve.

While the horse is confined to stall rest, or is in a very limited, controlled exercise phase, other therapeutic modalities should also be considered in conjunction with laser therapy. Each will benefit the injured area through mechanisms of relief of pain and swelling, a reduction in inflammation, and increased range of motion. The order in which you provide different multimodal therapeutic approaches is important. The effect of each modality on the injury must be understood in order to ensure that the beneficial effect of any earlier or concurrent treatment is not negated.

When dealing with a chronic problem, such as osteoarthritis, laser therapy is initially administered at a similar frequency as is used in acute cases. The level of recovery achieved must then be maintained through additional periodic administration of therapy sessions. This is referred to as the "maintenance phase" of therapy. Initially, treat daily, and then transition to two or three treatments a week until the therapeutic goal is reached. Treatments can then be spread out to the frequency required to maintain the same level of comfort for the patient. The frequency of treatments during the maintenance phase is unique to each individual case and is dependent on constant re-evaluation of the patient and adjustment to maintain response.

Multimodal Therapeutic Modalities

In a multimodal approach to rehabilitation, all available modalities in addition to laser therapy should be considered in order to facilitate a rapid recovery. It is important to understand how each of the other modalities affects the tissue and the symptoms, and the way it supports and promotes the healing process.

Cold Salt-Water Leg Spas

Cold salt-water leg spas are enclosed walk-in units in which the patient stands inside a watertight chamber that fills to the desired level with cold salt water (Figure 36.1). The water for the spa is stored in a holding tank and is kept at a temperature near freezing. Large quantities of Epsom and sea salt are mixed into the water, making it an almost supersaturated solution. In most spas, the water is constantly circulating to maintain even, cold temperatures around the legs.

The water level can be adjusted to any depth that is applicable to the injury, but is never filled higher than just below the forearms and gaskins. Filling the water to cover the forearms, gaskins, and above can result in a loss of core body temperature, due to the increased number of

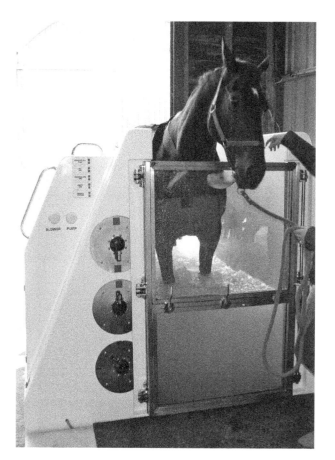

Figure 36.1 Patient standing in a cold salt-water leg spa.

blood vessels found in the muscle tissues above this height. There is predominately bone, tendon, and ligament tissue on the lower legs, and very little muscle tissue. This allows the equine species to stand in freezing temperatures, ice, and snow for prolonged periods. (This is unlike the lower extremities of humans, which have a much higher percentage of muscle tissue, limiting the amount and length of time that cold therapy can be applied in this species.) If the horse's injury is higher on the body, a hose attachment can be used to "spot treat" a higher problem (e.g., wounds, cellulitis, contusions) while maintaining the water in the unit at an appropriate level.

Cold salt-water leg spa treatment time is usually around 20 minutes. This is followed by a warm-up phase that allows the legs to return to normal temperature. The warm-up period may take a couple hours, depending on outside temperatures. Pain, inflammation, and swelling are addressed by the treatment in the spa (Zhang *et al.*, 2014). The near-freezing temperature of the water has an almost immediate analgesic effect (de Souza Bosco Paiva *et al.*, 2016). The extremely salty water acts like a "poultice," drawing out edema and swelling from the tissue. The submersion results in complete contact of the cold salt water with the entire surface of the legs. This allows the cold temperature to penetrate deeply, resulting in reduction of heat and inflammation all the way into the bone and hoof capsule. Cold salt water helps break the inflammatory cycle. With each treatment, there is a delay in time until the inflammation returns with reduced intensity.

During the warm-up phase, there is an increase in circulation. This warms the extremities and brings increased levels of oxygen to inflamed tissue. It is important not to shorten the warm-up phase by wrapping the legs or exercising, since doing so reduces the amount of time for which extra oxygen is available to the injury. Once the legs have warmed back up to normal body temperature, the process can be repeated if the injury is severe.

Cold salt-water spa sessions are limited to 20 minutes, since the legs cannot get any colder after that time. With most injuries, extending the period in the spa does not achieve better or faster results. The general protocol for frequency of treatments with acute injuries is daily while there is still detectable warmth within the injury and then every other day until resolution. Once the injury has repaired to the point that controlled exercise is added to the rehabilitation program, the cold spa should be carried out immediately after the exercise therapy is completed, to prevent heat and inflammation in the healing tissue. Doing more than one treatment a day can be advantageous for some acute problems, such as laminitis.

For acute injuries, using laser therapy in conjunction with cold salt-water therapy can help resolve pain, inflammation, and swelling much faster than either therapy used alone. When using both modalities on the same day for a horse that is still in the stall-rest or very limited hand-walking stage, the cold salt-water spa therapy should be carried out first, followed by laser therapy once the legs have had enough time to warm back up to normal body temperature. When the legs have returned to normal temperature, the beneficial effects of the spa are complete until the next spa session.

If the horse has progressed in its rehabilitation to including more exercise, laser therapy is applicable before the exercise to increase circulation and provide oxygen to the tissue (Levine *et al.*, 2015). Pre-exercise application of laser therapy helps warm up the tissue and allows it to be more flexible. The cold salt-water spa should be used directly after exercise to help reduce any inflammation caused by the exercise.

Hyperbaric Oxygen Therapy

Equine hyperbaric oxygen therapy (HBOT) chambers are walk-in units in which a horse breathes 100% oxygen at three times normal atmospheric pressure (Figure 36.2). The concept behind HBOT is very simple: it establishes a very high level of oxygen throughout the entire circulatory system, leading to increased oxygenation of damaged and healing tissues.

Oxygen in the blood is bound by hemoglobin, which is 97% saturated at standard atmospheric pressure. During HBOT, hemoglobin is saturated and blood can be hyperoxygenated by dissolving oxygen within the plasma. Because this oxygen is in solution, it can reach areas where red blood cells may not be able to pass due to their size. It can also provide tissue oxygenation in the event of impaired hemoglobin concentration or function (Kindwall, 2004).

During HBOT, the plasma can carry up to 20 times more dissolved oxygen to the tissues than it can under normal atmospheric pressure. This results in an increase of the oxygen levels in the tissue to as much as 15 times that possible with normal saturation at normal atmospheric pressure. Small or compromised capillaries, through which red blood cells cannot pass, due to their size, can deliver more oxygen to the tissue via the plasma. The diffusion of oxygen past the end of the capillaries is four times greater during increased pressurization (Boerema *et al.*, 1960). HBOT is a well-established treatment in the human field for decompression sickness, a hazard of scuba diving (Harvey, 1945). Other conditions treated with HBOT in the human field include serious infections, bubbles of air in blood vessels, and wounds that will not heal because of diabetes or radiation injury.

Physiologically, the effects of hyperoxygenation of the blood are significant. Vasoconstriction (Sukoff and Ragatz, 1982), angiogenesis (Knighton *et al.*, 1981), fibroblast proliferation and collagen synthesis (Hunt and Pai, 1972), and leukocyte oxidative killing (Park *et al.*, 1992) have all been reported. There is an increase in the

Figure 36.2 Patient entering a hyperbaric oxygen therapy (HBOT) unit. Image courtesy of The Equine Sanctuary Sports Therapy and Rehabilitation Center, Ocala, FL.

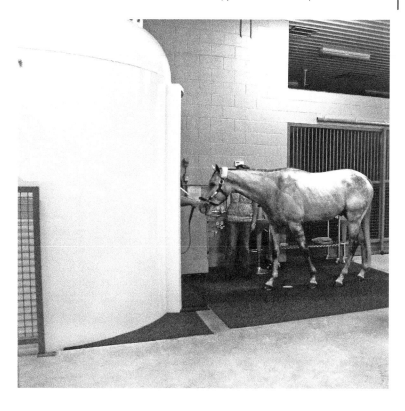

generation of oxygen free radicals, which oxidize proteins and membrane lipids and inhibit bacterial metabolic functions, making hyperoxygenation particularly effective against anaerobes. Additionally, there is evidence that HBOT alters the levels of pro-inflammatory mediators and may blunt the inflammatory cascade. More studies are needed to elucidate further this complex interaction. Thom *et al.* (2006) concluded that HBOT mobilizes stem cells through the stimulation of NO synthesis. The release of NO is also one of the many results of PBMT.

Since HBOT establishes a very high level of oxygen throughout the entire circulatory system, the resulting physiological effects make this a very useful modality for the treatment of quite a number of conditions and injuries. The most common cases presented for HBOT are wounds, blood-deprived tissue, chronic infections, osteomyelitis, colic surgery post-op, laminitis, gastric ulcers, colitis and other intestinal disorders, lung and abdominal abscesses, neonatal maladjustment syndrome (dummy foals), difficult dermatological disorders, and muscle, tendon, and ligament injuries.

Wound injuries that are difficult to manage (those that are infected, necrotic, and non-healing) benefit greatly from HBOT. These injuries have a damaged blood supply, depriving normal circulation to the tissue, and have had bacteria introduced into the body, which can result in infection. HBOT facilitates the delivery of oxygen-rich blood and plasma to this injured, oxygen-deprived tissue. The benefits are an initiation of angiogenesis, fibroblast proliferation, collagen synthesis, an inhibition of anaerobic bacterial metabolism, and a modulation of the inflammatory cycle.

HBOT sessions are cumulative in effect. The state of hyperoxygenation is temporary, but any positive changes that occur remain once the treatment ends. Treatment progress is retained, and therefore a number of treatment sessions are necessary to accomplish an accelerated healing of the condition.

A patient receiving PBMT before HBOT therapy will realize the following benefits:

- An increase in circulation and a vasodilation of the vasculature within the tissue, facilitating a higher level of perfusion of the hyperoxygenated blood and plasma.
- A reduction in inflammation and edema, allowing an increase in the level of perfusion of the hyperoxygenated blood within the tissues.
- An activation of fibroblasts, allowing an even higher level of activation during HBOT.
- An increased rate of collagen synthesis prior to the increases realized during HBOT.
- A down-regulation of cytokines and an up-regulation of growth factors.

Administering PBMT before a HBOT session is synergistic, in that the clinical response is greater than if each modality is used independently.

Along with the benefits of HBOT come safety concerns, both physically and physiologically. Several conditions and medications are contraindicated in pressurized chambers, and this can be limiting when assessing a patient for HBOT. Laser therapy provides many of the same physiological benefits, but with fewer contraindications. Wounds and contusions, skin, muscle, tendon, and ligament injuries, fractures, cellulitis, lymphangitis, and pharangitis all are applications for laser therapy in the rehabilitation process whether HBOT can be used concurrently or not. The use of PBMT and HBOT treatments during the same period is dependent on patient assessment and the degree of severity of the injury.

Targeted Pulsed Electromagnetic Field Therapy

Targeted pulsed electromagnetic field (tPEMF) technologies offer another scientific, evidenced-based modality for use in equine rehabilitation protocols (Figure 36.3). The effectiveness of tPEMF therapy has been well demonstrated by several experimental and clinical studies (Fini *et al.*, 2008; Ongaro *et al.*, 2011; Pipitone and Scott, 2001), and tPEMF therapy is widely used in human medicine (Markov, 2007; Ryang *et al.*, 2013). These devices have shown efficacy in accelerated wound and fracture repair, through stimulation of growth factors (Markov, 2007), relief of pain, inflammation, and edema, agonistic activity on adenosine, inhibition of prostaglandin synthesis, and release of endogenous opioids (Thomas *et al.*, 2007; Varani *et al.*, 2008).

The result of the mechanism of action is very similar to that of PBMT. These relatively simple devices generate short bursts of electrical current, which flow into injured tissue without producing heat or interfering with nerve or muscle function. Studies have shown that tPEMF modulates calmodulin-dependent NO/cyclic guanosine monophosphate (cGMP) signaling in cells that have a compromised metabolic rate (Pilla, 2012, 2015; Pilla *et al.*, 2011). Direct evidence of the immediate effect of tPEMF on NO production in a neuronal cell line challenged with lipopolysaccharide was reported by Pilla (2012). This release of NO clinically results in a relief of pain, modulation of the inflammatory reaction, angiogenesis, accelerated tissue healing, vasodilation, endorphin release, and a reduction in interleukin 1β (IL1β). These effects are very similar to those seen with the increased release of NO that occurs with PBMT. tPEMF can be utilized as a practical addendum to laser therapy. Their mechanisms of action differ, but their clinical results are very similar: they both provide relief of pain, modulation of the inflammatory cycle, and an increase in circulation.

PBMT and tPEMF are used synergistically along with standard wound care. The procedure is as follows. Clean and debride the wound and then apply PBMT at $8–10\,J/cm^2$ over the wound and all of the surrounding tissues. Apply an appropriate topical medication, dressing, and wrap. Over the next 24 hours, administer three to four tPEMF therapy sessions. These can be applied through the wrap and dressing. Continue this daily routine for 2–3 days. As healing begins, the time between bandage changes and PBMT can be increased to every 48 hours, but continue tPEMF three to four times a day. This routine is continued until the wound is healed.

Chronic musculoskeletal conditions will also benefit from a combination of PBMT and tPEMF. For example, the medical and management history of a 5-year-old thoroughbred with degenerative joint disease of both metacarpal-phalangeal joints might include multiple intra-articular injections, systemic analgesics and non-steroidal anti-inflammatory drugs (NSAIDs), ice wraps after any exercise, and cooling poultice wraps overnight. PBMT could be added after any work, and the day before and after a race. Bilateral PBMT should be applied to the superficial and deep flexor tendons, the suspensory ligaments, the carpus, and any palpable soreness in the shoulders and neck. tPEMF therapy could be applied to the metacarpal-phalangeal joint three times daily with wraps removed, with an additional session 4 hours before a race. Swimming might also be introduced twice a week to minimize the repetitive concussion on all limbs. With this multimodal regime, the horse would be expected to recover better after both work and racing.

Therapeutic Ultrasound

Therapeutic ultrasound is capable of significantly raising the temperature of specific deep-tissue targets. This focused application of heat is much more beneficial to the patient than the application of external heat to the skin. When it is used, the deep target tissue becomes warm. Therapeutic ultrasound is capable of heating deep tissues without elevating the temperature at the skin surface.

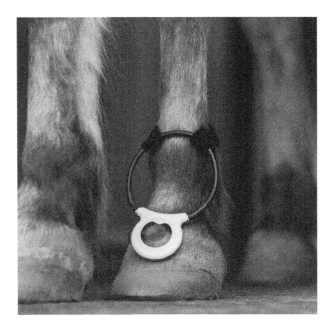

Figure 36.3 A tPEMF device in place over a patient's pastern.

Heat, being a form of energy, increases the metabolic activity within the cells. This increased activity causes an increase in oxygen demand locally. As a result, vasodilation occurs, in order to increase the amount of blood bringing oxygen and nutrients to the area. Membrane diffusion and enzymatic activity also increase, enabling oxygen consumption and removal of the waste products of injury, including prostaglandins, bradykinin, and histamine, all of which are implicated in nerve fiber sensitization and pain.

Therapeutic ultrasound should only be administered by someone properly trained in its usage, since the range between a healing temperature and a damaging temperature is only 5 °C: a tissue temperature of 40 °C is ideal for healing, yet heating above 45 °C will cause damage.

Therapeutic ultrasound has several beneficial applications, including softening of scar tissue, relief of deep muscle spasms, reduction of inflammation, and assistance in the healing of wounds (Avrahami *et al.*, 2015; Maura Junior Mde *et al.*, 2015). The versatility of this modality is limited, but it does have a beneficial effect on large muscle masses. PBMT has many more potential applications, with almost no danger of causing cellular damage. It stimulates the metabolic rate of the cell through a biochemical reaction, whereas therapeutic ultrasound stimulates cells with heat energy.

Underwater Treadmill

An underwater treadmill is a walk-in device for controlled exercise (Figure 36.4). The buoyancy and resistance of the water allow low-impact, high-resistance therapy or workouts for faster recovery and rehabilitation from injury, and for optimal training and conditioning. The modality increases strength, muscle tone, and range of motion, while limiting the concussion on the bones and soft-tissue structures. The use of underwater treadmill exercise for the training and rehabilitation of equine patients has become increasingly popular in recent years. It reduces loading on painful or healing structures, pain in joints with degenerative joint disease, edema, muscle spasms, joint stiffness, development of muscle atrophy, and time to complete recovery, and it increases resistance for muscles during exercise, tone in hypotonic muscle parts, muscle mass and strength, joint range of motion, soft-tissue extensibility, and cardiovascular fitness and endurance. Underwater exercise can continue when land exercise is restricted, reducing lay-up time.

Underwater treadmill exercise is controlled. Varying levels of water and different speeds of the treadmill belt affect how the horse's muscles and joints move and what areas are most utilized. At a lower water level, the horse will step up above the surface; as the level increases, the horse will continue to try to step above the water height, increasing range of motion in the muscles and joints (Figure 36.5). At hock depth, the horse performs full range of motion in all four legs. For many of the lower-leg soft-tissue injuries, lower water levels encourage the horse to move the recovering tissue in full flexion and extension, while reducing the concussion on the bones, joints, and tissue due to the rubber surface of the treadmill and the resistance of the water.

Figure 36.4 Underwater treadmill.

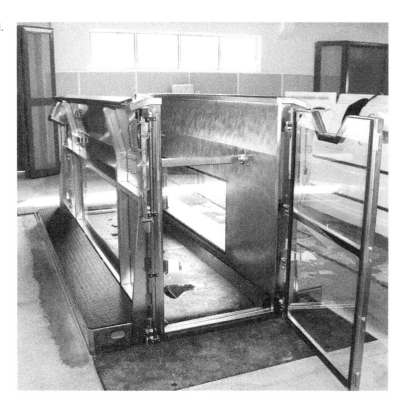

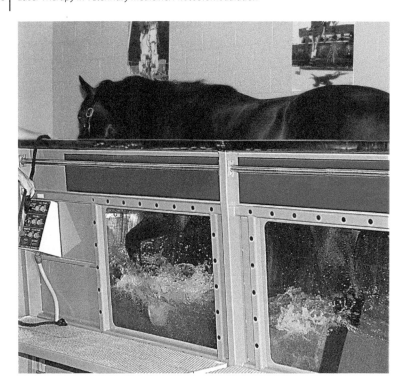

Figure 36.5 At a lower level of water, the horse will step up above the surface; as the level increases, the horse will continue to try to step above the water height, increasing its range of motion in the muscles and joints. Image courtesy of The Equine Sanctuary Sports Therapy and Rehabilitation Center, Ocala, FL.

As the water level increases even more, the horse begins to utilize different muscles in its body, reducing some of the range of motion in the joints, but requiring it to work harder against the resistance of the deeper water (Figure 36.6). Deeper water will further engage the core muscles, tightening the abdominal muscles, elevating the back muscles to lift up the torso, and using the hindquarters to propel forward through the water. For many performance horses, being able to start the exercise portion of their rehabilitation in the "round" frame that they use for their event allows them to return to their previous level of training and competition earlier, by strengthening them overall while supporting their still-fragile recovering tissue.

The underwater treadmill will also encourage the horse to take even strides with all four legs, promoting a balanced and proper gait. Many horses recovering from an injury will continue to limp on a recovering leg even after the pain has been resolved, possibly due to habit, or because of the formation of scar tissue that limits their range of motion. When working with a horse that has developed a shortened stride in one or more legs, it is important to slow down the underwater treadmill movement to allow equal and even strides. Once the horse is able to walk evenly, the speed of the belt can be increased to encourage a longer, more normal stride.

The water temperature and turbulence can be controlled in many underwater treadmills. Utilization of cold water will provide a small amount of analgesia, reduce swelling and edema, and increase energy expenditure as the patient tries to maintain core body temperature. The patient will create its own turbulence during movement, but many underwater treadmills are equipped with jets to create even more. The clinical benefit of these jets is unknown.

PBMT can be beneficial both before and after controlled exercise in an underwater treadmill. When PBMT is applied before exercise, it is essentially a warm-up of the muscle tissues, providing increased flexibility and endurance (Levine *et al.*, 2015). When applied after exercise, it provides a faster recovery of the tissues, combined with a relief of any pain subsequent to the exercise (Dos Reis *et al.*, 2014; Enwemeka *et al.*, 2004).

Swimming

Swimming exercise can be part of a training and conditioning program or a step in the rehabilitation process for horses recovering from injuries (Figure 36.7). Most equine pools are straight-line, round, or keyhole-design. In straight-line pools, the horse walks down a ramp into the water at one end, and then up another ramp at the other end to get out again (Figure 36.8). In round or keyhole-design pools, the horse walks down a ramp into the water, swims in a circle around the edge of the pool, and then exits up the same ramp by which it entered. Swimming is excellent cardiovascular exercise and allows a horse to work without any concussive forces on the musculoskeletal system. As a total-body workout, swimming improves muscle tone and fitness, and puts the joints through range of motion.

Figure 36.6 At higher water levels, the horse will begin to utilize different muscles in its body, reducing some of the range of motion in the joints, but working harder against the resistance of the deeper water.

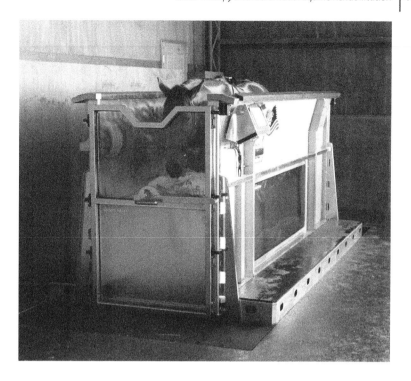

Figure 36.7 Patient swimming in a pool. Image courtesy of The Equine Sanctuary Sports Therapy and Rehabilitation Center, Ocala, FL.

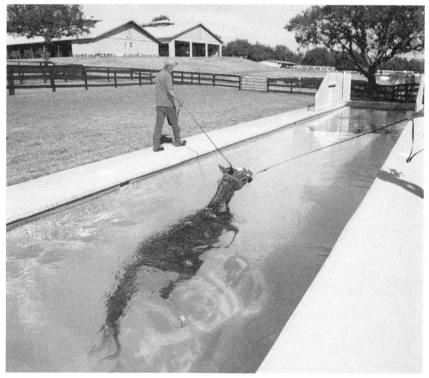

Though an appropriate exercise for many types of problems, swimming is not for every issue or patient. Like any form of exercise, it must be done properly in order to achieve a beneficial effect. Some horses are not natural swimmers. Others cannot swim properly, due to injury or lack of conditioning. If a horse struggles in the water, or is not able to swim evenly and with balance, there is the possibility of furthering the damage or creating new problems. While in the water, a horse is in an inverted frame, with the head and neck extending upward and the back hollowed out. This is not an ideal exercise posture for horses with back, sacroiliac, or stifle problems. It is possible to exacerbate these injuries with swimming. Due to this inverted frame, and the possibility of overextending the

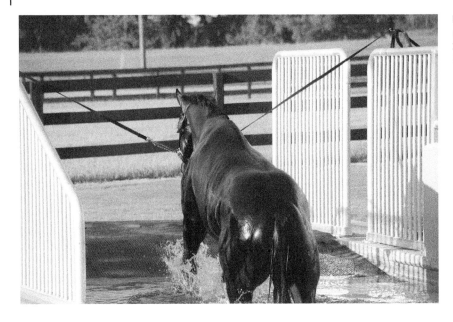

Figure 36.8 Patient exiting a straight-line pool. Image courtesy of The Equine Sanctuary Sports Therapy and Rehabilitation Center, Ocala, FL.

hindquarters, care should be taken that the horse does not further harm itself. Caution should also be exercised with horses with shoulder injuries: the swimming itself is usually not a problem, but exiting up the ramp can be difficult.

For horses that work in long, open frames, such as racehorses, barrel horses, and endurance horses, swimming is an excellent way to rehabilitate and strengthen them in the frame in which they compete in their discipline. For horses that are normally ridden in a more collected or round frame, such as jumpers, dressage horses, and English and Western performance horses, swimming may not be an appropriate way to rehabilitate them if there are other exercise options available, such as underwater treadmill.

At the beginning of a rehabilitation program for an injury that is acute and cannot tolerate any concussion-type exercise, swimming may be a good way by which to expend energy when a horse is too active in the stall. Once an injury has progressed enough to allow for a more concussive-type exercise, underwater treadmill exercise will be the better choice.

Case Studies

A multimodal rehabilitation approach utilized in conjunction with veterinary care and supervision ensures the best clinical outcome for the patient. Each case is unique and will have a rehabilitation program tailored to its individual needs. It is important for everyone on the staff involved with the rehabilitation protocol to assess the progress of the horse. The therapy technician must be vigilant to make sure that the horse is progressing as expected. Any increase in pain, heat, swelling, or lameness should be immediately reported to the veterinarian

for professional evaluation. Daily assessments should include making sure that temperature, pulse, and respiratory rate remain within normal ranges, along with the individual's temperament, appetite, and manure. Increases or decreases of heat in the affected tissue, pain upon palpation, or lameness upon moving should also be noted and reported. Frequent pictures, measurements of wounds, and temperature readings at an injury site allow the therapist, veterinarian, owner, and trainer to see changes and monitor progress.

The healing process is a fluid, constantly changing entity, and must be monitored closely to maximize results. Along with the daily progress assessments made by the therapist, the veterinarian should schedule re-checks and evaluate progress at specific intervals. At scheduled re-checks, the veterinarian should do a physical exam and utilize any appropriate diagnostic studies (ultrasound studies, radiographs, digital thermal imaging) needed to evaluate the patient's progress. Based on the findings at re-checks, the veterinarian should make any appropriate changes to medications and to the rehabilitation program.

To illustrate how PBMT is used with other technologies and exercise as part of multimodal rehabilitation, three case studies are detailed in this section. The wound case combines PBMT with HBOT and tPEMF, while the tendonitis and stress-fracture cases combine PBMT with cold salt-water leg spa therapy. All include controlled exercise as the rehabilitation progresses.

Laser Therapy and Multimodal Wound Management

The patient presented with a diagonal laceration and puncture wound over the left carpus with penetration into the carpometacarpal joint. The veterinarian cleaned, sutured, and dressed the wound with topical medication and a soft cast. Systemic antibiotics, anti-inflammatories, and pain-management medications were administered and daily bandage changes were schedule. Due to the expansive wrap immobilizing the limb, exercise was limited to stall rest or brief hand walking.

During the daily bandage change, PBMT was administered circumferentially throughout the entire carpus, using an off-contact delivery technique at a dosage of $10 J/cm^2$. The patient was weight bearing during these treatments, and no passive range of motion was attempted.

Daily HBOT sessions were conducted for 3 days and then every other day until the wound healed. tPEMF therapy was administered three times a day for the duration of the patient's rehabilitation.

By day 12, the wound has healing well with no sign of infection and the sutures were removed. Stall rest was continued with the addition of two 15-minute slow hand walks each day. Bandages continued to be changed daily and PBMT was administered every other day during bandage change. A tPEMF device embedded in the leg wrap was preprogrammed to treat for 15 minutes every 2 hours.

By day 18, healing was progressing, and hand walking was increased to 20 minutes twice daily, along with passive range-of-motion exercises. At this time, range of motion was 30% of normal. PBMT was administered during one of the two daily passive range-of-motion exercises. The patient's reduced pain level allowed on-contact administration throughout the entire anatomical structure, with particular attention to the carpometacarpal joint. The preprogrammed tPEMF device was still embedded in the leg wrap, providing 15 minutes' treatment every 2 hours.

On day 26, the patient had no sign of infection and almost full range of motion, and was discharged. If this wound had become infected, PBMT would have been administered more aggressively and HBOT treatment would have been daily instead of every other day.

Laser Therapy and Multimodal Tendonitis Management

The patient presented with significant bilateral swelling from the carpus to the fetlock throughout the superficial and deep flexor tendons. Ultrasounds did not reveal any lesions within the tendons.

For the first 30 days, exercise was limited to stall rest with controlled hand walking for 5–10 minutes, two to three times a day. Cold salt-water leg spa therapy was administered daily for 4 days, after which there was no more palpable heat in the legs, and then every other day, constantly checking for the presence of heat. Laser therapy was administered daily, on-contact, at $12 J/cm^2$ with a scanning technique for three consecutive days, then every other day for the next six treatments, and then twice a week until re-check at 30 days. A portion of the

laser therapy was administered while the patient was bearing weight on the leg, and the remainder while placing the leg through passive range-of-motion exercises (Figure 36.9). Standing wraps with cold poultice were applied each night.

At 30 days, a re-check indicated the condition was improving, with no clinically visible swelling or edema, and none seen in ultrasound images. For the second 30 days, a limited amount of controlled exercise was gradually added to the daily schedule. Hand walking increased to 20 minutes twice a day. Underwater treadmill therapy at hock depth was initiated for 10 minutes every other day, gradually increasing in duration when no swelling, pain, or heat was palpated. Before each controlled exercise session, laser therapy was administered on-contact, at a dosage of $12 J/cm^2$, while placing the tendons through passive range-of-motion exercise. A 10–15-minute cold salt-water spa session was administered directly after each exercise session. Bandages were applied over a cooling poultice for the first few days; then, just the poultice was applied following the spa session, left unwrapped to extend the benefits of the cold therapy.

At 60 days, hand walking increased to 25 minutes twice daily and underwater treadmill sessions were increased to daily, with a slow increase in speed. Laser therapy was administered twice a week at $12 J/cm^2$, on-contact while standing and while placing the tendons through passive range-of-motion exercise. During this time, the cold salt-water spa sessions were discontinued.

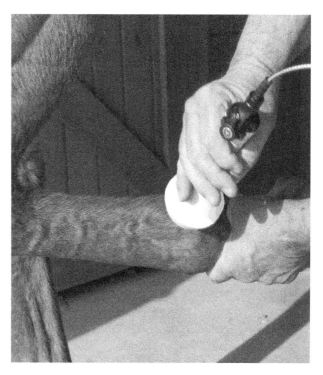

Figure 36.9 Treatment of the metacarpal area during passive range of motion.

On day 90, the patient appeared normal, and it was returned to conservative riding with a gradually increasing workload.

Laser Therapy and Multimodal Stress-Fracture Management

The patient presented with a dorsal cortical stress fracture of the left third metacarpal bone in the distal one-third of the bone. There was slight swelling throughout the metacarpal area, and the patient was 2/5 lame on left front. Surgical fixation was discussed, but the owner wanted to try physical therapy and rehabilitation.

For the first 30 days, exercise was limited to complete stall rest, with only a few minutes of hand walking in a grassy area each day. Cold salt-water spa sessions lasting 20–25 minutes were administered daily. Laser therapy was initiated on the day of presentation (3 days after the injury) and was continued daily for 6 days. These treatments were administered after the leg had warmed up following the daily cold salt-water spa session. A dosage of $15\,J/cm^2$ was applied off-contact due to the tenderness of the tissue, circumferentially and at right angles from just distal to the carpus to the fetlock. During the third daily treatment, on-contact administration was possible. After the sixth laser therapy session, treatments were transitioned to every other day. Support bandages were applied to both front legs using thick cotton quilts and cotton leg wraps.

On day 32, a radiograph revealed ossification all along the fracture line. Hand walking was increased to 30 minutes twice a day for 3 days, and then by a further 10 minutes per session each day. Cold salt-water spa sessions were administered for 20 minutes every other day. Laser therapy at a dosage of $15\,J/cm^2$ was administered twice a week after warm-up following the cold salt-water spa sessions.

On day 40, swimming for 20 minutes was added to the rehabilitation protocol. Swimming was immediately followed by a cold salt-water spa session, which was followed in turn by a laser therapy session after the leg had warmed up.

On day 54, the fracture was barely visible on radiograph and the patient was sound. The patient returned to training.

Conclusion

Equine rehabilitation is an expanding field that is rapidly changing as new physical therapy techniques and both diagnostic and therapeutic technologies are developed. The utilization of PBMT as the sole modality or in combination with other modalities provides an acceleration of the healing process. The use of this modality will only increase as new research into dosages, application techniques, optics, and clinical applications comes to light.

References

Abrahamse, H. and Hawkins, D. (2006) Effect of multiple exposure of low-level laser therapy on the cellular responses of wounded human skin fibroblasts. *Photomed Laser Surg.* **24**(24):705–714.

Anders, J. *et al.* (2015) Low-level light/laser therapy versus photobiomodulation therapy. *Photomed Laser Surg.* **33**(4):183–184.

Assis, L. *et al.* (2012) Low-level laser therapy (808 nm) contributes to muscle regeneration and prevents fibrosis in rat tibialis anterior muscle after cryolesion. *Lasers Med Sci.* **44**(9):726–735.

Avrahami, R. *et al.* (2015) The effect of combined ultrasound and electric field stimulation on wound healing in chronic ulcerations. *Wounds.* **27**(7):199–208.

Basso, F.G. *et al.* (2012). In vitro wound healing improvement by low-level laser therapy application in cultured gingival fibroblasts. *Int J Dent.* **2012**:719452.

Basso, F.G. *et al.* (2013) Biostimulatory effect of low-level laser therapy on keratinocytes in vitro. *Lasers Med Sci.* **28**(2):367–374.

Boerema, I. *et al.* (1960) Life without blood. A study of the influence of high atmospheric pressure and hypothermia on dilution of the blood. *J Cardiovascular Surg.* **1**:133–146.

Chow, R.T. *et al.* (2008) Efficacy of low-level laser therapy in the management of neck pain: a systemic review and meta-analysis of randomized placebo or active-treatment controlled trials. *Lancet.* **374**(9705):1897–1908.

de Jesus, J.F. *et al.* (2014) Low-level laser therapy on tissue repair of partially injured Achilles tendon in rats. *Photomed Laser Surg.* **32**(6):345–350.

de Jesus, J.F. *et al.* (2015) Low-level laser therapy in IL-1B, COX-2 and PGE2 modulation in partially injured Achilles tendon. *Lasers Med Sci.* **30**(1):153–158.

de Souza Bosco Paiva, C. *et al.* (2016) Length of perineal pain relief after ice pack application: a quasi-experimental study. *Women Birth.* **29**(2):117–122.

Dos Reis, F.A. *et al.* (2014) Effects of pre- or post-exercise low-level laser therapy (830 nm) on skeletal muscle fatigue and biochemical markers of recovery in humans: double-blind placebo-controlled trial. *Photomed Laser Surg.* **32**(2):106–112.

Enwemeka, C.S. *et al.* (2004) The efficacy of low-power lasers in tissue repair and pain control: a meta-analysis study. *Photomed Laser Surg.* **22**(4):323–329.

Fabre, H.S. *et al.* (2015) Anti-inflammatory and analgesic effects of low-level laser therapy on the postoperative healing process. *J Phys Ther Sci.* **27**(6):1645–1648.

Fini, M. *et al.* (2008) Effect of pulsed electromagnetic field stimulation on knee cartilage, subchondral and epyphiseal trabecular bone of aged Dunken Hartley guinea pigs. *Biomed Pharmacother.* **62**(10):709–715.

Hallstam, A. *et al.* (2016) Patients with chronic pain – one-year follow-up of a multimodal rehabilitation program at a pain clinic. *Scand J Pain.* **10**(10):36–42.

Harvey, E.N. (1945) Decompression sickness and bubble formation in blood and tissues. *Bull NY Acad Med.* **21**(10):505–536.

Hunt, T.K. and Pai, M.P. (1972) The effect of varying ambient oxygen tensions on wound metabolism and collagen synthesis. *Surg Gynecol Obstet.* **135**(4):561–567.

Karu, T. (2008) Mitochondrial signaling in mammalian cells activated by red and near-IR radiation. *Photochem Photobiol.* **84**(5):1091–1099.

Karu, T. *et al.* (2008) Primary and secondary mechanisms of action of visible to near-IR radiation on cells. *Phtomed Laser Surg.* **26**(6):593–599.

Kelly A. *et al.* (2012). Limb blood flow after class 4 laser therapy. *J Athl Train.* **47**(2):178–183.

Kindwall, E. (2004) A history of hyperbaric medicine. In: *Hyperbaric Medicine Practice*, 2 edn., pp. 1–20. Best Publishing, Flagstaff, AZ.

Knighton, D.R. *et al.* (1981) Regulation of wound-healing angiogenesis-effect of oxygen gradients and inspired oxygen concentration. *Surgery.* **90**(2):262–270.

Levine, D. *et al.* (2015) Effects of laser on endurance of the rotator cuff muscles. *Lasers Surg Med.* **47**(s26):44–45.

Lorenz H.P. and Longaker M.T. (2003) Wounds: biology, pathology, and management. In: *Surgery: Basic Science and Clinical Evidence*, pp. 191–208. Springer, New York.

Markov, M.S. (2007) Pulsed electromagnetic field therapy history, state of the art and future. *Environmentalist.* **27**:465–475.

Maura Junior Mde, J. *et al.* (2015) Assessing the biochemical changes of tendons of rats in an experimental model of tenotomy under therapeutic ultrasound and LEDs (625 and 945 nm) by near-infrared Raman spectroscopy. *Laser Med Sci.* **30**(6):1729–1738.

Merrick, D. *et al.* (2012). One-year follow-up of two different rehabilitation strategies for patients with chronic pain. *J Rehabil Med.* **44**(9):764–777.

Michael C.H. *et al.* (2012) Immediate effects of monochromatic infrared energy on microcirculation in healthy subjects. *Photomed Laser Surg.* **30**(4):193–199.

Midwood, K.S. *et al.* (2004) Tissue repair and the dynamics of the extracellular matrix. *Int J Biochem Cell Biol.* **36**(6):1031–1037.

Nguyen, D.T. *et al.* (2009) The pathophysiologic basis for wound healing and cutaneous regeneration. In: *Biomaterials For Treating Skin Loss*, pp. 25–57. CRC Press, Boca Raton, FL.

Ongaro, A. *et al.* (2011) Chondroprotective effects of pulsed electromagnetic fields on human cartilage explants. *Bioelectromagnetics.* **32**(7):543–551.

Park, M.K. *et al.* (1992) Oxygen tensions and infections: modulation of microbial growth, activity of antimicrobial agents, and immunologic responses. *Clin Infect Dis.* **14**(3):720–740.

Passarella, S. and Karu, T. (2014) Absorption of monochromatic and narrow band radiation in the visible and near IR by both mitochondrial and non-mitochondrial photoacceptors results in photobiomodulation. *J Photochem Photobiol B.* **140**:344–358.

Pilla, A.A. (2012) Electromagnetic fields instantaneously modulate nitric oxide signaling in challenged biological systems. *Biochem Biophys Res Commun.* **426**(3):330–333.

Pilla, A.A. (2015) Pulsed electromagnetic fields: from first messenger to healing. In: *Electromagnetic Fields in Biology and Medicine*, pp. 29–47. CRC Press, Boca Raton, FL.

Pilla, A.A. *et al.* (2011) Electromagnetic fields as first messenger in biological signaling: application to calmodulin-dependent signaling in tissue repair. *Biochim Biophys Acta.* **1810**(12):1236–1245.

Pipitone, N. and Scott, D.L. (2001). Magnetic pulse treatment for knee osteoarthritis: a randomized, double-blind, placebo controlled study. *Curr Med Res Opin.* **17**(3):190–196.

Plass, C.A. *et al.* (2012) Light-induced vasodilation of coronary arteries and its possible clinical implication. *Ann Thorac Surg.* **93**(4):1181–1186.

Ryang, We.S. *et al.* (2013) Effects of pulsed electromagnetic field on knee osteoarthritis: a systematic review. *Rheumatology.* **52**(5):815–824.

Silveira, P.C. *et al.* (2013) Effects of low-level laser therapy (GaAs) in an animal model of muscular damage induced by trauma. *Lasers Med Sci.* **28**(2):431–436.

Stadelmann, W.K. *et al.* (1998) Physiology and healing dynamics of chronic cutaneous wounds. *Am J Surg.* **176**(2A Suppl.):26S–38S.

Sukoff, M.H. and Ragatz, R.E. (1982) Hyperbaric oxygenation for the treatment of acute cerebral edema. *Neurosurgery.* **10**(1):29–38.

Thom, S.R. *et al.* (2006) Stem cell mobilization by hyperbaric oxygen. *Am J Physiol Heart Circ Physiol.* **290**(4):H1378–H1386.

Thomas, A.W. *et al.* (2007) A randomized, double-blind, placebo-controlled clinical trial using a low-frequency magnetic field in the treatment of musculoskeletal chronic pain. *Pain Res Manag.* **12**(4):249–258.

Ubbink, D.T. *et al.* (2015) Evidence-based care of acute wounds: a perspective. *Adv Wound Care (New Rochelle).* **4**(5):286–294.

Varani, K. *et al.* (2008) Characterization of adenosine receptors in bovine chondrocytes and fibroblast-like synoviocytes exposed to low frequency low energy pulsed electromagnetic fields. *Osteoarthr Cartil.* **16**(3):292–304.

Vasilenko, T. *et al.* (2010) The effect of equal daily dose achieved by different power densities of low-level laser therapy at 635 and 670 nm on wound tensile strength in rats: a short report. *Photomed Laser Surg.* **28**(2):281–283.

Versteeg, H.H. *et al.* (2013) New fundamentals in hemostasis. *Physiol Rev.* **93**(1):327–358.

Williams, J. (2004) Wound healing: tendons, ligaments, bone, muscles and cartilage. In: *Canine Rehabilitation and Physical Therapy*, pp. 100–110. Saunders, St. Louis, MO.

Wood, V. *et al.* (2010) Collagen changes and realignment induced by low-level laser therapy and low-intensity ultrasound in the calcaneal tendon. *Lasers Surg Med.* **42**(6):559–565.

Woodruff, L.D. *et al.* (2004) The efficacy of laser therapy in wound repair: a meta-analysis of the literature. *Photomed Laser Surg.* **22**(3):241–247.

Zhang, J. *et al.* (2014) Cryotherapy suppresses tendon inflammation in an animal model. *J Orthop Translat.* **2**(2):75–81.

37

High-Intensity Laser Therapy for the Equine Patient

Damiano Fortuna

Imaginalis S.r.l., Sesto Fiorentino (FI), Italy

Introduction

High-intensity laser therapy (HILT) is one of the natural evolutions of laser therapy. The goal of HILT is to promote tissue remodeling, tissue regeneration, and healing, especially in chronic, fibrotic lesions. Additionally, the use of high peak power makes it possible to reach deep-tissue lesions and tissues previously considered unreachable. These capabilities make HILT particularly useful in the treatment of musculoskeletal and other deep-tissue conditions in horses. The physical size of large food animals and some zoological species may make them potential candidates for HILT as well.

For many years, high-power lasers have been used in surgery. In the last decade, biostimulatory properties have been demonstrated. The HILT devices should be considered a particular subset of higher-power lasers, defined by the specific physical features of pulsed or superpulsed high radiance, with very energetic pulses. (Radiance is the radiant flux emitted, reflected, transmitted, or received by a surface per unit solid angle per unit projected area, and spectral radiance is the radiance of a surface per unit frequency or wavelength, depending on whether the spectrum is taken as a function of frequency or of wavelength. Historically, radiance is called "intensity" and spectral radiance is called "specific intensity." To simplify, radiance is the radiant energy emitted per unit time in a specified direction by a unit area of an emitting surface.)

The clinical efficacy of photobiomodulation therapy (PBMT) is related to many variables, such as the kind of lesion, the optical features of the target, the dose, the radiation frequency, the delivery system, and the spot size. With low-power devices (<500 mW), applications of several minutes are repeated at intervals of several days, often for months. The effects seen are primarily the result of a photochemical effect (Abergel *et al.*, 1987; Braverman *et al.*, 1989; Honmura *et al.*, 1992; Jimbo *et al.*, 1998). As laser power is increased (above 500 mW but below 30 W mean power), some photothermal effect may become present in addition to the photochemical effect experienced with lower-power devices. HILT devices are able to contribute photomechanical effects in addition to photothermal and photochemical effects.

The HILT Story

High-power neodymium-doped yttrium aluminum garnet (Nd:YAG) lasers first began being used for therapeutic purposes at the beginning of the 1990's (Parra *et al.*, 1992). They immediately showed promising results, especially in human sports medicine, even if their continuous emission represented a limitation from a safety point of view. The low water absorption of Nd:YAG light (1064 nm) results in very high photon distribution in the tissue (Palmer and Williams, 1974). Especially when compared to photons of other therapeutic laser wavelengths, Nd:YAG photons achieve good depth of penetration to lesions centimeters deep involving muscle, tendons, and joints.

Because of its ability to penetrate, the Nd:YAG laser met with favor among sports medicine physicians, at least in Europe. Moreover, it could be delivered through a flexible optical fiber, making it easy to use; at that time, the only other high-power laser on the market, the carbon dioxide laser, was delivered with an articulated mechanical arm.

Solid-State High-Intensity Lasers

Historically, the Nd:YAG solid-state laser has been the most used laser in HILT applications. Solid-state lasers, such as Nd:YAG, are characterized by the ability to emit a short pulsed beam with a duty cycle ≤1%. A duty cycle is described as a percentage of laser on time, in relation to pulse period (Barrett and Pack, 2006). Diode lasers have a duty cycle of 10–100%.

Light from a Nd:YAG laser is characterized by a wavelength of 1064 nm and is in the infrared band, not very far from the radiation of semiconductor lasers. The active medium is made of an artificial crystal of yttrium and aluminum (yttrium–aluminum garnet), which is also used for the production of artificial gems. The crystal is "doped" with impurities of neodymium, a rare soft silvery metallic chemical element that acts as an electron donor. The pumping system is a light source placed parallel to the crystal. Often, a multidiode laser of 808 nm is used as a "starter" for the Nd:YAG laser. A system of two concave mirrors, one of which reflects 98% and the other 100%, completes the base scheme of the Nd:YAG laser.

The radiation emitted is already collimated to the source; nevertheless, spots of various dimensions can be achieved depending on the intended use. In laser therapy, the laser beam is defocused to obtain spots of greater dimensions, generally 5–30 mm in diameter, to allow analgesic, anti-inflammatory, and tissue-regenerative effects.

Q-Switched Lasers for Therapeutic Applications

Q-switched lasers have also become available for therapeutic applications. Q-switching is a technique by which a laser can be made to produce a pulsed output beam characterized by extremely high (up to 1 GW) peak power, which is much higher than any other emitting modality (Früngel, 1965).

Q-switching is achieved by putting a variable attenuator inside the laser's optical resonator. When the attenuator is functioning, light, which leaves the gain medium, does not return, and lasing cannot begin. This attenuation inside the cavity corresponds to a decrease in the "Q factor" or quality factor of the optical resonator. A high Q factor corresponds to low resonator losses per round trip, and vice versa. The variable attenuator is commonly called a Q-switch when used for this purpose.

The most popular laser gain media for Q-switched devices are Nd:YAG and neodymium-doped yttrium vanadate (Nd:YVO4). While their properties for continuous-wave (CW) operation are overall quite similar, these media are rather different when used in Q-switched lasers. In general, Nd:YVO4 will allow for shorter pulses than Nd:YAG for any given repetition rate (Paschotta, 2006). The key advantages of Nd:YVO4 over other popular gain media such as Nd:YAG reside in its high gain, high diode-pump light absorption, and constantly polarized output (McDonagh and Wallenstein, 2007).

Biological Effects of Solid-State Lasers

In *Optical-Thermal Response of Laser-Irradiated Tissue*, Joseph T. Walsh writes, "If the light is absorbed in the material, then a number of vastly different processes can occur: the dominant ones are that the absorbed energy can drive chemical reactions, be re-emitted as light, or be converted into heat. In thermodynamic terms, the optical energy can increase the order in the system (e.g., drive a polymerization chemical reaction), minimally affect the system, or devolve into a less ordered state (e.g., random vibrations, i.e. heat)" (Walsh, 2011). In other words, the absorbed electromagnetic energy is transformed to other forms of energy, such as heat. The spectral distribution of the light due to the absorption process depends on the distribution, concentration, and absorption spectra of the absorptive elements. Absorptive elements are chromophores that can definitely affect light transmission and light absorption. A relationship between the absorption of light in a purely absorbing medium and the thickness of the medium is given by the Beer–Lambert–Bouguer law (IUPAC, 1997).

Chromophores and Absorption

The near-infrared window (also known as the optical window or therapeutic window) defines the range of wavelengths from 650 to 1350 nm, where light has its maximum depth of penetration in tissue (Smith *et al.*, 2009). Within the near-infrared window, scattering is the most dominant light–tissue interaction, and therefore the propagating light becomes diffused rapidly. Since scattering increases the distance travelled by photons within tissue, the probability of photon absorption also increases.

Chromophores are responsible for limiting light distribution and penetration into tissues (Anderson, 1981). The most prevalent natural chromophores are melanin, blood (oxyhemoglobin and deoxyhemoglobin), water, and fat (Figure 37.1). Absorption of photons by chromophores stops the path of the photons, but the concentration of photonic energy by chromophores can produce heat aggregation. Conversion of light into heat dictates a significant limitation for higher-power laser therapy devices, especially in equine practice, where black skin is very common.

These factors must be well analyzed and considered in making in the best choice of wavelength for a high-intensity laser. High-intensity laser application must be safe, with the lowest possible skin interaction, but, at the same time, it has to be capable of spreading in deeper targets during its journey.

Monochromatic light at 1064 nm represents an interesting wavelength that is characterized by the least possible absorption of light by the natural chromophores. In a 1998 study of light transmittances *in vivo* through African-American human skin, 1064 nm showed the best performance among the wavelengths most used in the laser therapy market (532, 632, 675, 810, 911, and 1064 nm) (Figure 37.2). "It was observed that the photons

Figure 37.1 Oxyhemoglobin, water, and melanin absorption coefficients at different wavelengths. The most prevalent natural chromophores are melanin (brown dotted line), the blood components oxyhemoglobin (blue dotted line) and deoxyhemoglobin (green line), water (brown line), and fat. Absorption of photons by chromophores stops the path of the photons, but the concentration of photonic energy by chromophores can produce heat aggregation. Monochromatic light at 1064 nm is characterized by the lowest possible absorption of light by the natural chromophores.

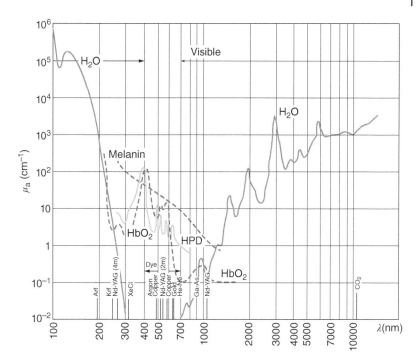

Figure 37.2 Transmittance of light through human skin in an African-American female. Among the wavelengths most used in laser therapy devices (532, 632, 675, 810, 911, and 1064 nm), 1064 nm shows the highest transmittance, which results in the deepest penetration.

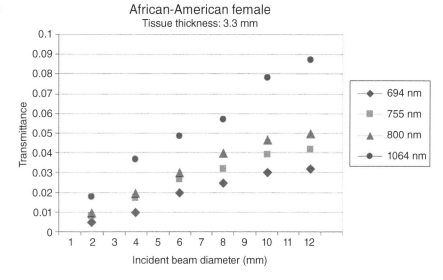

at 1064 nm penetrate deeper than the other colors studied for a given incident beam diameter, and the transmittance at the particular wavelength increases asymptotically with incident beam diameter" (Zhao and Fairchild, 1998). The low sensitivity of 1064 nm light toward the most common chromophores (oxyhemoglobin, water, and melanin) allows this wavelength to penetrate deeper than others that are usable in therapy.

Photochemical Effect

The absorption of photonic energy by the best-known chromophores (melanin, porphyrin groups, water) and by those that are less known (enzymes, cellular membranes) leads to the activation of the oxidative chain, with the mitochondrion as the main actor. The increase in adenosine triphosphate (ATP), RNA, and DNA found in tissues subject to laser irradiation is the basis of this theory (Haas *et al.*, 1994; Karu *et al.*, 1993, 1995, 2001; Manteĭfel' and Karu, 2004; Smolyaninova *et al.*, 1990, 1991). Other tissue effects, such as vasodilation (Claudry *et al.*, 1993), enhanced wound healing (Lyons *et al.*, 1987), and inhibited neuronal activity (Sato *et al.*, 1994; Tsuchiya *et al.*, 1994), have also been reported.

Photothermal Effect

A photothermal effect is the phenomenon produced by the photoexcitation of tissue, resulting in the production of thermal energy (heat). Increasing the cutaneous, intra-articular, and core temperatures of soft tissue is a useful adjunct for the treatment of musculoskeletal and soft-tissue injuries.

Heat, as a therapeutic intervention, decreases pain in joints and muscles, as well as in soft tissues. Most thermotherapies are designed to deliver thermal therapy to a target tissue volume with minimal impact on intervening or surrounding tissues. By increasing the temperature of the skin and soft tissue, the blood flow increases caused by vasodilatation, metabolic rate increases, and tissue extensibility will be made greater. Heat increases oxygen uptake and accelerates tissue healing. It also increases the activity of destructive enzymes such as collagenase and increases the catabolic rate.

Thermoreceptors, special temperature-sensitive nerve endings, are activated by changes in soft-tissue temperature. These receptors initiate nerve signals that block nociception (the pain signal process that results from a noxious stimulus) within the spinal cord (Mezawa *et al.*, 1988).

Topical modalities applied with physical support activate another type of specialized nerve ending called proprioceptors. Proprioceptors detect physical changes in tissue pressure and movement. Proprioceptor activity also inhibits the transmission of nociceptive signals to the brain. The activation of these receptors within the spinal cord reduces muscle tone, relaxes painful muscles, and enhances tissue blood flow (Scott *et al.*, 2004).

Thermal increase of the tissue depends on the quantity of energy delivered per unit volume. Pulsed emitting light, with a very low duty cycle, is the best strategy to pursue. The lower the duty cycle, the lower the thermal stress. High-intensity therapy lasers have a duty cycle in the range of 0.01–0.1%, whereas high-power diode lasers have a duty cycle ≥10%. A low duty cycle allows for long cooling times between pulses, which means the tissue is able to achieve physiological thermal relaxation before the next pulse. The thermal relaxation time is the time necessary for the irradiated tissue to lose 50% of its accumulated heat (Anderson and Parish, 1983).

Photomechanical Effect

Photomechanical effects are induced in tissue by lasers dispensing short-lasting impulses with high peak power. In surgery, photomechanical effects such as photoablation and photofragmentation are used, which require extremely high peak power levels (over 106 W) with an impulse length of nanoseconds. In physiotherapy, impulses of about 3000 W lasting about 100–200 microseconds are used, so they do not produce cytolysis. Nevertheless, impulses of this entity induce pressure waves with a stimulating effect in tissue.

From personal experience with these values in both animals (Fortuna *et al.*, 2001, 2002, 2004, 2005) and humans (Zati *et al.*, 2003, 2004, 2005a, 2005b), the author and his research colleagues have found considerable stimulatory effects on cartilage tissues. We have not been able to obtain the same effects with lower power levels. With the aim of increasing the photomechanical and biostimulatory action of the Nd:YAG laser, impulses with even higher power are under study.

Photomechanical laser–tissue interaction thus results in one of the most important effects of HILT: part of the energy is transferred into mechanical interaction at the tissue and cell level, resulting in a physiological therapeutic stimulus. This mechanical stimulus, appropriately called a "photoacoustic effect," has the ability to stimulate cell metabolism, proliferation, and differentiation (Fortuna and Masotti, 2010).

When a pulsed laser beam impacts a medium, an elastic pressure wave is immediately generated in the medium itself, propagating from the surface into the medium. Wave amplitude is directly related to light intensity, and inversely related to pulse duration time. It also depends on the light properties (wavelength) and the chemical–physical structure of the medium. The relationships between incident laser light and the photomechanical or photoacoustic effect generated in the tissue include: (i) a direct relationship between the intensity of the incident light and the intensity of the transitory mechanical deformation generated in the tissue; and (ii) a direct relationship between the pulse repetition frequency and the pulse duration (Fortuna and Masotti, 2010).

In conclusion, the shape of the acoustic wave is related to the shape of the laser pulse. The intensity of the mechanical effect may also depend on the optical, thermal, and mechanical features of the medium. When the peak pulse, the duty cycle, and the pulse repetition frequency are properly delivered, the photomechanical effect can result in substantial transitory modifications of the extracellular matrix (ECM), which can affect cell behavior.

An intimate connection exists between the ECM and cells, and in the case of cartilage, between the ECM and chondrocytes. Any spatial deformation of the ECM is therefore automatically transferred to the cells, as a mechanical stimulus. This specific absorption by the ECM is responsible for immediate tissue dilatation, followed by contraction, during the cooling phase. Such a transitory spatial deformation of the ECM is automatically transferred to the cells as a mechanical stimulus (Ragan *et al.*, 2000; Yasuda *et al.*, 1996).

The musculoskeletal system, which includes bones, cartilage, skeletal muscles and tendons, and ligaments, responds to mechanical stimulation with changes in metabolism, cytoskeletal organization, rate of proliferation, and state of differentiation during development (Grodzinsky *et al.*, 2000; Hall, 1979; Hunter *et al.*, 2002; Moonsoo *et al.*, 2001; Onodera *et al.*, 2005; Saitoh *et al.*, 2000; Wu *et al.*, 2001).

Fibrocytes, osteoblasts, and chondrocytes also respond to mechanical forces by changing their metabolism, their state of differentiation, and their proliferation, the response depending on the magnitude, frequency, and mode of mechanical stimulation (Elices and Hemle, 1989; Enomoto-Iwamoto *et al.*, 1997; Kumar *et al.*, 2003; Kurtis *et al.*, 2003; Li *et al.*, 2003; Loeser, 2000; Millward-Sadler *et al.*, 2000; Shakibaei *et al.*, 1995; Takahashi *et al.*, 1996).

High-Power Lasers: Continuous and Pulsed

Nd:YAG CW lasers were the first high-power lasers used in laser therapy (Parra *et al.*, 1992). They transmit high quantities of energy at very low light intensity (radiance). Thus, they do not provide an efficient solution. The chopped wave was introduced to improve heat dissipation in CW lasers, but transmittance could not be improved. The pulsed high-intensity Nd:YAG laser changed the scenario by allowing an increased light transmittance without increasing thermal risks.

Many high-power diode lasers are available for PBMT. They are characterized by high average power ($\leq 30\,W$) but very low intensity (kW/cm^2). Big pulses, characterized by high peak power and a high amount of energy per pulse, are useful for transferring high amounts of energy in accordance with the Beer–Lambert–Bouguer law. Increase of tissue temperature is directly correlated to the amount of energy supplied. Thus, the use of high-intensity (and especially Q-switched) lasers becomes indicated. High energy delivered according to this law is safe and allows for a sudden dramatic dilation of the energy throughout the tissue when the light is on, followed by a cooling beat when the light is off, which creates a photo-mechanical effect (Fortuna and Masotti, 2010).

Conclusion

The concept of HILT is actually quite simple: it involves high-power bursts of energy that are quickly pulsed deep into tissues. These short, high-power pulses produce photo-chemical and photomechanical effects in the tissues, while minimizing photothermal effects. This combination of laser–tissue interaction and effect can be especially useful when treating the larger and deeper tissue masses of horses. An interesting consideration that follows the successful use of HILT in horses is the potential indication for HILT use in larger food animals and zoological patients.

HILT should always be used in combination with a comprehensive injury rehabilitation protocol designed to achieve the most efficient return of musculoskeletal function. The addition of HILT can be important in recovery of tissue elasticity and strength, and in avoiding catastrophic relapses.

The inclusion and application of HILT should always be based on the recommendations of the device manufacturer. In general, HILT will be used daily during the first 1–2 weeks of rehabilitation in order to reduce inflammation, then every other day for 3–4 weeks to stimulate tissue remodeling and healing.

Each patient is different, and each injury is different. The individual HILT and rehabilitation program needs to be tailored to the patient's injury and monitored and adjusted as the injury responds to therapy.

References

Abergel, R. *et al.* (1987) Biostimulation of wound healing by lasers: experimental approaches in animal models and fibroblast cultures. *J Dermatol Surg Oncol.* **13**(2):127–133.

Anderson, R.R. (1981) The optics of human skin. *J Invest Dermatol.* **77**(1):13–19.

Anderson R.R. and Parish J.A. (1983) Selective photothermolysis: precise microsurgery by selective absorption of pulsed radiation. *Science.* **220**(4596):524–527.

Barrett, S.F. and Pack, D.J. (2006) Timing subsystem. In: *Microcontrollers Fundamentals for Engineers and Scientists*, pp. 51–64. Morgan and Claypool, San Rafael, CA.

Braverman, B. *et al.* (1989) Effects of helium-neon and infrared laser irradiation on wound healing in rabbits. *Laser Surg Med.* **9**(1):50–58.

Claudry, H. *et al.* (1993) Relaxation of vascular smooth muscle induced by low-power laser radiation. *Photochem Photobiol.* **58**(5):661–669.

Elices, M.J. and Hemle, M.E. (1989) The human integrin VLA-2 is a collagen receptor on some cells and a collagen/laminin receptor on others. *Proc Natl Acad Sci USA.* **86**(24):9906–9910.

Enomoto-Iwamoto, M. *et al.* (1997) Involvement of alpha 5 beta 1 integrin in matrix interactions and proliferation of chondrocytes. *J Bone Miner Res.* **12**(7):1124–1132.

Fortuna, D. *et al.* (2001) Nd:YAG laser in experimentally induced chronic degenerative osteoarthritis in chicken boiler, pilot study. *Proceedings of the 16th International Congress of Laser Medicine.* Firenze.

Fortuna, D. *et al.* (2002) Low level laser therapy (LLLT) ed efficacia clinica: studi in doppio cieco randomizzato a confronto. *Medicina dello Sport Min ed.* **55**:1–8.

Fortuna D. *et al.* (2004) High intensity laser therapy in transcutaneus treatment of cartilagineous lesions: experimental study. *Proceedings of the 5th Symposium of the International Cartilage Repair* Society – ICRS. Ghent.

Fortuna, D. (2005) High intensity laser therapy in the treatment of deep osteo-chondral defect. Pilot study in an animal model. *Osteoarthritis Cartilage.* **13**(Suppl. 1): S86–S87.

Fortuna, D. and Masotti, L. (2010) The HILT domain by the pulse intensity fluence (pif) formula. *Energy for Health.* **2010**(05):12–19.

Früngel, F.B.A. (1965) *Optical Pulses – Lasers – Measuring Techniques.* Academic Press, New York.

Grodzinsky, A.J. *et al.* (2000) Cartilage tissue remodeling in response to mechanical forces. *Annu Rev Biomed Eng.* **2**:691–713.

Haas, A.F. *et al.* (1994) Low energy helium-neon laser irradiation increase the motility of cultured human keratinocytes. *J Invest Dermatol.* **94**(6):822–826.

Hall, B.K. (1979) Selective proliferation and accumulation of chondroprogenitor cells as the mode of action of biomechanical factors during secondary chondrogenesis. *Teratology.* **20**(1):81–91.

Honmura, A. *et al.* (1992) Therapeutic effect of Ga-Al-As diode laser irradiation on experimentally induced inflammation in rats. *Lasers Surg Med.* **12**(4):441–449.

Hunter, C.J. *et al.* (2002) Mechanical compression alters expression and extracellular matrix synthesis by chondrocytes cultured in collagen I gels. *Biomaterials.* **23**(4):1249–1259.

IUPAC. (1997) *Compendium of Chemical Terminology*, 2 edn. (the "Gold Book"). Blackwell Scientific Publications, Oxford. Available from: http://goldbook.iupac.org/B00626.html (accessed November 30, 2016).

Jimbo, K. *et al.* (1998) Suppressive effects of low power laser irradiation on bradikinin evoked action potentials in cultured murine dorsal root ganglion cells. *Neurosci Lett.* **240**(2):93–96.

Karu, T. *et al.* (1993) Changes in oxidative metabolism of murine spleen following laser and superluminous diode (660–950 nm) irradiation: effects of cellular composition and radiation parameters. *Laser Surg Med.* **13**(4):453–462.

Karu, T. *et al.* (1995) Irradiation with He-Ne laser increases ATP level in cells cultivated in vitro. *J Photochem Photobiol B.* **27**(3):219–223.

Karu, T. *et al.* (2001) Cells attachment modulation by radiation from pulsed light diode (lambda 820) and various chemical. *Laser Surg Med.* **28**(3):227–236.

Kumar, V. *et al.* (2002) *Robbins Basic Pathology*, 7 edn., pp. 68–69. Elsevier, Amsterdam.

Kurtis, M. *et al.* (2003) Integrin-mediated adhesion of human articular chondrocytes to cartilage. *Arthritis Rheum.* **48**(1):110–118.

Li, K.W. *et al.* (2003) Microenvironment regulation of extracellular signal-regulated kinase activity in chondrocytes. *Arthritis Rheum.* **48**(3):689–699.

Loeser, R.F. (2000) Chondrocyte integrin expression and function. *Biorheology.* **37**(1–2):109–116.

Lyons, R.F. *et al.* (1987) Biostimulation of wounds healing in vivo by helium-neon laser. *Ann Plast Surg.* **18**(1):47–50.

Manteïfel', V.M. and Karu, T.I. (2004) [Increase in the number of contacts of endoplasmic reticulum with mitochondria and plasma membrane in yeast cells stimulated to division with He-Ne laser light.] *Tsitologia.* **46**(6):498–505.

McDonagh, L. and Wallenstein, R. (2007) Optimized pumping of neodymium-doped vanadate yields high-power lasers. *SPIE Newsroom.* doi:10.1117/2.1200707.0708.

Mezawa, S. *et al.* (1988) The possible analgesic effect of soft laser irradiation on heat nociceptors in the cat tongue. *Arch Oral Biol.* **33**(9):693–694.

Millward-Sadler, S.J. *et al.* (2000) Mechanotransduction via integrins and interleukin-4 results in altered aggrecan and matrix metalloproteinase 3 gene expression in normal, but not osteoarthritic, human articular chondrocytes. *Arthritis Rheum.* **43**(9):2091–2099.

Moonsoo, J. *et al.* (2001) Tissue shear deformation stimulates proteoglycan and protein biosynthesis in bovine cartilage explants. *Arch Biochem Biophys.* **395**(1):41–48.

Onodera, K. *et al.* (2005) Stepwise mechanical stretching inhibits chondrogenesis through cell-matrix adhesion mediated by integrins in embryonic rat limb-bud mesenchymal cells. *Eur J Cell Biol.* **84**(1):45–58.

Palmer, K.F. and Williams, D. (1974) Optical properties of water in the near infrared. *J Opt Soc Am.* **64**(8):1107–1110.

Parra, P.F. *et al.* (1992) Il Neodimio YAG defocalizzato nella sua evoluzione per un trattamento sempre più efficace dell'atleta infortunato. *Laser & Technology.* **2**(1):13–16.

Paschotta, R. (2006) Q-switched lasers: YAG versus Vanadate. Available from: https://www.rp-photonics.com/spotlight_2006_09_16.html (accessed November 30, 2016).

Ragan, P.M. (2000) Chondrocyte extracellular matrix synthesis and turnover are influenced by static compression in a new alginate disk culture system. *Arch Biochem Biophys.* **383**(2):256–264.

Saitoh, S. *et al.* (2000) Compressive force promotes chondrogenic differentiation and hypertrophy in midpalatal suture cartilage in growing rats. *Anat Rec.* **260**(4):392–401.

Sato, T. *et al.* (1994) Ga-Al-As laser irradiation inhibits neuronal activity associated with inflammation. *Acupunct Electrother Res.* **19**(2–3):141–151.

Scott, F. *et al.* (2004) The physiologic basis and clinical applications of cryotherapy and thermotherapy for the pain practitioner. *Pain Physician.* 7(3):395–399.

Shakibaei, M. *et al.* (1995) Changes in integrin expression during chondrogenesis in vitro: an immunomorphological study. *J Histochem Cytochem.* **43**(10):1061–1069.

Smith, A.M. *et al.* (2009) Bioimaging: second window for in vivo imaging. *Nat Nanotechnol.* **4**(11):710–711.

Smolyaninova, N.K. *et al.* (1990) Activation of synthesis of RNA in lymphocytes following irradiation by a He-Ne laser. *Radiobiologiia.* **30**(3):424–426.

Smolyaninova, N.K. *et al.* (1991) Effects of He-Ne laser irradiation on chromatin properties and synthesis of nucleic acids in human peripheral blood lymphocytes. *Biomed Sci.* **2**(2):121–126.

Takahashi, I. *et al.* (1996) Effects of expansive force on the differentiation of midpalatal suture cartilage in rats. *Bone.* **18**(4):341–348.

Tsuchiya, K. *et al.* (1994) Laser irradiation abates neuronal responses to nociceptive stimulation of rat-paw skin. *Brain Res Bull.* **34**(4):369–374.

Walsh, J.T. (2011) Basic interactions of light with tissue. In: *Optical-Thermal Response of Laser-Irradiated Tissue*, 2 edn., p. 13. Springer, New York.

Wu, Q. *et al.* (2001) Indian hedgehog is an essential component of mechanotransduction complex to stimulate chondrocyte proliferation. *J Biol Chem.* **276**(38):35290–35296.

Yasuda, T. *et al.* (1996) Possible involvement of RGD (Arg-Gly-Asp)-containing extracellular matrix proteins in rat growth plate chondrocyte differentiation in culture. *J Bone Miner Res.* **11**(10):1430–1437.

Zati, A. *et al.* (2003) Nuove prospettive fisiochinesiterapiche nel trattamento delle lesioni cartilaginee. *2° Congresso Nazionale GIRC.* Bologna.

Zati, A. *et al.* (2004) Trattamento della lombalgia causata da ernia del disco; confronto tra laser ad alta potenza, TENS e FANS. *Med Sport.* **57**(1):77–82.

Zati, A. *et al.* (2005a) Azione del laser Nd:YAG sulle lesioni cartilaginee: studio sperimentale sull'animale e studio clinico sull'uomo. Atti 33. *Congresso SIMFER.* Catania.

Zati, A. *et al.* (2005b) L'azione del laser di potenza HILT sulle lesioni cartilaginee articolari. Studio clinico e sperimentale a confronto. *Atti Ricerca Traslazionale.* Istituti Ortopedici Rizzoli, Bologna.

Zhao, Z.Q. and Fairchild, P.W. (1988) Dependance of light trasmission throug human skin on incident beam diameter at different wavelengths. *Proceedings of the SPIE 3254, Laser–Tissue Interaction IX.*

Part IX

Clinical Applications of Laser Therapy in Food Animal Practice

38

Laser Therapy in Food-Animal Practice

Julie Gard

Department of Clinical Sciences, Auburn University College of Veterinary Medicine, Auburn, AL, USA

Introduction

Food-animal medicine in the past has relied heavily on antibiotics and anti-inflammatories as aids in the prevention of infection of wounds, to decrease wound healing times, and for pain relief. However, as stated by the US Food and Drug Administration (FDA) in its document, "The Judicious Use of Medically Important Antimicrobial Drugs in Food-Producing Animals," antimicrobial resistance, and the resulting failure of antimicrobial therapies in humans, is a mounting public health problem of global significance (FDA, 2012). This phenomenon is driven by many factors, including the use of antimicrobial drugs in both humans and animals (FDA, 2012). Fear over the loss of effectiveness of drugs, especially those useful against bacteria, prompted the production of the FDA's document and the implementation of stricter regulations governing the utilization of all drugs in food-producing animals.

The FDA, along with the US Centers for Disease Control and Prevention (CDC) and the American Veterinary Medical Association (AVMA), has taken steps to help implement the judicious use of antimicrobials in humans and all animals (CDC, 2016). Proposed legislation currently before the United States Congress, the Preservation of Antibiotics for Medical Treatment Act, supports the elimination of the "non-therapeutic" use of antibiotic drugs considered important for human health in order to preserve their effectiveness and decrease the potential for development of antibiotic-resistant bacteria (House Rept. 1552). Additionally, the World Health Organization (WHO) completed a report in 2011 looking at antibiotic resistance in Europe from a food-safety perspective, which emphasized the need for prudent use of antimicrobials (WHO, 2011). A strain of completely resistant *Escherichia coli* was identified in June of 2016 at a slaughterhouse in Iowa (Washington Post, 2016).

The focus of these reports and this emphasis has been primarily on feeding antimicrobials and on parenteral administration of specific antibiotics known to stimulate bacterial-resistance genes, but the use of additional drug classes is a growing concern as well. Therefore, there is significant pressure to develop new alternative therapeutic applications that do not promote antimicrobial resistance or result in withdrawal times in food-producing animals.

Consumers are looking for products where no drugs, hormones, or antibiotics have been used in their production. This push has been manifested in the popularity of organically produced food. Laser therapy, now commonly called photobiomodulation therapy (PBMT), is an alternative therapy that can aid in healing and pain relief without consequential drug withdrawal. PBMT has been utilized in human and companion animal medicine for years to reduce pain caused by various conditions from traumatic injuries to chronic conditions such as arthritis. There have been multiple studies confirming its positive effects on the reduction and control of pain in humans and animals (Boerner *et al.*, 1996; Bjordal *et al.*, 2006; Cotler *et al.*, 2015; Moore and Calderhead, 1991; Sattayut and Bradley, 2012). Additionally, consumers are demanding changes in food-animal farming practices that focus on animal welfare. Therapies that promote healing and reduce pain do promote animal well-being, so PBMT is a practice that fits this category.

Laser therapy has historically been well received by owners of companion animals, but its use in food animals has been minimal. However, owners of food animals that are of higher value genetically, are organically produced, or are used as bucking stock are more open to PBMT. Utilization within the commercial animal sector will increase as familiarity with the equipment grows and consistent clinical results are clearly shown. The utilization of PBMT in food animals has lagged behind that in companion animals, but it is starting to be seen, especially in cattle, swine, camelids, sheep, and goats.

General Applications of PBMT in Food-Animal Medicine

The general applications of PBMT are similar to those in other species. Since there is a similarity in most conditions, it is easy to extrapolate the multitude of benefits seen in the equine species to cattle, swine, camelids, sheep, and goats. These applications include acute inflammatory conditions such as mastitis, post-operative edema, traumatic injuries, and chronic painful conditions such as osteoarthritis.

Traumatic injuries occur in all species and often necessitate cleansing, immediate surgical closure, or monitored second-intention healing. The standard of care includes antibiotic therapy, pain management, cleansing, debriding, and bandaging. Hydrotherapy, osmotic soaks, and poultices, along with systemic anti-inflammatory drug administration, are routinely instituted to manage edema within or surrounding a wound. PBMT has been shown in numerous case and clinical studies to decrease healing times by elevating blood flow to the injured site, increasing lymphatic drainage, and stimulating fibroblast migration into the site (Kuffler, 2016; Márquez Martínez *et al.*, 2008). Often, PBMT is utilized as an adjunctive therapy to promote healing of wounds. The blood supply to a wound is increased when PBMT is applied (Maegawa *et al.*, 2000). Increasing the blood supply and oxygenation is imperative to increasing wound healing and preventing secondary bacterial growth from bacteria such as *Clostridia* spp. that proliferate in an anaerobic environment. Cattle, sheep, goats, and horses are very predisposed to *Clostridia* diseases, so improving the circulation of traumatized tissue is preventative as well as therapeutic.

In cases of mastitis, such as with *E. coli*, endotoxins are released, causing severe inflammatory reactions and vasoconstriction. Mastitis is also an extremely painful condition. Dairy cows and dairy goats are the most predisposed to *E. coli* mastitis. Utilization of PBMT is quite beneficial in cases of mastitis, especially early in the course of the disease, as it minimizes the inflammatory reaction and increases the blood supply. Wang *et al.* (2014) investigated the effects of laser therapy on a rat model of lipopolysaccharide-induced mastitis and its underlying molecular mechanisms. They demonstrated that the number of polymorphonuclear cells in the mammary alveolus and the myeloperoxidase activity were decreased after laser therapy. These results suggest that laser therapy is beneficial in decreasing somatic cell count and improving milk nutritional quality in cows with an intramammary infection. PBMT has the added benefit, in food-animal patients, of having no withdrawal time.

Application Techniques Unique to Food-Animal Species

Food animals pose additional challenges beyond those encountered when treating companion animals with PBMT. Domesticated cattle, sheep, goats, and swine often do not mind human touch, and usually do not resist the contact of the therapy laser handpiece. However, food animals require different levels of restraint, even though they are domesticated. Beef cattle, especially bucking stock, are not as easy to handle as dairy cattle. Sedation may be necessary if an animal is extremely fractious, as is seen with bucking stock or in wildlife such as deer. Sedation may also be necessary if the animal is extremely sensitive around the area being treated, such as a post-operative area or an area such as the foot, which poses a hazard to the operator. Initiate laser therapy utilizing a non-contact technique to acclimate the patient to the sensation of the laser. Follow up with hand contact, and finally treat using an on-contact technique with the laser handpiece touching the skin.

Each food-animal species has unique considerations when applying PBMT. The presence of any organic debris, the thickness and color of the hair coat or wool, and the color and thickness of the skin and underlying tissues all need to be taken into account when determining the dosage to be administered, the power required for penetration, the administration technique, and the frequency of treatments. Cleaning of all organic debris within the area requiring treatment, even the lanolin in sheep's wool, is a stringent requirement before successful administration of PBMT.

The thickness of cattle hide can be problematic. Administration at a higher power level, utilizing longer treatment times, and treating more frequently is often necessary to achieve penetration to the target cells in cattle. The teat skin is an exception to this statement, and is much thinner than the rest of the hide, so it will require a lower power setting and a shorter treatment time. In sheep, the wool, and in goats, the hair can be problematic, and shaving may be necessary unless there is an objection from the client because it is a show animal. In short, there are unique conditions present in all species of food animal that require common sense and good judgment to ensure consistent clinical results.

Dosing

In the food-animal field, there is quite a variety of body types, body colors, hair coat lengths (e.g., sheep versus pigs), and hair coat colors. The goal of PBMT is to administer a safe dose to the skin, sufficient to penetrate through all of the unique anatomical structures of the patient that cause a loss of irradiance and produce a physiological response within the target tissues.

There is wide range of individual characteristics to consider. Examples are the umbilicus of the newborn lamb versus the lumbosacral spine of a 275 kg Duroc boar, post-umbilical herniation in a piglet versus spondylosis in a Holstein bull, and a laceration on the shoulder of an alpaca versus a laceration on the shoulder of an Angus bull. There are no scientific evidence-based research papers identifying specific dosages for any of the food-animal species. The mantra for the application of PBMT in any of the food animals is "dose to effect." The dosages recommended in Table 38.1 are based on a collection of anecdotal clinical cases and cross-species extrapolation. They are a general guide from which estimates of an appropriate dosage can be made on a case-by-case basis.

Table 38.1 Dosages for PBMT of food animals, by species. These dosages are a general guide from which estimates of an appropriate dosage can be made on a case-by-case basis. Re-evaluate before each therapy laser session and apply an appropriate dosage within the suggested ranges. If clinical improvement is not seen within three sessions, increase the dosage. Clipping of the hair coat greatly decreases the required dosage.

Species	Patient	Weight (lb)	Weight (kg)	Skin hair coat color	Dose (J/cm2) Superficial	Deep
Bovine (beef)	Adult	1200–1500	545–680	Black	10–15	15–25
				Light	8–10	12–20
	Yearling	450–650	205–295	Black	8–12	12–20
				Light	8–10	10–15
	Calf	60–75	27–34	Black	6–8	8–12
				Light	4–8	6–10
Bovine (dairy)	Adult	1200–1650	545–748	Black	12–20	20–23
				Light	10–15	15–25
	Yearling	400–800	181–362	Black	8–15	20–25
				Light	8–12	12–20
	Calf	60–85	27–39	Black	6–10	10–15
				Light	6–8	8–12
Camelid (llama)	Adult	250–450	113–205	Black/dark	8–10	10–12
				Light	6–8	8–10
	Cria	20–30	9–14	Black/dark	4–6	6–8
				Light	2–4	4–6
Camelid (alpaca)	Adult	110–190	50–86	Black/dark	6–8	8–12
				Light	4–6	6–10
	Cria	18–20	8–9	All	2–4	4–8
Caprine	Adult doe	140–170	63–77	Black/dark	6–8	8–12
				Light	4–6	6–8
	Adult buck	170–190	77–86	Black/dark	8–10	10–12
				Light	6–8	8–10
	Kid	4–120	2–54	Black/dark	2–8	4–10
				Light	2–4	4–6
Ovine	Adult	160–220	73–100	All	8–10	10–15
	Lamb	90	90	All	6–8	8–10
	Birth lamb	5–80	2–36	All	2–4	4–6
Porcine	Adult	280–500	127–227	All	8–10	10–20
	Shoat	20–120	9–54	All	4–6	6–8
	Pig	1–20	0.5–9.0	All	2–4	4–6

Some general dosing guidelines are applicable in almost all food-animal species. Increase the suggested dosage when:

- The animal has black pigmented skin and the hair coat cannot be clipped (e.g., black Angus show stock).
- Treating any of the bovine breeds with very thick skin. Thicker skin requires more energy to be administered so that an effective amount can reach the target tissues and produce a clinical response.
- Applying laser therapy to any of the ovine species that are not shorn. There is a great deal of energy lost within the thick, dense layer of wool, even with a baby lamb. Lanolin is also present, which will absorb a portion of the administered photons.
- There is an excessive amount of edema and swelling, as with mastitis and postpartum edema.
- The target cells are beneath thick layers of either adipose or muscle tissues.
- Applying laser therapy to areas where excessive granulation tissue has already formed.

Decrease the suggested dosage when:

- Treatment is applied directly over the bed of an open wound.
- Treating very young stock.

Numerous therapy lasers on the market are pre-programmed with software containing preset protocols for many different maladies in different species. Often, similar anatomical areas and circumstances exist between the equine or companion-animal protocol and that of food animals.

Most wound protocols are based on the area of the wound, and their application is therefore almost universal across species. Postoperative application of PBMT to surgical incisions is similar regardless of species. The use of pre-programmed software protocols for wounds and postoperative treatment of incisions can provide an initial dosage recommendation; adjustments can then be made during each subsequent re-evaluation.

Treatment of acute musculoskeletal injuries such as torn tendons and ligaments and of chronic conditions such as osteoarthritis and back pain in both bucking and breeding stock is highly beneficial. The equine or companion-animal software protocols for similar anatomical areas are a good place to start. Preset protocols for osteoarthritis in horses are very similar to those required for cattle, though an increase is usually warranted due to the thicker skin (increase the total dosage 25%). The equine preset protocols for the lumbosacral spine can be used for the treatment of both acute and chronic back pain in bucking stock and aged bovine breeding stock. Preset protocols for tendonitis and other soft-tissue injuries are comparable between species. Laminitis is not just a problem in the equine species, and since it is seen in the bovine, ovine, caprine, and porcine species, preset protocols for equine laminitis can be used here, too.

Conditions Responsive to PBMT in Food Animals

There are a number of acute conditions, such as mastitis, udder edema, traumatic injuries, foot rot, lacerations, and postoperative edema, as well as chronic conditions, such as osteoarthritis in stifle and fetlock joints, that benefit from PBMT.

Foot Conditions

Acute and chronic laminitis occurs not only in horses but also in cattle, sheep, goats, and pigs. Laser therapy can be applied as an adjunctive treatment in all of these cases. The laser beam should be directed at the coronary band around the foot, at the bulbs of the heel, and at the medial portion of the coronary band in the interdigital space for cattle, sheep, goats, and pigs.

A similar method is applied for the treatment of foot rot in cattle, except that the treatment area should include the entire pastern and the fetlock, and should continue more proximal if swelling has progressed to that level. Utilizing PBMT for cases of soft soles or abscess on the solar surface of the foot can be beneficial. Abscesses can be treated off-contact with a similar technique to that used for a wound in the equine species.

Mastitis and Udder Edema

Mastitis and udder edema are two inter-related conditions for which PBMT has been demonstrated to be efficacious (Wang *et al.*, 2014). In food animals, PBMT is used to treat mastitis and udder edema most commonly in dairy cattle and dairy goats.

Mastitis is an incredibly painful condition of the udder. The severity and frequency of mastitis in companion animals are quite low in comparison to those in dairy animals. Frequent milking or stripping of the udder is important in the treatment of this condition. PBMT can be utilized to reduce the pain, increase the blood supply and lymphatic drainage, and reduce the edema. This allows a more complete, less painful milking and stripping of the udder.

Most veterinary-specific therapy lasers with software protocols have a setting for "edema and swelling" that can be used on an udder with mastitis and edema. However, the udder can be quite large, so often the quarters will be treated separately. Additionally, the udder needs to be treated frequently: at least twice daily until the mastitis resolves. The ideal approach is to administer a portion of the PBMT dose immediately before milking, and the remainder after the quarter is completely empty. The liquid milk, before it is extracted from the quarter, is yet another layer of density that is photoabsorbing. When milk is present, it absorbs photons, and fewer reach the target tissue (mammary alveoli).

Administration of PBMT concurrently with massage is beneficial for the stimulation of milk let down, which is often inhibited by the pain associated with mastitis. Some laser therapy equipment emits its energy through optics contained within a rolling massage-ball handpiece. This is an ideal application handpiece for mastitis, since it combines the delivery of photonic energy with massage. If there are areas where hard, turgid, edematous tissue is present, these need to be treated at a higher dosage, administered at a higher power, more frequently, and for longer periods. Further research is warranted to determine whether PBMT administered to these tissues, using this massage technique, stimulates a release of oxytocin, further improving milk let down.

Dosages that are administered to the udder are governed by the color of the skin (black versus white), the hair coat length (long versus short or clipped), and the mass and density of the tissue. An udder with both black skin and hair will require a higher dosage, since the pigment is an incidental absorber of photons and will prevent some of the energy from penetrating to the target tissue. Immediately post partum, when the udder is usually very edematous, a higher dosage is also needed. Dosages for patients with shorter hair, lighter skin and hair color, and less dense udders should start at $12\,J/cm^2$. Dosages for patients with longer hair, dark skin or hair, or dense mammary tissue can be as high as $20\,J/cm^2$.

Reproductive Applications

The use of PBMT to increase fertility has not been thoroughly explored. However, anything that can be done to minimize lameness will increase fertility. It has been shown that lameness has a negative effect on conception rates (Bicalho *et al.*, 2007). Utilizing PBMT on the vulvar lips post partum to decrease swelling and/or on any lacerations of the vulvar lips would be beneficial. Metritis, vaginal or cervical prolapse, and post-castration edema are additional conditions that benefit from PBMT. Additional case studies and clinical research need to be performed with food animals to scientifically evaluate the benefits of PBMT in this area.

Swelling and Edema

Cattle, like horses, develop a significant amount of ventral edema, especially following wounds or suture lines located on the ventrum of the body. Livestock spend a great deal of time standing, adding to the amount of edema. Preputial lacerations in bulls are good examples of wounds that result in a collection of severe ventral edema surrounding them. Traditionally, hydrotherapy is often employed twice daily to help manage this swelling and edema. PBMT, in addition to the hydrotherapy, accelerates the reduction of swelling and edema. Fresh wounds on the prepuce should be treated off-contact, administering a dosage of $5–10\,J/cm^2$ twice daily, if possible, followed by $10–12\,J/cm^2$ on-contact to the surrounding margins of the laceration, to prevent or help relieve the accumulation of ventral edema. When the patient can tolerate on-contact therapy directly over the laceration, this administration technique should be used throughout the entire area of the wound and surrounding tissues. The benefits of administering PBMT to these types of lesion are vasodilation and an increase in the blood supply, increased lymphatic drainage, and relief of pain. Administer therapy for this type of edema and swelling twice a day for 3–4 days and then once a day until resolution.

Conclusion

PBMT is a primary or adjunctive therapy that can provide acceleration of wound healing and significant pain relief in all of the food-animal species. Additionally, utilization of PBMT does not require withdrawal times, because there is no drug residue within the tissues. This is extremely beneficial in the organic food-production industry, where the use of any drugs is strictly prohibited.

Utilization of PBMT will continue to grow in the food-animal industry as veterinarians, producers, and owners realize the multiple benefits this modality can provide.

References

Bicalho, R.C. *et al.* (2007) Visual locomotion scoring in the first seventy days in milk: Impact on pregnancy and survival. *J Dairy Sci.* **90**(10):4586–4591.

Boerner, E. *et al.* (1996) Double-blind study on the efficacy of the laser therapy. *Proc of SPIE.* **2929**:75–79.

Bjordal, J.M. *et al.* (2006) Low-level laser therapy in acute pain: a systematic review of mechanisms of action and clinical effects in randomized placebo-controlled trials. *Photomed Laser Surg.* **24**(2):158–168.

CDC. (2016) Antibiotic/Antimicrobial Resistance. Available from: https://www.cdc.gov/drugresistance/(accessed November 30, 2016).

Cotler, H.B. *et al.* (2015) The use of low level laser therapy (LLLT) for musculoskeletal pain. *MOJ Orthop Rheumatol.* **2**(5):pii:00068.

FDA (2012) Guidance for Industry: The Judicious Use of Medically Important Antimicrobial Drugs in Food-Producing Animals. Available from: http://www.fda.gov/downloads/AnimalVeterinary/GuidanceComplianceEnforcement/GuidanceforIndustry/UCM216936.pdf (accessed November 30, 2016).

House Rept. 1552. Preservation of Antibiotics for Medical Treatment Act of 2015. 114th Congress (2015–2016).

Library of Congress. Available from: https://www.congress.gov/bill/114th-congress/house-bill/1552 (accessed November 30, 2016).

Kuffler, D.P. (2016) Photobiomodulation in promoting wound healing: a review. *Regen Med.* **11**(1):107–122.

Maegawa, Y. *et al.* (2000) Effects of near-infrared low-level laser irradiation on microcirculation. *Lasers Surg Med.* **27**(5):427–437.

Márquez Martínez, M.E. *et al.* (2008). Effect of IR laser photobiomodulation on the repair of bone defects grafted with organic bovine bone. *Lasers Med Sci.* **23**(3):313–317.

Moore, K. and Calderhead, R.G. (1991) The clinical application of low incident power density 830 nm gallium aluminum arsenide diode laser radiation in the therapy of chronic intractable pain. *Int J OptoElectronics.* **6**(5):503–520.

Sattayut, S. and Bradley, P (2012) A study of the influence of low intensity laser therapy on painful temporomandibular disorder patients. *Laser Ther.* **21**(3):183–192.

Wang, Y. *et al.* (2014) Low-level laser therapy attenuates LPS-induced rats mastitis by inhibiting polymorphonuclear neutrophil adhesion. *J Vet Med Sci.* **76**(11):1443–1450.

Washington Post. (2016) Updated: Superbug found in Illinois and South Carolina. June 15. Available from: https://www.washingtonpost.com/news/to-your-health/wp/2016/06/14/superbug-found-in-second-pig-sample-in-u-s/(accessed November 30, 2016).

WHO. (2011) Tackling Antibiotic Resistance from a Food Safety Perspective in Europe. Available from: http://www.euro.who.int/en/publications/abstracts/tackling-antibiotic-resistance-from-a-food-safety-perspective-in-europe (accessed November 30, 2016).

Part X

Laser Therapy and Alternative and Regenerative Therapies

39

Laser Therapy and Acupuncture

Carolina Medina

Coral Springs Animal Hospital, Coral Springs, FL, USA

Acupuncture

Definition

Acupuncture is the insertion of fine, sterile needles into designated acupuncture points. These acupuncture points have been mapped out in several animal species and correspond to specific anatomical locations. There are about 400 acupuncture points in most animals. When acupuncture points are stimulated, physiologic responses occur. These physiologic responses are caused by the stimulation of both the central and the peripheral nervous systems.

Mechanisms of Action

Acupuncture stimulation releases endogenous substances such as beta-endorphins, dynorphins, enkephalins, serotonin, epinephrine, gamma aminobutyric acid, cortisol, and various hormones. The earliest scientific studies done on acupuncture stimulation focused on its analgesic effects. Endogenous opioid peptides were first discovered by Hughes (1975). Along the same time line, researchers discovered that acupuncture stimulation leads to an increased concentration of endogenous opioids in the serum and cerebrospinal fluid (CSF). One study showed that acupuncture increased endogenous opioids in the serum of human patients with soft-tissue pain, acute appendicitis, and peri-arthritis (Xi and Li, 1983). Another study revealed that acupuncture stimulation induced an increase in endogenous opioid concentration in CSF drained from the cerebroventricle in human patients suffering from brain tumors (Zhang *et al.*, 1980). Naloxone, an opioid antagonist, blocks the effects of acupuncture and decreases the pain threshold in acupuncture subjects (Mayer *et al.*, 1977). These were the first studies showing that endogenous opioids played a role in the mechanism of action of acupuncture analgesia.

Most acupuncture points are located in areas of low electrical resistance and high electrical conductance (Brown *et al.*, 1974; Reichmanis *et al.*, 1975; Urano and Ogasawara, 1978). Histological studies revealed that acupuncture points are located in areas where there are free nerve endings, arterioles, lymphatic vessels, and aggregation of mast cells (Pan *et al.*, 1986). Because of their anatomical location, stimulation of acupuncture points can lead to a variety of local effects, including an increase in local blood flow and circulation; release of Hageman's Factor XII, which activates the clotting cascade and complement cascade and causes a release of plasminogens and kinins; degranulation of mast cells, which releases histamine, heparin, and proteases; release of bradykinin, which leads to vasodilation; and production of local prostaglandins, which leads to smooth-muscle relaxation (Kendall, 1989a; Omura, 1975). The vasoactive effects that occur with acupuncture stimulation follow a specific sequence: first, there is a short vasoconstriction phase (lasting 15–30 seconds), then a quasi-control state (lasting 10 seconds to 2 minutes), and finally there is a vasodilation phase (lasting 2 minutes to 2 weeks) (Smith, 1994). This results in an enhanced local tissue immune status, improved local tissue perfusion, and muscle and tissue relaxation. Thus, pain relief occurs as a result of improved perfusion and muscle spasm relief caused by the local effects of acupuncture stimulation and somatovisceral reflexes (Kendall, 1989b).

Methods of Acupuncture Point Stimulation

There are nine techniques for the stimulation of acupuncture points. Dry needle and electro-acupuncture are the most common.

- **Dry needle:** The insertion of acupuncture needles into acupuncture points. These needles are typically left in place for approximately 20 minutes.
- **Electro-acupuncture:** The connection of electrical leads to dry needles and an electro-acupuncture unit. The unit can be set to a variety of frequencies; each stimulates a different pathway in the nervous system.

Laser Therapy in Veterinary Medicine: Photobiomodulation, First Edition. Edited by Ronald J. Riegel and John C. Godbold, Jr.
© 2017 John Wiley & Sons, Inc. Published 2017 by John Wiley & Sons, Inc.

Low frequency (1–20 Hz) predominantly stimulates A-delta fibers and releases beta-endorphins, meten-kephalins, and orphanins. High frequency (80–100 Hz) primarily stimulates C fibers which releases dynor-phins, and serotonergic fibers which releases seroto-nin and norepinephrine (Fry *et al.*, 2014; Melzack and Wall, 1965).

- **Acupressure:** The application of firm digital pressure to an acupuncture point for a specific length of time (e.g., 5 minutes).
- **Aqua-acupuncture:** The injection of a sterile liquid (e.g., saline, vitamin B12, lidocaine) into an acupuncture point. This causes constant stimulation of the point for an extended period (until the liquid is absorbed). It has the added benefit of imparting the medicinal properties of the liquid used.
- **Moxibustion:** The use of a Chinese herb called *Artemesia vulgaris* that is rolled into a cigar and burned just above the acupuncture point, without touching the skin. This is a warming technique that is therapeutic for older patients with chronic pain.
- **Gold implantation:** The injection of sterile pieces of gold, whether in a bead or wire form, into acupuncture points for permanent implantation. Gold implantation provides long-term stimulation in chronic conditions.
- **Pneumo-acupuncture:** The injection of air under the skin in the subcutaneous space to produce pressure and stimulate the acupuncture points, nerves, and muscles. Pneumo-acupuncture is used solely for muscle atrophy.
- **Hemo-acupuncture:** The insertion of a hypodermic needle into an acupuncture point that is located on a blood vessel in order to draw blood. Hemo-acupuncture releases heat, toxins, and fever, and can be applied in a similar fashion to leech therapy.
- **Laser acupuncture:** The use of laser therapy to emit light that penetrates the tissues and stimulates acupuncture points.

Laser Acupuncture

Laser acupuncture is becoming common practice in veterinary medicine. Acupuncture itself is relatively painless; however, there are certain patients that are very sensitive and do not tolerate the insertion of needles or will not sit still while the needles are left in place. There are also some clients who are intimidated by acupuncture because they think their pet will experience pain and so are reluctant to choose this treatment. For these instances, laser therapy is a suitable alternative, as it can be applied directly on the acupuncture points without needle insertion. Unlike traditional laser therapy, in which the energy emitted by the laser affects the metabolic processes of the target cells (photobiomodulation,

PBM), laser acupuncture affects neural response in a similar manner to needle acupuncture (de Oliveira and de Freitas, 2016). It is imperative that the practitioner is knowledgeable about the anatomical locations and clinical indications of acupuncture points, in order to maximize the benefits of laser acupuncture.

Acupuncture is superior to laser therapy for pain control (Chang *et al.*, 2014); however, the combination of laser therapy and acupuncture leads to improved pain relief, and so it is recommended when there is moderate to severe pain. This combination can also be used for other conditions besides pain, as the two therapies have similarities in their mechanisms of action. For example, both laser therapy and acupuncture improve circulation and stimulate cellular proliferation; therefore, both are beneficial for wounds. For wound care, proper cleaning and disinfection should be the first step, followed by laser therapy in and around the wound, and finally a "Circle the Dragon" acupuncture technique. This technique is performed by placing acupuncture needles all around the wound at a 45° angles and leaving them in place for 20 minutes. The synergistic effects of laser therapy and acupuncture are superior to either therapy alone.

Clinical Indications

There are a variety of clinical conditions that benefit from both laser therapy and acupuncture; many are similar. These include but are not limited to pain management, wound care, relief of trigger points, orthopedic conditions such as osteoarthritis, cranial cruciate ligament rupture, patellar luxation, hip and elbow dysplasia, and tendinopathies, as well as neurologic conditions such as intervertebral disk disease (IVDD), fibrocartilagenous embolism, cervical spondylomyelopathy, degenerative lumbosacral stenosis, polyneuropathy, and neuropraxia.

Safety Concerns

Overall, acupuncture is relatively safe, but there are a few precautions one should consider. It is imperative to note that electro-acupuncture is contraindicated in patients with a history of seizures, epilepsy, or cardiac arrhythmias, as well as those that have a pacemaker. Electro-acupuncture should be used with caution in patients with neoplasia and congestive heart failure. Acupuncture should never be performed directly into or around a tumor, into open wounds or scar tissue, or directly into skin that has severe dermatitis. In addition, there are certain acupuncture points that cause uterine contraction and induce parturition; therefore, these specific points are contraindicated in pregnancy that is not full-term. Laser therapy is also fairly safe; however, there are precautions and special considerations, as well as the contraindication of direct exposure to the retina through the pupil. For more details about therapy laser safety, see Chapter 4.

Research

Marques *et al.* (2015) evaluated laser acupuncture as an adjuvant for postoperative pain management in cats. In total, 20 cats undergoing ovariohysterectomy were sedated with intramuscular ketamine (5 mg/kg), midazolam (0.5 mg/kg), and tramadol (2 mg/kg). Prior to induction of anesthesia, the cats were randomly distributed into two groups: 10 received laser acupuncture at two points (bilateral ST-36 and SP-6) and 10 were in the control group and received no laser acupuncture. Anesthesia was induced using intravenous propofol (4 mg/kg) and maintained with isoflurane. Postoperative analgesia was evaluated by a blinded examiner for 24 hours following extubation using the Dynamic Interactive Visual Analogue Scale (DIVAS) and Multidimensional Composite Pain Scale (MCPS). Rescue analgesia was provided with intramuscular tramadol (2 mg/kg), and pain scores were reassessed 30 minutes after rescue intervention. If analgesia remained insufficient, a single dose of intramuscular meloxicam (0.2 mg/kg) was administered. Pain scores did not differ between groups. However, postoperative supplemental analgesia was required by significantly more cats in the control group (5/10) compared with the laser acupuncture group (1/10). Researchers concluded that laser acupuncture reduced postoperative analgesic requirements in cats undergoing ovariohysterectomy (Marques *et al.*, 2015).

Quah-Smith *et al.* (2010) performed a study to determine whether laser acupuncture has a biological effect, using functional magnetic resonance imaging (fMRI) to investigate the cerebral activation patterns caused by laser stimulation of relevant acupuncture points. They took 10 healthy human subjects randomly assigned into two groups: group 1 received laser acupuncture (808 nm, 25 mW) at four points (LIV-14, CV-14, LIV-8, HT-7), and group two received sham laser at a non-acupuncture point. The blood oxygenation level-dependent fMRI response was recorded from the whole brain on a 3 T scanner. Many of the laser acupuncture stimulation conditions resulted in different patterns of neural activity. Regions with significantly increased activation included the limbic cortex (cingulate) and the frontal lobe (middle and superior frontal gyrus). Laser acupuncture tended to be associated with ipsilateral brain activation and contralateral deactivation that cannot be simply attributed to somatosensory stimulation. The researchers concluded that laser stimulation of acupuncture points leads to activation of the frontal–limbic–striatal brain regions,

with the pattern of neural activity somewhat different for each acupuncture point. Differing activity patterns were demonstrated with different acupuncture point sites, suggesting that neurological effects vary with the site of stimulation (Quah-Smith *et al.*, 2010).

Yurtkuran *et al.* (2007) investigated the effects and minimum effective dose of laser acupuncture in stifle osteoarthritis to determine whether it is superior to placebo in the evaluation of clinical-functional outcome and quality of life. In this randomized, placebo-controlled, double-blind study, patients with stifle osteo-arthritis were selected. Group 1 (n = 27) received 904 nm laser therapy with a 10 mW/cm^2 power density, 4 mW output power, 0.4 cm^2 spot size, 0.48 J per session, and 120 second treatment time on the medial side of the stifle on the acupuncture point SP-9. Group 2 (n = 25) received placebo-laser therapy at the same place on the same point. Patients in both of the groups were treated 5 days per week (total duration of therapy was 10 days) and 20 minutes per day. The study comprised a 2-week (10 sessions) intervention. Participants were evaluated before treatment (baseline), after treatment (2nd week), and at the 12th week. The main outcome measures were as follows: pain on movement (pVAS), 50-foot walking time (50 foot w), knee circumference (KC), medial tenderness score (MTS), Western Ontario and McMaster Universities osteoarthritis index (WOMAC), and Nottingham Health Profile (NHP). In group 1, statistically significant improvement was observed in PVAS, 50 foot w, and KC. In group 2, statistically significant improvement was observed in PVAS, 50 foot w, and WOMAC. When the groups were compared with each other, the improvement observed in KC was superior in group 1 at the 2nd week (p = 0.005). The researchers found laser acupuncture to be effective in reducing periarticular swelling when compared with placebo laser (Yurtkuran *et al.*, 2007).

Schlager *et al.* (1998) conducted a double-blind, randomized, placebo-controlled study to investigate the effectiveness of laser acupuncture of point PC-6 on postoperative vomiting in children undergoing strabismus surgery. They randomly assigned 40 children into two groups: group 1 received laser acupuncture and group 2 received placebo laser. Laser acupuncture (670 nm, 10 mW) at PC-6 was administered 15 minutes prior to induction of anesthesia and 15 minutes after surgery. The incidence of vomiting was significantly lower in the laser acupuncture group (25%) than in the placebo group (85%). Schlager *et al.* (1998) concluded that laser acupuncture at PC-6 was effective at decreasing the incidence of postoperative vomiting.

Hayashi *et al.* (2007) performed a prospective controlled study to evaluate the use of electro-acupuncture combined with standard Western medical treatment versus Western medical treatment alone for treatment of thoracolumbar IVDD in dogs. They randomly assigned 50 dogs with signs of thoracolumbar IVDD to one of two treatment groups and classified them as having grade I–V neurologic dysfunction. Dogs in group 1 received electro-acupuncture combined with standard Western medical treatment; those in group 2 received only standard Western medical treatment. A numeric score for neurologic function was evaluated at four time points to determine the effects of treatments. Time (mean ± SD) to recover ambulation in dogs with grade III and IV dysfunction was significantly lower in group 1 (10.10 ± 6.49 days) than in group 2 (20.83 ± 11.99 days). Success rate (ability to walk without assistance) for dogs with grade III and IV dysfunction was significantly higher in group 1 (10/10 dogs) than in group 2 (6/9 dogs). Dogs without deep pain perception (grade V dysfunction) had a success rate (recovery of pain sensation) of 3/6 and 1/8 in groups 1 and 2, respectively, but the difference was not significant. Overall success rate (all dysfunction grades) for group 1 (23/26; 88.5%) was significantly higher than for group 2 (14/24; 58.3%). Researchers determined that electro-acupuncture combined with standard Western medical treatment was effective and that it resulted in a shorter time to recover ambulation and deep pain perception than did the use of Western treatment alone in dogs with signs of thoracolumbar IVDD (Hayashi *et al.*, 2007).

Draper *et al.* (2012) performed a prospective study to determine whether laser therapy and surgery for intervertebral disk herniation encouraged ambulation faster than surgery alone. They evaluated 36 dogs with acute paraparesis or paraplegia due to acute intervertebral disk herniation and gave them a modified Frankel score. Dogs with scores 0–3 were included in the study. Dogs were assigned to the control group (group 1) or the laser treatment group (group 2) based on alternating order of presentation. All dogs underwent surgery for their herniated disks. Dogs in group 1 did not receive laser therapy. Dogs in group 2 received postoperative laser therapy daily for 5 days, or until they achieved a modified Frankel score of 4. A 5 × 200 mW, 810 nm cluster-array laser was used. All dogs were scored daily by the investigators using the modified Frankel scoring system. The time to achieve a modified Frankel score of 4 was significantly lower in the low-level laser therapy group (median 3.5 days) than in the control group (median 14 days). Draper *et al.* (2012) concluded that low-level laser therapy in combination with surgery decreases time to ambulation in dogs with T3–L3 myelopathy secondary to intervertebral disk herniation.

Xie *et al.* (2005) evaluated the use of electro-acupuncture for the treatment of horses with signs of chronic thoracolumbar pain. There were 15 horses with signs of chronic thoracolumbar pain in this prospective study, which were randomly allocated to one of three treatment groups. Horses in group 1 received electro-acupuncture (once every 3 days for five treatments), those in group 2 received phenylbutazone (2.2 mg/kg PO, q12h for 5 days), and those in group 3 received saline (20 mL PO, q12h for 5 days). Thoracolumbar pain scores (TLPSs) were evaluated at baseline and after each treatment. Mean ± SD TLPSs in horses receiving phenylbutazone or saline solution did not change significantly during the study. After the third treatment, mean ± SD TLPS (2.1 ± 0.6) in horses receiving electro-acupuncture stimulation was significantly lower than baseline TLPS (6.0 ± 0.6). Mean ± SD TLPS in horses receiving electro-acupuncture stimulation was significantly lower than baseline in horses receiving phenylbutazone or saline solution from after the third treatment until 14 days after the last treatment. Xie *et al.* (2005) stated that electro-acupuncture was effective for the treatment of chronic thoracolumbar pain in horses. Their results provide evidence that three sessions of electro-acupuncture treatment can successfully alleviate signs of thoracolumbar pain in horses and that the analgesic effect can last at least up to 2 weeks.

La *et al.* (2005) investigated the effects of electro-acupuncture on nerve regeneration. The sciatic nerves (specifically at a location 5 mm above the stifle joint) of 15 rabbits were crushed by a Halsted straight mosquito hemostat with 8–11 N force for 60 seconds; then the rabbits were divided equally into three groups. Group 1 was treated with electro-acupuncture at acupuncture points GB-30 and BL-40 for 25 minutes daily for 7 days. Group 2 was treated with intramuscular administration of diclofenac 15 mg daily for 7 days. Group 3 was the control group and therefore was not treated. After treatment, the distal parts of the crushed nerve were examined under light microscope, the densities of normal myelinated fibers were determined, and the diameters of 20 normal myelinated fibers were measured for each rabbit. The results showed mean densities of 176.2 ± 5.953 in the electro-acupuncture group, 118.2 ± 10.878 in the diclofenac group, and 101.4 ± 8.548 in the control group. The mean values were significantly different between the electro-acupuncture and diclofenac groups ($p < 0.01$); highly significantly different between the electro-acupuncture and control groups ($p < 0.001$); and not significantly different between the diclofenac and control groups ($p > 0.05$). There were more small myelinated fibers (0–9 microns) in the electro-acupuncture group than in the diclofenac and control groups ($p = 0.0028$). La *et al.*'s (2005) results revealed and confirmed that electro-acupuncture promotes nerve regeneration while diclofenac does not.

In a study by Frederico *et al.* (2016), near-infrared laser was used to stimulate an acupuncture point in Wistar rats in order to determine whether results similar to manual acupuncture could be achieved. The authors wanted to examine the effects of laser (904 nm) application at "Zusanli" (ST-36) of the stomach meridian on the biodistribution of the radiopharmaceutical Na(99 m)TcO4. The rats were divided into a control group, which was not exposed to the laser at all, and an experimental group, which was exposed at ST-36 to the 904 nm laser at 1 J/min (40 mW/cm^2) for 1 minute daily. At day 8 after laser acupuncture, the rats were given the radiopharmaceutical Na(99 m)TcO4. After 10 minutes, the animals were all sacrificed and the thyroid glands were examined. The percentage of injected radiopharmaceutical was significantly increased in the thyroid glands of the experimental versus the control rats due to the stimulation of ST-36 by the laser. The study concluded that the stimulation of ST-36 does lead to biological phenomena that affect the metabolism of the thyroid gland (Frederico *et al.*, 2016).

Research continues to demonstrate the value of laser acupuncture. Attia *et al.* (2016) showed its effectiveness in alleviating oxidative stress and inflammation, improving antioxidant and energy metabolic status while suppressing disease activity in human patients with rheumatoid arthritis. The authors concluded that laser acupuncture is a promising treatment modality for reducing the pain and suffering of rheumatoid patients, because of its efficiency in inhibiting many of the main factors involved in the disease's pathogenesis. Dabbous *et al.* (2016) examined the value of laser acupuncture as an adjunctive therapy for spastic cerebral palsy in children. They found that laser acupuncture did have a beneficial effect on reducing spasticity and improving movement in these children.

References

Attia, A.M. *et al.* (2016) Therapeutic antioxidant and anti-inflammatory effects of laser acupuncture on patients with rheumatoid arthritis. *Lasers Surg Med.* **48**(5):490–497.

Brown, M.L. *et al.* (1974) Acupuncture loci: technique for location. *Am J Chin Med.* **2**(1):67–74.

Chang, W.D. *et al.* (2014) Analgesic effect of manual acupuncture and laser acupuncture for lateral epicondylalgia: a systematic review and meta-analysis. *Am J Chin Med.* **42**(6):1301–1314.

Dabbous, O.A. *et al.* (2016) Laser acupuncture as an adjunctive therapy for spastic cerebral palsy in children. *Lasers Med Sci.* **31**(6):1061–1067.

de Oliveira, R.F. and de Freitas, P.M. (2016) Laser therapy on points of acupuncture on nerve repair. *Neural Regen Res.* **11**(4):557–558.

Draper, W.E. *et al.* (2012) Low-level laser therapy reduces time to ambulation in dogs after hemilaminectomy: a preliminary study. *J Small Anim Pract.* **53**(8):465–469.

Frederico, E.H. *et al.* (2016) Laser stimulation of the acupoint "Zusanli" (ST.36) on the radiopharmaceutical biodistribution in Wistar rats. *J Biosci.* **41**(1):63–68.

Fry, L.M. *et al.* (2014) Acupuncture for Analgesia in Veterinary Medicine. *Topics Comp An Med.* **29**(2):25–32.

Hayashi, A.M. *et al.* (2007) Evaluation of electroacupuncture treatment for thoracolumbar intervertebral disk disease in dogs. *J Am Vet Med Assoc.* **231**(6):913–918.

Hughes, J. (1975) Isolation of an endogenous compound from the brain with pharmacological properties similar to morphine. *Brain Res.* **88**(2):295–308.

Kendall, D.E. (1989a) Part I: a scientific model of acupuncture. *Am J Acupuncture.* **17**(3):251–268.

Kendall, D.E. (1989b) Part II: a scientific model of acupuncture. *Am J Acupuncture.* **17**(4):343–360.

La, J.L. *et al.* (2005) Morphological studies on crushed sciatic nerve of rabbits with electro-acupuncture or diclofenac sodium treatment. *Am J Chin Med.* **33**(4):663–669.

Marques, V.I. *et al.* (2015) Laser acupuncture for postoperative pain management in cats. *Evid Based Complement Alternat Med.* **2015**:653270.

Mayer, D.J. *et al.* (1977) Antagonism of acupuncture analgesia in man by the narcotic antagonist naloxone. *Brain Res.* **121**(2):368–372.

Melzack, R. and Wall, P.D. (1965) Pain mechanisms: a new theory. *Science.* **150**(3699):971–979.

Omura, Y. (1975) Pathophysiology of acupuncture treatment. Effects of acupuncture on cardiovascular and nervous systems. *Acup Electrotherap Res.* **1**:51–140.

Pan, C. *et al.* (1986) *Research on Acupuncture, Moxibustion, and Acupuncture Anesthesia.* Springer-Verlag, New York.

Quah-Smith, I. *et al.* (2010) The brain effects of laser acupuncture in healthy individuals: a fMRI investigation. *PlosONE.* **5**(9):e12619.

Reichmanis, M. *et al.* (1975) Electrical correlates of acupuncture points. *IEEE Trans Biomed Eng.* **22**(6):533–535.

Schlager, A. *et al.* (1998) Laser stimulation of acupuncture point PC-6 reduces postoperative vomiting in children undergoing strabimus surgery. *Br J Anaesth.* **81**(4):529–532.

Smith, F.W.K. (1994) The neurophysiologic basis of acupuncture. In: *Veterinary Acupuncture Ancient Art to Modern Medicine*, p. 45. Mosby, St. Louis, MO.

Urano, K. and Ogasawara, S. (1978) A fundamental study on acupuncture point phenomena of a dog body. *Kitasato Arch Exp Med.* **51**(3–4):95–109.

Xi, Z.F. and Li, Q.S. (1983) Changes in serum levels of morphine-like substances during acupuncture therapy on patients with pain and its relationship to the curative effects. *Shanghai J Acupunct Moxibustion.* **1**:12–15.

Xie, H. *et al.* (2005) Evaluation of electro-acupuncture treatment of horses with signs of chronic thoracolumbar pain. *J Am Vet Med Assoc.* **227**(2):281–286.

Yurtkuran, M. *et al.* (2007) Laser acupuncture in knee osteoarthritis: a double-blind, randomized controlled study. *Photomed Laser Surg.* **25**(1):14–20.

Zhang, A.Z. *et al.* (1980). Endorphins and acupuncture analgesia. *Chin Med J (Engl).* **93**(10):673–680.

40

Laser Therapy in Veterinary Regenerative Medicine
Debra Canapp

Veterinary Orthopedic and Sports Medicine Group, Orthobiologic Innovations, Annapolis Junction, MD, USA

Laser Therapy in Veterinary Regenerative Medicine

Regenerative medicine refers to the methodology of stimulating, replacing, engineering, or regenerating a patient's cells, tissues, or organs, with the end goal of restoring or establishing normal function of the tissue treated. This relatively new field of translational medicine holds the potential to stimulate the body's own repair mechanisms to heal previously unrepairable tissues and organs. Regenerative medicine is on the forefront of newly developing technologies and treatments in veterinary medicine for multiple disease processes, especially in musculoskeletal and neurologic diseases and injuries (Bashir *et al.*, 2014). Once injured or affected by disease, some tissues are able to heal back to their original strength and resilience. Many of the current regenerative medicine applications are geared toward tissues that historically heal poorly or with scar tissue, such as tendons, ligaments, cartilage, and muscle.

Veterinary regenerative medicine currently focuses on harvesting the patient's naturally occurring reparative cells and molecules, concentrating them through either patient-side mechanisms or culture expansion, and then returning them to the precise location of injury. The most successful and popular regenerative medicine techniques are the use of platelet-rich plasma (PRP) and adult-derived stem cells, either alone or in combination.

Platelet-Rich Plasma Therapy

Platelets have been shown to recruit, stimulate, and provide a scaffold for stem cells (Braun *et al.*, 2014; Broeckx *et al.*, 2014; Cho *et al.*, 2011; Dohan *et al.*, 2008; Drengk

et al., 2009; Mishra *et al.*, 2009; Schnabel *et al.*, 2009; Torricelli *et al.*, 2011). Thus, PRP has been classified and used as a regenerative medicine therapy to aid in tissue healing. PRP, a fluid concentrate composed primarily of platelets and growth factors, is prepared from the patient's own blood sample. It has been shown to assist in healing by supplying growth factors, cytokines, chemokines, and other bioactive compounds (Boswell *et al.*, 2012). Many of these growth factors act individually or synergistically to help regulate cellular migration and proliferation, promote angiogenesis, promote matrix deposition in order to enhance tendon and wound healing, aid in cartilage health, and protect and counteract against the cartilage breakdown that is associated with osteoarthritis (Hsu *et al.*, 2013; McCarrel and Fortier 2009; McCarrel *et al.*, 2012; Mishra and Pavelko 2006; Patel *et al.*, 2013). Thus, PRP is becoming widely used in both human and veterinary medicine to aid in healing a wide range of tissues.

Recent studies have compared key parameters of the PRP products of well-known and commonly used commercial canine PRP systems and found variations in their composition (Carr *et al.*, 2014; Franklin *et al.*, 2015; Stief *et al.*, 2011). It is important (for both the patient and the practitioner) to look closely at the data, record product values, monitor treatment sites, and record all outcomes, in order to interpret and identify applications and any changes that may need to be discussed.

For osteoarthritis, PRP products are injected directly into the joint, with or without sedation; this technique requires advanced imaging (diagnostic ultrasound, digital radiography, or fluoroscopy) for guidance. Diagnostic ultrasound guidance is mandatory for soft-tissue injuries, as it ensures the accuracy of the injection – PRP is most effective when administered directly into the injury or lesion. Sedation is usually required for ultrasound-guided soft-tissue injections.

Stem-Cell Therapy

Stem cells are defined as the body's progenitor cells, from which all other cells are derived. Many studies have shown that mesenchymal stem cells, produced from adult stem cells, regenerate and heal injured tissue, decrease inflammation, and stimulate angiogenesis. They support healing, activate local tissue-resident stem cells, provide a scaffold for further healing of tissue, protect other tissue cells from death, and remodel and break down scar tissue (Grassel and Lorenz, 2014; Ham *et al.*, 2015; Mazor *et al.*, 2014; Sampson *et al.*, 2015; Wolfstadt *et al.*, 2015). In addition, several studies recently published in veterinary medicine show the benefit of stem-cell therapy when applied to the canine. These studies include stem-cell therapy as an adjunct to surgery in fragmented coronoid cases (Kiefer *et al.*, 2013), canine hip osteoarthritis (Cuervo *et al.*, 2014), and muscle and tendon strains (Case *et al.*, 2013).

The most widely used stem-cell therapy, autologous adult-derived mesenchymal cells, may be obtained from various sources in a patient's body. The most common places, based on research and clinical use, are the patient's bone marrow and adipose tissue. Stem cells from both sources have repeatedly shown the ability to differentiate into cartilage, bone, tendons, and ligaments. Previously, both bone marrow- and adipose-derived stem cells (ASCs) could be either processed on-site or shipped to an institution for processing, culture expansion, and banking for future use (Martinello *et al.*, 2011). With new Food and Drug Administration (FDA) guidelines released in December 2015, universities and institutions in the United States may be under new regulations that would potentially restrict certain stem-cell manipulations, expansion, and banking for commercial use. Further investigation into this is currently underway, and different criteria may be in place when publication of this textbook occurs.

Like PRP, stem-cell therapy is considered a minimally invasive procedure and is typically performed with or without the use of sedation, depending on the application and the location of the injection. A vast amount of energy is spent in exploring stem-cell engraphment and viability once cells have been embedded into a target tissue (Li *et al.*, 2016). Cell delivery techniques and biological vehicles are current areas of debate, and exploration is needed to find the best combination to ensure long-term stem cell survival, in order to increase the probability of tissue regeneration within the injured tissue (Zarembinski *et al.*, 2011).

Combination regenerative medicine therapy, combining PRP products with stem cells, regardless of their source, has become common among small-animal practitioners. Recent studies have shown that PRP recruits and stimulates stem cells, thereby supporting the notion that PRP should be combined with stem cells prior to injection (Figure 40.1). This method supports both activation and scaffold provision for the stem cells (Del Bue *et al.*, 2008; Carvalho *et al.*, 2013; Chen *et al.*, 2012; Manning *et al.*, 2013; Tobita *et al.*, 2013; Uysal *et al.*, 2012; Xie *et al.*, 2012; Yun *et al.*, 2014).

No matter the source or content of the product, ensuring that it is directly situated in the site of injury, through either ultrasound guidance or another assurance method, is one of the most important requirements for a successful outcome, followed by continued viability of the cell in its new environment.

Studies support regenerative medicine as an efficacious tool in managing numerous orthopedic conditions, including routinely occurring osteoarthritis and soft-tissue injuries. Soft-tissue injuries and osteoarthritis are extremely common conditions afflicting active, working, and sporting dogs, due to the repetitive forces placed on their joints. Micro-trauma to the tendons, ligaments, and articular surfaces of joints can occur, creating an environment favorable to osteoarthritic development. Once the degenerative cascade of osteoarthritis is initiated, its progression can be insidious. Therapies for this debilitating condition have focused on treating the symptoms or slowing the progression of the disease. Regenerative medicine therapy may not only treat symptoms and slow disease evolution, but also help to induce repair of the underlying damage that initiated the cascade. Regenerative medicine technology gives new hope for extending the career and improving the quality of life of our canine companions.

Rehabilitation Therapy following Regenerative Medicine Therapy

Rehabilitation therapy assists in tissue healing by decreasing inflammation, improving overall comfort, and eventually building muscle mass and increasing strength and range of motion. A well-structured, dedicated rehabilitation therapy program is recommended for at least 90 days following regenerative medicine therapy. Restricted activity and controlled exercise focused on maintaining muscle mass, not strengthening, is recommended for the first 8 weeks, in order to minimize additional inflammation. This protocol also allows the regenerative medicine treatment to focus on tissue regeneration and not removal of additional inflammation. Studies have shown that implanted stem cells remain in the tissue for approximately 8–10 weeks, depending on the target tissue (Bai *et al.*, 2011; Niemeyer *et al.*, 2008).

Rehabilitation therapy sessions often include manual therapies, standard isometric exercises, and laser therapy. Laser therapy, increasingly referred to as "photobiomodulation therapy" (PBMT), is recommended, as extensive literature supports the notion that light irradiation promotes stem-cell differentiation, proliferation, and viability. This will be explored extensively later in the chapter. Currently,

(a)

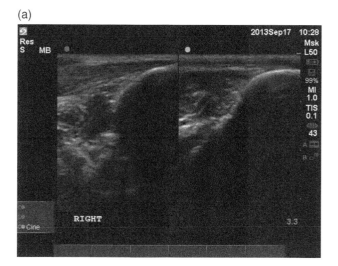

(b)

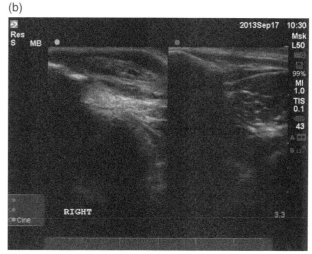

(c)

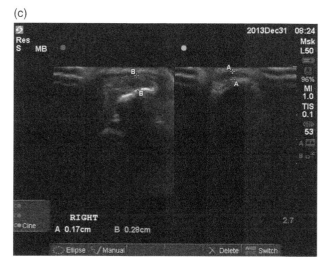

(d)

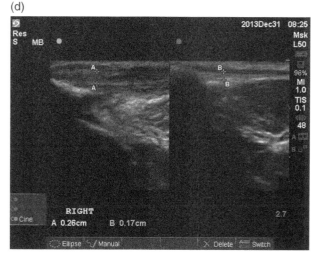

Figure 40.1 Initial ultrasound scans, (a) distal and (b) proximal, of a grade 2/3 patellar tendon strain, with normal comparison on the right. Scans of the same tendon, (c) cross-section and (d) longitudinal, 12 weeks post injection of stem cells and PRP and initiation of weekly laser therapy. Note the decrease in inflammation, decreased thickness of the patellar tendon, and improved fiber pattern when compared to the normal side, on the right.

all combination stem cell–PRP treatments performed at the author's veterinary practice are recommended to receive laser therapy weekly to twice weekly at the site of injection. A power density of 0.25 W/cm² (250 mW/cm²) and energy density of 5 J/cm² is used, with either a single wavelength between 600 and 900 nm or, preferably, multiple wavelengths (as seen in cluster probes), usually in the red to near-infrared range.

Underwater treadmill therapy is usually started 8 weeks after regenerative medicine treatment, due to its potential to add inflammation to the target tissues via water's strengthening techniques. Therapeutic ultrasound, shockwave therapy, neuromuscular electrical stimulation or trans-electrical neuromuscular stimulation, and non-steroidal anti-inflammatory drug (NSAID) usage are contraindicated within the first 8 weeks of regenerative medicine therapy, as their effects on stem cells and PRP have not been fully studied. Preliminary

reports suggest detrimental effects on transplanted cells (Nicpon *et al.*, 2015). Rehabilitation therapy should be performed weekly in conjunction with a well-structured and explicit home-exercise program.

Once the targeted tissue has regenerated, as confirmed by diagnostic ultrasound or arthroscopy, the rehabilitation program can advance to focus on strengthening and conditioning. When appropriate muscle mass has been attained, the canine patient is then cleared for re-training and return to sport or normal daily activity.

Regenerative Medicine and Photobiomodulation

Ultimately, regenerative medicine's purpose is to assist the patient's body in regenerating injured tissue back to its original condition. Laser therapy has also been proven to stimulate many different cell lines via positive, restorative mechanisms. However, there is a scarcity of studies on the action of laser therapy on mesenchymal stem cells, and even less data on the actual mechanism of action of laser therapy on adult stem cells (Ginani *et al.*, 2015). Nevertheless, a 2015 landmark review article on photobiomodulation (PBM), looking precisely at its effects of proliferation and differentiation of both human and animal derived stem cells, helps define the importance of power density and energy density on the end stem-cell response (Emelyanov and Kiryanova, 2015). This article, which will be explored further throughout this chapter, finds that the influence of wavelength does not appear to be insignificant. Elevated values of proliferation or differentiation are primarily seen in studies using high power densities, low energy densities, and short exposure times. The greatest differentiation is attained using laser irradiation protocols different from those necessary to achieve maximal proliferation of the same cells. The article concludes that increased power density and reduced energy density are the essential parameters needed to increase the overall positive stem-cell response (Emelyanov and Kiryanova, 2015). In general, there is an overall agreement that power density and energy density (with less importance placed on specific light wavelength, as long as it is in the red or near-infrared range) are the most important parameters with regards to the effects of PBM on stem cells and their use in regenerative medicine.

Unfortunately, all of these parameters are not always reported in every research article. In addition, when cited, they differ greatly from study to study, and often involve multiple different stem cell lines, species, and tissue origins. Using clinical research is important in determining when and how a tool can best be used to maximize its effectiveness. Researchers propose mechanisms that are involved in treating a broad spectrum of injuries or disease states so that clinicians may decide whether the combination and synergism of regenerative medicine and laser therapy might be useful in each individual case.

This treatment-method approach of evaluating the literature as a practice guide is often referred to as "evidence-based medicine." Using research aids clinicians in determining when a therapy is anticipated to have a benefit for the patient in question. The veterinarian then takes this information and uses his or her judgment as to when and where to apply the therapy. At times, there may be little support for the use of a particular treatment in a particular species.

Research regarding the use of regenerative medicine, specifically in canine musculoskeletal injuries, canine neurological injuries, or canine wound healing, is currently limited in the literature. For this reason, many protocols and indications are taken from the human or alternate mammal literature and applied to canine

patients. As stated before, much of the research on these alternative animal populations may be confusing, since the parameters and the power of the laser can vary from trial to trial. Use of these data across species has proven to be very successful clinically in the treatment of many musculoskeletal injuries seen in the canine. In spite of this experience, it is crucial for the veterinarian to be able to discern why a modality or treatment does or does not add benefit. This should be well documented in developing the ongoing treatment plan.

Despite the current lack of species-specific data or consistency in reporting details, key opinion leaders, residing in a broad range of well-respected disciplines, believe that PBM of stem cells is a valuable tool for boosting stem cell viability and proliferation. Extraordinary therapies will become available as a result of this intellectual drive and the promising synergism between regenerative medicine and laser therapy.

In Vitro Laser Therapy and Stem Cells

Many years of dedicated research into a wide range of light applications, light wavelength ranges, power densities, and exposures across several species and cell lines have paved the way for the useful clinical application we see today. Early research in laser therapy and adult stem cells suggested that laser therapy escalates the proliferation of stem cells, but the exact biological mechanisms responsible for this photobiostimulatory effect are not fully understood (Tuby *et al.*, 2007).

Huo *et al.* (2008) investigated the effect of a 635 nm diode laser with an output power of 60 mW at numerous dosages on rat-derived bone marrow-derived mesenchymal stem cells (BMSCs). This application of light demonstrated $0.5 \, \text{J/cm}^2$ to be an optimal energy density for the stimulation of cellular proliferation. At a higher $5 \, \text{J/cm}^2$ dose, the stem cells secreted both vascular endothelial growth factor (VEGF) and nerve growth factor. This dosage also facilitated myogenic differentiation. Huo *et al.* (2008) concluded that laser therapy stimulates proliferation, facilitates myogenic differentiation, and increases growth factor secretion in BMSCs. This study may provide data to support the preconditioning of BMSCs with laser light prior to implantation into the patient.

Abramovitch-Gottlib *et al.* (2005) irradiated BMSCs cultured *in vitro* with a 632.8 nm laser with an output power of 10 mW and a power density of $0.5 \, \text{mW/cm}^2$, using an increased exposure time of 10 minutes a day extended for 28 days. They found the laser irradiation had a biostimulatory effect on the conversion of BMSCs into bone-forming cells and induced ossification.

Mvula *et al.* (2008) investigated the other popular stem cell line, ASCs, using a 635 nm diode laser with an output power of 50.2 mW and a power density of $5.5 \, \text{mW/cm}^2$ at a one-time dose of $5 \, \text{J/cm}^2$. They evaluated the cells after

48 hours. Cell morphology did not change, but cell viability and proliferation were significantly increased.

Other studies looking at different cell populations, such as human dental pulp stem cells and cardiac stem cells, all show a positive effect of laser phototherapy, with improved cell growth, supporting the overall synergistic effect of progenitor cells and laser light irradiation (Eduardo *et al.*, 2008; Tuby *et al.*, 2007). Similar *in vitro* results are seen in the equine species, also. Equine peripheral blood mesenchymal stem cells incubated with growth factors and irradiated with laser light promoted differentiation into the tenocyte lineage (Gomiero *et al.*, 2016).

These cell-culture studies and prominent review articles support, in general, the notion that phototherapy can significantly "increase the initial number of stem cells before differentiation, thus increasing the number of differentiated cells for tissue engineering and regenerative and healing processes" (Ginani *et al.*, 2015). Yet, the issue remains that there is a deficiency in standardization of treatment parameters with regards to the wavelength, power density, radiation time, and polarization of light.

With reference to the wavelength used in these studies, the majority used the visible red spectrum in the 600–700 nm range. This is most likely due to the historical support from studies looking at the positive effects of these wavelengths on *in vitro* biostimulation of cells in general. Though there have been significantly fewer studies looking at the infrared range, results from Tuby *et al.* (2007) and Soleimani *et al.* (2012) show the positive proliferative and differentiation effects of an 810 nm wavelength on human bone-marrow cells.

One negative study by Bouvet-Gerbettaz *et al.* (2009) showed that the application of laser therapy in the near-infrared range (808 nm, 800 mW, 4 J/cm^2) on murine bone-marrow stem cells resulted in a lower number of colony-forming units (CFUs) when compared to non-treated cells. It was speculated by Ginani *et al.* (2015) that though it may have been the infrared spectrum that caused this result, the higher power could also have had an effect.

In Vivo Laser Therapy and Stem Cells

Regenerative medicine and PBMT are now also being looked at synergistically *in vivo*. Laser irradiation assisting in stem cell proliferation is a common area of research. A study looking at human ASCs transplanted into rats and treated with laser therapy with an 830 nm wavelength showed a significant increase in the number of human stem cells in the irradiated group compared to the non-irradiated group (Min *et al.*, 2015). Other studies looking at the effect of stem cells treated with light irradiation include a number of different applications in injury repair that could be translated to canines. In reference to wound therapy, one group looked at cultured

human adipose-derived mesenchymal stem cells treated with light from a light-emitting diode (LED) (660 nm, 10 mW/cm^2, 6 J/cm^2) prior to and following implantation into the wound beds of mice. The light-irradiated group appeared superior in many factors, including functional recovery (Park *et al.*, 2015a).

One of the few canine species-specific studies investigated the effect of canine ASCs on wound healing in athymic mice. When the ASCs were treated with laser therapy (632 nm, 17 mW, 1.2 J/cm^2, daily for 20 days), wound healing was enhanced (through increased neovascularization and regeneration of skin appendages) compared with the group receiving ASCs alone. In general, ASCs promoted skin regeneration through cell differentiation and secretion of necessary growth factors. In the ASC and laser-treated group, the survival of ASCs was increased by the fact laser therapy decreased cell apoptosis within the wound bed. In addition, the secretion of growth factors was increased in the ASC and laser-treated group compared with the ASC group (Kim *et al.*, 2012).

Vascularity within the area of stem cell injection or application, as seen in the previously cited studies, is often an important factor when looking at cell survivability. Stem cell survival inside the tissue needing treatment or repair is essential to their ability to aid in healing. In a recent study looking at human ASC implantation into ischemic mice limbs, the group that received both ASCs and LED light irradiation (660 nm, 50 mW/cm^2, 30 J/cm^2) showed an overall increase in ASCs due to the decreased cell death. The secretion of growth factors was also triggered in this group compared with the group receiving ASCs alone. The ASC and LED light group demonstrated enhanced treatment efficacy, including neovascularization and tissue regeneration. Laser Doppler blood perfusion images showed that blood perfusion of the treatment site was significantly improved by ASC and LED light treatment. These data suggest that LED light irradiation is an effective biostimulator of ASCs with regard to vascular regeneration and growth factors, showing improvement in the survival of implanted stem cells in ischemic limbs (Park *et al.*, 2015b).

Bone marrow-derived stem cells and laser therapies have also been explored. A recent study evaluated the effect of bone marrow aspirate (BMA), laser therapy, and their combination on bone healing in surgically created defects in rat calvaria. This study found the combination of BMA and laser therapy generated significantly greater bone formation compared to controls or either treatment alone (Fekrazad *et al.*, 2015; Nagata *et al.*, 2013).

The combination of laser therapy with regenerative medicine has also shown positive effects in neurologic injury. Once again, this is a necessary area for translational medicine within the canine community. In a study involving induced peripheral nerve-crush injuries in rats, laser therapy showed a synergistic effect when combined with transplantation of mesenchymal cells into the site of injury. This combined treatment provided greater functional recovery than either mesenchymal stem cell transplantation or laser therapy alone (Yang *et al.*, 2016). Another neurologic application demonstrated that applying laser light (660 nm, 50 mW, 10 minutes, single exposure) to adipose-derived rat stem cells elicited positive effects on stem cell differentiation, which in turn effectively treated ischemic stroke in rats, specifically improving motor function recovery when compared to controls and those receiving stem cells without laser irradiation (Shen *et al.*, 2015).

The use of stem cells stimulated by PBMT is expanding to new applications. Exploration into PBMT of stem cells while they are still *in situ* within the host has developed into ideas around preparing the body's resident stem cells to better react following injury. Mature mammalian cardiac tissue is known to have limited regenerative capabilities following acute injury. Early studies proposed that the photobiostimulation of autologous BMSCs might stimulate these stem cells to migrate to the infracted section of the heart and mitigate scarring. In one study, rats underwent myocardial infarction and had their exposed tibial bone marrow irradiated with laser light (804 nm, 10 mW/cm^2, 1 J/cm^2) for different time intervals. Infarct size and ventricular dilatation were significantly reduced in the rats receiving the laser treatment. The study concluded that laser irradiation applied *in situ* to the autologous bone marrow of rats following induction of myocardial infarction has promise in inducing BMSCs to move into the circulation and target the infracted heart and significantly reduce the scarring process post myocardial infarction (Tuby *et al.*, 2011).

In a similar, more recent January 2016 research article, irradiation of porcine long bones, targeting BMSCs, showed a significant reduction in scarring, enhancement of angiogenesis, and functional improvement in both the acute and long-term phase following induction of myocardial infarction (Blatt *et al.*, 2016). Another study found that mesenchymal stem cells harvested from wildtype mice and stimulated with laser therapy showed an increased ability to maturate toward a monocyte lineage, which in turn increased phagocytosis activity toward soluble amyloid beta (Aβ), an unwanted substance found in the brain of Alzheimer's disease (AD) patients. Using these preliminary data, the same team then looked at weekly laser therapy application to the bone marrow of an AD mouse model for 2 months, starting at 4 months of age (progressive stage of AD). Their findings showed an improved cognitive capacity and spatial learning as compared to sham-treated AD mice. Furthermore, postmortem histology disclosed a significant reduction in Aβ brain burden (Farfara *et al.*, 2015). These data could be useful in cognitive disorders, which are now seen more commonly in our canine patients due to their increased life spans.

In summary, these studies support the promise of synergism between PBMT and stem cells in a variety of applications, but they also show the diverse variability in treatment parameters. The review article by Emelyanov and Kiryanova (2015) nicely summarized the general effects of both power density and energy density in a graph pertaining to cell proliferation. Here, they illustrate the stages of change in cell response to laser stimulation. The data show a specific adaptation phase of the cells, or a prime treatment dosage. More importantly, they also defined a phase of photostress and photoshock, which illustrates that there is a threshold of irradiation, and that exceeding this threshold can cause damage to stem cells.

Laser Therapy and PRP

Recent studies have also looked at the effect of laser therapy with PRP alone. Achilles tendon injuries are commonly seen in our canine companions, and even more frequently in our canine athletes. In a study on rat Achilles tendon injury, the relative amount of type I collagen was significantly greater in the PRP plus 830 nm laser irradiation group, while the quantity of type III collagen was significantly greater in the PRP-only group, both compared to the irradiation-only group. The study concluded that PRP treatment combined with irradiation at 830 nm produced a larger number of fibroblasts and increased the concentration of type I collagen, thereby accelerating the healing of the injured tendon (de Carvalho *et al.*, 2015).

Similar findings were also noted when PRP and laser therapy were applied to rabbit Achilles tendon injuries using a wavelength in the visible-light spectrum. This study compared untreated injured tendons to irradiated injured tendons (650 nm diode laser, 30 mW, 1.8 J/cm^2, for 15 consecutive days) and to irradiated injured tendons injected with PRP. Though laser treatment had advantages over no treatment, the combination of PRP and laser light irradiation was even more efficient in decreasing tendon healing time (Allahverdi *et al.*, 2015).

Barbosa *et al.* (2013) combined 660 and 830 nm wavelengths at a dosage of 7 J/cm^2 applied to three points every other day for 13 days, in addition to PRP, in the treatment of Achilles tendon injury in rats. Their results showed that the deposition of collagen type I was higher with combined PRP and laser (660 and 830 nm) treatment, suggesting a faster regeneration of the tendon. These data are valuable for the canine world, since circumstances often create economic barriers to the use of stem cells in canine musculoskeletal injury. If these data can be translated, it would mean that canines could receive less expensive PRP treatment with the support of

(a)
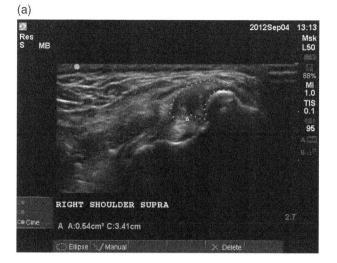

(b)
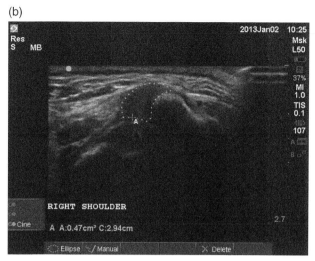

Figure 40.2 (a) Initial ultrasound scan, cross-section, of a supraspinatus tendon illustrating fibrous and calcified lesions within the outlined tendon. (b) Ultrasound scan, cross-section, 90 days post stem cell and PRP injection. Note the improved fiber pattern, decrease in inflammation and size of the tendon, and resolution of the fibrous and calcified lesions.

laser therapy, and thus reach a very healthy functional outcome for their tendon injury (Figure 40.2).

Conclusion

Regenerative medicine and laser therapy, separately, have been used to stimulate healing and help the body regenerate injured tissues back to their original conditions. Leading areas of interest now involve looking at both regenerative medicine and PBMT in the hope of discovering a superior healing approach across species. Current applications of this therapy are expanding, using translational evidence-based medicine, as explored in this chapter. Applications for sport-related conditions, neurologic injury, and wound healing in the canine include medial shoulder syndrome, shoulder tendinopathies, iliopsoas strain, Achilles tendon injury, early partial cranial cruciate ligament tear, carpal and tarsal ligament injuries, osteoarthritis, traumatic wound injury, intervertebral disk disease (IVDD), lumbosacral disease, and a wealth of other conditions seen routinely in canine patients. Continued emphasis on exploring this area of cutting-edge medicine, specifically for the canine patient, will be essential for our patients, veterinary medicine as a whole, and the world of translational medicine.

References

Abramovitch-Gottlib, L. *et al.* (2005) Low level laser irradiation stimulates osteogenic phenotype of mesenchymal stem cells seeded on a three-dimensional biomatrix. *Lasers Med Sci.* **20**(3):138–146.

Allahverdi, A. *et al.* (2015) Evaluation of low-level laser therapy, platelet-rich plasma, and their combination on the healing of Achilles tendon in rabbits. *Lasers Med Sci.* **30**(4):1305–1313.

Bai, X. *et al.* (2011) Tracking long-term survival of intramyocardially delivered human adipose tissue-derived stem cells using bioluminescence imaging. *Mol Imaging Biol.* **13**(4):633–645.

Barbosa, D. *et al.* (2013) Low-level laser therapy combined with platelet-rich plasma on the healing calcaneal tendon: a histological study in a rat model. *Lasers Med Sci.* **28**(6):1489–1494.

Bashir, J. *et al.* (2014) Mesenchymal stem cell therapies in the treatment of musculoskeletal diseases. *PM R.* **6**(1):61–69.

Blatt, A. *et al.* (2016) Low-level laser therapy to the bone marrow reduces scarring and improves heart function post-acute myocardial infarction in the pig. *Photomed Laser Surg.* **34**(11)516–524.

Boswell, S.G. *et al.* (2012) Platelet-rich plasma: a milieu of bioactive factors. *Arthroscopy.* **28**(3):429–439.

Bouvet-Gerbettaz, S. *et al.* (2009) Effects of low-level laser therapy on proliferation and differentiation of murine bone marrow cells into osteoblasts and osteoclasts. *Lasers Surg Med.* **41**(4):291–297.

Braun, H.J. *et al.* (2014) The effect of platelet-rich plasma formulations and blood products on human synoviocytes. *Am J Sports Med.* **42**(5):1204–1210.

Broeckx, S. *et al.* (2014) Regenerative therapies for equine degenerative joint disease: a preliminary study. *PLoS ONE.* **9**(1):e85917.

Carr, B.J. *et al.* (2014) Canine platelet rich plasma systems: a multicenter, prospective analysis. *Proceedings of the*

American College of Veterinary Surgeons Surgery Summit. October 15–18. San Diego, CA.

Carvalho, A.M. *et al.* (2013) Equine tendonitis therapy using mesenchymal stem cells and platelet concentrations: a randomized controlled trial. *Stem Cell Res Ther.* **4**(4):85.

Case, J.B. *et al.* (2013) Gastrocnemius tendon strain in a dog treated with autologous mesenchymal stem cells and a custom orthosis. *Vet Surg.* **42**(4):355–360.

Chen, L. *et al.* (2012) Synergy of tendon stem cells and platelet-rich-plasma in tendon healing. *J Orthop Res.* **30**(6):991–997.

Cho, H.S. *et al.* (2011) Individual variation in growth factor concentrations in platelet-rich plasma and its influence on human mesenchymal stem cells. *Korean J Lab Med.* **31**(3):212–218.

Cuervo, B. *et al.* (2014) Hip osteoarthritis in dogs: a randomized study using mesenchymal stem cells from adipose tissue and plasma rich in growth factors. *Int J Mol Sci.* **15**(8):13 437–13 460.

de Carvalho, P.K. *et al.* (2016) Analysis of experimental tendinitis in rats treated with laser and platelet-rich plasma therapies by Raman spectroscopy and histometry. *Lasers Med Sci.* **31**(1):19–26.

Del Bue, M. *et al.* (2008) Equine adipose-tissue derived mesenchymal stem cells and platelet concentrations: their association in vitro and in vivo. *Vet Res Commun.* **32**(1):S51–S55.

Dohan Ehrenfest, D.M. *et al.* (2008) Classification of platelet concentrates: from pure platelet-rich plasma (P-PRP) to leukocyte- and platelet-rich fibrin (L-PRF). *Trends Biotechnol.* **27**(3):158–167.

Drengk, A. *et al.* (2009) Influence of platelet-rich plasma on chondrogenic differentiation and proliferation of chondrocytes and mesenchymal stem cells. *Cells Tissues Organs.* **189**(5):317–326.

Eduardo, F.P. *et al.* (2008) Stem cell proliferation under low-intensity laser irradiation: a preliminary study. *Lasers Surg Med.* **40**(6):433–438.

Emelyanov, A.N. and Kiryanova, V.V. (2015) Photomodulation of proliferation and differentiation of stem cells by the visible and infrared light. *Photomed Laser Surg.* **33**(3):164–174.

Farfara, D. *et al.* (2015) Low-level laser therapy ameliorates disease progression in a mouse model of Alzheimer's disease. *J Mol Neurosci.* **55**(2):430–436.

Fekrazad, R. *et al.* (2015) The effects of combined low level laser therapy and mesenchymal stem cells on bone regeneration in rabbit calvarial defects. *J Photochem Photobiol B.* **151**:180–185.

Franklin, S.P. *et al.* (2015) Characteristics of canine platelet-rich plasma prepared with five commercially available systems. *Am J Vet Res.* **76**(9):822–827.

Ginani, F. *et al.* (2015). Effect of low-level laser therapy on mesenchymal stem cell proliferation: a systemic review. *Lasers Med Sci.* **30**(8):2189–2194.

Gomiero, C. *et al.* (2016) Tenogenic induction of equine mesenchymal stem cells by means of growth factors and low-level laser technology. *Vet Res Commun.* **40**(1):39–48.

Grassel, S. and Lorenz, J. (2014) Tissue engineering strategies to repair chondroal and osteochondral tissue in osteoarthritis: use of mesenchymal stem cells. *Curr Rheumatol Rep.* **16**(10):452.

Ham, O. *et al.* (2015) Therapeutic potential of differentiated mesenchymal stem cells for treatment of osteoarthritis. *Int J Mol Sci.* **16**(7):14 961–14 978.

Hsu, W.K. *et al.* (2013) Platelet-rich plasma in orthopaedic applications: evidence-based recommendations for treatment. *J Am Acad Orthop Surg.* **21**(12):739–748.

Huo, J.F. *et al.* (2008) In vitro effects of low level laser irradiation for bone marrow mesenchymal stem cells: proliferation, growth factor secretion and myogenic differentiation. *Lasers Surg Med.* **40**(10):726–733.

Kiefer, K. *et al.* (2013) Autologous and allogeneic stem cells as adjuvant therapy for osteoarthritis caused by spontaneous fragmented coronoid process in dogs. *VOS Proceedings 2013. 40th Annual Conference of the Veterinary Orthopedic Society*. March 9–13. Canyons Resort, UT.

Kim, H. *et al.* (2012) Enhanced wound healing effect of canine adipose-derived mesenchymal stem cells with low-level laser therapy in athymic mice. *J Dermatol Sci.* **68**(3):149–156.

Li, X. *et al.* (2016) Improving cell engraftment in cardiac stem cell therapy. *Stem Cells Int.* **2016**:7168797.

Manning, C.N. *et al.* (2013) Controlled delivery of mesenchymal stem cells and growth factors using a nanofiber scaffold for tendon repair. *Acta Biomater.* **9**(6):6905–6914.

Martinello, T. *et al.* (2011) Canine adipose-derived-mesenchymal stem cells do not lose stem features after a long-term cryopreservation. *Res Vet Sci.* **91**(1):18–24.

Mazor, M. *et al.* (2014) Mesenchymal stem-cell potential in cartilage repair: an update. *J Cell Mol Med.* **18**(12):2340–2350.

McCarrel, T. and Fortier L. (2009) Temporal growth factor release from platelet- rich plasma, trehalose lyophilized platelets, and bone marrow aspirate and their effect on tendon and ligament gene expression. *J Orthop Res.* **27**(8):1033–1042.

McCarrel, T.M. *et al.* (2012) Optimization of leukocyte concentration in platelet-rich plasma for the treatment of tendinopathy. *J Bone Joint Surg Am.* **4**(19):e143(1–8).

Min, K.H. *et al.* (2015) Effect of low-level laser therapy on human adipose-derived stem cells: in vitro and in vivo studies. *Aesthetic Plast Surg.* **39**(5):778–782.

Mishra, A. and Pavelko T. (2006) Treatment of chronic elbow tendinosis with buffered platelet-rich plasma. *Am J Sports Med.* **34**(11):1774–1778.

Mishra, A. *et al.* (2009) Buffered platelet-rich plasma enhances mesenchymal stem cell proliferation and chondrogenic differentiation. *Tissue Eng Part C Methods.* **15**(3):431–435.

Mvula, B. *et al.* (2008) The effect of low level laser irradiation on adult human adipose derived stem cells. *Lasers Med Sci.* **23**(3):277–282.

Nagata, M.J.*et al.* (2013) Bone marrow aspirate combined with low-level laser therapy: a new therapeutic approach to enhance bone healing. *J Photochem Photobiol B.* **121**:6–14.

Nicpon, J. *et al..* (2015) The effect of metamizole and tolfenamic acid on canine and equine adipose-derived mesenchymal stem cells (ASCs) an in vitro research. *Pol J Vet Sci.* **18**(1):3–11.

Niemeyer, P. *et al.* (2008) Survival of human mesenchymal stromal cells from bone marrow and adipose tissue after xenogenic transplantation in immunocompetent mice. *Cytotherapy.* **10**(8):784–795.

Park, I.S. *et al.* (2015a) Vascular regeneration effect of adipose-derived stem cells with light-emitting diode phototherapy in ischemic tissue. *Lasers Med Sci.* **30**(2):533–541.

Park, I.S. *et al.* (2015b) Enhancement of ischemic wound healing by spheroid grafting of human adipose-derived stem cells treated with low-level light irradiation. *PLoS ONE.* **10**(6):e0122776

Patel, S. *et al.* (2013) Treatment with platelet-rich plasma is more effective than placebo for knee osteoarthritis: a prospective, double-blinded, randomized trial. *Am J Sports Med.* **41**(2): 356–364.

Sampson, S. *et al.* (2015) Stem cell therapies for treatment of cartilage and bone disorders: osteoarthritis, avascular necrosis, and non-union fractures. *PM R.* **7**(4 Suppl.):S26–S32.

Schnabel, L.V. *et al.* (2009) Mesenchymal stem cells and insulin-like growth factor-I gene- enhanced mesenchymal stem cells improve structural aspects of healing in equine flexor digitorum superficialis tendons. *J Orthop Res.* **27**(10):1392–1398.

Shen, C.C. *et al.* (2015) Corrigendum to "Low-level laser stimulation on adipose-tissue-derived stem cell treatments for focal cerebral ischemia in rats." *Evid Based Complement Alternat Med.* **2015**:278951.

Soleimani, M. *et al.* (2012) The effects of low-level laser irradiation on differentiation and proliferation of human bone marrow mesenchymal stem cells into neurons and osteoblasts: an in vitro study. *Laser Med Sci.* **27**(2):423–430.

Stief, M. *et al.* (2011) Concentration of platelets and growth factors in canine autologous conditioned plasma. *Vet Comp Orthop Traumatol.* **24**(2):122–125.

Tobita, M. *et al.* (2013) Periodontal tissue regeneration by combined implantation of adipose tissue-derived stem cells and platelet-rich plasma in a canine model. *Cryotherapy.* **15**(12):1517–1526.

Torricelli, P. *et al.* (2011) Regenerative medicine for the treatment of musculoskeletal overuse injuries in competition horses. *Int Orthop.* **35**(10):1569–1576.

Tuby, H. *et al.* (2007) Low level laser irradiation promotes proliferation of mesenchymal and cardiac stem cells in culture. *Lasers Surg Med.* **39**(4):373–378.

Tuby, H. *et al.* (2011) Induction of autologous mesenchymal stem cells in the bone marrow by low-level laser therapy has profound beneficial effects on the infarcted rat heart. *Lasers Surg Med.* **43**(5):401–409.

Uysal, C.A. *et al.* (2012) Adipose-derived stem cells enhance primary tendon repair: biomechanical and immunohistochemical evaluation. *J Plast Reconstr Aesthet Surg.* **65**(12):1712–1719.

Wolfstadt, J.I. *et al.* (2015) Current concepts: the role of mesenchymal stem cells in the management of knee osteoarthritis. *Sports Health.* **7**(1):38–44.

Xie, X. *et al.* (2012) Comparative evaluation of MSCs from bone marrow and adipose tissue seeded in PRP-derived scaffold for cartilage regeneration. *Biomaterials.* **33**(29):7008–7018

Yang, C.C. *et al.* (2016) Synergistic effects of low-level laser and mesenchymal stem cells on functional recovery in rats with crushed sciatic nerves. *J Tissue Eng Regen Med.* **10**(2):120–131.

Yun, J.H. *et al.* (2014) Effects of bone marrow-derived mesenchymal stem cells and platelet-rich plasma on bone regeneration for osseointegration of dental implants: preliminary study in canine three-wall intrabony defects. *J Biomed Mater Res B Appl Biomater.* **102**(5):1021–1030.

Zarembinski, T.I. *et al.* (2011) The use of a hydrogel matrix as a cellular delivery vehicle in future cell-based therapies: biological and non-biological considerations. Available from: http://www.intechopen.com/books/regenerative-medicine-and-tissue-engineering-cells-and-biomaterials/the-use-of-a-hydrogel-matrix-as-a-cellular-delivery-vehicle-in-future-cell-based-therapies-biologica (accessed November 30, 2016).

Part XI

Integrating Laser Therapy into Veterinary Medicine

41

Successful Implementation and Marketing of Laser Therapy

Diane J. Miller

The Animal Athlete, Newark, DE, USA

Introduction

You now have a therapy laser or are considering purchasing one. This non-invasive product can have a huge impact on the way you practice medicine. However, simply introducing a laser will not automatically grow your business. Like anything in your practice, laser therapy is a business segment that needs to be nurtured in order to grow and flourish. Can it be done? Absolutely! Can you realize a significant revenue stream within a year? Absolutely! However, it will depend on how well you integrate laser therapy into your practice and build an infrastructure to support it. Numerous articles have appeared in veterinary trade publications and journals recently, detailing the implementation, integration, and economics of laser therapy (Andersen, 2014; Arp, 2009a, 2009b; Reeder, 2015; Tremayne, 2012; Zimlich, 2015). Despite the success stories featured in these articles, expecting your laser therapy business to grow without any planning or effort is unrealistic and sets you up for failure.

The business model for laser therapy is quite different from other traditional veterinary practice business models. We usually price an item based on a percentage markup or a flat dollar increase. That model makes sense for us. It is easy to handle in our practice-management software, it is something that we are familiar with, and it relates to most aspects of the practice. Laser therapy does not fit this model. Laser therapy, through the process of photobiomodulation (PBM), provides potential benefits in a vast array of disorders and conditions. The previous chapters have detailed the science, the mechanisms, and the many applications of PBM. All patients presented with pain, inflammation, or a process requiring healing may be candidates for laser. These attributes indicate that laser therapy will become part of multiple treatment protocols, and this can be rather intimidating when you are trying to integrate this modality in to your practice.

When I lecture about how to "Maximize Patient Care and Grow Your Bottom Line with Laser Therapy," I stress that thinking in terms of traditional marketing is a mistake. The world of direct mail, newspaper advertising, and yellow page ads is gone. These media are a waste of marketing dollars. The return on these methods is so low that the time to a breakeven point is measured in months, not days – if it ever comes.

If you look at laser therapy with a myopic view of traditional marketing techniques, you will have a difficult time implementing and maintaining a solid laser therapy foundation. Instead, look beyond your everyday experiences, and learn from other business models that are disconnected from the veterinary industry. Look at other unique businesses and see how they set up their infrastructure and pricing, how they handle customer service and other related business aspects. Their ideas may require some modification to fit the veterinary practice environment, but it will be well worth the effort.

In this chapter, you will see examples of different business strategies that will give you a better understanding of the elements you need to consider. There are many paths up the mountain, and these are in no way the only options. These concepts have been used by thousands of laser therapy practices, including companion, specialty, mixed, feline-only, equine-only, and mobile. Each has implemented these ideas and achieved results.

Pricing

One of the first questions to cross everyone's mind is, "How should I charge for laser therapy?" There is not a single answer that will satisfy the needs of all practices. Keep in mind that there are many options. However, if you follow the guidelines in this section, you will be able to develop a model that will work in almost any practice.

Pricing Guidelines

Avoid using subjective descriptions as pricing classifications (e.g., acute versus chronic). This is the first mistake

Laser Therapy in Veterinary Medicine: Photobiomodulation, First Edition. Edited by Ronald J. Riegel and John C. Godbold, Jr.
© 2017 John Wiley & Sons, Inc. Published 2017 by John Wiley & Sons, Inc.

most practices make. Using subjective descriptions guarantees that at some time there will be an error in estimating. "My dog has a reoccurring problem with otitis. Is this acute or chronic?" Unless there are absolute definitions established, you are setting yourself up for confusion.

All staff must be able to give the same estimate every time; therefore, pricing components and parameters must be consistent. The worst-case scenario is that clients come in for the same condition on different occasions, find the condition interpreted differently by staff, and are invoiced for different amounts for the same therapy. If a client is provided two different prices depending on who gave the estimate, there is a problem not with the staff, but with your pricing model.

Clients must be able to follow your pricing structure. Every time a client comes in for a laser therapy session, they need to understand what they are being billed for and how the fee was determined. Since photobiomodulation therapy (PBMT) can be included in multiple treatment protocols, a client may see a laser therapy fee for different species, different conditions, and different treatment durations.

Do not micromanage your pricing model. It is easy to get carried away and develop models that consider the condition, the length of treatment, and the species being treated. This can get out of hand very quickly. If the pricing model is confusing enough for your own staff to make errors, then you can imagine what it looks like to your client.

One of the biggest problems is pricing by species. Since they are smaller patients, the application of laser therapy to feline, avian, and exotic species takes less time. However, you will need an additional technician in the room to restrain such patients. Thus, therapy time is short, but the expenses associated with that time are high. When applying laser therapy to a canine, the treatment time will be greater, but the dog will likely be more cooperative, and the owner will be able to hold the leash while the dog lies or stands for the treatment. Therefore, the treatment time is longer but the expenses for that time is lower. These two scenarios thus even out in terms of revenue and expenses. As you devise a pricing structure, delve deeper into the process and consider the total expense associated with a treatment before assigning a fee.

Select a model that allows for the least number of practice-management software codes. It should not take your staff an exorbitant amount of time to locate the appropriate code and charge a client the correct amount. You should be able to develop a pricing structure with approximately 15 codes that will cover the majority of scenarios.

Core Pricing Structure

Notice in the following two examples how the fees are calculated by numbers rather than words ("acute versus chronic"). This means the fee determination is a numeric calculation and not a subjective interpretation.

1) **Core pricing by treatment site:** This model is based on the number of sites, body parts, or areas to be treated. The "Initial Site" charge is always billed. This is a higher fee, since it will cover the expenses associated with the services. Pricing for this is US$25–40 depending on the practice and the demographics. In addition, there are associated charges for "Additional Sites." This is a quantity field that depends on the number of sites treated. The fee is usually 50% of the "Initial Site" fee. By adding the "Additional Sites" to the "Initial Site," you calculate the total fee.

2) **Core pricing by block of time:** For some practices, mimicking their appointment schedule enables them to manage, book, and coordinate their laser therapy business. If the practice operates on 20-minute appointments, it is helpful to know that you can roughly treat two sites in a 20-minute block of time. The fee or charge for the first 20 minutes is approximately US$40, which covers the therapy of up to two sites. If the prescribed treatment protocol is more than two sites then the client will be charged for additional 20-minute blocks of time. As with the "by site" example, the additional slots of time will be at a reduced rate, usually about 50% of the initial fee.

The other pricing categories that will need to be taken into consideration are: post-surgical applications, dental applications, pre-paid bundles of three, six, nine, and twelve, and redeemed pre-paid sessions. The pricing for these will vary depending on your core pricing strategy.

The most significant takeaway is that it is imperative to minimize the chance of different estimate interpretations. Clients should not be confused about what they are being billed for each time their animal has laser therapy, regardless of the species or condition.

Internet, Website, and Social Media Marketing

Traditional marketing venues are no longer valid. The standard marketing tools for the promotion of our businesses, products, and services used to be newspaper advertising, yellow pages, and direct mail. Over the last 10 years, the Internet and social media have replaced these outdated tools. The continued investment of advertising dollars in older venues must be evaluated carefully, with hard core returns established and monitored.

Your website is a critical extension of you and your practice. Free, cookie-cutter sites are not sufficient long-term. Be cautious and look critically at the layout and photos being used on your site. If stock photos are supplied by the web designer then you stand the risk of them appearing on other sites.

One of the best marketing tools is photos of patients in laser-safe goggles. These are fun to see, eye-catching, and an excellent promoter of your laser therapy business. When clients see these cute pet photos, their immediate reactions are, "Why are they wearing them?" and, "I want a photo with my pet!" When using photos of pets receiving laser therapy in goggles at your practice, clients see familiar "landmarks." This makes the photos personal and unique to your practice, while showcasing this innovative treatment modality.

Search the Internet and look at a variety of websites, not just veterinary, to see what looks good and what doesn't from the perspective of the reader. Then, design your website with those thoughts in mind. It takes time and effort to build this important marketing tool.

Consider the audience when creating your website. For example, there needs to be different content for new versus existing clients. New clients need a lot more information about the practice itself. They have little or no experience or relationship with you. Therefore, you need to provide them with detailed information about your practice: who, what, when, and where. You should critically evaluate this information and ask yourself, "Why should they come to you?" That your practice is "nice" or "close" is not enough. Looking at your practice from this myopic perspective is not going to assist you in gaining or retaining clients. Your website will often provide a potential new client's first impression of your practice. It must be a fair and accurate representation.

The flip side is that your information also needs to appeal to existing clients. It is frustrating to view webpages that give line-item lists of services, with no additional information: Laser Therapy, Geriatrics, Wellness, Diagnostics, Laboratory, Surgery, Boarding, and Grooming often appear as a list of services. This type of information does not provide any significant medical or technical knowledge to your client. A line item like "Laser Therapy" requires additional information and clarification. You should link "Laser Therapy" to a whole page of technical information and sub-pages with testimonials, photos, and success stories. If it is important enough to mention, then it is important enough to provide technical and substantive information on. If sufficient information is not given, a client may perceive your practice as being lazy, as not having the knowledge, or as providing only a minimal version of the service. Remember, a client's perception is your reality.

Another by-product of inadequate web design is that you force clients to look elsewhere to obtain technical medical information. This leads your clients to other sites: your veterinary competition, blogs loaded with personal opinion wrapped up as authority, self-professed experts with a beautiful webpage. When you encourage browsing, clients may receive information that is inaccurate, medically dangerous, or contrary to your practice's philosophy regarding quality of care. Do not open the door to clients leaving your website to obtain additional information.

Your website is used to display information that is relatively static, whereas Facebook and other social media are primarily used to disseminate information that is rapidly changing. Social media, in some form, is a marketing must for today's practice. To use social media effectively, you need to make regular updates and posts. New videos of patients receiving treatments, pictures, and testimonials keep people involved.

Appeal to your clients' egos. Having their pet posted on your Facebook page wearing laser-safe goggles and getting their laser therapy treatment will generate a buzz. It will become a contest to see which pet's picture receives the most "likes." Client ego is good for your business if you execute it correctly and adhere to a regular posting schedule. Interspersing those postings with links to YouTube channels and technical and medical information about laser therapy and its benefits will not only keep clients engaged but will educate them before they even walk through your door.

Many laser therapy equipment manufacturers have YouTube channels and other sources of information that you can link to on Facebook and your website. By linking to appropriate information, you encourage clients to become self-educated, informed, and updated. Guiding them to accurate information regarding PBMT and its applications can help emphasize your own practice philosophies about the technology.

Regardless of which social media channels you decide to use, they must be monitored regularly to ensure that posts, comments, and tags are professional and appropriate. By regularly monitoring outside comments, you can also respond promptly to provide any necessary clarification.

The Internet is the communication tool of the future, and is critical to promoting your laser therapy business. Create laser therapy content on your website and in your social media platform that encourages visitors to submit emails, pet information, and questions, all of which can increase identification of laser therapy candidates. Making the most of the Internet by creating these tools and incentives will identify patients that can benefit from laser therapy and will increase the success of your marketing tactics.

Daily Communication Opportunities

If laser therapy is a new business segment for your practice, you have to spend the time and effort to develop, cultivate, and integrate it into your day-to-day activities. When you're busy practicing, it is easy to remain within your comfort zone and avoid that which is new; therefore, you will need to develop specific actions that effectively develop, cultivate, and integrate this new treatment modality into your practice. These actions can be anything from tagging appointments as laser opportunities to developing base protocols integrating laser therapy into the standard treatment of common conditions.

We are so busy in our day-to-day operations within our practices that we operate in a basic stimulus-response mode. Whatever situation presents itself to us in the moment is what we address. Rarely do we look past this and take an "aerial view" of what our day and our interactions look like. Unfortunately, when busy, we miss dozens of opportunities to integrate laser therapy into our treatment protocols and to educate our clients about this technology.

Every interaction with a client can be a laser opportunity: an opportunity to communicate who you are, how laser therapy differentiates you from other practices, how laser therapy impacts the quality of medicine you provide, and how laser therapy can benefit pets.

The 3P's of Communication

When a client comes in for an appointment, there are multiple opportunities to start the communication and education process. Effective communication requires that we Prepare for it, Provide it, and Personalize it.

Prepare

In veterinary practice, there is never enough time to educate clients about services and products. Especially when dealing with laser therapy, the education curve is significant, since this is a relatively new treatment modality. Staffing is stretched, and we often fall behind in appointments rather than get ahead of the schedule, so having time to discuss the features and benefits of laser therapy with each client is not always possible.

Preparing clients with rudimentary information about laser therapy before they come to the practice can help in effectively communicating with them during the visit. Some of the most effective tools for this process are the Internet and other electronic information channels. Websites and social media, email blasts, and on-hold messaging are examples.

Collecting email addresses is a vital component of preparing your clients, and should be a priority. Email is a free communication tool that allows you to share a whole new dimension of information. Email gives you the ability to embed links to videos, send targeted, market-specific information, and link recipients to your website. You can communicate with substantive information and allow recipients to review the material at their convenience, while reducing advertising expenditures drastically.

Provide

Provide clients with quality information during their visit to the practice. Use this time to educate them with detailed information, photos, videos, testimonials, and presentations. Information displays should include not only what's on the walls, but also the materials present throughout the lobby and exam rooms.

A practice is not a repository of expired magazines. These publications have no positive impact on your business. If it seems there is neither the staff nor the time to educate your client base about medical and technical issues, then don't encourage clients to read materials that provide no medical or business benefit. All publications, materials, and displays should have some value to the business and practice.

Develop laser therapy literature with a list of conditions that PBMT can be used for on one side, and text about your laser therapy services on the other. Laminate this resource and place it on chairs throughout the lobby. Usually, when a client picks something up from a chair before sitting, they will look at it. They should first see the list with their pet's condition included, then flip the document over to read about laser therapy and how it can help. You have thus prepared them with laser therapy information prior to getting them into the exam room. This has the opportunity to impact your business; outdated, non-related magazines do not.

Personalize

Personalize the information you provide: "What does laser therapy mean for my pet?" Translate materials and communications into impact statements for the client.

Achieve client compliance by taking pictures and videos of pet treatments. This can be a huge asset on multiple levels. In essence, you are making the intangible tangible in the client's mind. Developing an infrastructure that incorporates photos and videos into laser therapy treatment protocols will be a substantial business asset and will make the laser therapy experience very personal. Re-creating a client experience via photos or videos is invaluable. For example, videos are essential when getting new clients to accept laser therapy for osteoarthritis, and when documenting improvement of a pet's quality of life through laser therapy follow-up maintenance sessions.

Appointment Process Touch Points

The entire appointment process and patient visit offers multiple opportunities to Prepare, Provide, and Personalize communications (Figure 41.1).

Published Practice Information (Prepare)

Regularly updating information on social media and ensuring that your website is informative provides the first touch point of the appointment process. By using

Figure 41.1 Appointment process touch points.

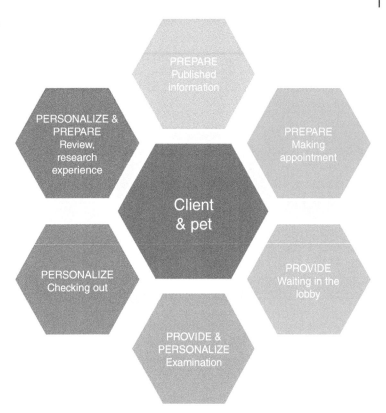

Internet communication tools, you can highlight technical products and services like laser therapy. This allows clients to learn and experience technical aspects before coming to the practice.

Sending email blasts that link clients directly to online portals can help educate them at their convenience. Many therapy laser manufacturers have technical information posted on their websites and YouTube channels. They often show unique case studies with wonderful results that can encourage your clients to consider PBMT as a treatment option for their pet. Links like these help fill the information gap. Creating links within emails requires minimal effort and creates an entirely new quality communication tool. Email is a free marketing tool that becomes available when a concerted effort is made to collect and continually update email addresses.

Making the Appointment (Prepare)

Analyze how an appointment is processed and how a patient visit is routed through your practice. Take into consideration what materials and steps are used from the moment the client enters the building through their exit. Create reminders along the pathway for staff, and tools they can use to encourage clients to accept laser therapy as an option.

Tagging appointments when they are made allows your staff to be prepared for a laser opportunity before the client walks through the door. Tagging can involve noting the appointment in the practice software, highlighting travel sheets, placing notices on examination room doors, and distributing brochures to clients when they check in. Each of these actions is designed to remind the staff and the client of laser therapy as a treatment option during the appointment.

Lobby (Provide)

Many practices keep Christmas pictures and cards posted year round. Yes, it gives a warm, fuzzy feeling, but these displays don't create income to pay staff salaries, the electric bill, or the lease. Limit this season-specific display to the month of December. During the remaining months, a more appropriate use of the space is to display pictures of laser therapy patients with their goggles on. This will create excitement and initiate questions, and can have a positive impact on your practice revenue. There is nothing wrong with warm and fuzzy, but there has to be a practice pay off as well. Look critically at all of your materials and how they can increase your business. Don't sacrifice warm and fuzzy: complement it.

Exam Room (Provide and Personalize)

Videos are a critical component of successful laser therapy client acceptance. They do not have to be lengthy, nor do they have to win any Academy Awards.

When documenting osteoarthritis, for example, videos need to present the animal in multiple motion states and be consistent in format. Videos should be taken in the same location within the practice and should consist of the same motion exercises. Record patients as they walk up and down a hallway in a frontal and posterior view, then while they are sitting, lying down, and getting up. These views will enable a client to see their pet's progress in multiple motion states during the course of multiple therapy sessions.

By recording videos, comparisons can be drawn as treatment progresses. Seeing the first video prior to commencing laser therapy and comparing it to the latest session will present a dramatic benefit picture for the client. This successful progression creates client compliance to continue with additional laser therapy treatments. Without videos, you are asking clients to remember what a pet looked like several weeks ago. They will likely not remember all the subtle progress that has been made.

An additional benefit is that the video becomes a sales tool for others considering laser therapy. When you describe laser therapy to them and present videos of other pets with similar circumstances, they're able to visualize what you are trying to accomplish, and you stand a better chance of getting them to accept laser therapy as part of their treatment program.

Checking Out (Personalize)

Invoices are the one communication tool that every client walks out of the practice with. Rather than considering this document a business by-product, think of it as a valuable means of communication. Placing a label on the bottom of the invoice with information about laser therapy, or a special offer, can promote the technology and turn an unread or unacknowledged document into a marketing opportunity. Staff should point out this additional information to the client in order to maximize invoices as a new revenue-generating tool.

Developing a Medical Infrastructure

Creating Base Protocols

Developing base protocols and integrating laser therapy into them will not only increase your laser therapy business, it will also increase revenue from additional services. Make a habit of integrating laser therapy into three new protocols every quarter, so that an increasing number of protocols are in place that include laser therapy and are consistent for your entire team.

As an example, consider how your practice manages a wound of unknown origin. This common feline presentation may go undetected for a period of time before an abscess is noted. Your practice already has a standard-of-care base protocol for treating this presentation. It may include clipping, cleaning of the wound, application of laser therapy, and application of systemic and topical antibiotics. Veterinarians don't ask permission to clip

and clean wounds. We come from a position of power and automatically say we are going to do so. However, after that, we often want to apologize and explain away what we wish to do.

What we should explain to the pet owner is this: "We are going to clip and clean the wound (obvious reason, we usually do not explain further), we are going to apply PBMT to it (this will help to reduce pain, inflammation, and speed healing), and we will provide you an antibiotic to help combat the infection (obvious reason)." The client hears a coherent treatment plan that makes sense.

When you develop protocols in this fashion, the client has an understanding of all of the components necessary to improve their pet's health and speed their healing. The more confident the practice is in providing a medical treatment protocol, the more likely the pet owner will comply.

Though we would like for clients to act solely in their pet's best interest, we know that sometimes they take actions based on their own convenience or needs. Include comments that emphasize the impact of your protocol on their time and convenience. This will personalize the plan and get a more positive response to your treatment suggestions. If you use a long-acting antibiotic injection, saying, "This is because after day 2, I know you cannot pull the cat out from underneath the couch without getting sliced and diced" creates a picture of the impact it will have on them. Money becomes less of a deciding factor and convenience has a greater value. The resulting benefit is that the cat gets the antibiotic you ultimately wish to prescribe.

Creating base protocols using this approach will increase overall service revenue, while providing pets with quality medical care that meets your standards.

One Voice and One Message

Veterinarians have different preferences for drugs, treatment protocols, and other medical techniques. In general, this diversity has minimal impact on the day-to-day operations of a practice. When introducing laser therapy into the business model, however, there must be a united consensus on when and where this technology should be applied. Failure to achieve such a consensus can result in client distrust of medical recommendations and erode confidence in the practice as a whole.

For example: I am a client of Dr. A. My pets have been seeing him for years, and he has recommended laser therapy for a variety of conditions. We have used laser therapy for wounds, otitis, and hotspots. We have used it in addition to cytology, cleaning, and topical medication. Dr. A is on vacation and my pet has an otitis issue. I go to see Dr. B at the same practice. I do not expect any surprises. However, we get to the end of the appointment and there has been no mention of laser therapy. When I ask Dr. B about this, she responds, "It's not necessary;

you should be all right without it." As a client, I hear one of two messages, and neither of them is good. The first is that Dr. A has been padding the bill and I have been getting laser therapy when it is unwarranted. The second is that Dr. B is not practicing quality medicine. Neither of these messages is acceptable.

When you are introducing a new treatment protocol that includes laser therapy, it is imperative that the practice team is united and provides the same message. By developing these treatment protocols, you will provide clients with a uniform message and quality of care.

Advise with Conviction

Clients look to us as experts with all the answers who can provide a course of action that is guaranteed to be a success. That is far from the case. Diagnosis and treatment is a complicated puzzle. Sometimes, the pieces do not fit until you get further in, and then you find they do not add up to a whole picture. However, we set ourselves up to have clients refuse our recommendations when we start with an expression of apology.

Our everyday language consists of qualifying words such as "try," "could," "would like to," and "maybe." When we use these words, our clients hear, "The treatment may or may not work," "This is unnecessary," or "I want you to pay for something unnecessary." This applies not only to laser therapy, but to every treatment protocol and client interaction. By using these words, we set ourselves up for client refusal, as they do not support the quality of medicine to which our clients and their pets are entitled.

As when changing any longstanding habits, there must to be a concerted effort to remove these words from our everyday business vocabulary. We do our clients and their pets a disservice if we do not medically advise with conviction.

Everybody on Board

Describing laser therapy to a client can be an overwhelming task. Defining and explaining PBMT can be daunting. Nonetheless, clients do need some explanation of what laser therapy is, why it is referred to as "PBMT," how it works, and what its benefits are for their pet. Developing a standardized message about laser therapy for the entire practice is very important in getting clients to accept it, and is not nearly as intimidating as it sounds.

One of the basic analogies to use in explaining PBMT is to photosynthesis. Regardless of the educational background of your client, they know about photosynthesis. Using photosynthesis as an analogy is helpful for the layperson: "Sunlight hits a plant and through the process of photosynthesis the plant grows." We can take this a step further, and use the same idea in describing laser therapy: "We have found that when certain wavelengths of light come in contact with human or animal cells, their activity is stimulated. This activity reduces inflammation, reduces

pain, and speeds healing." Though this definition is simplistic, it does help the client have a basic understanding of what is happening to their pet. More technical and scientific information can be given if the client requests it. Brochures from your laser therapy equipment manufacturer, links to your webpage (containing additional links to technical and scientific information), case studies, or a simple one-page handout with detailed information can be provided.

Regardless of how you approach laser therapy education with your client, it is critical that the entire team has a fundamental grasp of the core message and its impact. Each member will have a unique mode of delivering or of talking about laser therapy, but the core medical and technical information must be consistent.

Communication Tools

There are many existing communication tools currently in use in practices that we underutilize as marketing tools. These are often free, or through the economies of scale, have minimal costs associated with them. They provide additional marketing exposure for products and services such as laser therapy. Some of these tools do require additional infrastructure design and support in order to incorporate them into laser therapy marketing, but these changes should become part of your business practices. These existing communication tools include invoices, vaccine reminders, email blasts, on-hold messaging, social media, and activities within the practice.

To successfully use communication tools, there are specific considerations that should be addressed with every marketing effort. The days of "just placing an ad" or "donating to a club" are long gone. Calculated evaluations should take place for each and every marketing endeavor, in order to decide whether or not to do it again.

Know the Goal

You must have a goal in order to evaluate success. If you are investing resources, you should know what you hope to gain. Is it clients sending you laser therapy success stories? More photos of patients in goggles? More commitments for laser therapy bundles? Greater acceptance of laser therapy as an exam-room treatment option? There may be instances where the goal is not monetary but rather increased awareness. Regardless, the goal should be determined before initiating marketing using a communication tool.

Monitor Success

Any laser therapy marketing endeavor requires a quantitative measure of success. At minimum, one should know the breakeven point and be able to calculate the return on investment. Data should be tracked, monitored, and regularly evaluated.

Make Information Audience-Appropriate

The audience determines the marketing message. The type of information used to communicate laser therapy to your clients can be based on specific conditions. Marketing to clients with senior pets presenting an osteoarthritis-related condition should be different from marketing to clients whose patients have hot spots. Communications cannot be everything to everyone, or they end up being nothing at all.

Include a Call to Action

Marketing messages need to provide a reason or incentive for a client to take action. This incentive could be in the form of discounts, information, opportunities, or something else. The call to action should require a client to partake of a product or service within a specified time frame. Examples are encouraging clients to schedule an appointment for a free laser therapy assessment or purchasing six laser therapy sessions and getting one free.

Establish a Reasonable Time Frame

Ensure that the client has a reasonable time frame within which to take action and avail themselves of the marketing offer. In most cases, the time frame should be no less than 30 days and no more than 90. Fewer than 30 days may not allow enough people to become aware of your laser therapy offer and take action. More than 90 allows too much time to elapse before clients have to decide, contributing to a lack of urgency.

Targeting Elite Markets

Do not limit your target market. There are many different market segments that can appreciate and utilize laser therapy. Some will require added investigation to locate, but most special-interest groups and clubs can easily be found via the Internet. The examples in this section should make you look at your clients and community differently.

Pet Insurance

Clients with pet insurance are often more willing to try something non-traditional, as long as it is covered by their plan. We surveyed the 11 known pet insurance companies in the United States at the time of writing, and 10 reimbursed for laser therapy (a supplemental "rehabilitation" or "premium" policy may be required). Knowing this, your practice should be recommending pet insurance programs that reimburse for laser therapy,

and identifying clients with insurance in the practice-management software. Ensuring that clients know their insurance covers laser therapy is good for both the practice and the pet. The pet insurance industry has changed, and the reimbursement process usually no longer affects billing and payment for the practice. The biggest win with pet insurance is that pets can receive the care and services that the veterinarian recommends. Money does not become a limiting factor for the acceptance of recommended treatments.

Performance Animals

Performance animals are animal athletes. Some of the more common canine performance activities are agility, field trial, flyball, and Schutzhund. Dogs performing these very strenuous, endurance-oriented programs can receive a tremendous benefit from the regular administration of laser therapy. Pre- and post-event laser therapy sessions can provide a warm-up and assist with recuperation (Borsa *et al.*, 2013). Since dogs participating in these sports are often costly, and owners have invested considerable time and money in them, keeping them physically fit and injury-free is a priority. The importance of laser therapy in the care of canine athletes is detailed in Chapter 20.

Figure 41.2 depicts a performance dog competing in Schutzhund. In pictures of the protection and obedience work shown, you can envision the speed as the dog approaches the helper, and the momentum as it takes the grip and follows through. Note the body positioning, especially of the spine. Look at the curve of the dog's spine and the location of its rear quarters in relation to its shoulders. PBMT is truly a benefit to these animals, as it allows them to maintain their level of performance. The same is true of the physical demands and needs of police and military dogs.

Laser therapy is equally important to equine athletes. The physical stress on performance horses and their propensity for injury are significant. Incorporating laser therapy into an equine practice is easy, since portable, battery-powered devices are available. The new higher-power lasers allow deep penetration into tissues and reasonable treatment times even in large horses.

Service Dogs

Service dogs work across a diverse list of fields, including detection disciplines (explosives, cadaver, drug), handicap assistance, military, police, and search and rescue. Creating a laser therapy program for service dogs helps them minimize injuries, facilitates their recuperation, and keeps them on the job. It is a benefit to the animal and to the community to keep these dogs working. If you do not have a program or plan to offer laser therapy for service dogs, make it a priority to develop one.

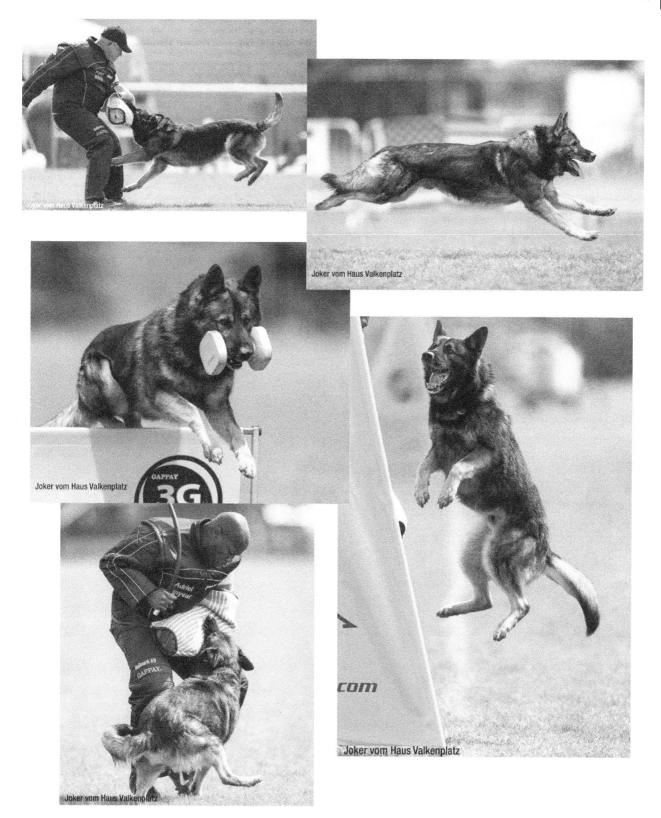

Figure 41.2 A performance dog competing in Schutzhund.

Conclusion

Effective integration of laser therapy into the veterinary practice requires a business plan. Most successful practices have looked at the individual marketing components and outlined steps with action items to ensure that key elements are addressed. The goal is to have a laser therapy program that is self-sustaining, meshes with existing processes, and elevates the quality of patient care. Be realistic and self-critical in your marketing efforts. Traditional marketing channels are no longer effective. Continuing to invest time and money with minimal results is not a sound business strategy. Constant vigilance is needed to weed out marketing programs that are ineffective.

To successfully integrate laser therapy, you will need to step outside the box and be daring, looking at other successful professions and adapting their marketing techniques to fit veterinary medicine. With focused efforts, much can be accomplished that will not only increases your laser therapy business, but also provide patients with increased quality of care.

References

Andersen, D. (2014) Vets say why they use laser therapy. *Vet Pract News*. August 20.

Arp, D. (2009a) Lasers financially therapeutic, too. *Vet Pract News*. April 17.

Arp, D. (2009b) Spreading the warmth. *Vet Pract News*. August 31.

Borsa, P.A. *et al.* (2013) Does phototherapy enhance skeletal muscle contractile function and postexercise recovery? A systematic review. *J Athl Training.* **48**(1):57–67.

Reeder, J. (2015) Fired up about lasers. *Trends*. December.

Tremayne, J. (2012) Lasers offer a therapeutic plan for pain. *Vet Pract News*. August 6.

Zimlich, R. (2015) Two practices shine light on laser therapy in the veterinary business model. *Vet Econ*. June 1.

42

The Role of Veterinary Technicians and Nurses in Laser Therapy

Renaud Houyoux[1] and Laura Kortelainen[2]

[1] *Companion Animal Health, Newark, DE, USA*
[2] *Evidensia Finland, Järvenpää, Finland*

Veterinary Technicians

The veterinary technician has a crucial role in all aspects of laser therapy in veterinary medicine. Educating the client, administering and documenting treatments, adjusting treatment protocols and time frames, and keeping the attending veterinarian apprised of the patient's progression are all important tasks the technician must undertake and oversee in order to provide optimal care for the patient.

The therapy laser is a technician's tool. Laser therapy is prescribed by the veterinarian, and it is the technician's responsibility to fill the prescription.

The technician must ensure that all patients with applicable conditions are given the opportunity to benefit from this modality. If it is painful, inflamed, or needs to be healed, it is a candidate for laser therapy (Farivar *et al.*, 2014; Fulop *et al.*, 2010; Karu, 1999; Pryor and Millis, 2015). The dedicated technician will keep his or her ears trained to listen for any word with the suffix "-itis," an indication that the patient may be a candidate for laser therapy.

It is crucial to have a key technician who will oversee the use of the laser and nurture other team members to make sure this modality is used to its fullest potential. This technician often has a dual role, also serving as the Laser Safety Officer for the practice. This title makes them responsible for the safe use of the therapy laser and ensuring that all persons handling the laser are properly trained (Barat, 2006; Oleson, 2016).

The ability to think outside the box and to be adaptive to different situations is a crucial requirement of the effective laser technician. For example, while it is not recommended that serial treatments be performed on active growth plates (de Oliveira *et al.*, 2013), it is not contraindicated to administer a single palliative treatment to an acute epiphysitis case (Oliveira *et al.*, 2012; Son *et al.*, 2012), or to treat a puppy with active epiphyses

for parvoviral enteritis abdominal pain. An example of the "adapt and overcome" mantra might be where a patient is sensitive to the use of needles in acupuncture. Photonic energy could instead be administered to the acupuncture points, often with the same results as needling (de Oliveira and de Freitas, 2016) (e.g., in the treatment of point P6 to prevent nausea in a patient undergoing chemotherapy treatments: see Figure 42.1; Lorenzini *et al.*, 2010).

Laser therapy has a bright and promising future. The veterinary technician plays an important role in its continued development. As our knowledge and understanding of its mechanisms continue to grow, technicians will be able to apply this modality to patients more efficiently and comprehensively.

The Technician's Role in Client Communication and Preparation

Just as in many other aspects of veterinary medicine, the entire veterinary team must have a unified, core message for the client about laser therapy. As when explaining the benefits of good dental care, it is usually the responsibility of the veterinary technician to explain to the client the basics of laser therapy. The veterinary technician often introduces the term "photobiomodulation therapy" (PBMT) (Anders *et al.*, 2015) and explains how this non-invasive, non-pharmacological modality will benefit a patient with pain, inflammation, or a need for tissue healing and normalization (Chung *et al.*, 2012).

When a client hears the term "laser," they will more than likely think of those medical lasers with which they are most familiar: the surgical and invasive lasers. Like surgical lasers, therapy lasers produce a coherent, cohesive, and collimated beam of light. That is where the likeness ends. Surgical and therapeutic lasers operate with greatly different wavelengths and power densities. The different combinations of these parameters determine the effect that laser light has on organic tissues. With a

Laser Therapy in Veterinary Medicine: Photobiomodulation, First Edition. Edited by Ronald J. Riegel and John C. Godbold, Jr.
© 2017 John Wiley & Sons, Inc. Published 2017 by John Wiley & Sons, Inc.

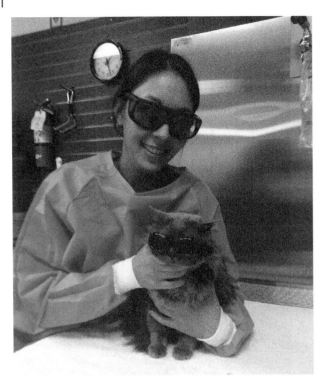

Figure 42.1 Chemotherapy patient prior to treatment with a laser therapy acupuncture protocol to prevent nausea. Chemotherapy follows laser therapy.

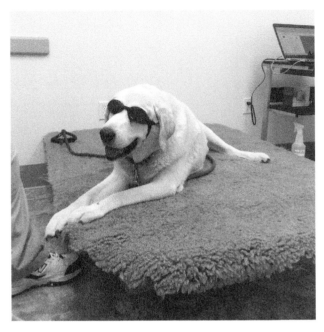

Figure 42.2 Relaxed and comfortable patient eager to begin a laser therapy session.

surgical laser, the energy is absorbed by the tissues, and the tissues are ablated (vaporized) through a photothermal effect. With therapy lasers, the energy is absorbed by the tissues, producing a photochemical effect that results in photobiomodulation (PBM).

Very few clients will be interested in learning about the physics of laser therapy. It is usually counterproductive to go into the details of population inversions, metastable states of electrons, and how photons share properties of both waves and particles with clients who simply want to seek a non-invasive approach to healing their precious companion who is in pain or physically debilitated.

The easiest way to get across to clients the concept of PBM is to make it analogous to other processes of light interaction with tissues that are commonly known and understood by lay people, such as photosynthesis in plants or vitamin D synthesis. These are similar enough that the correlation can be made, allowing the client to grasp the concept of PBM and thus feel much more comfortable and compliant as they proceed with the treatment.

It can be challenging to convey to a client that laser therapy is a scientific and evidence-based modality. If the technician is able to get across, in lay terms, how it works, the client will perceive the value of the modality and will be much more likely to accept laser therapy treatments.

Patient Preparation and Habituation

Veterinary patients are much more adaptive creatures than are humans. Whereas humans tend to dwell on things and over-rationalize, animals live in the moment and take everything as is, without wasting any time feeling sorry for themselves or questioning why things are the way they are. It is a victory for us as medical professionals, and for the patients entrusted to our care, if we as technicians can make a moment minimally painful and potentiate the body's ability to heal more quickly and effectively.

The patient needs to be assessed as an individual, taking into account breed, age, predispositions, pre-existing conditions, lifestyle, and current medical modalities, including any pharmaceuticals the patient is receiving. It makes sense that a young and otherwise healthy patient will be able to respond more effectively and more quickly than a geriatric patient, which may have pre-existing conditions already taxing its body's energy and its overall ability to function and repair itself.

Patients will very quickly habituate to laser therapy treatments; they quickly learn that these sessions are non-invasive and relatively short. It is not uncommon for a client to report that their dog is actually eager to come in for a treatment (Figure 42.2). Patients quickly correlate a palliative response to therapy. They often visibly relax during treatment, and actually offer access to the treatment site, or lean into the therapy laser handpiece as the treatment is administered. Successive treatment sessions become more relaxed as the patient's pain is reduced and the client comes to appreciate how his or her companion is able to resume historical behaviors that had been lost due to injury or the progression of osteoarthritis and degenerative joint disease.

Some patients with extreme pain or advanced chronic disease may require an extended habituation to treatment. They may be too sensitive in the early part of treatment to allow direct contact of the handpiece to the treatment site, movement of joints through range of motion, or a massage technique. As long as the patient is improving, it is acceptable to allow them to respond as an individual, and to give them the time they need to reach their peak plateau of response and habituation. No two patients or conditions are alike. The treatment plan, just like the administration of the treatment, needs to be tailored to the specific needs and responses of the patient as an individual.

Short-Term versus Chronic Treatment in Phases

The specific condition being treated will determine the frequency and duration of ongoing treatments. Laser therapy treatments have a cumulative effect; they build upon one another. For acute, curable conditions (e.g., otitis externa, a snakebite wound), a series of treatments should be administered until complete resolution is achieved. A different approach can be taken when treating a chronic condition such as osteoarthritis. Chronic conditions are by nature incurable, but they can be managed and maintained, and their degenerative nature can be altered to be less aggressive and progressive. Since we cannot completely cure most chronic conditions, the goal is to promote comfort and mobility, realizing that each patient will have an individual peak plateau response.

There are multiple ways to design a treatment plan for patients presenting with either an acute or a chronic condition. While it is possible to underdose a patient with an inadequate total target dose (the total amount of energy delivered to the target tissues), or to carry out treatment inappropriately, it is difficult, if not impossible, to overdose a patient. Damaged cells repairing themselves via PBM will only respond when the metabolic rate is less than normal. Healthy tissue cannot become "super tissue" through PBM. The best way to treat a patient is to re-evaluate at each presentation and adjust the treatment plan accordingly.

If there is any level of pain, it needs to be addressed. When a patient presents with pain, it is appropriate to treat daily until a clinical response is noted. If the patient is in intractable pain, it is advantageous to treat more often, such as twice daily. Once a clinical response is noted, an every-other-day treatment frequency is recommended until resolution, or until a peak plateau in response is achieved. With chronic conditions, the cumulative effect of multiple treatments will then enable a tapering in treatment frequency to maintain the peak plateau response.

With chronic conditions, the frequency of treatment should be tapered once the patient has reached the initial therapeutic goal. With tapering, ongoing treatment phases are designed with increased times between treatments. As long as the patient does not have any setbacks, this tapering can continue.

Prevention of setbacks while maintaining a clinical effect is the key to effective tapering. Regardless of the planned treatment time frame, the client must understand that the patient needs to return immediately if there are any setbacks. The plan is only a plan; the patient needs to be treated as an individual. This is where each patient's unique physical status, daily routine and lifestyle, and potential secondary diseases come into play. No two patients are alike; treat the individual appropriately.

Fortunately, only a small percentage of patients are beyond the reach of therapy. With an appropriate treatment plan, tailored for the individual, a clinical response and improvement are usually noted.

Technician Treatment Tips and Techniques

Administering laser therapy treatments is actually an art when you consider the intricacies involved. The laser technician should adapt and individualize their technique for each patient. Even though treatments are usually short in duration and do not hurt, we can't take away all the years of regular veterinary visits, which may have included rectal temperature checks, blood draws, or other uncomfortable procedures. The savvy technician will assume a non-threatening body language and tone of voice, and help the patient relax during the treatment.

Done correctly, the treatment should be comfortable and not cause any pain. Treatments are non-invasive, require no sedation, and can be done on an outpatient basis in a relatively short amount of time. The client can be present during treatments, and can take an active role.

Laser therapy treatments should be exactly what the name implies: therapeutic. So should be the setting in which they are conducted. Design a setting that is as therapeutic psychologically as is the physiological effect on the tissues. If possible, use a room specifically designed for therapy laser treatments. Make it a quiet and comfortable environment for the patient, the technician, and the client.

Small patients can be treated on a table, bringing them up to a comfortable level for the technician. Treatments for larger patients can be done either on the floor or on a raised platform large enough for the patient, technician, and client (Figure 42.3). Regardless of where the patient is treated, it should be able to lie on a very comfortable surface with good footing. Thick fleece liners, which can be cut to any shape, are ideal, and provide good traction and enhanced comfort for all involved.

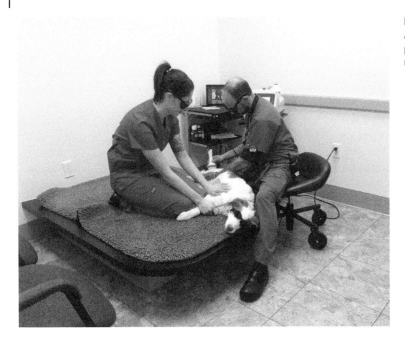

Figure 42.3 Laser therapy patient being treated on a padded, raised platform that is comfortable for patient, technician, client, and assisting staff members.

Manage the environment to create a relaxed, comfortable experience. Soft, natural lighting will provide a calming sensation during the treatment. Aromatics may be calming, but be careful with their use since some clients may respond negatively to certain odors. Natural, soothing sounds (such as birds chirping or a babbling brook) can be played at a low level. Have treats and catnip on hand as well; patients are easily bribed. Treats provide an extra touch of care and empathy to patients and clients. The perception of the client will go a long way to ensuring their willingness to comply with ongoing treatment recommendations.

Occasionally, a client will report that a patient suffering from a chronic condition seemed a little stiffer the afternoon or evening after the first few treatments. This is actually a positive sign of response, indicating that the patient's tissues are being affected by PBM. Typically, these symptoms are low-grade and transient, do not cause severe pain, and do not last more than 24 hours. If they are noted early in the treatment phase, it is encouraging, since it points to the patient's physical ability to respond.

When given the option, it is always more efficient to make light and steady contact with the tissues in order to maximize photon transmission into them (Figure 42.4). However, there will be times when a contact technique will not be possible, such as with an intraoperative treatment of a sterile surface like a closed cystotomy incision or an anastomosis site (Kirkby *et al.*, 2012). When not in contact with the tissue, the laser technician may choose to increase the total target dose by 20–40% to account for surface scatter of photons.

Treating the appropriate target site is, of course, necessary. The nearby healthy tissues should be treated as

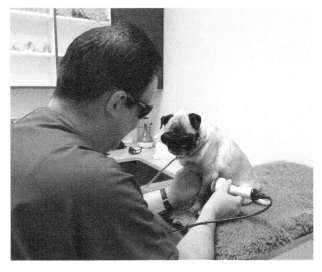

Figure 42.4 Laser therapy being administered with the handpiece perpendicular to and in contact with the target tissues.

well. In order to do this, the laser beam needs to make a full excursion over the affected area, as well as the nearby healthy tissue margins. Proper illumination of the target tissues and nearby healthy tissues will ensure an optimal response from the patient. The handpiece needs to be perpendicular to the target tissues to ensure a uniform beam spot on the tissues being treated.

When treating limbs or any part of an extremity, treatment should be administered in a circumferential manner to ensure complete photon penetration into the tissue. If the patient will allow it, joints should be moved through a passive range of motion while treating. With severely affected and painful patients, this may not always be possible during initial treatments. Most patients will habituate to treatments and reach a comfort level where they will allow some degree of motion. Putting a joint through a passive range of motion ensures that the photonic energy reaches all of the target tissues and intra-articular surfaces. Monitoring of these sites by taking goniometric measurements at presentation and during ensuing treatments can be an effective tool in documenting the patient's progress.

When treating an extremity, it is also recommended to perform a separate treatment to the spinal nerve root segments innervating that limb. Treating this site will optimize the treatment done on the extremity by reducing the transmission of painful stimuli (Chow *et al.*, 2007).

Laser therapy should always be applied to any secondary, tertiary, and compensatory sites. For example, when treating the hip joint, it is helpful to palpate the pectineus muscle, which originates on the pubic crest and inserts on the medial shaft of the femur. It is useful to assess how tight, sensitive, or reactive the pectineus muscle is to palpation. Often, a patient having hip discomfort will have compensatory pain in the pectineus muscle, which will be very tight and reactive, even to the lightest of palpation. Continuing to palpate this muscle as further treatments are carried out can be a useful tool by which to assess the patient's progress.

Another example of a compensatory site that should be treated in any hind-limb musculoskeletal disorder is the iliopsoas muscles. The iliopsoas muscles originate from the ventral aspect of lumbar vertebrae L2–L7 and insert on the lesser trochanters, and are frequent sites of compensatory pain.

With all treatments, the laser technician should be mindful of the need to monitor the patient for any reactivity or sensitivity to specific trigger points in the tissues being treated. If the patient does exhibit a focal sensitivity, special attention should be paid to that area. Monitoring decreased reactivity to previously sensitive trigger points is another good way to measure the patient's progression in response to laser therapy treatments.

Treatment Documentation by the Technician

Just like all medical treatments, each laser therapy treatment needs to be included in the patient's medical record. The most efficient way of doing this is to design a form that is incorporated in the patient's daily record. This form should include specifics such as the date of treatment, the name of the laser technician, the attending veterinarian, and treatment specifics (sites being treated, power, time, the target dose delivered to each site). It is also important for this form to include the technician's notes about the patient's progress or response to treatments. Notes about the patient's progress are crucial, since they allow all of the practice's

technicians to have current information, regardless of who is administering the treatment. Documenting the patient's progress helps determine the need for further treatments and at what time intervals they should be applied, and it can be used by the attending veterinarian to declare resolution of a condition.

Documentation of laser therapy treatments in the patient's medical record is as imperative with laser therapy, as with all other modalities in veterinary medicine. If it is not documented, it did not happen. It is the technician's responsibility to make it happen.

The Veterinary Technician's Role in the Evolution and Future of Laser Therapy

While there remains much to learn about laser therapy, it has proven to be valid, safe, and effective when used appropriately (Mandel and Hamblin 2012). As the science continues to develop, so will our understanding of its potential, and we will learn to fully harness the power of PBMT. The accomplished technician will be wise to stay at the forefront of this dynamic and rapidly evolving aspect of veterinary medicine. Technicians should also monitor continuing technological developments that facilitate patient evaluation while undergoing laser therapy. Examples are digital thermal imaging units and stance analyzers. Just as technicians have played a significant role in the advancement of laser therapy, so too can they play a significant role in the incorporation of allied technologies.

This is a unique and exciting time to be a veterinary technician. Laser therapy gives us a non-invasive tool that can actually heal tissues instead of simply attenuating symptoms of underlying disease. It is the experienced technician's responsibility to pass on knowledge about laser therapy to newcomers in our ranks, and to help ignite the spark of motivation and innovation integral in furthering this technology as it continues to develop.

There is a point in each technician's career when it is their duty to ensure the torch is being passed on. Though the experience we gather as we work through the years belongs to us as individuals, the knowledge that we gain does not. This knowledge must be shared for the benefit of our patients and the medical community as a whole. With veterinary medicine, knowledge is power. It is the seasoned technician's Hippocratic Oath and duty to share this knowledge and power for the benefit of the patients entrusted to their care.

Veterinary Nurses

Though their titles, background and training, and points of interest may vary, veterinary nurses join veterinary technicians in using laser therapy to achieve the same result: helping to improve the lives of their patients. This portion of the chapter gives an international perspective on the important role veterinary nurses play in laser therapy around the world.

Laser therapy offers huge opportunities to veterinary practices when the technology is implemented and properly used (Reeder, 2015). Nurses are vital to the success of laser therapy. They are instrumental in its implementation in the practice and in the development of practice procedures for laser use. Nurses should have the responsibility of overseeing laser training for the staff. They should help establish both scheduling procedures and fee structures. Since nurses know the clients and customer base, they can help plan and target marketing. With their knowledge of the practice's information-technology system, nurses can ensure proper laser record keeping and effective communication about laser therapy with clients. In addition, since nurses administer laser therapy to patients, they have the one-on-one opportunity to positively affect the lives of patients and their owners (Jergler, 2013).

The Nurse's Role in Laser Therapy Training

Your practice has decided to invest in a therapy laser. You have thought through the indications you are going to use it for, researched your patient records, and identified candidates for therapy. You have established a scheduling process that will allocate enough time to administer this therapy to your patients. The staff has heard about laser therapy, and is now excited to have a new technology. The next important step is training.

Organized training needs to be established before the first laser therapy treatment. With proper training, all staff will have the necessary information and the basic principles for everyday use. It is important that the entire staff has the right attitude and believes in the usefulness of laser therapy. If anyone has any doubts about the technology, they should be addressed during initial training so that everyone supports its successful implementation.

In every practice, there should be a person who is responsible for the laser, ensures everyone is properly trained, and maintains all the information about laser therapy in one place that is accessible to everyone (Figure 42.5). This important role is usually filled by a veterinary nurse.

The head laser nurse makes sure that everyone knows proper safety instructions and the basics about the laser. They keep the laser user manual updated with the latest information. The manual should include short guidelines on how to treat everyday conditions, as well as all of the email exchanged between the practice and the laser supplier, so that all the information is readily available. A single document should be prepared, in the practice's native language, containing short, basic rules for the laser (indications, contraindications, fees, and treatment plans), and kept with the laser for staff reference. Interesting cases and basic information about laser therapy should be collected in an additional notebook for the coffee room, so that everyone on the staff can study it during their coffee break.

An initial training for the entire staff should be organized by the supplier. Commit all of the staff to whatever time the supplier requests for training. This ensures that all will benefit from the training. Encourage staff to make a list of questions before training, to ask them during training, and to write down the answers. The supplier should also provide all material in a written format for future reference.

If the practice staff is large (e.g., 10 or more veterinarians and nurses), the initial training may include only a portion of it. Those who are trained will become the laser VIPs, responsible for guiding and training other

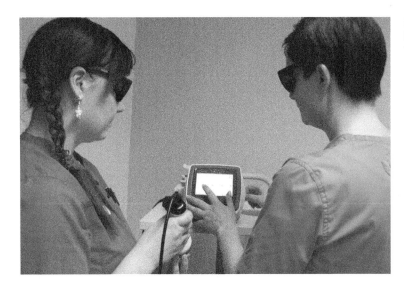

Figure 42.5 In most practices, a veterinary nurse will be responsible for being sure everyone is properly trained in the use of the therapy laser.

staff members. Whether or not staff members will actually be using the laser, they should be trained and have a good knowledge of the basics of laser therapy. This is the best way to ensure that all of the staff is familiar with laser therapy and can recommend it to clients.

Those responsible for the administration of laser therapy to patients should be able to deliver good customer service and ensure an overall good experience for both patients and clients. They are crucial to success when the practice first uses this new technology. They should also be willing to continue to learn more about laser therapy and to think of new ways to market it.

Training Tools

Have a written training plan with the following suggested steps:

1) Basic laser therapy training for everyone on the staff, conducted by the laser supplier.
2) Basic training on the specific therapy laser device to be used in the practice for everyone on the staff, conducted by the laser supplier.
3) Training on the indications for laser therapy. All staff should know the patients and conditions for which laser therapy is indicated. All should know how laser therapy fits into the overall management of a condition: when, how frequently, and how many times the condition may be treated. This training should be started by the laser supplier and continued by the head laser nurse.
4) Laser VIP hands-on training. This will include detailed information about the therapy laser device, its use, and specific treatment techniques for those who will be administering treatments. Initial laser VIP training is conducted by the laser supplier and is then continued by the head laser nurse.
5) Advance training for VIPs after they have used the laser for several months. This important step in training will help answer questions that arise from early use of the therapy laser. Advanced VIP training may be provided by the laser supplier or by the head laser nurse.
6) Continuing education. All staff should receive updates about laser therapy. Laser VIPs should have access to laser therapy seminars, webinars, and written educational material.
7) New staff training. After laser therapy is implemented, new staff members who join the team will require appropriate training by the head laser nurse. Staff who will not be using the laser should receive basic training, and those using the laser should receive basic and hands-on training.

Identify less experienced nurses who may need to be mentored before treating patients. Be sure all who are administering laser therapy are comfortable and secure with anatomy. A good knowledge of anatomy, of how best to treat different anatomical areas, and of how to read patients and their reaction to laser therapy comes with experience. Laser VIPs who have gained this experience can help those who have not. Observations during actual patient treatments are helpful, as are demonstrations using staff pets.

An additional, very effective way to educate staff members about laser therapy is to encourage them to treat their own animals. Practice policies about laser therapy fees for staff members should facilitate this. After treating their own animals, staff members can tell clients about the experience and the results of the treatments.

Scheduling Laser Therapy

It is important to plan when laser patients will be treated during the daily schedule. Laser therapy for patients with acute conditions normally requires little time, so these patients can be treated during an outpatient visit. Treating patients with chronic conditions often takes longer, and laser therapy sessions must be scheduled when a laser nurse will be available. In larger practices, to ensure that adequate staff is available, it may be necessary to have a nurse whose only responsibility is to work with laser therapy patients.

If the patient is going to receive more than one treatment, be sure that all future treatments are scheduled before the end of the first visit. Assign and collect fees for all of the future visits at this time. This is helpful to clients, since it lets them know when future treatments will be and how much they will cost, and they will not have to go through a lengthy checkout after subsequent treatment sessions.

When establishing a system for scheduling laser therapy sessions, include guidelines that will ensure the laser device is available for use when the treatment is to be administered. With so many potential patients, some with acute conditions scheduled on short notice during outpatient visits, the therapy laser needs to be easily moved from one location to another. Trolleys, with adequate storage for therapy laser equipment, cleaning supplies, and manuals, are recommended.

A plan for who will talk to the client about laser therapy should also be established. Staff members who book appointments, either in person or over the phone, should mention laser therapy during the booking process. When checking patients in, the receptionist should tag or flag the files of patients with conditions for which laser therapy is indicated. This alerts the exam-room nurse to begin talking about laser therapy in the room, give the client written material to read, and remind the veterinarian that the patient is a potential laser therapy case.

Making the Client and Patient Experience Excellent

As in any phase of veterinary practice, good people skills are useful for the nurse who administers the laser treatments. Clients are often present during laser therapy treatments. With treatments lasting anywhere from 5 to 20 minutes, small talk can help make the session more comfortable and the client more secure (Figure 42.6). It is good to have a very social, outspoken laser nurse.

Not all staff members are adept with small talk, especially in the author's area of Northern Europe. Help the staff make small talk with proper training about laser therapy, and by practicing the phrases they will use when talking about it. Each staff member will have a different style, but all should speak with the same basic laser terminology. A radio or soft music in the laser room can help avoid awkward quiet moments during extended sessions.

During laser treatments, one of the nurse's roles is to explain what happens, why, and how it affects the patient. The veterinarian may have detailed this to the client when prescribing laser therapy, but there is more time during treatment, and clients tend to be more focused on the information being communicated (Andersen 2014).

Clients usually have many questions about laser therapy, so nurses should be prepared with answers to the most common ones:

- How does it feel? Does it hurt?
- Is it dangerous?
- Why are we wearing safety glasses? What happens if we don't wear them?
- Who can administer laser therapy?
- How long does it take?
- Can the pet move around normally after treatment?
- When will we see the effects? How will we know it has helped?
- Why do not all veterinarians have laser therapy?
- Are there different kinds of laser?
- Can humans receive laser therapy?
- Can you laser me?

The location where laser therapy treatments are administered should be quiet and peaceful. Short treatments may be administered in the exam room, but for longer treatments, patients and their owners should be moved to a designated area for increased comfort. Regardless of treatment location, be sure there is non-slippery flooring, a blanket, towel, or mat for dogs, and a bed for cats. Smaller patients can be comfortably treated on a table. Larger patients should be treated on the floor, or on a short raised platform.

During treatments, nurses should explain to the owners that each laser nurse will have a slightly different style of treatment. Handpiece movement speed may vary, the order in which areas are treated may vary, and positioning may vary. Be sure clients are comfortable with these variations and understand that they will not affect the treatment results.

Records and Owner Instructions

Laser nurses are responsible for recording treatment parameters in the patient's record. For each laser therapy treatment, the record should include the condition, the target tissue, the protocol used, the power setting, the handpiece used, and any patient-specific parameters entered in the therapy laser's software. The software in newer therapy lasers may allow patient treatment details to be stored and retrieved for convenience, but all of that information should also be in the medical record.

Since some therapy laser treatments are administered during sessions in which the patient is not examined by a veterinarian, it is important for the laser nurse to evaluate the patient, record their progress in the medical record, and note any client concerns. This can help the

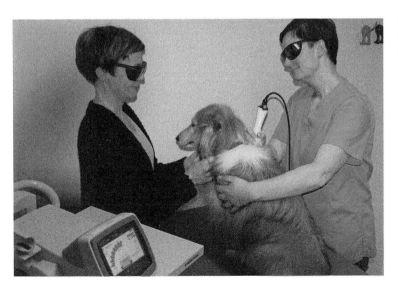

Figure 42.6 Patient and owner with a veterinary nurse for a short therapy laser treatment. Nurses should be able to answer clients' most common questions.

attending veterinarian respond to any such concerns and know when it is time to adjust the treatment schedule.

Give the client clear, written, take-home instructions after the visit. Prepare basic information for them, in which laser therapy is explained (this can be the same information used when prescribing laser therapy). Include detailed instructions about the patient's care at home and what the client should expect. Nurses are usually responsible for preparing this information, going over it with the client, making sure they understand it, and making sure they leave with it.

Nurses can also facilitate client compliance with the use of emails and text messages. Monitoring patient progress or reminding the client of the next scheduled laser therapy session is easy with digital communication.

Marketing Tips for Nurses

The practice should include laser therapy as a fixed element of many routine protocols (Zimlich, 2015). Marketing of laser therapy is much easier when it is part of the practice's standard of care. Making laser treatment a standard element of castrations and sterilizations is a good way to establish it as a standard within the practice.

The rationale for laser therapy being a standard of care can be communicated in a number of ways:

- Pictures and videos of patients that include before-and-after images.
- Pictures of patients wearing laser-safe goggles (protective eyewear).
- Video clips showing how the laser is used.

- Laser evenings with demonstrations, trial treatments, and laser information.
- Direct emails targeting owners of pets with specific conditions, such as osteoarthritis.
- Co-operation with local kennel clubs and special-interest groups.

Regardless of who in the practice manages marketing, nurses play a big role in promoting laser therapy.

Nurses can communicate their own experience with laser therapy and share the stories of patients they have helped. Owners also love to talk about their own good experiences with laser therapy, and clients love to read about patient success stories on the practice's Web pages. Since nurses are present when patients are treated, they can help share the stories on social media. Though most owners are pleased to be included, be sure to obtain their permission before posting their images online.

Conclusion

Veterinary technicians and nurses play an essential role in laser therapy. They should be involved in planning for and implementing laser therapy in the practice. They help train other staff members and can become a vital communication resource for clients. It is their responsibility to be adept in administering treatments and guiding the patient and client through their scheduled therapeutic regimen. With proper training, technicians and nurses can help ensure that laser therapy is administered utilizing a proper and consistent technique, individualized protocols, and effective client communication.

References

Anders, J. *et al.* (2015) Low-level light/laser therapy versus photobiomodulation therapy. *Photomed Laser Surg.* **33**(4):183–184.

Andersen, D. (2014) Vets say why they use laser therapy. *Vet Pract News.* August 20.

Barat, K. (2006) Laser safety officer or advisor. In: *Laser Safety Management*, p. 9. Taylor & Francis, Boca Raton, FL.

Chow, R.T. *et al.* (2007) 830 nm laser irradiation induces varicosity formation, reduces mitochondrial membrane potential and blocks fast axonal flow in small and medium diameter rat dorsal root ganglion neurons: implications for the analgesic effects of 830 nm laser. *J Peripher Nerv Syst.* **12**(1):28–39.

Chung, H. *et al.* (2012) The nuts and bolts of low-level laser (light) therapy. *Ann Biomed Eng.* **40**(2):516–533.

de Oliveira, R.F. and de Freitas, P.M. (2016) Laser therapy on points of acupuncture on nerve repair. *Neural Regen Res.* **11**(4): 557–558.

de Oliveira, F. *et al.* (2013) Helium-neon laser therapy interferes with epiphyseal plate growth in the femur and tibia of rabbits. *Photonics Lasers Med.* **2**(4):349–354.

Farivar, S. *et al.* (2014) Biological effects of low level laser therapy. *J Lasers Med Sci.* **5**(2):58–62.

Fulop, A. *et al.* (2010) A meta-analysis of the efficacy of laser phototherapy on pain relief. *Clin J Pain.* **26**(8):729–736.

Karu, T. (1999) Primary and secondary mechanisms of action of visible to near-IR radiation on cells. *J Photochem Photobiol B.* **49**(1):1–17.

Jergler, D. (2013) Staffs embrace laser therapy. *Vet Pract News.* November 14.

Kirkby, K. *et al.* (2012) The effects of low-level laser therapy in a rat model of intestinal ischemia-reperfusion injury. *Lasers Surg Med.* **44**(7):580–587.

Lorenzini, L. *et al.* (2010) Laser acupuncture for acute inflammatory, visceral and neuropathic pain relief: An experimental study in the laboratory rat. *Res Vet Sci.* **88**(1):159–165.

Mandel, A. and Hamblin, M. (2012) A renaissance in low-level laser (light) therapy - LLLT. *Photon Lasers Med.* **1**(4):231–235.

Oleson, S. (2016) Laser Safety Officer Information. Available from: https://www.lia.org/subscriptions/safety_bulletin/laser_safety_info/#The Laser Safety Officer (accessed November 30, 2016).

Oliveira, S. *et al.* (2012) Low-level laser on femoral growth plate in rats. *Acta Cir Bras.* **27**(2):117–122.

Pryor, B. and Millis, D.L. (2015) Therapeutic laser in veterinary medicine. *Vet Clin North Am Small Anim Pract.* **45**(1):45–56.

Reeder, J. (2015) Fired up about lasers. *Trends.* December.

Son, J. *et al.* (2012) Bone healing effects of diode laser (808 nm) on a rat tibial fracture model. *In Vivo.* **26**(4):703–709.

Zimlich, R. (2015) Two practices shine light on laser therapy in the veterinary business model. *Vet Econ.* June 1.

43

Return on Investment for a Therapy Laser

David J. Fenoglio

Augusta Animal Clinic, Indianapolis, IN, USA

Introduction

My practice is a classic example of the clinical and economic success of laser therapy in veterinary medicine. I invested in a therapy laser in 2009 and have enjoyed the positive impact that a new technology can have on patients, clients, and practice staff. The investment I made for my solo companion-animal practice has produced a very positive return, both clinically and financially.

In clinical practice, veterinarians are always performing services for their clients and patients. These services should be performed with the patient's well-being as a top priority. Keeping up with new technology and purchasing capital medical equipment is paramount to performing services and achieving successful outcomes.

Veterinary business owners make financial decisions every day. One decision that requires careful analysis is the purchase of capital equipment. New equipment is generally quite expensive; therefore, the return on investment (ROI) must be considered. ROI is a performance measure used to evaluate the efficiency of an investment. It measures the amount of return gained relative to the investment's cost.

To calculate ROI, the benefit (or return) of an investment is divided by its cost, and the result is expressed as a percentage or ratio. Simply put, the ROI is the economic gain versus the economic cost, or the net profit from the investment. The economic cost of equipment includes the initial cost of purchasing the equipment itself, the cost of maintenance, and the cost of labor required for the equipment's use.

Other factors should also weigh in the decision to invest in capital equipment, among them its medical necessity, its potential frequency of use, its ease of use, and the learning curve for using it. New equipment may affect employees and staffing needs. It may affect attitude and morale, and the image of the practice.

Some equipment is a necessity for the operation of a clinical practice. A good example is surgical instrumentation, without which a practice cannot function. Other equipment is optional. In the latter case, it is important to consider the potential ROI before purchase.

The questions a business-minded veterinarian should ask about a therapeutic laser are: "Do I think laser therapy is medically necessary for a progressive veterinarian?" and "Is a therapy laser a good investment for my practice?" The first question has been answered in all the preceding chapters. This chapter will answer the second.

Yes, laser therapy is a good investment for practices. Multiple examples of practices that have realized a positive ROI will be given here, examples of fee structures will be detailed, and ROI calculations will be demonstrated.

The fees mentioned in this chapter represent examples of what is being charged for laser therapy in the United States but should not be construed as being recommendations. The discussion of fees is included so that those considering investing in a therapy laser will have some idea about the possible ROI. Each practice should establish its own appropriate fee structure.

ROI for a Therapy Laser in My Own Companion Animal Practice

After practicing for 30 years, I was looking for something new that would set my practice apart from others in the area. I needed a new technology to re-energize me and get my burners fired up again. As a practice owner, I was stuck in a stale daily routine and wanted to revive the excitement I had earlier in practice. First and foremost, the revival needed to be effective and to help my patients. Second, it needed to be profitable.

Laser Therapy in Veterinary Medicine: Photobiomodulation, First Edition. Edited by Ronald J. Riegel and John C. Godbold, Jr.
© 2017 John Wiley & Sons, Inc. Published 2017 by John Wiley & Sons, Inc.

At that time, I was also looking for a better way to manage patient pain and wanted to do so without having to rely solely on medications. I started researching what I had heard was a "new" approach to pain management: laser therapy. I initially had doubts and questions. Was laser therapy effective? Did it really work? How long did it take to work? What was the learning curve for using the therapy laser? I read about it, and talked to pain-management specialists and therapy laser vendors, and it quickly began to make sense for me. It was non-invasive, comforting to the patient, and effective, and it had an easy learning curve. Equally importantly, it could be profitable.

I did my homework on different therapy laser companies and the equipment each supplied. I wanted a company that supplied excellent equipment and customer support, and could assist with marketing support. I found a company I was comfortable working with and purchased my first therapy laser in March 2009.

I started using our therapy laser immediately, primarily for geriatric dogs with osteoarthritis pain. I saw results when patients showed decreased pain and improved mobility and function. I then progressed to using laser therapy for any condition involving pain, inflammation, swelling, and healing. I continued to see positive results, became very excited, and started using it more and more for various maladies. My burners had been re-ignited.

By September 2009, 6 months after purchase, my therapy laser had paid for itself. My investment had been returned. In the well-known words of Dave Ramsey, the American financial author, radio host, and motivational speaker (www.daveramsey.com), I was "debt free."

I increased my practice revenue by using laser therapy as an adjunct to other treatment modalities, maximizing its effectiveness. My patients were happy, my clients were happy, and by having a new technology, I was separating myself from other practices and attracting new patients by word of mouth. Unlike many other pieces of equipment, which require long-term maintenance costs, the only cost of using my therapy laser after the first 6 months was the cost of labor. I have now used a therapy laser for over 7 years without any repair or maintenance costs.

Laser therapy treatments can be safely and easily administered. My staff members have been to several continuing-education courses on laser therapy and have been trained and certified by the American Institute of Medical Laser Applications (AIMLA; www.aimla.org). Administering laser therapy is now second nature to them. Treatment sessions keep them involved in hands-on patient care and in communication with our clients.

I tell clients my plan of treatment and the expected results, and explain why the addition of laser therapy will expedite these results. I rarely have a client refuse the addition of laser therapy to a patient's management protocol. Often, I will administer a short sample application of the laser light to the client to alleviate any concerns that the pet will feel any pain from laser therapy treatment.

My fee structure is simple. Induction- and maintenance-phase packages are sold as six-packs for US$300 and are pre-paid in order to ensure client compliance and encourage return visits. These packages include a US$60 discount, so the client is essentially paying for five treatments and getting the sixth for free. I prescribe the original protocol and laser therapy settings, and the technician then administers the treatments. After the sixth and last treatment of the pre-paid package, I consult with the client at no charge, talk about the patient's progress, and decide with the client whether we are going to continue using laser therapy. At this point, most clients (90–95%) tell me they see noticeable improvement, elect to continue laser therapy, and purchase another package of six treatments. Treatments in the second package are usually used to transition to less frequent maintenance-phase treatments. The fees for individual treatments that are not part of a package are US$45–60, depending on the time required.

I also use the therapy laser on all of my surgical patients as part of our post-op pain-management protocol. The additional fee for laser therapy for pain management is US$15–20. Occasionally, I will elect to reduce or not charge laser therapy fees in order to facilitate owner compliance. Because my therapy laser is paid for, and the only cost for its use is staff time spent administering laser treatments, I can be flexible about fees when it is used on patients owned by clients with financial constraints.

In 7 years, I have grossed more than US$98 000 in laser therapy fees. That figure does not include all of the times I have used the therapy laser when the fee is built in to an overall protocol fee so that there is not a line item for laser use. Built-in laser use fees would easily add another US$10 000 of revenue, for a total return of more than US$108 000 on an US$18 000 investment.

Not wanting to lease and pay interest, I paid for my therapy laser with cash. Without considering the cost of 6 months of loss of use of my cash investment, or the cost of labor for administration of laser therapy treatments, and using the formula mentioned at the start of the chapter for calculating the return on an investment, my ROI has been approximately 500%. My clinic is a one-veterinarian practice and is located in an area where the median household income in 2014 was 21% below the median household income for the entire United States (QuickFacts 2015).

My question about a therapy laser being a good investment for my practice has been more than answered. Based on my ROI figures, I firmly believe that my therapy laser is the best piece of capital equipment I have purchased in 33 years of practice ownership.

Because of the success I have had with laser therapy, I upgraded to a newer and more powerful device in 2015. The increased power level reduced the time of many treatments and thus reduced the cost of labor for delivering them. The more sophisticated device software allowed us to expand the number of different conditions we were treating. I expect a rapid ROI on my second therapy laser.

ROI for a Therapy Laser in Other Companion Animal Practices

John Godbold, Jr., DVM of Stonehaven Veterinary Consulting in Jackson, TN, a co-editor and contributing author of this book, has lectured worldwide on laser therapy in veterinary medicine, and has contributed articles and chapters to various publications. He is another small-animal practitioner from a one-veterinarian practice in which laser therapy was very successful, both clinically and financially. Dr. Godbold's practice, Stonehaven Park Veterinary Hospital, is in an area where the median household income in 2014 was 29% below the median household income for the entire United States (QuickFacts 2015).

In an email communication in November 2015, Dr. Godbold noted that the economic demographics of a practice's area, or the actual fees for laser therapy, are less important to a positive ROI than being sure the device is used as often as possible. That means treating many diverse conditions. Data from Dr. Godbold's practice (Box 43.1) demonstrate that the therapy laser can be used as part of the management of a diverse range of conditions.

Dr. Godbold feels the most important factor for a quick ROI on a therapy laser is having the technology become part of standard treatment protocols. Just as lab work and radiographs have become parts of standard protocols, so too should laser therapy. Acute otitis? Just as cytology, cleaning, and medications are a standard part of therapy, so should laser therapy be. Pyotraumatic dermatitis? Just as clipping, cleaning, and medications are

---

Box 43.1 **Distribution of all conditions treated with laser therapy at Stonehaven Park Veterinary Hospital, Jackson, TN.**

Post-Procedure Pain Management
40%

Acute Conditions
24%

Chronic Conditions
36%

---

part of standard therapy, so should laser therapy be. Adding laser therapy to standard protocols removes unnecessary deliberation about whether or not to include it in the management of a condition. When it is part of a standard protocol, laser therapy is automatically prescribed by the veterinarian, automatically administered by a staff member, and universally accepted by clients. When part of a standard protocol, laser therapy becomes a standard of care.

According to Dr. Godbold, it is important for everyone in the practice to be trained in laser use, as well as to have one person who can be the laser point person and answer questions. "All should know something about it, and some should know all about it." He maintains that it's important to establish a core message about laser therapy that all staff members can communicate. That message should address the "why" question that clients have: "Why are you prescribing laser therapy?" The core message should be as simple as: "We want to reduce pain and inflammation and speed the healing process in a safe and effective way that is not invasive, so we are going to treat your pet with laser therapy."

From a profitability standpoint, Dr. Godbold notes that it is not a good business model for the veterinarian to spend 15 minutes administering a treatment that results in an average fee of US$40–45. But that is a good use of time for a staff member or technician. The ROI for a therapy laser can best be achieved when treatments are administered by staff members (Arp, 2009b).

Jeffrey J. Smith, DVM, CCRP from Middletown, CA, a contributing author of this book, agrees that therapy lasers are an excellent investment. Dr. Smith owns the multi-veterinarian Middletown Animal Hospital and All Valley Equine, and is also an independent laser consultant. In a November 2015 email communication, Dr. Smith observed that most one-doctor practices generate about US$3000 in laser fees in the first month of use. Most have a lease payment of US$500–600 a month over 48–60 months. The result is a positive cash flow of US$2400 a month while the lease is being paid. Dr. Smith stated that he had consulted with a three-doctor practice that generated US$9000 in laser fees in its first month, and that many practices pay off their laser in the first year.

Dr. Smith's own fee structure assigns fees based on the length of the treatment session. When sold as a package of six treatments, each session is:

- 1–10 minutes: US$25–30 (US$150–180 total)
- 11–20 minutes: US$40 (US$240 total)
- 21–30 minutes: US$50 (US$300 total)
- 31–40 minutes: US$60 (US$360 total)

Individual treatments that are not part of a package of six are US$10 more per session. Dr. Smith treats every post-op and post-dental case with the laser, and adds

US$10 for these treatments as part of the procedure. With the fees Dr. Smith uses, treating two large arthritic dogs through an initial series of six sessions generates enough fee income to make a monthly lease payment. That is a scenario that is easy for most clinics.

Dr. Smith maintains that part of the success of laser therapy comes from this being a completely new revenue stream for a practice. According to Dr. Smith, there are clients who want this type of drug-free, surgery-free, non-invasive therapy for their pets. Laser therapy joins rehabilitation, physical therapy, and other non-pharmacological methods of addressing pain that clients understand and want for their animals.

Arp (2009a) reported on the financial success of therapy lasers in two practices. Integrity Animal Hospital, located in a semi-rural area in Kingsland, GA, is an example where a therapy laser can have a significant effect on the economics of practice. Don Nunn, DVM, the owner of the practice, reported to Arp that his practice's therapy laser fees ranged from US$20 to US$40 per session, and with more than 500 treatment sessions during the first 9 months, this generated sufficient income to pay for his therapy laser during that time.

Arp reported similar success by Bob Cohn, DVM of North Laurel Animal Hospital in Laurel, MD. As detailed by Arp, Dr. Cohn added a therapy laser to his practice in 2009, and fees from his first month of use exceeded his first year of lease payments. Arp noted that Dr. Cohn, like others, offers packages of six laser therapy treatment sessions for US$265–285.

In a more recent review of laser therapy's role in the veterinary business model, Zimlich (2015) noted the same positive economic impact that Arp reported in 2009. In her article, Zimlich emphasized the importance of establishing laser therapy as a standard in practice. As an example of the importance of this approach, Zimlich detailed the success of Jennifer Johnson, VMD, CVPP, the owner of Stoney Creek Veterinary Hospital in Morton, PA and a contributing author of this book. Following her investment in a therapy laser in 2010, Dr. Johnson experienced a 3% increase in revenue and US$85 000 in profits from laser therapy services. According to Zimlich, Dr. Johnson accomplished that by adding laser therapy as a practice standard for all surgery patients and using it for a diverse range of other conditions. Dr. Johnson's purchase lease had a 4-year payment plan to cover the US$30 000 cost. Zimlich reported that Johnson was able to pay off the entire balance in a year.

Another recent review of why lasers are a worthwhile investment for veterinary practices reported on the success of Deborah Fegan, DVM, owner of Big Creek Pet Hospital in Cleveland and Olmstead, OH (Reeder 2015). According to Reeder, Dr. Fegan purchased a therapy laser in 2014 and realized a very positive return on her investment, with monthly therapy laser income of US$2600 and monthly lease payments of US$450. Reeder also noted the fee structure used by Big Creek Pet Hospital: "The first month of unlimited laser therapy on two pain sites is US$260 versus individual sessions for US$24. Packages for subsequent months, when the animal will need less frequent treatment, are reduced to US$140" (Reeder 2015).

Reeder reported another positive ROI by Ayers Animal Hospital in Huntington, WV. Following a US$27 000 investment in a therapy laser, the practice generated US$31 000 in laser fees in the first year. Reeder quoted Elaine Kern, veterinary technician and office manager for the practice, saying the therapy laser was "the best investment we have made" (Reeder 2015).

ROI for a Therapy Laser in an Exotic-Animal Practice

In addition to being a clinical and financial success in companion-animal practices, laser therapy has had a positive impact on patients and profits in less traditional practices. Robert D. Ness, DVM, owner of Ness Exotic Wellness Center in Lisle, IL and a contributing author of this book, purchased his first therapy laser in 2010. In an email communication in November 2015, Dr. Ness noted that the unit paid for itself in 6–8 months following frequent use (two to four times daily). Dr. Ness's usual fees are US$48 per session or US$260 for pre-paid package of six sessions.

Most of the laser therapy treatments at Ness Exotic Wellness Center are administered during a technician appointment following the initial visit with the doctor, who prescribes the treatment protocol for the case. Dr. Ness realized US$120 000–140 000 total revenue in his first 5 years of using the therapy laser. This is an excellent return on his initial investment.

ROI for a Therapy Laser in a Mobile Practice

Erin O'Leary, DVM, of Cary, NC, owns a mobile laser therapy practice serving all species and is a contributing author of this book. Her HEAL Mobile Veterinary Service takes the therapeutic benefits of laser technology to pets in their home, office, or veterinary clinic. In an email communication in November 2015, Dr. O'Leary stated that within the first 3 years of purchasing her therapy laser, she was averaging 15–20 appointments per week and was able to pay off her investment.

Dr. O'Leary began by charging a modest fee for each anatomical area treated, as well as a mileage fee for her travel distances. This became too complicated, and she did not like clients having to decide whether to treat an additional anatomical area based on costs. So after about a year, she changed her fee structure to a set fee (laser and travel cost incorporated into one fee), and she charges extra if the patient is outside of a 30-mile radius or if the visit is an extended session (as is usually the case with horses or arthritic dogs with multiple affected joints). Her current fees are US$35 for the initial consult and US$80 per laser therapy session. She adds a US$25 fee for travel outside of a 30-mile or 30-minute range. Her fees are based on the average fees practices in her area charge, with an addition for the mobile visit.

Dr. O'Leary considered packages of multiple treatments for a pre-paid fee when she started, but decided not to offer them because the distances she had to travel to patients and the number of anatomical areas patients required treating were so variable. She still does not offer packages, but she is considering them again because of their effectiveness in guaranteeing income and in keeping clients involved with the patient's long-term care.

Dr. O'Leary's practice is mobile and 100% laser therapy: a model for effective delivery of laser therapy to patients, and an excellent example of the investment in a therapy laser giving a positive return.

ROI for a Therapy Laser in Equine Practice

Ron Riegel, DVM, Marysville, OH, a co-editor and contributing author of this book, has a background in equine practice, and was one of the early pioneers of laser therapy in veterinary medicine. Dr. Riegel first began using laser therapy in his mixed yet predominantly equine practice in 1979. Since then, he has seen the technology grow, expand, and become a standard of care in all types of veterinary practice. Dr. Riegel has facilitated the development of laser therapy in veterinary medicine through his work in practice as well as his work as an author, consultant, and speaker.

In an email communication in November 2015, Dr. Riegel explained that therapy lasers give a rapid and positive ROI in equine practice but that any consideration of fees for equine laser therapy is complicated due to the many different fee schedules and pricing systems in equine practice. As Riegel explained, fees for laser therapy when treating equine patients vary depending on the geographical location, the discipline of the equine patient, and whether one is charging by the anatomical area, by the disorder being treated, or by the time required to treat.

Examples of equine laser therapy fees are shown in Boxes 43.2–43.5. These examples include a range of fees averaged from multiple practices located in different geographical locations within the United States.

Box 43.2 Laser therapy schedule of fees for equine acute injuries.

Time and frequency of treatment determine cost. Fees are assigned per treatment or area.
- Wound: US$30–40
- Tendon/soft-tissue injury: US$40–45
- Individual joint: US$40 (for large joints, add an additional US$10–20)
- Thoracic, lumbar, or sacral spine: US$150–300
- Lumbosacral area: US$60–90
- Fetlock, pastern, or hoof: US$40–50

Box 43.3 Laser therapy schedule of fees for equine performance maintenance protocols.

Fees are unique to each discipline, for laser therapy administered prior to an event or as an accelerated recovery protocol after an event or a hard training workout.

Hunter/Jumper
Back, hind quarter: US$200–300

Reiner
Back, stifles and hocks: US$175–250

Cutter
Fore limbs and lumbosacral area: US$150–175

Standardbred
Lumbosacral area, stifles, and hocks: US$150–225

Thoroughbred
Knees, tendons, and fetlocks: US$150–250

Dressage
Poll, back, and lumbosacral area: US$175–300

Box 43.4 Laser therapy schedule of fees for unique equine applications.

Post intra-articular injection, joint maintenance: US$50–60
- Acute laminitis, both front feet: US$100–125
- Post extracorporeal shockwave therapy: US$50–80
- Acupuncture therapy: US$75–200, or US$6–8 per point
- Acupuncture performed along with an area treatment: US$5 per point

---

Box 43.5 Laser therapy schedule of fees for equine applications based on professional's time.

Administration by Technician
Blocks of 15 minutes: US$20–45

Administration by Veterinarian
Blocks of 15 minutes: US$45–60

As is frequently the case in other types of practice, equine practitioners often bundle or package laser therapy sessions and include discounts for pre-payment. Packages of four treatments are typically discounted by 10% and packages of six sessions by 15%. Just as in other types of practice, equine clients are more compliant when they pre-pay for services.

Dr. Riegel concluded that there are a variety of fee structures that can be used, but regardless of the structure, the most important factor is that the therapy laser unit, having so many diverse applications, be used multiple times every day. This reinforces Dr. Godbold's premise that the frequency of use is more important in generating revenue than the actual fee assigned for the service.

Calculating Potential ROI for a Therapy Laser

Calculation of a potential ROI in a therapy laser can easily be done using figures appropriate for the practice type, location, and economic demographics. Estimates of an average laser use fee and an average number of daily uses allow a quick calculation of projected laser revenue. See Boxes 43.6 and 43.7.

Practices should consider a range of fees and frequencies of therapy laser use in order to establish a realistic

---

estimation of laser therapy revenue. Projected revenue can then be compared to the investment required to purchase the therapy laser, and a potential ROI can be calculated. As calculations are made, it is clear that the less important factor is the laser use fee, and the more important is the frequency of use.

Conclusion

Looking back on nearly 40 years of clinical practice, I am amazed at how much veterinary medicine has evolved. We have gone from using a practice business model in which our primary income was derived from vaccinations, spays, neuters, and retail sales, to one that relies on other profit centers. Formerly profitable activities in practice have become less profitable, but other sources of revenue and profit have emerged. Examples of new revenue sources are in-house blood analyzers, enhanced dental care, geriatric programs, rehabilitation programs, underwater treadmills, and acupuncture pain relief. Laser therapy joins these as a significant new revenue source.

Veterinary medicine will continue to evolve. With better technology, we have new ways to fulfill the oath we take when we become veterinarians and technicians. Though the actual wording of the oath varies across the world, the commitment we make is universal, and is represented by the oath used in the United States: "As a member of the veterinary medical profession, I solemnly swear that I will use my scientific knowledge and skills for the benefit of society. I will strive to promote animal health and welfare, relieve animal suffering, protect the health of the public and environment, and advance comparative medical knowledge. I will practice my profession conscientiously, with dignity, and in keeping with the principles of veterinary medical ethics. I will strive continuously to improve my professional knowledge and competence and to maintain the highest professional and ethical standards for myself and the profession" (AVMA 2015).

I believe laser therapy helps us fulfill the commitment we make when we take the oath. Laser therapy does promote animal health and welfare, and reduces animal suffering. Laser therapy does improve the quality of patients' lives. The benefits to our patients are well established; for these alone, we should make the investment and incorporate laser therapy into our practices. Equally well established is the financial benefit of incorporating laser therapy. Yes, therapeutic lasers help our patients; they also generate a significant amount of revenue, resulting in a healthy return on the investment we make in them.

> **Box 43.6 Laser therapy revenue projection using modest laser fees and assuming infrequent use.**
>
> **Average fee: US$30**
>
> **Three Patients a Day Treated with Laser Therapy**
> Per day: US$90
> Per week: US$450
> Per month: US$1935
> Per year: US$23 200

> **Box 43.7 Laser therapy revenue projection using average laser fees and assuming more frequent use.**
>
> **Average fee: US$45**
>
> **Six Patients a Day Treated with Laser Therapy**
> Per day: US$270
> Per week: US$1350
> Per month: US$5805
> Per year: US$69 660

References

Arp, D. (2009a) Lasers financially therapeutic, too. *Vet Pract News.* April 17.

Arp, D. (2009b) Spreading the warmth. *Vet Pract News.* August 31.

AVMA. (2015) Veterinarian's Oath. Available from: https://www.avma.org/KB/Policies/Pages/veterinarians-oath.aspx (accessed November 30, 2016).

QuickFacts. (2015) United States census information. Available from: http://www.census.gov/quickfacts/table/PST045215/00 (accessed November 30, 2016).

Reeder, J. (2015) Fired up about lasers. *Trends.* December.

Zimlich, R. (2015) Two practices shine light on laser therapy in the veterinary business model. *Vet Econ.* June 1.

Index

Note: Page numbers in *italics* represent figures; those in **bold**, tables.

Laser Therapy in Veterinary Medicine: Photobiomodulation, First Edition. Edited by Ronald J. Riegel and John C. Godbold, Jr.
© 2017 John Wiley & Sons, Inc. Published 2017 by John Wiley & Sons, Inc.